AF760072

POCKETBOOK OF

SURGERY

SIXTH EDITION

POCKETBOOK OF SURGERY

Edited by

Michael S. Delbridge MBChB(Hons) MD FRCS(Eng)

Consultant Vascular and Endovascular Surgeon,
Norfolk and Norwich University Hospital,
Norwich, UK

Wissam AL-Jundi MBBS MSc MEd MBA FRCS

Consultant Vascular and Endovascular Surgeon,
Norfolk and Norwich University Hospital,
Norwich, UK

ELSEVIER

ELSEVIER
First edition 1996
Second edition 2001
Third edition 2006
Fourth edition 2011
Fifth edition 2017

Copyright © 2025 by Elsevier Inc. All rights are reserved, including those for text and data mining, AI training, and similar technologies.

Publisher's note: Elsevier takes a neutral position with respect to territorial disputes or jurisdictional claims in its published content, including in maps and institutional affiliations.

No part of this publication may be reproduced or transmitted in any form or by any means, electronic or mechanical, including photocopying, recording, or any information storage and retrieval system, without permission in writing from the publisher. Details on how to seek permission, further information about the Publisher's permissions policies and our arrangements with organizations such as the Copyright Clearance Center and the Copyright Licensing Agency, can be found at our website: www.elsevier.com/permissions.

This book and the individual contributions contained in it are protected under copyright by the Publisher (other than as may be noted herein).

Notices

Practitioners and researchers must always rely on their own experience and knowledge in evaluating and using any information, methods, compounds or experiments described herein. Because of rapid advances in the medical sciences, in particular, independent verification of diagnoses and drug dosages should be made. To the fullest extent of the law, no responsibility is assumed by Elsevier, authors, editors or contributors for any injury and/or damage to persons or property as a matter of products liability, negligence or otherwise, or from any use or operation of any methods, products, instructions, or ideas contained in the material herein.

ISBN: 978-0-323-93579-1
978-0-323-93624-8

Senior Content Strategist: Alexandra Mortimer
Content Project Manager: Shruti Raj
Design: Matthew Limbert
Illustration Manager: Rupa Rai
Marketing Manager: Belinda Tudin

Printed in India

Last digit is the print number: 9 8 7 6 5 4 3 2 1

Working together to grow libraries in developing countries
www.elsevier.com • www.bookaid.org

Contents

Preface

The authors of the fifth edition (MSD and WAJ) are grateful to the publishers, Elsevier Ltd, for the invitation to produce the sixth edition of the *Pocketbook of Surgery*. All the chapters have had input from specialists in the field to ensure that everything is up-to-date. We, ourselves, have written the general chapters.

It has now been 20 years since the first edition was published; much has changed in that time, and all the chapters have been updated. The authors of each chapter were given a brief to write material that is medical student friendly, as well as suitable for MRCS candidates. In particular, it was decided to emphasise certain points, and to this end we have added 'hints and tips' placed in boxes throughout the chapters. We hope that the readership will find these useful.

The aim of this small volume, however, remains the same: namely, to provide a concise and didactic account of the essential features of the more common surgical disorders. The book covers fundamental principles along with providing basic information on aetiology, diagnosis and management, including preoperative and postoperative care. It will give the student some idea of history taking, what physical signs to elicit, the differential diagnosis and what investigations to order and how to treat the patient. The text covers the field of general surgery but aims to cover the basic needs of undergraduates and those in the early years of postgraduate training, as far as the surgical specialties are concerned.

We are assured that in these days of self-directed, student-centred, problem-based learning led by medical educationalists, there is still a place for a small book offering a didactic approach to the acquisition of surgical knowledge. Read in conjunction with *Pocketbook of Differential Diagnosis*, it will provide almost everything the undergraduate needs to know and also sufficient information for the postgraduate studying for the MRCS. We hope the book will continue to help you on the wards and in the clinics and will provide the necessary information for success in examinations.

Mike and Wissam

Acknowledgements

Pocketbook of Surgery has been going for over 20 years now, and the list of contributors has become extremely long. Both Wissam and I would like to thank all the contributors, both old and new, for making the book as popular as it is. We would also like to thank the support of the publishers for continuing the book over so many years.

Mike and Wissam

Contributors

Wissam Al-Jundi, MBBS MSc MEd MBA FRCS
Consultant Vascular and Endovascular Surgeon Vascular Surgeon, Norfolk and Norwich University Hospital, Norwich, UK

Eleanor Atkins, FRCS
SPR, Department of Vascular and Endovascular Surgery, Norfolk and Norwich University Hospital, Norwich, UK

Neil Baillie, PhD MB BCh BAO BSc (Hons) FRCSI FRCS(ORL-HNS)
Assistant Professor of Otolaryngology – Head and Neck Surgery, University of Toronto, Canada; Staff Otolaryngologist and Neurotologist, Toronto General Hospital, Toronto, Canada

Akshdeep Bawa, MBBS MS Orth FRCS T & O
Locum consultant Trauma and Orth, Norfolk and Norwich University Hospital, UK; BOA Council Member (SAS rep)

Yusuf Bayrak, MD
Associate Staff Physician of Thoracic Surgery, Cleveland Clinic Abu Dhabi, United Arab Emirates

Gopal Bhatnagar, MD FRCSC
Clinical Professor of Medicine, Lerner College of Medicine Case Western Reserve University Chair Heart, Vascular and Thoracic Institute Cleveland Clinic, Abu Dhabi, United Arab Emirates

Katherine I. Bridge, MBChB(Hons) MRCS(Eng)
Clinical Research Training Fellow in Vascular Surgery, University of Leeds and Yorkshire and Humber Deanery, UL

Michael S. Delbridge, MBChB(Hons) MD FRCS(Eng)
Consultant Vascular and Endovascular Surgeon, Norfolk and Norwich University Hospital, Norwich, UK

Richard England, MBChB FRCS Ed (Paed Surg)
Consultant Paediatric Surgeon, Department of Paediatric Surgery, Jenny Lind Children's Hospital, Norwich, UK

Laszlo Göbölös, MD PhD FACS FESC FACC FGHA
Clinical Professor of Surgery, Cardiac Surgery, HVI, Cleveland Clinic Abu Dhabi, Abu Dhabi, United Arab Emirates

Bhaskar Kumar, MD FRCS
Associate Professor, Upper Gastrointestinal Surgeon, University of East Anglia, Norwich, UK; Consultant Upper Gastrointestinal Surgeon, Norfolk and Norwich University Hospitals, NHS Trust, Norwich, Norfolk, UK

Manar Malki, FRCS (Urol)
Consultant Urologist and Robotic Surgeon, Urology Department, Frimley Health NHS Foundation Trust, Frimley, Surrey, UK

Cecilia McCormick, MD BS
Specialist Registrar Clinical Oncology, Norfolk and Norwich University Hospital, Norwich, UK

Alastair Mckelvey, FRCOG MB BCh BAO
Consultant and Associate Professor, Fetal and Maternal Medicine, Norfolk and Norwich Hospitals University Trust, Norwich, UK

Bahar Mirshekar-Syahkal, MBBChir MA(Cantab) PhD FRCS PGDipMedEd
Specialty Registrar, Breast Surgery, Norfolk and Norwich University Hospitals, Norwich, UK

Diaa Othman, Sr. FRCS Plast. UK
Consultant Plastic Surgeon, Plastic Surgery, Dr Sulaiman Al Habib Hospitals Group, Riyadh, Saudi Arabia

Simon Pain, MB BChir FRCS
Consultant Breast & Endocrine Surgeon, Department of Surgery, Norfolk & Norwich University Hospital, Norwich, UK

Andrew T. Raftery, BSc MBChB(Hons) MD FRCS(Eng) FRCS(Ed)
Retired Clinical Anatomist; Formerly Consultant Surgeon, Sheffield Kidney Institute, Sheffield Teaching Hospitals NHS Foundation Trust, Northern General Hospital, Sheffield; Member (formerly Chairman), Court of Examiners, Royal College of Surgeons of England; Formerly Member of Panel of Examiners, Intercollegiate Specialty Board in General Surgery; Formerly Member of Council, Royal College of Surgeons of England; Formerly Honorary Clinical Senior Lecturer in Surgery, University of Sheffield, Sheffield, UK

Mark A. Rochester, MA MD FRCS(Urol)
Consultant Urological Surgeon, Norfolk & Norwich University Hospital, UK; Honorary Associate Professor, University of East Angila, UK

Tarek P. Sunna, MD FABNS, FEBNS, FRCS(Ed), FACS
Minimally Invasive, Oncology & complex Spine Surgeon, Head of Neurosurgery Division, Aman Hospital, Doha, Qatar; Adjunct Assistant Professor, American University of Beirut Medical Center, Lebanon

Teresa Diago Uso, MD
General Surgery, Liver Transplant, Cleveland Clinic Abu Dhabi, United Arab Emirates

Paul Timmons, MBChB MRCOG
Sub-Specialty Fellow - Maternal Fetal Medicine, Obstetrics and Gynaecology, Norfolk and Norwich University Hospitals NHS Foundation Trust, Norwich, UK

Marcus J.D. Wagstaff, BSc MBBS PhD FRCS(Plast) FRACS
Specialist Plastic and Reconstructive Surgeon, Head of Unit of the Adult Burns Service at the Royal Adelaide Hospital (RAH), Associate Professor affiliated with the University of Adelaide Faculty of Health and Medical Sciences, Australia

Abbreviations

AAA	abdominal aortic aneurysm
ABC	airway, breathing and circulation
ABG	arterial blood gases
ABPI	ankle–brachial pressure index
AC	alternating current
ACC	adenoid cystic carcinoma
ACE	angiotensin-converting enzyme
ACTH	adrenocorticotrophic hormone
ADH	antidiuretic hormone
A&E	accident and emergency
AF	atrial fibrillation
AFP	α-fetoprotein
AI	aromatase inhibitor
AIDS	acquired immunodeficiency syndrome
AIN	anal intraepithelial neoplasia
ALND	axillary lymph node dissection
ALT	alanine transaminase
ANF	antinuclear factor
AOM	acute otitis media
AP	anteroposterior
APC	argon plasma coagulation
APTT	activated partial thromboplastin time
AR	angiotensin II receptor
ARBs	angiotensin II receptor blockers
ARDS	acute respiratory distress syndrome
ARF	acute renal failure
ARS	acute rhinosinusitis
ASA	American Society of Anethesiologists
ASD	atrial septal defect
AST	aspartate transaminase
ATG	antithymocyte globulin
ATLS	advanced trauma life support
ATN	acute tubular necrosis
AV	arteriovenous
AVM	arteriovenous malformation
AXR	abdominal X-ray
BAPRAS	British Association of Plastic, Reconstructive and Aesthetic Surgeons
BBB	bundle branch block
BCG	bacille Calmette–Guérin
BCS	breast conservation surgery
BEVAR	branched endovascular aneurysm repair
BMI	body mass index
BOA	British Orthopaedic Association
BP	blood pressure

BPH	benign prostatic hyperplasia
BTS	blood transfusion service
BXO	balanitis xerotica obliterans
CABG	coronary artery bypass graft
CAI	chronic allograft injury
CAPD	continuous ambulatory peritoneal dialysis
CBD	common bile duct
CC	craniocaudal
CCF	congestive cardiac failure
CCU	coronary care unit
CD	cluster of differentiation
CDH	congenital dislocation of the hip
CEA	carcinoembryonic antigen
CML	chronic myeloid leukaemia
CMV	cytomegalovirus
CN	cranial nerve
CNI	calcineurin inhibitor
CNS	central nervous system
COPD	chronic obstructive pulmonary disease
CPB	cardiopulmonary bypass
CPET	cardiopulmonary exercise testing
Cr	creatinine
CRF	chronic renal failure
CRP	C-reactive protein
CRS	chronic rhinosinusitis
C&S	culture and sensitivity
CSF	cerebrospinal fluid
CSOM	chronic suppurative otitis media
CT	computerized tomography
CTC	computerized tomography colonography
CTPA	computerized tomography pulmonary angiogram
CVA	cerebrovascular accident
CVP	central venous pressure
CVVH	continuous venovenous haemofiltration
CXR	chest X-ray
DBD	donation after brain death
DCD	donation after circulatory death
DCIS	ductal carcinoma *in situ*
DDH	developmental dysplasia of the hip
DIC	disseminated intravascular coagulation
DM	diabetes mellitus
DMSA	dimercaptosuccinic acid
DP	dorsalis pedis
DPL	diagnostic peritoneal lavage
DSA	digital subtraction angiography
DTPA	diethylenetriamine pentaacetic acid

DU	duodenal ulcer
DVT	deep venous thrombosis
DWI	diffusion weighted imaging
EBUS	endobronchial ultrasound
ECD	expanded criteria donor
ECF	extracellular fluid
ECG	electrocardiogram
EEG	electroencephalogram
EMD	electromechanical dissociation
EMG	electromyography
EMSU	early morning specimen of urine
ENT	ear, nose and throat
ePTFE	expanded polytetrafluoroethylene
ERCP	endoscopic retrograde cholangiopancreatography
ESR	erythrocyte sedimentation rate
ET	endobronchial tube
EUA	examination under anaesthesia
EUS	endoscopic ultrasound
EVAR	endovascular aneurysm repair
FAST	focused abdominal sonography for trauma
FBC	full blood count
FDPs	fibrin degradation products
FEV_1	forced expiratory volume (1 second)
FEVAR	fenestrated endovascular aneurysm repair
FFP	fresh frozen plasma
FMTC	familial medullary thyroid cancer
FNAC	fine needle aspiration cytology
FOBs	faecal occult bloods
FRS	fungal rhinosinusitis
GA	general anaesthetic
GCS	Glasgow Coma Scale
GI	gastrointestinal
GORD	gastro-oesophageal reflux disease
GP	general practitioner
GSW	gunshot wound
GTN	glyceryl trinitrate spray
GU	genitourinary
GVH	graft-versus-host disease
HBsAg	hepatitis B surface antigen
HBV	hepatitis B virus
HCC	hepatocellular carcinoma
HCG	human chorionic gonadotrophin
HCO_3	bicarbonate
Hct	haematocrit
HCV	hepatitis C virus

5HIAA	5-hydroxyindoleacetic acid
HIV	human immunodeficiency virus
HLA	human leukocyte antigen
HPV	human papilloma virus
HRT	hormone replacement therapy
HSV	highly selective vagotomy
HTA	Human Tissue Authority
HVA	homovanillic acid
ICP	intracranial pressure
IGTN	ingrowing toenail
IHD	ischaemic heart disease
IJV	internal jugular vein
IL-2	interleukin-2
IMPDH	inosine monophosphate dehydrogenase
INR	international normalized ratio
ITP	idiopathic thrombocytopenic purpura
ITU	intensive therapy unit
IUD	intrauterine device
i.v.	intravenously
IVC	inferior vena cava
IVDU	intravenous drug user
IVU	intravenous urography
JAK-3	Janus kinase-3
JVP	jugular venous pressure
KCCT	kaolin cephalin clotting time
KUB	kidney ureter bladder (plain X-ray)
LA	left atrium
LAD	left axis deviation
LBBB	left bundle branch block
LCIS	lobular carcinoma *in situ*
LCP	Liverpool Care Pathway
LDH	lactate dehydrogenase
LDN	laparoscopic donor nephrectomy
LE	lupus erythematosus
LFTs	liver function tests
LH	luteinizing hormone
LHRH	luteinizing hormone releasing hormone
LIF	left iliac fossa
LMWH	low molecular weight heparin
LP	lumbar puncture
LUQ	left upper quadrant
LUTS	lower urinary tract symptoms
LV	left ventricle
LVF	left ventricular failure

TLSO	thoracolumbar support orthosis
TNF-α	tumour necrosis factor-α
TNM	tumour, node, metastasis
TPN	total parenteral nutrition
TPO	thyroid peroxidase
TRA	traumatic rupture of the aorta
TRAB	thyroid receptor antibodies
TSH	thyroid stimulating hormone
TURP	transurethral resection of the prostate
UADT	upper aerodigestive tract
UC	ulcerative colitis
U&Es	urea and electrolytes
UHMWPE	ultra-high molecular weight polyethylene
UO	urine output
URTI	upper respiratory tract infection
USg	ultrasound guided
USS	ultrasound scan
UTI	urinary tract infection
VAB	vacuum assisted biopsy
VDRL	venereal disease research laboratory
VF	ventricular fibrillation
VMA	vanillylmandelic acid
V/Q	ventilation/perfusion ratio
VSD	ventricular septal defect
VT	ventricular tachycardia
VTE	venous thromboembolism
WCC	white cell count
WLE	wide local excision
ZES	Zollinger–Ellison syndrome
ZN	Ziehl–Neelsen

Terms and Definitions

Students starting a surgical firm will be introduced to a number of terms and definitions which, it is often taken for granted, they will have heard before. As a useful reminder, these are listed below.

Terms

Angio- Relating to (blood) vessels, e.g. angiogram – contrast imaging of an artery; cholangiogram – contrast imaging of the bile ducts.

Antegrade Going in the direction of flow, e.g. antegrade pyelogram – injection of contrast medium under imaging control into the renal pelvis percutaneously to delineate a distal obstruction.

Chole- Related to the biliary tree or bile, e.g. cholelithiasis – gallstones; cholecystectomy – removal of the gall bladder; choledochoscopy – examination of the bile ducts with an instrument.

-cele A cavity containing gas or fluid, e.g. hydrocele – collection of fluid between the layers of the tunica vaginalis of the testes; lymphocele – a localized collection of lymph; galactocele – a cavity containing milk in a lactating breast.

-docho- Related to ducts, e.g. choledochoscopy – examination of the bile ducts with an instrument; mammadochectomy – removal of the lactiferous ducts of the breast (for duct ectasia).

-ectasia Related to dilatation of the ducts, e.g. mammary duct ectasia – abnormal dilatation of the lactiferous ducts with periductal inflammation; sialectasia – dilatation of salivary gland ducts.

-ectomy Cutting something out, e.g. appendicectomy, gastrectomy, parotidectomy.

-gram An imaging technique using radio-opaque contrast medium, e.g. angiogram – visualization of the arterial tree; venogram – visualization of veins, e.g. to look for deep vein thrombosis; cholangiogram – to visualize the bile ducts.

Lith- Stone, e.g. pyelolithotomy – removal of a stone from the renal pelvis by opening the renal pelvis; cholelithiasis – gallstones.

-oscopy The inspection of a cavity, tube or organ with an instrument, e.g. cystoscopy – inspection of the bladder; laparoscopy – inspection of the abdominal cavity; colonoscopy – inspection of the colon; endoscopy – general term for inspection of internal organs.

-ostomy Opening something into another cavity or to the outside, e.g. colostomy – an opening of the colon onto the skin; gastroenterostomy – an opening of the stomach into the small bowel.

-otomy Making an opening in something, e.g. laparotomy – exploring the abdomen; cystotomy – opening the bladder.

Per- Going through a structure, e.g. percutaneous – going through the skin.

-plasty Refashioning something to alter function, e.g. pyloroplasty – to relieve pyloric obstruction; ileocystoplasty – to enlarge the bladder with a piece of ileum; angioplasty – to widen an obstruction in an artery.

Pyelo- Relating to the pelvis of the kidney, e.g. pyelogram – contrast imaging showing the renal pelvis; pyelonephritis – inflammation of kidney and renal pelvis.

Retrograde Going in a reverse direction against flow, e.g. endoscopic retrograde cholangiopancreatogram (ERCP) – retrograde injection of contrast medium up the common bile duct via cannulation of the papilla of Vater via a duodenoscope; retrograde pyelogram – injection of contrast medium in a reversed direction up the ureter to delineate the ureter and renal pelvis.

Trans- Going across a structure, e.g. percutaneous transluminal angioplasty – going through the skin and across an obstructed lumen in an artery to widen it and improve distal blood flow.

Some Important Definitions

Abscess A localized collection of pus.

Aneurysm An abnormal dilatation of an artery.

Cyst A fluid-filled cavity.

Fistula An abnormal communication between two epithelial surfaces (endothelial in the case of an arteriovenous fistula), e.g. colovesical fistula – between the sigmoid colon and the bladder, occurring usually as a complication of diverticulitis, carcinoma, or Crohn's disease.

Gangrene Death of tissue.

Sinus A blind-ending track communicating with an epithelial surface, e.g. pilonidal sinus where the 'sharp' end of hairs burrow into the skin.

Ulcer A break in the continuity of an epithelial surface.

Varix An abnormal dilatation of a vein.

Biochemical Values

VENOUS BLOOD: ADULT REFERENCE VALUES

Analyte	Reference Values
Acid phosphatase (unstable enzyme)	0.1–0.4 i.u./L
Alanine aminotransferase (ALT) (glutamic-pyruvic transaminase (GPT))	10–40 i.u./L
Alkaline phosphatase	40–100 i.u./L
Amylase	50–300 i.u./L
α_1-Antitrypsin	2–4 g/L
Ascorbic acid – serum	23–57 µmol/l 0.4–1.0 mg/dL
Ascorbic acid – leucocytes	1420–2270 µmol/L 25–40 mg/dL
Aspartate aminotransferase (AST) (glutamic-oxaloacetic transaminase (GOT))	10–35 i.u./L
Bilirubin (total)	2–17 µmol/L
Caeruloplasmin	1–2.7 µmol/L
Calcium (total)	2.12–2.62 mmol/L
Carbon dioxide (total)	24–30 mmol/L
Chloride	95–105 mmol/L
Cholesterol (fasting)	3.6–6.7 mmol/L
Copper	11–24 µmol/L
Creatinine	55–150 µmol/L
Creatinine clearance	90–130 mL/min
Creatine kinase (CK) – males	30–200 i.u./L
Creatine kinase (CK) – females	30–150 i.u./L
Ethanol – marked intoxication	65–87 mmol/L
Ethanol – coma	109 mmol/L
Ferritin – males	6–186 µg/mL
Ferritin – females	3–162 µg/mL
α-Fetoprotein	2–6 u/mL
γ-Glutamyl transferase:	
(γ-GT) – males	10–55 i.u./L
(γ-GT) – females	5–35 i.u./L
Glucose (fasting)	3.9–5.8 mmol/L
Immunoglobulins (Ig): IgA	0.5–4.0 g/L (40–300 i.u./L)
Immunoglobulins (Ig): IgG	5.0–13.0 g/L (60–160 i.u./L)
Immunoglobulins (Ig): IgM – males	0.3–2.2 g/L (40–270 i.u./L)
Immunoglobulins (Ig): IgM – females	0.4–2.5 g/L (50–300 i.u./L)
Iron – males	14–32 µmol/L
Iron – females	10–28 µmol/L
Iron binding capacity (total)	45–72 µmol/L

Analyte	Reference Values
Iron binding capacity (saturation)	14–47%
Lactate	0.4–1.4 mmol/L
Lactate dehydrogenase (LDH)	100–300 i.u./L
Lead	0.5–1.9 µmol/L
Magnesium	0.75–1.0 mmol/L
5′-Nucleotidase	1–11 i.u./L
Osmolality	285–295 mOsm/kg
Phosphatase; *see* acid and alkaline	
Phosphate	0.8–1.4 mmol/L
Potassium	3.3–4.7 mmol/L
Proteins – total	62–82 g/L
Proteins – albumin	36–47 g/L
Proteins – globulins	24–37 g/L
Proteins – electrophoresis (% of total): Albumin 52–68 Globulin α_1 4.2–7.2 α_2 6.8–12 β 9.3–15 γ 13–23	
Sodium	132–144 mmol/L
Triglyceride (fasting)	0.6–1.7 mmol/L
Urate – males	0.12–0.42 mmol/L
Urate – females	0.12–0.36 mmol/L
Urea	2.5–6.6 mmol/L

Haematological Values

Analyte	Reference Values
Bleeding time (Ivy)	Up to 11 min
Body fluid (total):	50% (obese)–70% (lean) of body weight
Intracellular	30–40% of body weight
Extracellular	20–30% of body weight
Blood volume:	
Red cell mass, men	30 ± 5 mL/kg
Red cell mass, women	25 ± 5 mL/kg
Plasma volume (both sexes)	45 ± 5 mL/kg
Erythrocyte sedimentation rate (Westergren)	0–6 mm in 1 h normal
	7–20 mm in 1 h doubtful
	>20 mm in 1 h abnormal
Fibrinogen	1.5–4.0 g/L
Folate – serum	2–20 µg/L
Folate – red cell	>100 µg/L
Haemoglobin – men	13–18 g/dL
Haemoglobin – women	11.5–16.5 g/dL
Haptoglobin	0.3–2.0 g/L
Leucocytes – adults	4.0–11.0 × 10^9/L
Differential white cell count:	
Neutrophil granulocytes	2.5–7.5 × 10^9/L
Lymphocytes	1.0–3.5 × 10^9/L
Monocytes	0.2–0.8 × 10^9/L
Eosinophil granulocytes	0.04–0.4 × 10^9/L
Basophil granulocytes	0.01–0.1 × 10^9/L
Mean corpuscular haemoglobin (MCH)	27–32 pg
Mean corpuscular haemoglobin	30–35 g/dL concentration (MCHC)
Mean corpuscular volume (MCV)	78–98 fl
Packed cell volume (PCV) or haematocrit:	
Men	0.40–0.54
Women	0.35–0.47
Platelets	150–400 × 10^9/L
Prothrombin time	11–15 s
Red cell count – men	4.5–6.5 × 10^{12}/L
Red cell count – women	3.8–5.8 × 10^{12}/L
Red cell life span (mean)	120 days
Red cell life span T½(^{51}Cr)	25–35 days
Reticulocytes (adults)	10–100 × 10^9/L
Vitamin B_{12} (in serum as cyanocobalamin)	160–925 ng/L

Emergencies

Chapter 1

Introduction to Surgery

Marcus J.D. Wagstaff • Andrew T. Raftery

CHAPTER OUTLINE

The practice of surgery today involves not only technical skills but also a whole range of other skills, such as communication skills, delivery of informed consent, breaking bad news and bereavement counselling. Surgical practice must be evidence-based, and surgeons must conduct regular audits as well as be aware of their accountability in patient care.

APPROACH TO THE PATIENT

Most patients are quite happy to be seen and examined by medical students. Their usual attitude is: 'Doctors have to learn, don't they?' Some patients, however, resent being seen by students, some understandably because they are shy and embarrassed by their condition, but others because they do not feel they should be treated as 'guinea pigs'. The latter are almost certainly those who in subsequent years will complain that doctors have failed to make the correct diagnosis, and one wonders exactly how they consider medical students should learn.

Bedside manner is extremely important. It is important to establish rapport with patients so that they can trust you. Before approaching any patient on the ward, always ask the nurse in charge of the ward if you can see the patient. It may be that the patient is not well enough to be seen and examined repeatedly by students. When approaching the patient, introduce yourself with a handshake and let the patient know who you are: 'My name is John Smith. I am a medical student. Would you mind if I talk to you and examine you?' Always attend the ward at a sensible time and try to avoid disturbing the patients during their rest period. Always examine the patient with a colleague or a nurse present (chaperone). Do not carry out intimate examinations such as rectal or vaginal examinations except under strict supervision.

In the outpatient clinic, there will usually be notices displayed that students may be present during the consultation. Patients are told that if they do not wish to see students, they should inform the nurse in charge of the outpatient clinic. It is our practice always to ask the accompanying nurse to check with the patients whether they mind seeing students before they are brought into the consultation room. Always take plenty of time to take a history from the patient. Never rush, or you may miss important points in the history. Always wash your hands both before and after examining a patient.

TAKING A HISTORY

The importance of taking a clear history cannot be overemphasised. Success in examinations will depend on the ability to take a clear and concise history in a fixed period of time. Always allow yourself plenty of time to take a full history. Develop a method of taking it, trying not to write and talk to the patient at the same time. Although as students you will not normally write the patient's history in the notes, you should get used to recording it so that you know exactly how to record it in the notes when you become a qualified doctor. Initially you should record the following:

- Full name (if the patient is wearing an identification band on the wrist, check that the name corresponds with that given to you by the patient.)
- Address
- Sex
- Age
- Ethnic group
- Marital status
- Occupation.

Make sure that you record the date and time of the examination. You will need to do this so that you can record subsequent progress.
The remainder of the history should be taken in the following order:

1. *The presenting complaint*. Ask what symptoms the patient is complaining of. If there is more than one complaint, list them in the order in which they are most troublesome to the patient. It is important that you document what the patient says, not what the diagnosis is, i.e. presenting complaint is pain in the right lower abdomen – not appendicitis.
2. *The history of the presenting complaint*. Record the full details of the main complaint or complaints. Allow the patient to give a full record of complaints relating to a particular system and then ask any remaining questions that you may have about the abnormal system. For example, if the patient complains of indigestion, nausea and vomiting, make sure that as part of the history of the presenting complaint, which clearly relates to the alimentary tract, you ask all other questions in this section about the alimentary tract, e.g. bowel habit, abdominal distension, jaundice.
3. *Systematic enquiry*. Once you are satisfied that you have obtained the full history of the presenting complaint and have asked all pertinent questions about the abnormal system, you should ask direct questions about other systems. These are laid out below:
   a. *Alimentary system*. Appetite. Change in diet. Change in weight. Nausea. Difficulty in swallowing. Regurgitation. Heartburn. Flatulence. Indigestion. Vomiting. Character of the vomit, e.g. coffee grounds, blood, bile, faeculent. Abdominal pain. Abdominal distension. Change in bowel habit. Characteristics of the stool. Rectal bleeding. Change of skin colour, e.g. pallor of anaemia, jaundice.

b. *Respiratory system*. Cough. Sputum – character of sputum, e.g. purulent, haemoptysis. Dyspnoea. Wheezing. Hoarseness. Chest pain.
c. *Cardiovascular system*. Chest pain. Dyspnoea. Paroxysmal nocturnal dyspnoea. Orthopnoea. Palpitations. Ankle swelling. Cough. Dizziness. Intermittent claudication. Rest pain. Temperature or colour changes of hands and feet. Oedema.
d. *Nervous system*. Blackouts. Fits, loss of consciousness. Fainting attacks. Tremor. Weakness of limbs. Paraesthesia. Disturbances of smell, vision or hearing. Headaches. Change of behaviour.
e. *Musculoskeletal system*. Pain in joints. Swelling of joints. Limitation of movement. Muscle pain. Muscle weakness. Disturbance of gait.
f. *Genitourinary system*. Frequency of micturition. Hesitancy. Poor stream. Dysuria. Colour of urine, e.g. haematuria. Thirst. Polyuria. Symptoms of uraemia – headache, drowsiness, fits, vomiting, peripheral oedema. Loin pain. Date of menarche or menopause. Menstruation. Dysmenorrhoea. Previous pregnancies and their complications. Breast symptoms – pain, lumps. Impotence. Dyspareunia.

4. *Past medical history*. Previous illnesses, operations or accidents. Diabetes. Rheumatic fever. Tuberculosis. Asthma. Hypertension. Sexually transmitted disease.
5. *Family history*. Cause of death of close relatives, e.g. parents, brothers and sisters. Enquire particularly about cardiovascular disease and malignancy. Check for familial illnesses, e.g. adult polycystic kidney disease.
6. *Social history*. Occupation – check fully the details of the occupation and make sure you understand exactly what the patient does. For example, if the patient has worked in the dyeing industry and is complaining of painless haematuria, a likely diagnosis is bladder cancer. If the patient has worked in the building industry in the past and presents with chest symptoms, there must be a possibility of asbestos-related malignancy. Housing. Travel abroad. Leisure activities. Marital status. Sexual habits. Smoking. Drinking. Eating habits.
7. *Drug history*. Check the patient's present medication. Make particular enquiries about steroids, anticoagulants and the contraceptive pill. Ask about recreational drugs. Ask about allergies, especially to antibiotics. Ask specifically, 'Does any drug bring you out in a rash?'

HINTS AND TIPS

When you gain more experience in taking a history, you may want to move away from a systems review. A systems review is a good way to start, but when you are more experienced, it is better to present symptoms in a more positive and practical way. An example is presenting a surgical case to an anaesthetist. Rather than listing shortness of breath (SOB) and chest pain in a systems review, present it as what distance on the flat they get SOB. Can they climb a flight of stairs or do they stop halfway to the top? Can they lie flat? Do they have a glyceryl trinitrate (GTN) spray – if so, how often do they use it? After this 'end of the bed' assessment, a colleague will have a far better idea about the patient.

History of Pain

It is important that you accurately assess the nature of the patient's pain. When taking the history, you need to ask the following questions:

- Where is the pain?
- When did the pain begin?
- What is the nature of the pain?
- Does anything make the pain better or does anything make the pain worse?
- Are there any associated symptoms?
- Have you had a similar pain before?
- Do you have any idea what is causing the pain?

Taking a pain history can be facilitated by remembering the mnemonic '**SOCRATES**':

- **S**ite: where did the pain start and is it still in the same place or has it moved?
- **O**nset: was the onset sudden, e.g. peritonitis, or gradual, e.g. the colicky pain of small bowel obstruction?
- **C**haracter: e.g. dull, vague, cramping or colicky, sharp, burning
- **R**adiation: e.g. loin to groin as in ureteric colic
- **A**ssociated factors: e.g. vomiting, diarrhoea, fever, affect of movement, affect of micturition
- **T**iming: is the pain constant or intermittent, e.g. the pain of peritonitis is constant while the pain of colic comes and goes? Ask how long the pain lasts if it is intermittent.
- **E**xacerbations and relieving factors: ask the patient what makes the pain better and what makes it worse. For example, the pain of peritonitis is eased by lying still whereas the pain of colic makes the patient move about in an attempt to get comfortable.
- **S**everity: it is often difficult to determine the severity of the pain. Ask the patient to attempt to grade the pain on a system of 1–10, 10 being the most severe. However, the patient may tell you that it is the worst pain they have ever had or, in the case of a female, you can judge it if they tell you that the pain is worse than labour pain.

Always ask the patient if they have had a similar pain before; e.g. if a patient has had biliary colic before, they will be able to tell you if they think it is biliary colic again. Similarly, a patient who has had previous myocardial infarct will be able to tell you whether the symptoms are similar on this occasion. It is always worth asking the patient if they have any idea what the pain is due to, as friends or family members may have had similar pains.

EXAMINATION OF A LUMP

History

1. When did the patient first notice the lump?
2. What brought the lump to the patient's notice, e.g. pain?
3. Is the lump symptomatic?
4. Has there been any change in size?
5. Does the lump ever disappear, e.g. a hernia may disappear on lying down or a sebaceous cyst may discharge and settle down only to fill up again at a later date?

6. Are there any other lumps on the body of similar nature, e.g. lipomas or neurofibromata may be multiple?
7. Does the patient know of any cause for the lump, e.g. trauma?

Examination

- *Site*: describe this in exact anatomical terms. It is best to measure it from a fixed bony point.
- *Shape*: e.g. is it spherical, does it have an irregular outline?
- *Size*: measure this accurately using a tape measure.
- *Surface*: is it smooth or irregular?
- *Edge*: is the edge of the lump clearly defined or indistinct?
- *Colour of overlying skin*: e.g. red and inflamed suggesting an inflammatory lesion.
- *Temperature*: is the skin overlying the lump hot or of normal temperature?
- *Tenderness*: is the lump tender?
- *Composition*: is the mass solid, fluid or gas? Check for consistence, fluctuation, fluid thrill, translucency, pulsation, compressibility and bruits.

Consistency. A lump may vary from soft to bony hard. A simple scale of consistence is suggested: soft, e.g. subcutaneous lipoma; firm, e.g. Hodgkin's lymph node; hard, e.g. carcinoma of the breast; stony hard or bony hard, e.g. ivory osteoma of the skull.

Fluctuation. Demonstration of this sign indicates a fluid-filled cavity. Pressure on one side of a fluid-filled cavity causes the other surface to protrude because an increase in pressure within a cavity is transmitted equally and at right angles to all parts of its wall. The test should be carried out in two planes at right angles to each other.

Fluid Thrill. This detects the presence of free fluid in a cavity. A percussion wave can be conducted across the fluid. Tap one side of the lump and feel the transmitted vibration at the opposite extremity. This is a classical sign of ascites, and to prevent a thrill being transmitted through the abdominal wall, a second person should place the edge of their hand along the abdomen, midway between the percussing and palpating hands.

Translucency. If a swelling transilluminates, it must contain clear fluid. Use a bright torch in a darkened room. Lumps that classically transilluminate brilliantly are hydroceles, cystic hygroma in children and joint ganglia.

Resonance. Solid and fluid-filled lumps are dull to percussion. Gas-filled swellings are resonant, e.g. distended obstructed bowel.

Pulsatility. Rest your hand on every lump and make sure that it does not pulsate. If a pulse is present, distinguish between transmitted pulsation through a lump and an expansile pulsatile lump, i.e. an aneurysm. To do this, place a finger of either hand on opposite sides of the lump. If the fingers are pushed up and down in the same plane, it is a transmitted pulsation. If they are pushed upwards and apart, it is a true expansile pulsation, i.e. aneurysm.

Compressibility. Try to empty a lump by gentle pressure and see if it refills spontaneously. This is the sign of compressibility, e.g. strawberry naevus, sapheno-varix.

Bruit. Listen over the lump. A systolic bruit may be heard over an aneurysm or a vascular goitre associated with thyrotoxicosis. A continuous machinery bruit may be heard over an arteriovenous fistula.

Reducibility. This is a property of herniae. The lump may be gently compressed and reduced to the cavity in which it is normally contained. It will reappear by coughing or gravity (standing up).

Relation to Surrounding Structures. Assess the mobility of the lump. Is it attached to the skin or is it attached to deep structures? Is it within the peritoneal cavity or the abdominal wall? Tensing the abdominal muscles by raising the head and shoulders will allow you to distinguish.

Regional Lymph Nodes. Always remember to palpate the regional lymph nodes.

Surrounding Tissues and Extremities. If the lump is on a limb, make sure that it is not interfering with the normal function of the limb, such as pressure on a nerve or interference with distal circulation, e.g. a popliteal artery aneurysm associated with distal ischaemia, or pressure on the common peroneal nerve.

General Examination

Always remember to examine the whole of the patient, e.g. a lump in the breast may not only be associated with axillary lymphadenopathy but may be associated with a pleural effusion, and a malignant melanoma on the leg may be associated with hepatomegaly.

> **HINTS AND TIPS**
>
> If you are having difficulty in deciding the origin of a lump, it is a good idea to consider the anatomy of the area and consider the tissues present in the area, from superficial to deep, and then to think what pathology can affect those tissues, e.g. a common lesion in the skin is a sebaceous cyst, a common lesion in the subcutaneous fat is a lipoma, if there is an artery present in the deeper tissues, the swelling may be an aneurysm. Examples of this reasoning are demonstrated more fully for lumps in the groin in Chapter 13.

EXAMINATION OF AN ULCER

Definition

An ulcer is a break in the continuity of an epithelial surface. Many ulcers are occult in the gastrointestinal (GI) tract and, unfortunately, many of these tend to be malignant. However, ulcers on the skin and in the oral cavity are easily noticed by the patient.

History

1. When did the patient first notice the ulcer?
2. What first made the patient notice the ulcer, e.g. was it painful or did it start as a different sort of lesion and then become ulcerated, e.g. malignant melanoma?
3. What are the symptoms of the ulcer?
4. Has the ulcer changed since it first appeared, e.g. has there been a chronic venous ulcer on the leg which has previously healed and then broken down again?
5. Has the patient ever had any other ulcers?
6. Is there any obvious cause for the ulcer, e.g. trauma?

Examination

Record accurately the site and size of the ulcer. Check for colour, tenderness, increased temperature, base, edge, depth, discharge and surrounding tissues. Check the state of the local lymph nodes and carry out a general examination.

Base. Usually slough or granulation tissue. Some ulcers have a characteristic base, e.g. ischaemic ulcers often contain no granulation tissue but may contain black necrotic tissue, or tendons or bone may be seen in the base of the ulcer. Syphilitic ulcers have a classic slough that looks like a wash leather.

Edge. Classically, five types are described. These are shown in Figure 1.1 together with their usual aetiologies.

Depth. Record this accurately in millimetres.

Discharge. This may be serous, sanguineous or purulent. It may be necessary to remove slough from the base of an ulcer to accurately assess it.

Surrounding Tissues. Are the surrounding tissues pink and healthy? Is the innervation normal, e.g. neuropathic ulcer associated with diabetes? Are there black satellite nodules around the ulcer, e.g. malignant melanoma?

Examine the Local Lymph Nodes.

Carry out a General Examination.

CLASSIFICATION OF DISEASE

When initially starting your surgical training, your knowledge will be limited. You will, therefore, find it difficult to reach a diagnosis. To do this you should go through a broad classification of the aetiology of disease as shown in Table 1.1. This is sometimes known as the 'surgical sieve'. Ask yourself, is this lesion congenital (usually easy to decide) or is it acquired? If it is acquired, go through the 'sieve' and try and decide which classification it belongs to. As you learn more pathology and more surgery, you will still find this classification suitable when trying to reach a differential diagnosis. It is a good idea when you are first learning, with every disease, lump or ulcer you meet, to sit down and go through the 'surgical sieve' and decide which of these groups it belongs to.

EVIDENCE-BASED MEDICINE

Evidence-based medicine is the conscientious, explicit and judicious use of current best evidence in making decisions about the care of individual patients. Evidence-based medicine combines the individual doctor's expertise and the best available external evidence when making decisions about the patient's healthcare.

Evidence-based medicine is a lifelong process that involves:

- Asking clinical questions
- Tracking down the best evidence
- Assessing the evidence
- Applying the results in practice
- Evaluating subsequent performance.

Evidence-based medicine has the following advantages:

- It offers an objective way to determine and maintain consistently high quality and safety standards in medical practice.
- It helps speed up the process of transferring clinical research findings into clinical practice.
- It has the potential to significantly reduce the cost of delivery of healthcare.

External evidence includes research from basic medical sciences, patient-centred clinical research, randomised trials and meta-analyses. Patient-centred clinical research looks at the accuracy and appropriateness of diagnostic tests, the use of prognostic

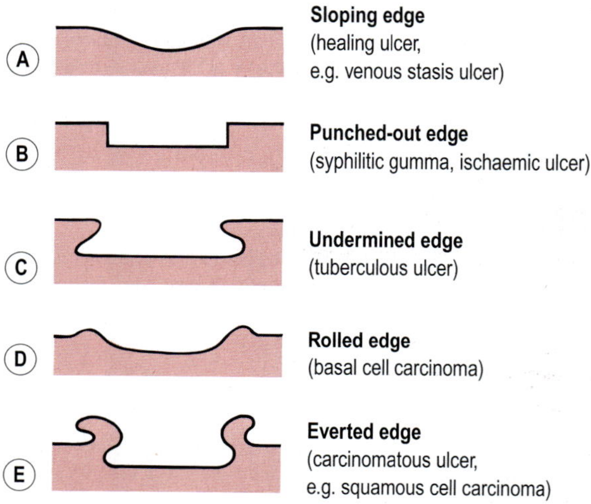

FIGURE 1.1
Common types of ulcer edge.

TABLE 1.1

CLASSIFICATION OF DISEASE ('SURGICAL SIEVE')
Congenital
Acquired
Traumatic
Inflammatory:
• Physical stimuli • Chemical stimuli • Infection
Neoplastic:
• Benign • Malignant
Degenerative
Vascular
Endocrine/metabolic
Autoimmune
Iatrogenic
Psychogenic

indicators and the effectiveness and safety of treatments. External clinical evidence may invalidate previously accepted tests and treatments, replacing them with new ones that are more accurate, effective and safe. Without the current best evidence, surgical practice risks becoming out of date, to the detriment of patient care.

Evidence may be available from individual randomised trials or via meta-analysis of several trials such as those published in the Cochrane Database of Systematic Reviews.

CLINICAL GOVERNANCE IN SURGICAL PRACTICE

Clinical governance is a framework through which healthcare organisations are accountable for continually improving the quality of their services and safeguarding high standards of care by creating an environment in which excellence in clinical care will flourish.

The purpose of clinical governance is to ensure a systematic approach to maintaining and improving the quality of patient care. It embodies three main areas:

1. Recognisable high standards of care
2. Transparent responsibility and accountability for those standards
3. A drive for improvement through constant monitoring of standards.

Clinical governance covers organisational systems and processes for monitoring and improving services including:

- Education and training
- Clinical audit
- Clinical risk management
- Clinical effectiveness
- Research and development
- Openness.

Effective clinical governance addresses those structures, systems and processes that ensure quality and accountability, thus ensuring proper management of an organisation's operations and delivery of service in an open and transparent setting. In doing so, it ensures continual improvement of patient care with a commitment to quality and the prevention of clinical errors.

CLINICAL AUDIT

Clinical audit is a continuous cycle of quality improvement that seeks to improve patient care and service delivery through systematic review of care against explicit criteria and the implementation of change. The clinical audit process is known as the audit cycle. This involves observation of existing practice, the setting of standards, comparison between observed and set standards, implementation of change and reaudit of clinical practice (Figure 1.2). The main components of the audit cycle are:

- Choosing a topic
- Reviewing current standards or agreeing on standards
- Accurate collection of data on current practice
- Use of data to compare with standards
- A system for implementing change to make improvement
- Reaudit to ensure practice has improved.

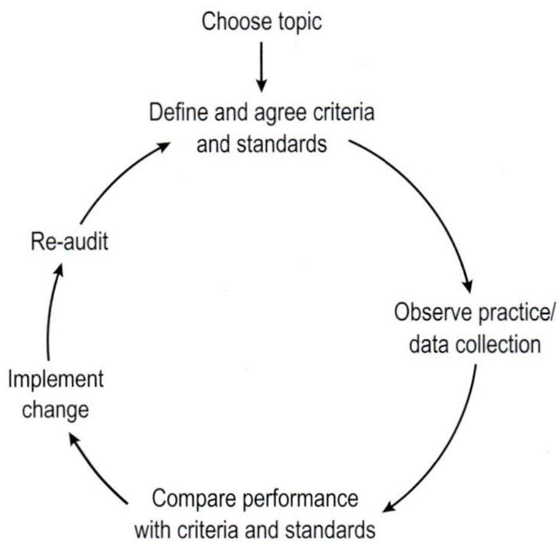

FIGURE 1.2
The audit cycle.

Benefits of undertaking clinical audit include:

- Improvements in clinical practice benefiting patient care and service delivery
- Meeting evidence-based best practice
- Minimising error
- Developing local guidelines/protocols
- Reducing adverse clinical incidents, complaints and claims.

Clinical audit is used to compare current practice with evidence of good practice. It basically asks the question, 'Are we actually doing what we think we are doing?' Clinical audit can:

- Identify major risk, resource and service development implications
- Reinforce implementation of evidence-based practice
- Influence improvements to individual patient care
- Provide assurance on the quality of care.

When considering topics to audit, the following may be a useful guide; high-risk practice, cost-effectiveness, patient concerns, local concerns, conforming to international guidelines, new treatments or procedures.

Types of audit vary from basic clinical audit, e.g. morbidity/mortality, to national audit, e.g. National Confidential Enquiry into Patient Outcome and Death (NCEPOD). Whatever the subject audited, the following are essential requirements:

- Accurate high-quality data collection
- Recognition of variation in case mix
- Clearly defined outcome measures
- Appropriate statistical analysis

- A system for introducing change
- Re-evaluation of the system after change.

How does *audit* differ from *research*?

- Research:
  - Aims to establish best practice
  - Aims to generate new knowledge
  - Is theory driven
  - May involve a completely new treatment.
- Audit:
  - Aims to evaluate how close actual practice is to best practice
  - Aims to improve service delivery
  - Is practice based
  - Never involves a completely new treatment.

MEDICOLEGAL ISSUES

When a patient pursues a claim of negligence against an individual or trust, they must establish three elements:

1. The doctor owes a duty of care to that individual.
2. A breach of that duty has occurred that falls below the required standard.
3. That this breach of duty was responsible for the harm that has resulted in the claim (causation). Causation may be accepted on a balance of probability of >50% that the actions of the defendant caused the harm.

Breach of duty has historically been tested against the Bolam principle (Bolam *vs.* Friern Hospital Management Committee 1957), where the doctor is not guilty if he has acted in accordance with a practice accepted as proper and responsible by a responsible body of medical professionals skilled in that particular art. Although there may be a body of professional opinion opposing the view, as long as it can be considered acceptable practice to a group of doctors of similar standing, the action may not form a breach of duty.

More recently, the case of Bolitho *vs.* City & Hackney Health Authority (1997) led to the House of Lords deciding that if professional opinion called in support of a defence case was not capable of withstanding logical analysis, the court would be entitled to hold that the body of opinion was not reasonable or responsible. This means that a court can overrule a body of professionals supporting a defendant through the Bolam principle if it feels that their argument does not follow logical reasoning.

With the exception of minors, patients have 3 years from the time of injury, or recovery from mental illness if present at the time of injury, to bring a case to court. There can therefore be a considerable time lag prior to representation in court. It is therefore vital to maintain high standards of thorough and contemporaneous note-keeping.

Civil Procedure Rules require a Letter of Claim to be sent to the defendant and a response drawn. Particulars of Claim and Negligence are then prepared by the plaintiff, which are defended with any statements as a formal defence. If the case is to proceed, the court will hear expert opinions on each area of disagreement. If no agreement is formed, the case will go to trial.

Compensation may be awarded by the courts as 'general' damages for pain and suffering and 'special' damages for actual amounts such as claim expenses, need for care, loss of income, etc.

CONSENT

Informed consent is required for all invasive procedures. Consent should be obtained by the person who is actually going to carry out the procedure or certainly by somebody who is suitably trained and qualified and has sufficient knowledge of the proposed treatment. It is probably best that consent for major procedures is obtained either by the consultant or with the consultant present. It is good practice that consent should be obtained for any procedure that can have a complication.

For consent to be valid, the patient must have the capacity to:

1. Be able to comprehend and retain the information relevant to the decision in question
2. Believe that information
3. Weigh that information in the balance to arrive at a decision.

Consent should be informed, i.e. the patient should be given the full information about:

- The procedure
- The reasons for carrying it out
- Any alternative treatments
- Benefits of the procedure
- Adverse effects or complications
- The outcome without any treatment.

Consent must be voluntary, i.e. not the result of coercion by medical staff, relatives or friends.

Minors between the ages of 16 and 18 are presumed to have capacity to consent in English law. If a doctor feels that a child under 16 has the intelligence and maturity to comprehend the risks and benefits of an intervention (Gillick competence), the patient may consent against parental wishes. Children under 16 who are not Gillick competent may not withhold or give consent; parents must act on their behalf. Patients over 16 with fluctuating capacity (e.g. under the influence of drugs affecting mental state) should be given the opportunity to consent when lucid, if management of their medical condition can wait until then. Otherwise, doctors may consent on their behalf.

Consent may be verbal or written. Consent forms provide some evidence that the process of consent has taken place but are not themselves legal documents that prove that consent is valid.

Risks of operation may be general or specific to the operation. The general risks include the risks of anaesthesia and the risks of any operation, e.g. haemorrhage, wound infection, deep vein thrombosis. Examples of specific complications are recurrence after inguinal hernia repair, recurrent laryngeal nerve palsy after thyroid surgery, facial nerve palsy after superficial parotidectomy.

It is generally accepted that complications should be explained to the patient when they arise at a rate of 1% or greater. However, any devastating complication which may occur and has an incidence of less than 1% should be explained to the patient, e.g. paraplegia after aortic cross-clamping.

The degree of information to be conferred to a patient continues to evolve through debate in English law. Consent issues challenged by a claimant are tested in English law against the elements of negligence. Rulings have been led by legal precedent. In Sidaway *vs.* Bethlem Royal Hospital (1985), a patient undergoing cervical cord decompression was not warned against a 1–2% risk of spinal cord injury, which she subsequently suffered. Although she claimed she would not have undergone surgery if she had been warned, a responsible body of surgical opinion would also not have warned a patient of the risk, and therefore the court ruled for the doctor on the basis of the Bolam test.

Since then, in Chester *vs.* Afshar (2004), surgery for back pain resulted in cauda equina syndrome, the possibility of which the patient was not informed of prior to surgery. The judges ruled that failure to inform had violated her right to choose. The patient may, however, have still opted for this surgery; therefore it is debated that it is difficult to establish causation if the failure to inform may not have changed the outcome, i.e. the patient's choice for surgery.

Any move away from Bolam towards a Bolitho-style ruling by the English courts has not yet led to a deviation from the 'prudent doctor test' where it is a matter of clinical judgement by the doctor as to the degree of information to be given to the patient. However, in an Australian case (Rogers *vs.* Whitaker, 1992), a patient underwent surgery to her blind right eye but suffered a 1:14,000 complication of sympathetic ophthalmia leading to blindness in her functional left eye. She successfully claimed, as the court ruled that the doctor had failed to answer her questions with proper care and skill, and if the risk had been disclosed, the plaintiff would not have had the operation. This approach to disclosure of all relevant information is called the 'prudent patient test'.

BREAKING BAD NEWS

Breaking bad news to patients and their relatives is almost a daily occurrence. Most medical schools provide tutorials on 'breaking bad news' as part of the course, and much experience may be obtained in role-play in such tutorials. However, there is no substitute for the real thing, and it is appropriate for a medical student to sit in when bad news is actually being broken to relatives or patients. A doctor who is explaining the bad news should always check with the patient or the relatives that it is appropriate for a medical student to be present at the time. It is understandable that some patients' relatives may find this obtrusive.

When we think of the nature of breaking bad news, we usually think in terms of explaining to someone that they have an inoperable condition. However, for some patients' relatives it is merely bad news that the patient actually requires surgery or that, as a result of curative surgery, the patient, for example, needs a permanent colostomy. Usually, however, breaking bad news involves explaining inoperable and incurable cancer and the need to face death. A problem then arises about how much the patient needs to know and in some cases, whether the patient actually needs to know at all. The answer to the latter is that the patient should always be told. Unless the patient is fully aware of the facts, it is difficult to deal with subsequent management, particularly explaining palliative treatment, e.g. radiotherapy or the fact that the patient requires hospice care.

Occasionally, relatives request that the patient is not told. This is not appropriate and should be explained to the relatives, particularly the fact that if the patient finds out by other means (and the patient surely will, maybe even through a careless word on a ward round), then trust is lost between patient and relative and patient and doctor. It is well recognised that most patients are told less than they would actually like to know. Occasionally, even the medical professional will rationalise reasons for not wanting to tell the patient, e.g. the patient would not want to know. In fact, most patients are intelligent and shrewd, and when you actually sit down to explain the bad news to them, you will realise that they have already half suspected it and many will thank you for being honest with them. Always remember that patients have many affairs that they wish to put in order, and also explaining to them honestly about life expectancy will enable them to decide if further unpleasant palliative therapy is worthwhile.

It is always difficult to know how and what to tell the patient. It is probably best not to do this on a busy ward round but to take time to go back to the bed with the nurse who is looking after the patient, sit down and take time to explain. There is a balance to explaining bad news which is somewhere between giving a long explanation skirting round the problem without actually indicating how bad the problem is and the brusque honesty approach ('You have got incurable cancer and less than 3 months to live'). Do not leave the bedside immediately after giving bad news and, worse still, do not indicate that somebody else will come back shortly and re-explain what you have already said. It is best to wait a while to give patients a chance to ask any questions. If they do not have any at the time, indicate that you will come back later when they have had a chance to let the bad news sink in and when they may have thought of some questions that they wish to ask. It is important to allow sufficient time to talk to patients and to talk to them sensitively and also indicate that you are prepared to talk to members of the family and explain things fully to them. Some patients would be grateful if members of the family are present when bad news is broken.

Accepting terminal illness often takes time and involves a number of well-defined stages, although not all of these may occur in a particular patient. These include:

- Shock and numbness
- Denial
- Anger
- Grief
- Acceptance.

It is important that every member of the team knows exactly what has been explained to the patient and also that the family doctor is aware. Over the days following the breaking of bad news, the patient and relatives may often have numerous questions, and time must be taken to sit down and provide the answers.

DEATH AND THE CERTIFICATION OF DEATH

When you are qualified, you will be required to diagnose death. The patient is pulseless, apnoeic, and has fixed, dilated pupils. Auscultation reveals no heart sounds or breath sounds. If the patient is on a ventilator, brain death may be diagnosed even though the heart is still beating. The preconditions and the criteria for testing for brain death are explained in Chapter 19. Do not forget that after death, organs and tissue may be donated for transplantation purposes. Any solid organ and tissues may be removed from a ventilated brain-dead patient, but remember that kidneys may be removed within 30 min of death and other tissues such as cornea, bone, skin and heart valves may be removed within 24 h of death.

Certification of death is important and should be carried out as soon as possible after death. This is not the same as certifying (or diagnosing) death but is the official documentation of the patient's cause of death that must be delivered, usually by the next of kin, to the Registrar of Births and Deaths within 5 days of the death. In practice, death certification should normally be carried out on the day after death to allow the patient's relatives to make the funeral arrangements as soon as possible. Only a doctor who has seen the patient within 14 days prior to the death can legally fill in the certificate. In some cases, e.g. where the patient has died postoperatively, or after an emergency admission, or accident, the coroner must be informed. If in any doubt, it is always best to ring the coroner and discuss the case. If the coroner decides to take the case, the associated department will deal with the certification of death.

BEREAVEMENT COUNSELLING

Explaining the death of loved ones to their relatives is never easy. It is best that the medical student attends a course in bereavement counselling and also, during attachments to both medical and surgical firms, accompanies the houseman or consultant who is explaining the death to relatives. The circumstances of death may cause different emotional reactions in relatives: some react with shock, others with anger and guilt, the latter being common emotions. Anger may be directed towards the deceased, other family members or the medical profession involved in the patient's care. Support offered to the family both during the patient's illness and at the time of the patient's death not only helps them to cope better but may also reduce the likelihood of future problems. Religious beliefs and cultural background may influence reactions, and some individuals may resort to alcohol, drugs or denial as a way of coping with loss. In such cases, the help of bereavement counsellors should be sought.

Chapter 2

An Introduction to Surgical Techniques and Practical Procedures

Katherine I. Bridge

CHAPTER OUTLINE

There are a number of basic techniques and principles that are part of the 'stock-in-trade' of any surgeon. It is vital that students and surgical trainees are familiar with these, as they provide the basic skills required to effectively care for the surgical patient, to be a useful assistant and, with time, to become an independent surgeon.

SURGICAL INCISIONS

When choosing an incision, the following points should be considered:

- *Access*: the incision must be appropriately placed, large enough and capable of extension.
- *Orientation*: if possible, along the lines of skin tension (Langer's lines) or skin creases. This leads to minimal distortion and better healing.
- *Healing potential of tissues*
- *Anatomy of underlying structures*, e.g. the avoidance of nerves
- *Good cosmetic result*
- *Abdominal incision*: the common abdominal incisions and their indications are shown in Figure 2.1A. Rarer abdominal incisions are shown in Figure 2.1B. Paramedian incisions are rarely used nowadays but are included, as their scars are still seen on the abdominal wall of the older patient. The site of incisions can be useful clues as to the surgical history of a patient who is unable to recall what operations they have had in the past!

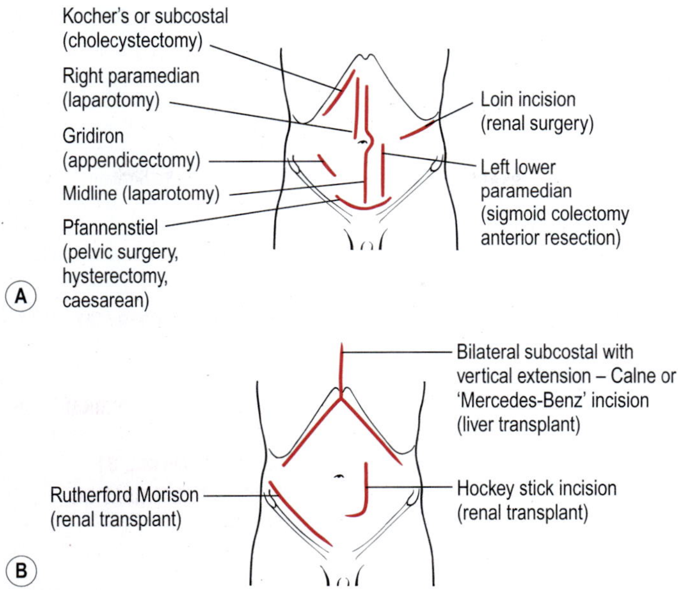

FIGURE 2.1

Abdominal incisions. (**A**) Common incisions, (**B**) rarer incisions.

HINTS AND TIPS

Remember that the incision is the only part of the operation that the patient will see. It does not matter how beautiful the internal sutures are, if the external appearance does not reflect this, they may not be happy! Making a note of skin creases and planning where to make the incision before applying surgical drapes can help with this.

SUTURES

Students are usually introduced to suturing in a clinical skills laboratory and during their A&E attachment. There is a wide range of suture materials, broadly divided into absorbable and nonabsorbable, natural and synthetic, braided and monofilament.

Absorbable

These are plain catgut (natural monofilament); chromic catgut (natural monofilament); polyglycolic acid (synthetic braided – Dexon); polyglactin (synthetic braided – Vicryl); polydioxanone (PDS, synthetic monofilament); and poliglecaprone (Monocryl – synthetic monofilament). The strength of absorbable sutures declines according to the material, catgut being the quickest to lose strength. (Catgut sutures are no longer available in the UK because of their theoretical potential for transmitting spongiform encephalopathy and the fact that there are adequate supplies of acceptable alternative synthetic sutures.)

Nonabsorbable

These include silk (natural braided); linen (natural braided); wire (stainless steel, usually monofilament); nylon (synthetic monofilament – Ethilon); polypropylene (synthetic monofilament – Prolene); and expanded polytetrafluoroethylene (ePTFE, expanded monofilament). Nonabsorbable sutures retain strength indefinitely and are used where strength is needed until repair is completed naturally, e.g. abdominal incisions and hernia repair. Nonabsorbable sutures are often used for skin closure – synthetic monofilament used in subcuticular fashion giving the best cosmetic result.

Natural Sutures

These are catgut, silk and linen, but their use is declining. Catgut is cheap but of variable strength. Silk handles well but, as with linen, elicits a strong inflammatory reaction.

Synthetic Sutures

Types include Dexon, Vicryl, Monocryl, PDS, nylon, polypropylene and ePTFE. They are more expensive than natural sutures but cause little tissue reaction. The degree of strength and absorbability can be controlled in manufacture.

Monofilament

These include catgut, polydioxanone, wire, polypropylene and nylon. They are smooth and pass easily through tissues and cause less tissue reaction. The disadvantage is that they are stiff, slippery and difficult to knot.

Braided (Polyfilament)

These include polyglycolic acid, polyglactin, silk, nylon and linen. They handle well, but interstices harbour bacteria.

Wire

This is useful for closing the sternum in cardiac procedures and for orthopaedic procedures. It is strong, inert, but subject to breakage and handles poorly.

Gauge

Gauge (G) is the calibre of the suture and is expressed in numbers. Originally, the finest gauge was '1' and the heaviest '4', but with the development of finer sutures, a scale of '0s' was developed, wherein the more the 0s, the finer the suture, e.g. '0', '00' (2/0), '000' (3/0). The finest suture is 10/0 and is used in eye surgery. The gauge used depends on the strength required, number of sutures, type of suture material being used and cosmetic requirements.

Needles

Needles are cutting or round-bodied. They come in a variety of shapes and lengths and may be straight or curved. Cutting needles are usually triangular in cross-section and are useful for skin, tendon and breast tissue. Round-bodied needles are oval or round in cross-section. Round-bodied needles are useful for gastrointestinal (GI) tract and vascular anastomoses.

Methods of Suturing

Sutures may be interrupted, continuous, vertical mattress, horizontal mattress or subcuticular. The different methods of suturing are illustrated in Figure 2.2. The choice depends on the site and nature of the operation and surgeon's preference. Interrupted

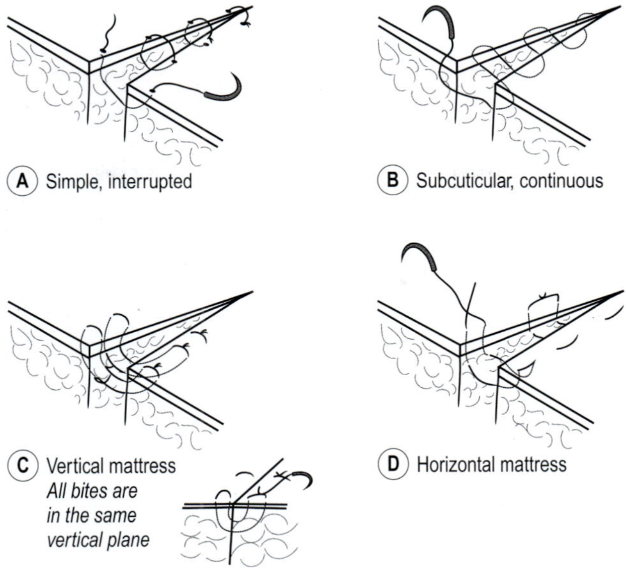

FIGURE 2.2

Methods of wound closure.

sutures may be used if there is a risk of infection, where some individual sutures may be removed to allow drainage. Subcuticular sutures may be used to give good cosmetic results, especially when using synthetic monofilament. Synthetic absorbable subcuticular sutures (e.g. Vicryl) may be used in children to avoid the trauma of suture removal.

Removal of Sutures

The timing is a balance between strength of healing and a good cosmetic result. Some areas are better vascularised under less tension, and therefore heal quicker than others. The following is a rough guide for the time of removal for different areas: face and neck (3–4 days); scalp (5–7 days); limbs (10–14 days); hands and feet (10–14 days); and abdomen (8–10 days).

Alternatives to Sutures

Alternatives include clips and staples. Michel clips appose the skin edges but do not penetrate the skin, and cosmetic results are good. Preloaded disposable staples have largely replaced Michel clips. Cosmetic results are excellent. Stapling devices are also available for GI anastomoses. Simple wounds in children can be closed with adhesive strips (Steri-Strips). Increasingly, skin glue (e.g. Dermabond) is used to close small, superficial incisions and lacerations and can generally be used for skin incisions/wounds that would previously have required 5/0 sutures, such as on the scalp. It is water resistant and removes the need for suture removal. It is most often used in children and in the emergency department, although a number of surgeons are starting to use skin glue to close the small wounds that result from laparoscopic ports. Scalp lacerations in children can also be closed using hair adjacent to the wound edges as 'sutures'. The hairs are knotted across the wound.

DRAINS

Drains are used prophylactically to drain anticipated collections, e.g. haematomas, bile leaks, urine leaks, or therapeutically to remove collections of pus, blood or other body fluids. Most drains consist of latex-based material or silicone. Red rubber tube drains are still used occasionally. Red rubber and latex drains form better tracks than silicone by exciting more tissue reaction. Drainage may be open or closed, suction or nonsuction.

Open Drainage

This is drainage by capillary action or gravity into dressings or stoma bags. Drainage may depend on the position of the patient. Sepsis is commoner with open drains.

Closed Drainage

This is drainage into a bag or bottle attached to the drain. Usually it is a suction system, although it may be passive, working on the syphon system. Sepsis is less common with closed systems.

Suction Drains

These help to collapse down potential spaces as well as draining blood and other fluids. They are usually closed systems, and therefore the risk of sepsis is less. Sump drains are open drains used in connection with suction. Sump drains contain an air inlet lumen to prevent blockage with soft tissue. Sepsis is a risk with sump drains.

Nonsuction Drains

These are used mainly intraperitoneally to drain gastrointestinal and biliary anastomoses. They are usually left for up to 5 days. They are usually rubber, polyvinyl chloride (PVC) or Silastic. If prolonged drainage is necessary and there is need for a tract to be established, rubber drains should be used, as they stimulate fibrosis.

Complications of Drains

- Sepsis: commoner with open drains
- Failure: especially suction drains which draw fat or omentum into the side holes
- Pressure or suction necrosis of the bowel leading to leakage of the intestinal contents with peritonitis
- Rarely, erosion into a vessel with haemorrhage.

HINTS AND TIPS

The contents of a drain can be extremely useful when assessing an unwell patient postoperatively. Outputs into a drain should be monitored by nursing staff in a similar way to urine output and recorded on input–output charts. Do not be fooled into a false sense of security by an empty drain! This can mean one of three things: there is nothing to drain, the drain has been emptied (and may have been full 5 min prior to your arrival – check the chart) or that the drain is not working. If, for example, you suspect that a patient is bleeding, but the drain is empty, it is safer to assume that the drain is not working than it is to assume that the patient is not bleeding.

STOMAS (-OSTOMIES)

Colostomy

A permanent colostomy usually opens onto the anterior abdominal wall in the left iliac fossa (LIF). It is flush with the skin, and the contents of the bag are usually formed faeces. It is most commonly created following an operation for abdominoperineal resection of the rectum. A temporary colostomy in this position is usually consequent on a Hartmann's procedure. Colostomies may occasionally be seen in the upper abdomen, either to the right or left of the midline, when they are defunctioning colostomies fashioned in the transverse colon to protect a distal anastomosis, although defunctioning ileostomies are preferred nowadays.

HINTS AND TIPS

If a patient with a colostomy presents with symptoms of obstruction, be sure to examine the stoma properly. Occasionally, constriction due to scarring at the site of the stoma can be the cause of obstruction rather than anything more sinister. In the case of a colostomy, you should be able to insert a finger into the stoma and assess the stool in the same way as you might perform a rectal examination on a patient without a colostomy.

Ileostomy

An ileostomy is usually in the right iliac fossa (RIF). It is *not* flush with the skin but overhangs as a 'spout' for about 2.5 cm. This is so that the liquid small bowel content, rich in pancreatic enzymes, does not come into contact with the skin of the abdominal wall, resulting in tryptic digestion of the skin. The contents of the bag are fluid and are of the consistency of porridge. An ileostomy usually results from total colectomy with excision of the rectum (panproctocolectomy) for ulcerative colitis. Defunctioning loop ileostomies are used to protect distal anastomoses.

Urostomy (Ileal Bladder)

A urostomy is usually in the RIF. It is a blind-ended loop of ileum and looks not dissimilar to an ileostomy, i.e. it is not flush with the skin edge but looks like a 'spout'. The ureters have been transplanted into the ileal loop. Urine drains from the ileal loop. It is usually created following total cystectomy for carcinoma of the bladder.

Mucous Fistula

In some operations it may be necessary to bring out both ends of the bowel, e.g. ischaemic bowel, to assess viability. One end will be the functioning draining stoma (either ileostomy or colostomy) and the other end will be the functionless stoma, termed a 'mucous fistula'. In paediatric/neonatal surgery, contents from the stoma are sometimes 'recycled' down the mucous fistula to encourage distal bowel development prior to a delayed anastomosis.

LOCAL ANAESTHESIA

Local anaesthetics are frequently used in hospitals (and in the community) for minor surgical procedures as well as adjuncts to other forms of anaesthesia in more complex operations. Knowledge of local anaesthesia is therefore vital for any surgeon in training, as many of these minor procedures can be done by a junior surgeon without supervision. Only local anaesthetic infiltration will be described in this chapter, as other local anaesthetic techniques, such as regional nerve blocks and spinal and epidural anaesthesia, are the province of the anaesthetist.

Some operations will require only very small amounts of anaesthesia, while others (e.g. repair of an inguinal hernia) may reach the maximum safe dose. Local anaesthetics reversibly block nerve conduction by inactivating sodium channels, blocking electrical depolarisation. Smaller nerve fibres are more sensitive than larger nerve fibres, so pain and temperature sensation are lost first, followed by proprioception, touch and pressure and motor impulses. This explains why the patient may feel pressure but no pain, and loss of motor function occurs later.

HINTS AND TIPS

When using local anaesthetic for minor surgical procedures, remember to tell the patient that it is normal to feel pressure, pulling and movement, but that they should not feel any pain. A patient who is expecting to feel nothing may become alarmed if they can feel pressure, even if the anaesthetic is working perfectly well!

Types of Local Anaesthetic

Three main types of local anaesthetic are available: lidocaine, bupivacaine and prilocaine – lidocaine being the most widely used.

Lidocaine. Rapid onset, short duration. Comes in three strengths: 0.5% (5mg/mL), 1% (10mg/mL), 2% (20mg/mL). The upper dose limit for lidocaine is 3mg/kg (plain), 7mg/kg (with 1:200,000 adrenaline).

Bupivacaine. Slower onset, longer duration. Comes in two strengths: 0.25% (2.5mg/mL), 0.5% (5mg/mL). Upper dose limit is 2mg/kg (both plain and with adrenaline).

Prilocaine. Rapid onset, shorter duration than lidocaine. Comes as 1% solution (10mg/mL). Upper dose limit is 6mg/kg.

Local anaesthetics may be mixed with 1 in 200,000 adrenaline. Adrenaline is included as a vasoconstrictor. It diminishes local blood flow, slows the rate of absorption of the local anaesthetic and prolongs its local effect. Adrenaline should be used in low concentration, e.g. 1 in 200,000 (5 μg/mL). The total dose of adrenaline should not exceed 500 μg.

Adrenaline must not be used where there are 'end' arteries, i.e. never on the digits or penis. It is also inadvisable to use it on other extremities, i.e. the nose, nipple or lobe of the ear. Addition of adrenaline does not increase the safe dose of bupivacaine, and there is little point in using it for infiltration with bupivacaine except to reduce bleeding. As adrenaline has a shorter half-life than bupivacaine, it does not ultimately protect against systemic bupivacaine toxicity. The safe dose of bupivacaine therefore is unaffected by the presence of adrenaline. Adrenaline is used, however, for its vasoconstrictive effect to reduce local bleeding. Local anaesthetic techniques should only be performed where adequate resuscitation facilities are available. Local anaesthetics should not be injected into inflamed or infected tissues where they are largely ineffective and may be responsible for further spread of infection.

Complications

- Injection site: pain, haematoma, direct nerve trauma (with delayed recovery of sensation), infection
- With adrenaline: ischaemic necrosis (digits and penis)
- Systemic effects: idiosyncratic or allergic reactions (rare)
- Toxicity.

Toxicity

This may be due to excess dosage, inadvertent intravenous injection or premature release of a Bier's block (intravenous regional anaesthesia) cuff. Toxic effects include light-headedness, tinnitus, circumoral and tongue numbness, nausea, vomiting, visual disturbances, fits, CNS depression leading to coma, arrhythmias and cardiovascular collapse.

TOURNIQUETS

Tourniquets are used in limbs where a bloodless field is required or to limit blood loss. They can also be used for a Bier's block (i.v. local anaesthetic for the manipulation of upper limb fractures). The principles of use of tourniquets include:

- Empty the limb of blood (this can be performed by elevation, Esmarch bandage or rubber 'sleeve-like' appliances which both aim to empty the limb of blood).
- The tourniquet is placed at the proximal end of the limb (layers of crepe bandage are used underneath the cuff to protect the skin).
- For upper limb surgery an inflation pressure of 200 mmHg (or 50–75 mmHg above patient's systolic blood pressure) is used and for lower limb surgery 250–350 mmHg (100–150 mmHg above patient's systolic blood pressure).
- One hour is the recommended inflation time for upper extremity surgery and 1.5–2 h for lower extremity surgery. The tourniquet should be deflated for 10 min after the maximum recommended time, after which the tourniquet may be reinflated for another full period.

Complications of tourniquet use include:

- Nerve injury – associated with pressure
- Emboli – use of tourniquet may lead to formation of a deep vein thrombosis (DVT) and pulmonary embolism (PE)
- Sickle crisis – in susceptible patients the buildup of potassium, lactate, etc. may precipitate a sickle crisis
- Compartment syndrome – prolonged ischaemia may lead to reperfusion injury and swelling of muscles
- Post-tourniquet syndrome – consists of nonpitting oedema, sensory loss, muscle weakness and stiffness. This may last up to a month
- Burns – can occur if alcohol-containing skin preparations get under the tourniquet
- Raised core temperature and increased plasma viscosity – these events are known to occur after tourniquet use, but their clinical significance is uncertain
- Increased postoperative pain.

HINTS AND TIPS

Tourniquets are used very commonly in operations of the extremities. Important safety points to remember are:

- Use the correct size, with adequate padding.
- Keep the duration of inflation to a minimum, and time the period of inflation accurately.
- Use the minimum pressure required to achieve the desired effect (this can be titrated to the patient's blood pressure).
- Avoid multiple inflation and deflations.
- Remember the contraindications – history of DVT/PE, peripheral vascular disease, sickle cell disease.

Postoperatively, be cautious of bleeding. Remember, the tourniquet was probably still on when the first layer of the dressing was applied. The first signs of bleeding may not appear until the patient is back on the ward!

DIATHERMY

Surgical diathermy is an invaluable tool in providing haemostasis but can also be used to cut tissues. It involves high-frequency alternating current (AC). There are a number of important points to understand regarding surgical diathermy:

- Diathermy used in surgery is very high frequency (400 kHz–10 MHz) and uses high current intensity (as high as 500 mA can be used). However, home electricity is capable of inducing ventricular fibrillation (VF) (as much as 100 mA is sufficient); this is due to the much lower frequency of around 50–60 Hz.
- Monopolar. This is the most common type of diathermy. An AC is produced and passed to an electrode with a small surface area (the diathermy tip). Current is passed to the tissues as heat. The current passes through the body tissue and completes the circuit by returning to a much larger surface plate, i.e. the indifferent electrode plate which is usually placed on the patient's thigh (Figure 2.3A). Good contact is essential. Current recommendations to improve contact include shaving hair from the skin where the plate is placed and using disposable self-adhesive diathermy plates. Monopolar diathermy is most widely used for operative haemostasis, but there is wide dispersion of coagulating and heating effects, which makes it unsuitable for use near nerves and other delicate structures.
- Bipolar. There is no need for a plate and uses much less power. The two active electrodes are the tips of a pair of forceps (or between the blades of a pair of scissors). Current flows between the tips of the forceps and thus only affects the tissues between them (Figure 2.3B). Bipolar diathermy is used for finer surgery where greater precision is required. There is minimal tissue damage around the point of coagulation and therefore safety in relation to nearby nerves and blood vessels.
- Coagulation. This involves sealing blood vessels. The AC output is pulsed, and haemostasis occurs by a combination of cellular dehydration and protein denaturation.

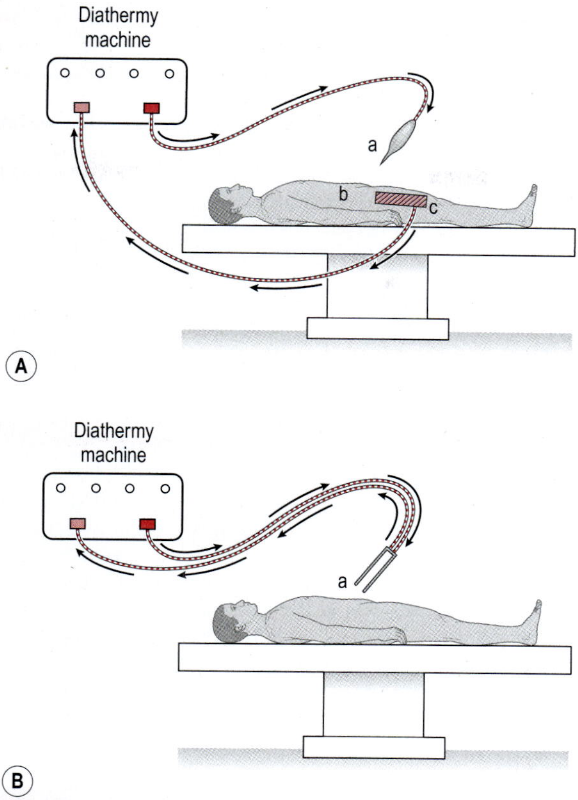

FIGURE 2.3

(**A**) Monopolar diathermy. Current passes through the fine instrument tip (a), through the patient (b) and returns via the large indifferent electrode (c). (**B**) Bipolar diathermy. Current passes between the tips of the forceps (a) and coagulates tissue grasped between the tips. It does not pass through the patient.

- Cutting. In this form, the AC output is continuous and forms an arc between the diathermy and the tissue. The heat generated is sufficient to cause water to explode into steam. A combination of cutting and coagulation is often referred to as 'blend'. Cutting diathermy is mainly used for dividing large muscle masses, e.g. thoracotomy and transverse abdominal incisions.
- Fulguration. A form of coagulation in which a higher voltage is used that creates sparks which arc from the diathermy to the tissues and create charring of the tissue.

Complications of diathermy include:

- Electrocution. Very low risk with modern equipment.
- Explosion. Rare – can occur with pooling of alcohol-based skin preparations or with colonic gases.
- Burns. Most common problem. Can occur with faulty application of the patient plate. Patient is earthed by touching a metal object (e.g. drip stand), faulty insulation on the diathermy wires, accidental activation and accidentally touching another metal object while activating diathermy (e.g. retractor).
- Interference with pacemakers. Diathermy activation may result in no pacing or the pacemaker reverting to a fixed rate. Bipolar diathermy is considered safe to use. If monopolar diathermy must be used, the patient plate should be sited as far away as possible from the pacemaker.
- Channelling. The use of diathermy in tissues with narrow channels or pedicles can lead to the current being 'channelled' through a short surface area and thus high heat production. Examples of this would be in a child's penis during circumcision or along the spermatic cord with operations on the testicle. Bipolar diathermy is safe to use.
- Direct coupling. The active diathermy comes into contact with another metal instrument (e.g. camera) that is touching tissues (e.g. bowel) and results in a burn.
- Capacitance coupling. Very rare with modern ports. Occurs when ports have a plastic portion to anchor them into the abdomen. When a current is applied through an insulated instrument within a metal tube (e.g. port), some electrical charge is transferred to the cannula. If the port is entirely metal, there is no problem, as the charge will dissipate through the abdominal wall over a large area of contact. If a plastic collar is present, this will prevent discharge and potentially lead to burns on adjacent tissue. Diathermy injury during laparoscopic surgery may also occur with accidental activation, faulty insulation of equipment and retained heat in the instrument.

HINTS AND TIPS

The use of a monopolar diathermy is commonly delegated to the assistant surgeon to use direct coupling to coagulate structures held in the forceps of the primary surgeon. Ensure that you can see the whole length of the diathermy tip before you press the button to activate it; it is very easy to catch the edge of the skin and cause a burn whilst concentrating on the forceps held by the operating surgeon!

LASER

Laser stands for **L**ight **A**mplification **S**timulated **E**mission of **R**adiation. Lasers work by energy being directed at a lasing medium. This excites atoms into a higher energy state. Photons are emitted as electrons fall from the excited to a ground state. These photons are amplified by being reflected between two mirrors. A small amount of laser light is allowed to emerge, and this forms the laser beam. This beam vaporises tissues and coagulates small vessels. A number of lasing mediums are used, usually gaseous (e.g. carbon dioxide, argon), but crystals are also used (**N**eo**d**ymium, **Y**ttrium, **A**luminium and **G**arnet – **NdYAG**). The lasing medium determines the wavelength and the wavelength determines the depth of absorption and thus clinical effect. Lasers are used in a number of surgical specialties such as destroying tumours of the gastrointestinal tract (GIT), e.g. oesophageal, urinary bladder and female genital tract, and for lithotripsy of renal stones. They are used in ophthalmology to destroy thickened lens capsules with cataracts. They are classified according to the degree of danger in their use (class I to class IV).

Potential risks involved with lasers include:

- Risk to patient – burning of normal tissue can lead to perforation, e.g. in the oesophagus.
- Risk to operator – the laser can damage the eyes or skin.

A number of safety measures should therefore be adhered to:

- Appropriate local personnel. A laser safety officer and laser protection adviser should be nominated to draft safety protocols and ensure that they are followed.
- All lasers should be labelled with their hazard category.
- All personnel using or involved in the use of lasers should wear eye protection.
- An appropriate environment with minimal reflective surfaces should be provided for laser use.

LAPAROSCOPIC SURGERY

Laparoscopy has been in use by gynaecologists for many years in diagnosing pelvic disorders and for sterilisation by tubal ligation. It is now being used more widely in other branches of surgery, particularly for minimally invasive surgery. Laparoscopy may be either diagnostic or therapeutic.

Diagnostic Laparoscopy. For biopsy of lesions, staging of cancers, e.g. gastric and pancreatic, and increasing diagnostic accuracy in the acute abdomen.

Therapeutic Laparoscopy. Widely practised, the most common operation being cholecystectomy. Other procedures include appendicectomy, inguinal hernia repair, division of adhesions, colonic resection, Nissen fundoplication for gastro-oesophageal reflux disease, nephrectomy, splenectomy. Laparoscopic operations may need to be converted to 'open' surgery if difficulties are encountered, e.g. gross adhesions, poor visualisation of the operation site, slow progress with the operation, uncontrollable haemorrhage.

Technique

Usually performed under general anaesthesia. A pneumoperitoneum is created by introducing carbon dioxide under controlled pressure. This may be done by direct visualisation of the peritoneal space by an open cut-down technique made below the umbilicus (Hassan technique), with the first port (used for the telescope and camera) inserted under direct vision at the umbilicus and insufflation initiated through this port once it is in place. The use of a Veress (insufflation) needle is still popular, but it requires gas to be insufflated without confirmation of the correct location of the needle tip. To perform procedures, additional puncture sites are required (secondary ports). Trocars are inserted at these sites under direct laparoscopic vision to prevent injury to the viscera. Various instruments are then introduced through these port sites. Basically, these instruments may be divided into those for visualisation, grasping, retraction, dissection, ligation/suturing and retrieval.

HINTS AND TIPS

The instruments used in laparoscopic surgery vary in diameter; for example, the camera and laparoscopic stapling devices are often larger in diameter compared with graspers, hooks and diathermy. Ensure that the ports inserted are large enough for the equipment you intend to use!

Instruments introduced through port sites include scissors, diathermy hooks and clip applicators. Some operations are described as 'laparoscopic assisted', where the major dissection is performed laparoscopically and subsequently a small incision is made in the abdomen to deliver the specimen. 'Hand-assisted' laparoscopy requires a small incision to insert the operator's hand to assist with dissection and delivery of the specimen. Retrieval bags may be introduced into the peritoneal cavity to aid the delivery of specimens, the aim being to prevent the spread of infection, seeding of tumours, or to prevent disruption of the specimen when it is pulled out through an abdominal incision. The operation is performed by the operator with one or more assistants who control the camera or manipulate the ports, the progress of the operation being observed on video monitors.

HINTS AND TIPS

As the junior surgeon, you are likely to be tasked with directing the camera. Remember that the surgeon can only see what is on the screen. Try to keep the area under operation in the centre of the screen; to do this, you will need to follow the actions of the primary surgeon and not just remain in one place. Sometimes difficult visualisation can be improved by using an angled camera, e.g. cameras angled at 45° are commonly used in bariatric surgery and pelvic surgery. Being a good assistant requires practice; a few hours spent on laparoscopic training devices outside of the operating theatre can help you to refine your camera skills!

Robotic laparoscopic surgery is now becoming more common, particularly in specialties such as paediatrics and urology, where the robot provides an increase in the level of precision that can be achieved, compared with conventional laparoscopic instruments. The surgeon does not scrub up but sits inside the control station (often located within the same operating theatre, although there is the scope for remote surgery) and directs the 'limbs' of the robot whilst watching the operation on a 3D video screen. One disadvantage is the increase in operating time; setting up the robot and ensuring all the instruments are in place means that the length of anaesthetic is increased before the operating has even begun.

Complications

These include:

- Dangers of pneumoperitoneum; needle/trocar injury to bowel or blood vessels; compression of venous return predisposing to DVT and PE; subcutaneous emphysema; shoulder tip pain (irritant effect of carbon dioxide producing carbonic acid locally and irritating the diaphragm with referred pain to the shoulder tip); pneumothorax (rare); and pneumomediastinum (rare)

- Inadvertent injury to other structures either by dissection or diathermy or inappropriate application of clips, e.g. damage to the bile duct in cholecystectomy; uncontrollable haemorrhage
- Complications related to duration of anaesthesia, which may be longer for laparoscopic procedures than for open procedures. The diaphragm is splinted by abdominal inflation, and this may result in cardiorespiratory complications.
- Herniation at port sites with possible subsequent strangulation.

VENOUS ACCESS

Venous access may be required for simple venepuncture or insertion of a cannula. Suitable sites are veins on the back of the hand or the antecubital fossa. The foot veins may also be used if there are no suitable veins in the arm, but these should be approached only in an emergency in a diabetic patient! However, injections should not be given into veins in the antecubital fossa, in case of accidental puncture of the brachial artery, which is immediately deep to the veins and separated from them only by the bicipital aponeurosis. In children and patients with needle phobia, EMLA cream (containing 2.5% lignocaine and 2.5% prilocaine) may be applied and left for 45–60 min to anaesthetise the skin. It should be wiped off before cannulating. The following steps are required in the procedure:

PROCEDURE

SIMPLE VENEPUNCTURE/INSERTION OF A CANNULA

- Choose the site.
- Place a tourniquet or sphygmomanometer (inflated to just below diastolic pressure) above the site.
- Swab with alcohol.
- Advance cannula until flashback of blood.
- Release tourniquet or sphygmomanometer.
- Withdraw needle leaving cannula in the vein.
- Connect infusion.

When removing the needle or cannula, raise the arm and compress the site for about 1 min to prevent bruising.

If no other site is available for venous access in an emergency, a venous cut-down may be required. This should only be used if it is not possible to gain venous access elsewhere, despite the use of ultrasound. A cut-down is usually carried out at the ankle where there is a constant vein, i.e. the great saphenous vein lying immediately anterior to the medial malleolus.

PROCEDURE

VENOUS CUT-DOWN

- Prepare skin and drape.
- Infiltrate with local anaesthetic.
- Make an incision over the vein.
- Dissect the vein from other structures, e.g. the saphenous nerve in association with the great saphenous vein at the ankle.
- Ligate the distal end of the vein and put a suture sling around the proximal end.
- Make an incision in the vein.
- Insert a large-bore cannula into the vein and ligate proximally to secure cannula in the vein.
- Attach infusion.
- Close wound and apply dressing.

CENTRAL VENOUS CATHETERISATION – INTERNAL JUGULAR VEIN

Indications for internal jugular vein cannulation include the determination and monitoring of central venous pressure and establishing a route for intravenous therapeutic agents. Complications include pneumothorax, carotid artery damage and haematoma. A clotting screen should be checked before starting the procedure. Nowadays, it is rare to insert a central venous catheter without ultrasound guidance.

PROCEDURE

CENTRAL VENOUS CATHETERISATION – INTERNAL JUGULAR VEIN

- Patient is prepared with head tilted 15° down and turned to the opposite side.
- Infiltrate the skin with local anaesthetic at the level of the thyroid cartilage (three fingers' breadth above the medial end of the clavicle), lateral to the carotid artery pulse.
- Site of entry is at the apex of the triangle formed by the two heads of the sternocleidomastoid and the clavicle.
- Using an 18G 'finder' needle, enter the apex of the triangle keeping lateral to the pulse of the carotid artery. (Most central venous pressure (CVP) lines are inserted under ultrasound guidance.)
- Insert the needle at 30° angle and aim for the ipsilateral nipple.
- Once in the vessel, remove the syringe, hold the thumb over the needle to avoid air embolism.
- Insert guidewire.
- Make a small nick in the skin where the guidewire enters.
- Advance dilator over guidewire.
- Remove dilator.
- Place catheter over guidewire.
- Remove guidewire and aspirate blood and flush all three ports of cannula.
- Suture to skin.
- Arrange chest X-ray (CXR) to check position.

BLOOD GAS SAMPLING

Vessels of choice are the radial artery (immediately lateral to the tendon of flexor carpi radialis just above the wrist), the brachial artery (immediately medial to the biceps tendon at the elbow) or the femoral artery at the midinguinal point (halfway between the anterior superior iliac spine and the pubic symphysis). For radial artery cannulation, always check the patency of the ulnar artery (Allen test).

PROCEDURE

BLOOD GAS SAMPLING

- Swab site with alcohol.
- Use a 2 mL heparinised syringe (usually prefilled syringes are available).
- Expel air from syringe.
- Advance at 60–90° into the artery (it may help to rest the wrist on a bag of saline). The artery may have been transfixed, so it may be necessary to withdraw the needle slowly until blood fills the syringe.
- Obtain 2 mL of blood and cap the syringe immediately.
- Compress puncture site for 3–5 min.
- Empty syringe of any air bubbles and send to laboratory immediately for analysis. If there is any delay, place the syringe on ice.

URINARY CATHETERISATION (MALE)

A Foley catheter is inserted into the bladder. For adults a 12–14 F gauge should be used. For children a 8–10 F gauge should be used.

PROCEDURE

URINARY CATHETERISATION (MALE)

- Wash hands, put on sterile gloves and arrange contents of catheter pack on sterile tray.
- Place patient in supine position.
- Drape with sterile towels with penis exposed.
- Grasp penis with sterile swab, retract foreskin and clean the urethral opening and glans with antiseptic solution.
- Squeeze lignocaine gel into urethra and allow time for it to work.
- Remove catheter from pack and insert fully into bladder to ensure that balloon is in bladder. *Do not use force.*
- Check that there is urine flow from catheter.
- Inflate balloon with sterile water, 5–10 mL.
- Withdraw catheter to lodge against bladder neck.
- Remember to replace foreskin to avoid paraphimosis.
- Attach drainage bag.

Chapter 3

Investigative Procedures

Andrew T. Raftery • Michael S. Delbridge

CHAPTER OUTLINE

This chapter describes various investigative procedures commonly used in surgery. The procedures are described briefly, together with their indications and possible complications.

CONVENTIONAL RADIOLOGY

Radiographs penetrate differentially through tissues of the body, resulting in different exposure of the silver salts in the radiograph film. On a plain radiograph, gas and fat absorb few X-rays and consequently appear dark, while bone and calcified defects are poorly penetrated and appear white or radio-opaque.

- A *plain* radiograph is one where no contrast medium is administered to the patient, e.g. routine chest X-ray (CXR).
- A *contrast* study involves administration of a contrast medium, which outlines or delineates the structure under study, e.g. barium in gastrointestinal (GI) studies or iodinated benzoic acid derivatives in arteriography.

Plain Films

Chest X-ray (CXR)

Always check the name of the film and the right and left markers. Make sure the whole chest and diaphragm are clearly visible on the film. When interpreting a CXR, it is always useful to have a system to use. It prevents you from forgetting to look for things and is useful when you are likely to be stressed, for example in an examination. An easy one to remember is '**S**ome **B**ody **P**inched **M**y **F**luffy **T**oy **D**inosaur':

- **S**oft tissues – look for surgical emphysema, mastectomy.
- **B**ones – count the ribs to rule out a cervical rib; look for rib notching secondary to coarctation of the aorta; bony metastases; rib fractures. If the CXR is taken for trauma, look at the nonthoracic bones – you might pick up on a fractured humerus.

- **P**leura – look for pneumothorax, pulmonary vascular pattern, consolidation, collapse, carcinoma.
- **M**ediastinum – look at the aorta – is there any evidence of a thoracic aneurysm? – assess the cardiothoracic ratio or heart size (maximum width of heart divided by maximum 'bony' (rib-to-rib) diameter of chest should be <50% in normal adults).
- **F**oreign bodies – this can be anything from medical devices, e.g. endotracheal tube, nasogastric tube; swallowed coins; knives and bullets.
- **T**rachea – check that the trachea is central.
- **D**iaphragm – check for diaphragmatic elevation; check for free air under the diaphragm on erect CXR which would suggest perforation of a hollow viscus.

Abdominal X-ray (AXR)

Check the name and the right/left markers. Is the film supine or erect (all AXRs will be AP)? A system for remembering what to look for in an AXR is '**B**ig **C**uddly **S**panish **G**iants **A**gain':

- **B**ones, e.g. bony metastases, hip and pelvic fractures, osteoarthritis of the hips.
- **C**alcifications – calcified calculi (kidney, ureter, bladder – 85% of renal calculi are radio-opaque); gallbladder (10% of gallstones are radio-opaque); look for abnormal calcification, e.g. atherosclerotic vessels, 'eggshell' outline of an aortic aneurysm, pancreatic lesions, phleboliths, uterine fibroids and lymph nodes.
- **S**oft tissues and solid organs – the liver and spleen are difficult to see. An enlarged bladder may be seen. The kidneys are usually visible in outline. Look for the psoas shadow – absence may indicate retroperitoneal pathology.
- **G**as pattern – look for free air under the diaphragm to suggest perforation of a hollow viscus; look at the air in the small and large bowel, e.g. small and large bowel obstruction; look for air in abnormal places, e.g. air in biliary tree with cholecystoduodenal fistula and gallstone ileus, air in bladder with colovesical fistula.
- **A**rtefacts – these include drains, grafts, swallowed (and rectally inserted!) foreign bodies.

Plan radiographs of the limbs and skull are dealt with in Chapters 4, 18 and 19.

> **HINTS AND TIPS**
>
> When asked to look at an AXR or CXR, start off by saying, 'This is a CXR/AXR of Mr Jones. It was taken on a particular date and is well/poorly penetrated. It is/is not rotated' (only applies for chest films). You should comment on the type of CXR view; the standard is a PA view. In patients who are unwell the X-ray plate is placed behind them (e.g. sitting on a trolley) and the beam is AP. In an AP view the heart will be larger, thus making it harder to comment on cardiomegaly.

Contrast Studies

Gastrointestinal Tract

Barium Meal. This investigation is used less commonly now in view of the increased use of endoscopy. Barium suspension is given orally together with sodium bicarbonate tablets to give a barium/air double-contrast study. The progress of barium is checked by screening, with image intensification being used to show a moving image on a TV monitor. Areas of interest are noted and radiographs taken. The patient should not have any solid food overnight, but sips of water are allowed prior to the investigation. A study is useful for diagnosis of pharyngeal lesions, e.g. pharyngeal pouch; oesophageal lesions, e.g. carcinoma, reflux, achalasia; stomach lesions, e.g. ulcers and carcinoma; and duodenum, e.g. duodenal lesions ulcer and pyloric stenosis.

Barium Enema. Barium suspension is administered rectally. Rectal and lower sigmoid lesions should have first been excluded by sigmoidoscopy. Air is usually insufflated to give a double-contrast picture. Buscopan, an anticholinergic agent, may be given i.v. to relax the bowel during the investigation. This is an unpleasant investigation, and the patient should be forewarned.

Strict bowel preparation is required prior to barium enema. A laxative should be administered the evening prior to the enema, and the occasional rectal washout is required if there is evidence of residual faecal loading. The study is useful for diagnosis of bowel carcinomas, polyps, diverticular disease and inflammatory bowel disease. Fine mucosal abnormalities may be missed on barium enema, and colonoscopy should now be considered the first-line investigation for large bowel lesions.

HINTS AND TIPS

Barium enema should not be performed within 7 days of a rectal biopsy because of the risk of perforation.

Barium Follow-Through or Small Bowel Enema. Barium may be swallowed and followed through the small bowel into the colon. Alternatively, a duodenal tube may be positioned under radiographic control and barium injected into the duodenum and followed through the small bowel (a small bowel enema). This is useful for the diagnosis of Crohn's disease and small bowel tumours.

HINTS AND TIPS

Barium should be avoided in the following situations:

- If there is a significant risk of peritoneal leakage, e.g. assessing the integrity of an anastomosis. Barium causes an intense peritoneal irritation and adhesion formation, and water-soluble contrast media should be used in preference when checking an anastomosis, e.g. Gastrografin.
- In bowel obstruction, as the barium may rest at the site of a partial obstruction, solidify and cause a partial obstruction to become complete.

Biliary Tree

Ultrasound. Ultrasound is now the first-line test for diagnosis of gallstones. It will also show a dilated biliary tree but will rarely pick up stones in the common bile duct due to the fact that the lower end of the common bile duct is likely to be obscured by gas from the transverse colon.

Magnetic Resonance Cholangiopancreatography (MRCP). MRCP is now the initial imaging test of choice for biliary tree abnormalities, e.g. obstruction. It is a noninvasive method for imaging the biliary and pancreatic ducts. The technique does not require intravenous contrast material and uses specialised MRI sequences (i.e. heavily T2-weighted) to make the fluid in the ducts appear bright while the surrounding organs and tissues are suppressed and appear dark. Heavily T2-weighted images give excellent anatomical detail. MRCP may be used as a screening examination in patients with a low or intermediate probability of choledocholithiasis; with failed or incomplete endoscopic retrograde cholangiopancreatography (ERCP); to demonstrate variations in ductal anatomy; to demonstrate postoperative anatomy (e.g. biliary-enteric anastomoses, sclerosing cholangitis); and to demonstrate complications of chronic pancreatitis (e.g. ductal dilatation, strictures).

Endoscopic Retrograde Cholangiopancreatography (ERCP). Contrast medium is injected retrogradely through the ampulla of Vater via a side-viewing duodenoscope. The technique is described more fully in the section on endoscopy, below.

Percutaneous Transhepatic Cholangiography (PTC). This is used for diagnosis of obstructive jaundice. A long fine needle (22G Chiba) is passed percutaneously into the liver until a duct is pierced, witnessed by the aspiration of bile. Contrast is then injected to outline the biliary tree.

Complications include haemorrhage, bile peritonitis, cholangitis and septicaemia. This technique, however, has been largely superseded by MRCP.

HINTS AND TIPS

Jaundiced patients and/or patients with liver disease often have abnormal clotting. Ensure that the patient has a recent INR. If elevated, they may need vitamin K or FFP prior to the procedure.

Operative Cholangiogram. At operation for cholecystectomy, the ducts should be checked for stones. Contrast is injected via a cannula inserted into the common bile duct via the stump of the cystic duct, and radiography is carried out or the image intensifier used. The diameter of the ducts, presence of filling defects and failure of contrast to pass into the duodenum are significant.

T-Tube Cholangiogram. If the common bile duct has been explored to exclude or remove stones, a latex T-tube is usually inserted. The horizontal bar of the T is in the duct and the vertical bar is brought out through the skin. Contrast is injected down the T-tube 8–10 days postoperatively to check for any residual stones, biliary leakage or stenosis prior to removal of the tube. There should be free flow of contrast medium into the duodenum and no filling defects.

Urinary Tract

Intravenous Urography (IVU). Intravenous contrast is administered, which is excreted by the kidneys and eventually delineates the renal pelvis, ureters and bladder. A plain film is taken first so that any opacities seen can be compared with the films after contrast administration. It is useful for the diagnosis of obstruction, tumours, infection, congenital abnormalities and trauma. The only contraindication is allergy to the contrast medium. Caution must be exercised in diabetes mellitus, renal failure, multiple myeloma and cardiac failure.

HINTS AND TIPS

When looking at the plain film of an IVU, it is useful to know the course of the ureter to identify possible stones. The hilum of the kidney is around L2, and the ureter courses along the tips of the L2–5 transverse processes. It crosses the pelvis at the sacroiliac junction and enters the bladder just above the ischial spine.

Cystography. The patient is catheterised and the bladder filled with contrast medium. Bladder leaks, tumours, vesicoureteral reflux and diverticulae can be diagnosed. A post-micturition film will diagnose residual urine. This technique has largely been superseded by ultrasonography.

Urethrography. A water-soluble contrast medium is injected per urethra. Ruptures of the urethra, strictures or tumours may be seen.

Retrograde Pyelography. This is carried out via cystoscopy by passing a ureteric catheter into each ureteric orifice. Clear views of the ureter and pelvicalyceal system are obtained. This test is used in patients with impaired renal function with poor concentration of contrast or if incomplete filling of the collecting structures is seen on IVU. The ureteric catheter may be left in situ to allow drainage of an obstructed system and for renal function tests to normalise prior to operative procedures.

Antegrade Pyelography. The pelvicalyceal system of the kidney is punctured with a fine 22G needle. Contrast is injected and allows accurate assessment of the ureter and pelvicalyceal system, as well as assessing drainage.

Vascular System

Arteriography. Contrast medium is injected directly into the lumen of an artery. The catheter is usually introduced via the Seldinger wire technique into a suitable and easily accessible artery. The femoral artery at the groin is the usual portal of entry, although the brachial and axillary artery may be used. A careful history of allergies to contrast media needs to be ascertained. A clotting screen should be carried out prior to vascular radiology. With a catheter in situ, water-soluble contrast medium is injected directly into the artery and images recorded in rapid sequences. Stenosis, thrombosis, embolism or aneurysm can be demonstrated. Complications include haemorrhage at the puncture site, dislodgement of atheromatous plaques, embolism, thrombosis.

Digital Subtraction Angiography (DSA). DSA is now commonly used. Vascular images may be obtained with lower concentrations of contrast medium. The digital images are processed by subtracting unnecessary background, e.g. bones, and enhancing contrast between the tissues. Where high resolution is not needed, the contrast can be given intravenously into a fast-flowing vein, e.g. via a central line or into the femoral vein, and the arteries imaged when the contrast reaches them. These studies are known as intravenous digital subtraction angiography (IVDSA) or digital intravenous angiogram (DIVA). Diagnostic angiography is rarely performed nowadays, computerised tomography (CT) or MR angiography being preferred.

Venography. Contrast is injected into a superficial vein, i.e. a vein on the dorsum of the foot in the lower limb, and a tourniquet is placed around the ankle to direct the contrast into the deep veins. Lower limb venography is used to confirm or exclude deep vein thrombosis (DVT) or to investigate deep venous insufficiency, i.e. it would demonstrate the site of incompetent perforating veins. This technique has been largely superseded by Doppler ultrasound and MR venography.

ULTRASONOGRAPHY

Ultrasound works on the principle that the ultrasound emitted as a pulse from a transducer travels at constant velocity into tissue and is reflected by varying amounts from different tissue interfaces and travels back to the receiver at the same speed. The transducer is a piezoelectric crystal that both transmits and receives the ultrasound. The time required for the pulse to travel to the interface and back can be used to determine the depth of that interface. An image of the slice of the body is obtained by directing a narrow beam of high-energy sound waves into the body and recording the manner in which the sound is reflected by different structures. Sound is transmitted well through any fluid but poorly or not at all through air or bone. Returning echoes are electronically converted into a video image on a monitor, the resulting picture being a wedge-shaped slice of the area of interest.

Advantages

- It does not employ ionising radiation and therefore produces no biological injury in the tissues.
- Any plane can be employed to examine the region of interest.
- It is less expensive than CT or MRI.
- It can be used at the bedside if the patient is too ill to be moved.

Dimensions of organs or lesions can be measured and the volume of the bladder and the left ventricle can also be assessed. Stones cause marked changes in acoustic impedance with almost complete reflection of ultrasound, showing echogenic foci with fan-shaped acoustic shadowing.

Very little preparation is necessary. For pelvic ultrasound the bladder should be full, providing a fluid-filled nonreflective medium for the ultrasound to reach the pelvic organs. The patient should be starved for biliary ultrasound to allow the gallbladder to fill with bile and to minimise gas shadows.

Ultrasound is noninvasive, painless, safe and cheap in comparison with CT and MRI, although it does not produce as sharp an image.
Ultrasound may be used for the following:

- Assessment of abdominal masses
- Distinguishing solid from cystic lesions, e.g. renal carcinoma from a renal cyst
- Assessment of liver secondaries
- Detecting stones in the gallbladder or urinary bladder
- Measuring the size of lesions, e.g. the diameter of an abdominal aortic aneurysm or the width of a dilated bile duct
- Guided biopsy, e.g. biopsy of liver secondary or other mass
- Guided drainage, e.g. of localised collections of fluid or subphrenic or pelvis abscesses.

Disadvantages

Although limitations are few, lesions of the lower end of the common bile duct and head of the pancreas may be obscured by bowel gas. Bone completely reflects ultrasound, and the method is therefore useless for studying organs encased by bone, e.g. brain and spinal cord. In addition, ultrasound interpretation is operator dependent, and a retrospective review of images may not be possible.

DOPPLER ULTRASOUND

Doppler ultrasound is used in vascular monitoring to study blood flow. A beam of ultrasound is directed at a vessel using a special probe. Ultrasound is reflected from the red cells, which cause a frequency shift related to their velocity. The shift can be heard as a noise or recorded as a waveform or sonogram. The faster the flow of red cells past the probe, the higher the sound pitch. The Doppler probe is coupled to the skin with acoustic gel and angled towards the direction of arterial flow. Stenoses and occlusions cause diminished signals distal to a proximal obstruction.

Uses of Doppler Ultrasound

Measurement of Systolic Pressure in Peripheral Arteries. A sphygmomanometer cuff is applied to occlude the artery. The probe is placed over the artery (dorsalis pedis, posterior tibial in the case of the lower limb), the tourniquet is slowly released and the pressure recorded when a signal is picked up. This pressure is compared with a normal brachial pressure, i.e. the ankle/brachial pressure index. The normal value is 1.0–1.2.

Other methods include analysis of waveforms to assess stenoses and occlusions.

Duplex Scanning

This combines real-time B-mode imaging with a pulsed Doppler spectral analysis of flow velocity pattern. Blood vessels are identified by their characteristic B-mode images with prominent wall echoes and dark sonar-lucent lumina. Calcified plaques show bright echoes with acoustic shadowing behind. The pulsed Doppler beam is placed in the centre of the identified vessel, and the spectral analysis allows classification of the degree of stenosis. Duplex scanning may be applied to analyse carotid disease, lower extremity arterial disease, intestinal arteries, renal arteries and venous thromboses. Colour coding of flow direction may give further information.

COMPUTERISED TOMOGRAPHY (CT)

CT produces cross-sectional images of the body, taking a series of transverse slices through the body. Sensitive X-ray detectors measure the X-ray attenuation through the patient in a large number of different directions, and a fast digital computer then uses the measurements to compute an image. These images are displayed on a screen and subsequently recorded on film. CT scanning may be used in conjunction with contrast medium enhancement. This may be given i.v. to show, for example, hepatic tumours, renal parenchyma and collecting system, aorta and IVC. It may enhance brain lesions when the blood–brain barrier is breached. Contrast may also be given by mouth or enema to outline the GI tract.

A new generation of spiral CT scanners is in use. The patient passes quickly through the scanner, and a volume of data is obtained and analysed. Scanning is performed in a single breath-hold, decreasing motion artefact and allowing accurate timing of intravascular contrast enhancement. Images are superior to conventional CT. Specific applications include CT angiography and imaging of pulmonary emboli (CTPA).

Advantages

CT has many uses but is the investigation of choice in head injuries. It is also useful for studying the retroperitoneum, pancreas, mediastinum and lungs. It can be used for staging tumours, e.g. lymphomas, and can be used for guided biopsy.

CT Angiography. Scan is performed simultaneously with high-speed contrast media injection. It may be used for visualising vessels anywhere in the body. Specific uses include:

- Examination of the pulmonary arteries in suspected pulmonary embolism
- Visualising blood flow in the renal arteries in suspected renal artery stenosis
- Assessment of prospective kidney donors to visualise the arterial anatomy of the kidney
- Identification of aortic aneurysms
- Identification of aortic dissection
- Identification of DVT.

CT Urography. Multidetector CT urography is a single examination that allows evaluation of potential urinary tract calculi, renal parenchymal masses and both benign and malignant urothelial lesions. Upper tract urothelial malignancies, including small lesions <5 mm in diameter, can be detected with high sensitivity. It is useful in the assessment of haematuria and also trauma to the urinary tract.

CT Colonography (CTC). CTC is a noninvasive alternative to conventional colonoscopy. By combining CT technology with sophisticated software, CTC creates 2D and 3D images of the colon. The procedure is faster, easier and more comfortable for the patient than conventional colonoscopy. It is used for detection of polyps, diverticulae and colorectal cancer. However, if an abnormality is found, specimens cannot be taken, so conventional colonoscopy must be performed to obtain a tissue diagnosis.

MAGNETIC RESONANCE IMAGING (MRI)

MRI is also known as NMR. MRI is based on the fact that certain atomic nuclei placed in a magnetic field and acted on by a suitable radiofrequency pulse undergo changes in their energy states, which result in the emission of measurable radio signals. The signals are then manipulated in a computer to provide sectional radiographic images. No ionising radiation is involved. The procedure is noninvasive and can be carried out as an outpatient procedure. It is relatively time consuming, with extensive studies taking in excess of 1 h. MRI gives high soft tissue contrast, and the body can be imaged in coronal, sagittal or transverse planes.

Advantages

The technique is particularly useful for studies of the central nervous system (CNS; lipids have a high hydrogen content), soft tissues of the pelvis, soft tissue tumours and orthopaedic problems. Magnetic resonance angiography is also being increasingly used to assess the heart, renal arteries and peripheral vessels. MRCP can also be used to image the biliary tract.

Disadvantages

These include high cost, limited availability, low patient throughput, poor detail of bone and calcified tissues, and image artefacts from respiratory and cardiac movements and bowel peristalsis. The patient is in the 'tube' for long periods, and it is difficult to monitor the ill patient. Contraindications include patients with cardiac pacemakers and cranial surgery with metal clips.

POSITRON EMISSION TOMOGRAPHY (PET)

PET is an imaging technology that produces a 3D image or picture of functional processes within the body. The system detects a pair of gamma rays emitted by a positron-emitting radionuclide that is introduced into the body on a biologically active molecule, usually a sugar. The most common form of tracer used is flurodeoxyglucose (FDG), a glucose analogue. The concentrations of tracer image then give tissue metabolic activity in terms of glucose intake. Images of the tracer concentration in 3D space within the body are then reconstructed by computer analysis. PET scans are increasingly read alongside CT scans, a combination giving both anatomic and metabolic information. Modern PET scanners are integrated with high-end multidetector row CT scanner. PET scanning is advantageous in the management of malignancy, as it can often detect tumours before structural changes are seen on CT or MRI. Its extreme sensitivity makes it possible to detect cancers at their earliest stages and to outline their exact locations. It is useful in follow-up looking for cancer recurrence and monitoring the effectiveness of chemotherapy and other treatments. It is also useful in neurological diseases such as Alzheimer's disease and has been used in the diagnosis of infected prosthetic vascular grafts.

Advantages

Advantages of PET scanning include more detailed diagnostic information not available from other investigations such as CT or MRI, shorter time for definitive diagnosis, earlier detection of disease with the need for less invasive diagnostic procedures, precise staging of disease, and improved monitoring of recurrences and more effective assessment of results of chemotherapy. Its ability to distinguish between benign and malignant tumours can result in the avoidance of unnecessary surgery.

Disadvantages

These include high cost and limited availability. The radioactive component used in PET scanning means that there are only a limited number of times a patient can undergo this procedure.

MAMMOGRAPHY

A mammogram is a soft tissue radiograph of the breast. The tissues constituting the breast have a very low inherent contrast. Soft tissue mammography depends on the fact that tumour tissue is denser than breast tissue, particularly in an older patient (age 40+), where glandular tissue has been replaced by fat. The study is uncomfortable and somewhat undignified for the patient, since compression of the breast is essential to 'spread' the breast over the film cassette, to immobilise the breast and reduce the radiation dose. A radiolucent, translucent compression plate is used. Two projections are usually taken – superoinferior and mediolateral. For screening programmes, two projections are used on the first attendance and one projection only on follow-up, unless the patient is symptomatic, and then two projections are used. Careful viewing of the film under high-intensity light with magnification is essential. An infiltrating radio-opaque mass is suggestive of malignancy, but fine-stippled calcification (like salt grains scattered on the film) strongly suggests the diagnosis. Mammography is used for the following:

- To assess palpable lumps
- To exclude lumps in other symptomatic patients, e.g. painful breasts
- Screening.

If a nonpalpable lump is picked up on mammography, preoperative localisation with wires is undertaken via mammography. The wire is left in the breast and acts as a guide to the surgeon to the location of the radiological abnormality. When the specimen of breast tissue has been removed, it is submitted for radiography to confirm that the abnormal area has in fact been excised.

RADIOISOTOPE SCANNING

A suitable tracer agent is given intravenously or orally. The tracer agent is a substance taken up by the target tissue. This substance is combined with a radioactive label, the most commonly used being technetium-99m (^{99m}Tc). A gamma camera is placed over the area of interest and simultaneously collects and counts the level of radioactivity. Dynamic imaging involves measuring the changing level of radioactivity over a period of time and storing this in a computer for later analysis. Renal blood flow measurement is an example of dynamic imaging. The following are applications of radioisotope scanning which are used in clinical practice.

Bone Scans

Phosphates labelled with technetium are tracer agents. The tracer is taken up in areas of increased bone deposition and resorption. Uptake occurs in sites of infection, secondary tumour and acute arthritis. Indications for bone scanning include suspected bony secondaries, suspected osteomyelitis, abnormal biochemical profiles suggesting bone disease, e.g. raised calcium or alkaline phosphatase.

Renal Scans

Two isotopes are commonly used, i.e. MAG3 and DMSA. MAG3 is excreted dynamically through the kidney while DMSA remains in cortical tissue. They are useful in assessing asymmetrical renal function. Dynamic computer analysis allows assessment of renal blood flow as well as excretory activity. Practical applications include investigation of renal artery stenosis and also differentiating ATN, renal ischaemia and obstruction in transplanted kidneys.

Lung Scanning

This is important in the diagnosis of pulmonary embolism (PE), although it is being somewhat superseded by CTPA. Emboli obliterate areas of pulmonary arterial circulation, but ventilation remains intact. A V/Q scan is usually carried out. The perfusion scan involves the injection of radioactive particles small enough to temporarily block a small number of pulmonary capillaries. Technetium-labelled albumin microspheres are usually used. A ventilation scan using an inert radioactive gas, e.g. xenon, is performed simultaneously. The scans are compared. Areas that are ventilated and not perfused suggest embolism. Areas that are perfused but not ventilated suggest consolidation or collapse.

Scanning for Infection

Ultrasonography or CT scanning will locate a collection of pus, but in equivocal cases, white cell scanning may help. The patient is bled and the white cells separated. These are then labelled with indium-111 (^{111}In) and reinjected. The body is then scanned and areas of interest noted. The test is useful in patients with pyrexia of unknown origin or septicaemia where other methods have failed to locate an area of sepsis.

Screening for GI Bleeding

The patient's own red cells are labelled with technetium and reinjected. The abdomen is scanned at intervals over the next 24h. The investigation reveals only the general area of bleeding, e.g. stomach, right or left colon, rather than the exact site.

ENDOSCOPY

Endoscopy implies examination of part of the body through an instrument. This may be through a natural orifice, e.g. oesophagoscopy or sigmoidoscopy, or through a surgically created hole, e.g. laparoscopy or arthroscopy. Endoscopy may be carried out with a rigid instrument, e.g. oesophagoscopy or sigmoidoscopy, the latter two being the most commonly used rigid endoscopy instruments. More recently, fibre-optic instruments have become more sophisticated and more widely used, e.g. gastroscopy, colonoscopy.

USE OF ENDOSCOPES

Rigid Endoscopes

Sigmoidoscopy. This is probably the most commonly used rigid endoscope. It is 25 or 30 cm long. Examination is usually carried out in the left lateral position. The position of a lesion is usually indicated by measuring its distance in centimetres from the anal verge. Biopsies may be taken with long forceps inserted through the scope.

Oesophagoscopy. This has largely been superseded by the flexible instrument. The rigid one, however, remains useful for removing large foreign bodies from the oesophagus.

Cystoscopy. The rigid instrument has been widely used for many years but has now been largely superseded by the flexible scope. The rigid instrument remains useful for retrograde ureteric catheterisation. Transurethral resection of the prostate has been carried out for many years via the rigid cystoscope.

Laparoscopy. This technique was widely used by gynaecologists but is now being more widely used by the general surgeon, particularly for minimally invasive surgery. A cannula is introduced into the peritoneal cavity and the peritoneal cavity distended with carbon dioxide gas. It is useful not only for diagnosis and biopsy but also in many operative procedures that are now being carried out with it in all branches of surgery.

Flexible Endoscopes

Gastroscope (Oesophago-Gastro-Duodenoscope). This is used with intravenous sedation and a pharyngeal local anaesthetic spray. A clear view can be obtained of the oesophagus, stomach and duodenum, and with a side-viewing scope the ampulla of Vater may be clearly seen. It is used for the identification and biopsy of lesions; tracing sources of GI haemorrhage; injection of oesophageal varices; lasering of bleeding lesions; dilatation of oesophageal strictures; and cannulation of the ampulla of Vater for ERCP. With the technique of ERCP a diathermy wire can be used down the gastroscope for dividing the sphincter of Oddi and allowing stones to pass out into the GI tract.

Colonoscopy. It is possible to inspect the whole of the colon after adequate bowel preparation. Biopsies can be carried out. Polyps can be removed by a wire snare or diathermy. Routine follow-up of patients having had previous carcinomas resected or ulcerative colitis can be carried out, avoiding the need for repeated barium enemas.

Bronchoscopy. Narrow fibre-optic bronchoscopes can be passed under local anaesthetic. They are mainly used for diagnostic purposes but can also be used postoperatively for removing mucous plugs that have caused segmental collapse.

Other Flexible Scopes. These include cystoscopes, sigmoidoscope and choledochoscopes (for inspecting the common bile duct at open surgery to assess for stones, tumours, etc.)

Advantages and Disadvantages of Endoscopy

Advantages

- Usually well tolerated. No need for general anaesthetic, and therefore can be used on the elderly and unfit patients.
- Any lesion can be directly visualised and biopsy taken under direct view.
- Flexible endoscopy is safer than rigid endoscopy.

Disadvantages

- Perforation of a hollow viscus
- Tissue samples are usually small due to the size of the biopsy channel.
- Sterility of the instrument is paramount to offset the risk of HIV or hepatitis B.

Complications

The main complications include perforation, haemorrhage at the site of biopsy or operative procedure and pulmonary aspiration. Cardiovascular complications may be related to the medication.

TISSUE DIAGNOSIS

Biopsy

This is removal of a piece of tissue from the living to provide a diagnosis. *Incisional biopsy* is the surgical removal of a piece of accessible tissue. *Excisional biopsy* is the complete removal of a discrete lesion without a wide margin and without it being considered curative of the disease. Biopsies may be performed in a number of ways (Figure 3.1).

Cytology

Specimens obtained by scraping or fine-needle aspiration are spread on a slide and stained. The earliest example of this technique was cervical smears stained by the Papanicolaou technique.

Cytological diagnosis requires a skilled pathologist. The method must be both specific and sensitive. False positives and false negatives may occur. Cytological diagnosis is useful in the following situations in general surgery:

- Aspiration of ascites or pleural effusions
- Aspiration of solid masses, e.g. breast, thyroid, pancreas or lymph nodes.

INTERVENTIONAL RADIOLOGY

Interventional radiology has increased markedly over the past two decades. The areas listed below have seen advances in interventional radiology.

Tissue Diagnosis

- Automated Tru-Cut needle biopsy under ultrasound or CT control, e.g. liver biopsy
- FNAC: a 22G needle can usually be safely passed through most organs to aspirate the suspicious lesion under ultrasound or CT control, e.g. lesions in the head of the pancreas.

Biliary Tract

In obstructive jaundice caused by malignant compression, either intrinsic (cholangiocarcinoma) or extrinsic (nodes at porta hepatis), the site can be accurately located by

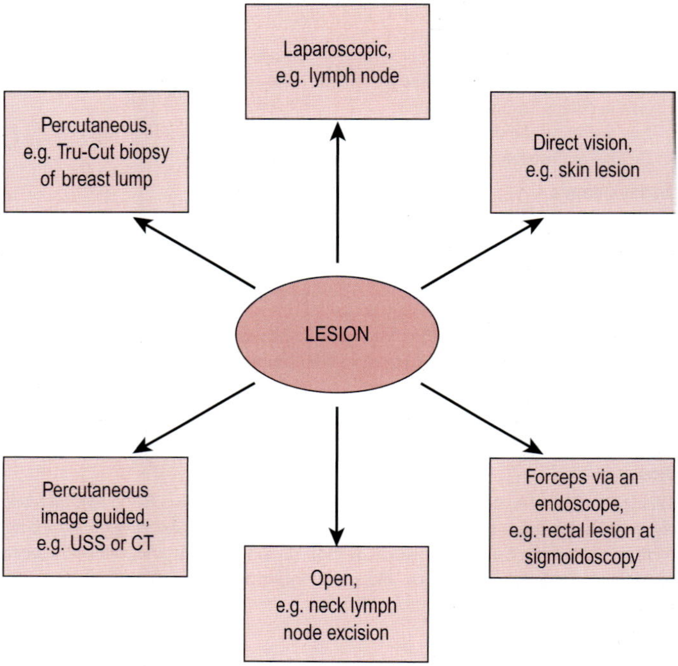

FIGURE 3.1
Ways of performing biopsy.

PTC and treated by stenting. A guide wire is passed through the stenosis and the stenosis dilated, following which a stent is passed over the guide wire to lie across the stenosis. This procedure may also be carried out at ERCP and is likely to be associated with fewer complications by the latter method.

Urinary Tract

The renal pelvis can be punctured by percutaneous insertion of a needle under ultrasound or CT control. The tract can be dilated to allow tubes to be inserted, and this allows for removal of stones from the renal pelvis or the insertion of nephrostomy tubes to drain the kidney prior to definitive treatment of a distal obstruction. The procedure is known as percutaneous nephrostomy.

Vascular System

Percutaneous Transluminal Angioplasty (PTA) and Stenting. Arteriography is carried out by the Seldinger technique. A flexible guide wire is then passed across the stenosis. Next, a catheter with a rigid plastic inflatable balloon is placed along the guide wire to lie within the stenosis and its position is checked under the image intensifier. The balloon is inflated to dilate the stenosis. Measurement of pressures above and below the site of the dilatation is used to assess the success of the procedure. The complications include arterial rupture, embolism, thrombosis or dissection. It is also possible to percutaneously insert a stent across the dilated stenosis. This is usually performed if a residual stenosis exists after balloon dilatation or to deal with a complication i.e. vessel rupture or dissection. A vascular surgeon should always be available to deal with any complications that may arise.

Thrombolysis. Systemic thrombolysis carries dangers of haemorrhage, e.g. GI or cerebral, and local thrombolysis is safer. Arteriography is carried out to confirm the diagnosis. The tip of a catheter is then placed within the clot and a thrombolytic agent, e.g. streptokinase, urokinase or tissue plasminogen activator, is infused directly into the clot. Radiography is repeated at 8–12h intervals to check progress. At each radiograph the catheter is advanced further into the dissolving clot. The technique can be used for clotted bypass grafts (without significant neuro-muscular deficit), thrombosed AV fistulas and central DVTs, i.e. ilio-femoral and axillary. When the clot is cleared, any stenoses demonstrated radiologically may be submitted to angioplasty/stenting if suitable.

Embolisation. This is suitable for highly vascular tissues, e.g. arteriovenous malformations, or to treat lesions not amenable to surgery, e.g. liver metastases or extensive renal carcinoma. The main arterial supply is identified via arteriography and a catheter placed within it. An occlusive material is then injected. Suitable agents include gelatin foam or minute steel coils. Embolisation is being increasingly used to arrest haemorrhage following trauma or from the GI tract.

Prevention of Pulmonary Emboli. Recurrence of pulmonary emboli in the presence of adequate anticoagulation is an indication for interrupting the IVC. It is possible to insert a filter in the cava percutaneously via the internal jugular vein or femoral vein. A commonly used filter is the Greenfield, which is shaped like a shuttlecock and is held closed with a special introducing catheter. This catheter is inserted through a sheath in the femoral vein. It is positioned in the inferior vena cava below the renal veins and released. The feet of the filter hook into the vein wall to prevent it from being dislodged.

Endovascular Aneurysm Repair. This is an area that has seen perhaps the greatest advances. Aneurysms of the abdominal (EVAR) and thoracic (TEVAR) aorta can be repaired through small incisions to access the common femoral arteries. More complex grafts known as FEVAR and BEVAR can also be used to repair aneurysms unsuitable for standard grafts or those that involve the visceral vessels.

Chapter 4

Shock and Trauma

Michael S. Delbridge • Wissam Al-Jundi

CHAPTER OUTLINE

SHOCK

Shock is defined as an abnormality of the circulatory system that results in inadequate organ perfusion and tissue oxygenation. Five types of shock may be encountered in surgical practice: hypovolaemic, septic, cardiogenic, neurogenic and anaphylactic.

Hypovolaemic Shock

This is due to decreased circulating blood volume.

Causes. These include:

- Haemorrhage, e.g. trauma, haematemesis, ruptured aortic aneurysm
- Dehydration, e.g. severe vomiting or diarrhoea, third space loss in inflammatory conditions
- Burns resulting in massive loss of serum.

Classification. The blood volume of a 70kg man is approximately 5L or 80mL/kg. Hypovolaemic shock can be divided into four categories, depending on the amount lost:

I. <750mL or <15%
II. 750–1500mL or 15–30%
III. 1500–2000 mL or 30–40%
IV. >2000 mL or >40%.

Symptoms and Signs. The symptoms and signs relate to the amount of blood lost:

I. Minimal symptoms
II. Tachycardia >100 bpm, tachypnoea, decreased pulse pressure, pale, sweaty, cold peripheries
III. Classic symptoms of shock – tachycardia >120 bpm, hypotension, tachypnoea, pallor, cold peripheries, decreased conscious level, oliguria
IV. Immediate threat to life – tachycardia >140 bpm, hypotension (unobtainable diastolic), pallor, cold peripheries, unconscious (>50%), anuria.

Management. Shock is a surgical emergency and needs rapid treatment:

1. Ensure an adequate airway. Deliver 100% oxygen by mask. If comatose, intubate.
2. Keep the patient recumbent and elevate the foot of the bed.

3. Establish vascular access with two large-bore intravenous catheters – ideally in the antecubital fossa. If the cause of shock is haemorrhage, take blood for crossmatching. Also take blood for haemoglobin, haematocrit, U&Es and assess base deficit. The latter is a good indicator of the severity of haemorrhagic shock, e.g. base deficit of -10 mEq/L or less is expected in class IV patients. Restore circulating volume with crystalloid initially and with plasma expanders or blood as indicated. Class II and above tend to require blood transfusion. It is vital for survival to give blood products at a low ratio of packed RBCs to plasma and platelets early in the management of class III and IV shock.
4. Compression of any obvious external haemorrhage, i.e. stab wound to the groin.
5. Insert a central venous line to monitor central venous pressure (CVP) and to assess the response to fluid administration.
6. Insert a urinary catheter to monitor urinary output.
7. Establish basic observations of temperature, pulse, BP, respiratory rate and level of consciousness and urinary output.
8. The underlying cause of the shock should be ascertained and definitive treatment planned.
9. Administer tranexamic acid within 3h of injury. A bolus dose of 1g is given over 10min followed by 1g infusion over 8h.

Failure of resuscitation may be due to persistent massive haemorrhage. Surgical intervention is often necessary.

HINTS AND TIPS

The anterior cubital fossa is the preferred site of vascular access. Try to pick a site for cannulation where the vein bifurcates, as here it will be fixed more to the fascia and will move less, making cannulation easier. Alternative sites include the cephalic vein at the wrist, the long saphenous vein (LSV) at the ankle or ultrasound-guided puncture of a central vein. If you are really struggling, the back of the wrist may provide the site for a last attempt – veins are easy to see, as there is less subcutaneous tissue (but it is painful!). Intraosseous cannulas are now available for adults too in really extreme cases.

Septic Shock

Septic shock is part of the SIRS. Sepsis is defined as SIRS with a confirmed source of infection. Severe sepsis is sepsis with one or more organ dysfunction. Septic shock is defined as hypotension and hypoperfusion despite adequate fluid resuscitation. Septic shock is uncommon in trauma unless there has been a delay in presentation.

Causes. Septic shock is due to the release of a number of proinflammatory mediators such as IL-1, IL-6, TNF-α, PAF and the eicosanoids; and as a result of bacterial endotoxins (lipopolysaccharides). Septic shock is usually due to Gram-negative organisms such as *Escherichia coli, Klebsiella* and *Pseudomonas,* although peptidoglycans and teichoic acids in Gram-positive bacteria can also have similar effects. The pathophysiology underlying shock in septic patients includes:

- Peripheral vasodilation
- ↑ Vascular permeability (third space loss)
- Peripheral arteriovenous shunting
- Myocardial depression due to toxic effects on heart
- Uncoupling of oxidative phosphorylation and anaerobic respiration leading to severe metabolic acidosis.

Symptoms and Signs. There may be an obvious source of infection, together with a predisposing condition. The patient may be confused and restless; initially the skin is hot and flushed and the pulse characteristically 'bounding'. Vasoconstriction and the classic signs of shock may develop later.

Management. This is urgent and involves resuscitation, identification of the source of sepsis, appropriate antibiotic therapy and any necessary surgery to eradicate the focus of infection.

1. Ensure adequate airway and ventilation. Give high-flow oxygen.
2. Restore circulating volume with plasma expanders while monitoring the venous pressure and urine output.
3. Obtain FBC, U&E, LFTs, clotting screen, ABG, serum lactate, cultures of blood, sputum, urine and any drainage fluid.
4. Commence intravenous antibiotics. This will depend on a number of factors. These include:
    a. *Site of sepsis* – from the patient history and clinical examination, a best-guess site of sepsis can usually be ascertained, i.e. gastrointestinal (GI), respiratory, urinary and secondary to intravascular lines.
    b. *Previous antibiotics* – a patient who develops septic shock after prophylactic antibiotics is likely to have infection from a resistant organism, and thus use of a different antibiotic is essential.
    c. *Length of time in hospital* – organisms in the community and nosocomial organisms differ greatly; a patient admitted from the community with septic shock from a respiratory infection will require different antibiotics to a patient from ITU who has been in hospital for 4 weeks.
    d. *Local resistance* – depending on whether the patient is ward-based or on ITU, the likely infecting organism and likely antibiotic resistance will differ. This is also true from hospital to hospital. In these situations, it is best to consult the on-call microbiologist. They will be able to give advice on the likely organisms responsible and on the most appropriate antibiotic therapy.
5. Carry out appropriate surgical intervention, e.g. drainage of abscess, peritoneal lavage.
6. Further supportive measures may be required, e.g. inotropic agents, ventilation.

HINTS AND TIPS

Do not be afraid to give several litres of fluid rapidly in septic patients. They will have lost litres in third space losses – this is no time for a litre of normal saline over 8h! Also make sure the antibiotics are given; do not just write them up and leave the patient. It has been shown that time to first dose of antibiotics can be crucial to survival in septic patients.

Complications. Sepsis and septic shock can progress to MODS and multiorgan failure syndrome (MOFS). Patients with MODS often present with sequential failure of organs, lung–liver–intestine–kidney; this may present as acute respiratory distress syndrome (ARDS), abnormal LFTs, ileus and renal failure. With continued illness, organ dysfunction progresses to organ failure. Mortality with one-organ failure is around 30%. This rises to 100% with four-organ failure.

Cardiogenic Shock

Cardiogenic shock or 'pump failure' is due to a loss of myocardial contractility.

CAUSES. These can be divided into compressive, obstructive or functional. All lead to problems with myocardial function and an inadequate cardiac output.

- Compressive – external forces compress the heart and great vessels leading to impairment of diastolic filling, a decrease in stroke volume and consequent hypotension. Causes include cardiac tamponade, positive pressure ventilation, tension pneumothorax and abdominal compartment syndrome.
- Obstructive – occurs when intravascular obstruction, excessive stiffness of arterial walls and microvascular blockage place an undue stress on the heart. It may be right- or left-sided. Tension pneumothorax is the commonest traumatic cause, but other causes include valvular stenosis, pulmonary embolism (PE) and ARDS.
- Functional – the heart itself is not functioning efficiently. This may be due to arrhythmias or impaired muscle function after contusion or infarction.

Symptoms and Signs. The traumatic causes will be discussed later in the chapter. Cardiac causes may present with chest pain and collapse. There may be a past history of cardiac problems or presence of risk factors, i.e. diabetes. Patients may be dyspnoeic with signs of pulmonary oedema. The patient may also display the classic signs of shock, i.e. pale, clammy, tachycardia, hypotension. PE may present similarly (→Ch. 5).

Investigations. Urgent investigations include portable chest X-ray (CXR), FBC, U&E, cardiac enzymes, D-dimers, ABGs, ECG.

Management

1. ABC – high-flow oxygen administration and i.v. access
2. Place patient in most comfortable position, i.e. sitting up with pulmonary oedema.
3. Pain relief, e.g. diamorphine
4. Drugs – consider aspirin (if myocardial infarction (MI)), furosemide (if pulmonary oedema), inotropic agents.
5. Correct arrhythmias.
6. Correct U&Es and acid–base abnormalities.
7. Cardiac monitoring (preferably on CCU)
8. CVP monitoring – avoid fluid overload.
9. Consider angioplasty for MI in the postop setting, as thrombolytic therapy is contraindicated.
10. Surgery for valvular abnormalities
11. Consider aortic balloon pump in extreme circumstances.

Neurogenic Shock

Neurogenic shock is due to impaired descending sympathetic pathways in the spinal cord; this results in loss of vasomotor tone and sympathetic innervation to the heart. This leads to pooling of blood in the lower limbs. Although neurogenic shock can occur with spinal injury, it is *not* synonymous with spinal shock; this refers to the flaccidity and areflexia seen after a spinal injury. Neurogenic shock also occurs from certain nervous stimuli, i.e. fright – this leads to a sudden dilation of the splanchnic vessels and a bradycardia – the transient hypotension may lead to collapse.

Symptoms and Signs. The classic sign of neurogenic shock in the trauma patient includes:

- Bradycardia – due to loss of sympathetic tone
- Hypotension – there is no narrowed pulse pressure
- No vasoconstriction of peripheries.

Treatment

- ABC
- Maintain spinal immobilisation.
- Vasopressors may be needed to maintain blood pressure.
- Atropine – if significant bradycardias occur.

In the nontrauma setting, neurogenic shock is self-limiting.

HINTS AND TIPS

NEVER assume hypotension in a trauma patient is due to neurogenic shock. Hypovolaemia is by far the commonest cause.

Anaphylactic Shock

Anaphylactic shock is a type I hypersensitivity reaction occurring in response to a previously sensitised antigen. Shock occurs as a result of vasodilation and increased vascular permeability. In surgical practice this may follow administration of drugs or radiological dyes. In the community it may follow wasp or bee stings or ingestion of certain foods, i.e. peanuts.

Symptoms and Signs. Generalised urticaria, wheezing, laryngeal oedema, hypotension, loss of consciousness.

Management

1. ABC and call for help.
2. Remove the cause.
3. Give i.v. fluids, i.e. normal saline.
4. 0.5 mL of 1:1000 adrenaline i.m. (given in the anterolateral aspect of middle third of the thigh and can be repeated after 5 min)
5. Chlorpheniramine 10 mg i.v.
6. Hydrocortisone 100 mg i.v.

HINTS AND TIPS

UK Resuscitation Council updated guidance in 2021 emphasised the importance of giving i.m. adrenaline when anaphylaxis is suspected, while chlorpheniramine and hydrocortisone are no longer part of the algorithm for managing anaphylaxis. The latter drugs are more relevant for milder forms of allergic reactions, e.g., rash.

The importance of an adequate drug and sensitivity history cannot be overemphasised. Always make sure before giving parenteral injections that resuscitation equipment and drugs are available. Remember the strength of adrenaline used is 1:1000 for i.m. administration BUT 1:10,000 for i.v. use. i.v. adrenaline should only be given by a specialist in the field who has experience in giving the drug intravenously.

TRAUMA

Trauma is the main cause of death in people under the age of 35 years. Mortality can be greatly reduced by appropriate handling of the injured in the following three settings:

1. Emergency medical teams capable of going to the scene of an accident
2. A transportation system capable of rapid transport to a specified trauma centre
3. A trauma centre with trained personnel who are capable of rapidly assessing the injuries with facilities capable of handling a large number of trauma cases with trained teams.

Initial Assessment of the Trauma Patient

Prehospital Care. In the prehospital phase, the same priorities exist in terms of ABCs; there is particular emphasis on airway control with restriction of cervical spine motion, adequate breathing or ventilation and control of external bleeding. The key is to limit time on the scene and to transfer the patient to the nearest appropriate hospital. Communication with the local hospital allows advanced warning to assemble the trauma team.

Initial Assessment and Resuscitation. This should follow ATLS guidelines. Initial assessment is divided into a primary survey where immediately life-threatening injuries are assessed and treated. This is followed by a secondary survey, which is a head-to-toe assessment that aims to find other injuries and to take a more detailed history. This does not begin until the primary survey is completed, resuscitation is well established and the patient has normal vital signs.

Primary Survey

This process constitutes the **ABCDE** protocol of ATLS:

- **A**irway maintenance with restriction of cervical spine motion – ensure a clear airway. The mouth and upper airway should be inspected for foreign bodies; these should be removed. If the patient has an airway problem, there are a number of airway adjuncts (see later).
- **B**reathing – check for chest movements, asymmetry of movements, respiratory rate, abrasions or bruising over the chest, cyanosis, use of accessory muscles,

distension of neck veins. Examine the chest for pain, crepitations (indicating subcutaneous emphysema), auscultation, percussion and palpation of the trachea
- **C**irculation and haemorrhage control – i.v. access should be gained with two large-bore cannulae (12–14G) in the antecubital fossa. Two litres of Hartmann's solution should be rapidly infused. Obvious haemorrhage can be treated with compression dressings. Tourniquets are effective in massive exsanguination from an extremity but carry a risk of ischaemic injury to that extremity. Use a tourniquet only when direct pressure is not effective and the patient's life is threatened.
- **D**isability – in the primary survey a rapid assessment of neurological status is made. This includes assessment of pupillary size and level of consciousness. The level of consciousness can be remembered by the mnemonic **AVPU**:
    - **A**lert
    - Responds to **V**ocal stimuli
    - Responds to **P**ainful stimuli
    - **U**nresponsive.
- **E**xposure and environmental control – the patient should be fully undressed and examined from head to toe (secondary survey). The patient's temperature must be monitored and hypothermia prevented by covering with warming blankets and use of warmed i.v. fluids.

During the primary survey and in tandem with examining the patient, certain adjuncts are used, including ECG, pulse oximetry, BP and respiratory rate, insertion of NG tube and urinary catheter (as required); also, the patient is provided with adequate analgesia.

Secondary Survey

The secondary survey is a head-to-toe evaluation of the trauma patient, i.e. a complete history and physical examination, including a reassessment of all vital signs. Each area of the body should be completely examined. A full neurological examination is carried out, including Glasgow Coma Scale (GCS) determination (Table 4.1).

History. This is obtained from the patient (if possible), ambulance staff or other witnesses. A mnemonic to help remember this is to take an **AMPLE** history:

- **A**llergies
- **M**edications – taken regularly and those given at the scene of the accident
- **P**revious illnesses – prior surgery and current comorbidities
- **L**ast meal
- **E**vents surrounding injury – mechanism of injury, blood loss at scene, etc.

Examination. A full examination is carried out during the secondary survey looking for head injuries, maxillofacial injuries, cervical spine injuries, chest injuries, abdominal and perineal injuries, musculoskeletal injuries and neurological trauma. Typical injury patterns include:

- Frontal impact – injuries to diaphragm, cervical spine, flail chest, myocardial contusion, pneumothorax, TRA, ruptured liver and spleen, possible dislocation of hip or knee
- Side impact – injuries to cervical spine, flail chest, pneumothorax, TRA, diaphragmatic tear, ruptured liver, ruptured spleen, ruptured kidney, fractured pelvis or acetabulum

TABLE 4.1
GLASGOW COMA SCALE (GCS)

Responses	Score
Eye-Opening Response	
Spontaneous	4
To voice	3
To pain	2
None	1
Best Verbal Response	
Orientated	5
Confused	4
Inappropriate speech	3
Incomprehensible speech	2
None	1
Best Motor Response	
Obeys commands	6
Localises pain	5
Withdraws to pain	4
Flexion to pain	3
Extension to pain	2
None	1
Total	3–15

A score of 3 indicates a severe injury with a poor prognosis. A score of 13–15 indicates minor injury with a good prognosis.

- Rear impact – cervical spine injury
- Pedestrian – head injury, TRA, abdominal visceral injury, fractured lower limb and pelvis
- Fall from a height – calcaneal fracture, tibial plateau fracture, pelvic or acetabular fracture, lumbar spine compression fracture, TRA, pneumothorax, head injury.

Investigations. The timing of the investigations depends on the clinical state of the patient. These include: blood grouping and crossmatch, FBC, U&E, amylase, LFT, glucose, beta-human chorionic gonadotrophin (β-HCG; in women of child-bearing age) and arterial blood gas. X-rays in the primary survey include chest and pelvis X-ray. FAST is an imaging modality often performed during the primary survey to identify an abdominal source of bleeding in a hypotensive patient. All other X-ray images, computerised tomography (CT) scans, contrast studies, etc. are obtained depending on the stability of the patient and the presence of other injuries. As a rule, these would be obtained as part of the secondary survey when the immediate threat to life has been treated and the patient is stable.

Head Injury (→ Ch. 19)

Primary brain damage occurring at the time of injury cannot be repaired. Management should be aimed at preventing secondary injury.

Management. The management of specific head injury is dealt with in the section on Neurosurgery (→ Ch. 19), but the basic principles are outlined here.

Treat hypoxia, hypercapnia, hypovolaemic shock and anaemia to prevent further neurological deterioration. Primary neurological management is identification and rapid treatment of localised lesions and intracranial haemorrhage, cerebral debridement and prevention of raised ICP.

Hypotension in adults is not due to intracranial blood loss. However, in children, significant blood loss can occur in head injuries and can be responsible for hypotension. The scalp should be examined for lacerations and boggy wounds. Observation should be made for bleeding and cerebrospinal fluid (CSF) leakage from the ear and nose. The cranial nerves should be checked and the limbs examined. Assessment of head-injured patients include skull X-rays and CT scan; indications for these are detailed in Chapter 19.

HINTS AND TIPS

Immediate management depends on severity. The presence of abnormal pupillary reflexes, asymmetrical motor signs or deteriorating level of consciousness is an indication for immediate treatment.

Immediate measures in severe head injury includes:

- ABC
- Intubation
- Ventilate with 100% oxygen – prevention of secondary brain injury
- Intravenous mannitol can be given to produce a diuresis and reduce cerebral oedema.
- Maintain normovolaemia.
- Monitor ABGs and maintain normocapnia.
- Immediate transfer to theatre for burr holes and evacuation of haematoma.

Less urgent management is required where there are focal lesions without brainstem compression and with an unconscious patient without focal neurological signs.

Thoracic Trauma

Blunt and penetrating thoracic trauma is responsible for 25% of deaths due to trauma, but less than 20% of patients require thoracotomy for the treatment of their injuries.

Management. Thoracic injuries can be divided into those that are immediately life-threatening or potentially life-threatening.

Immediately life-threatening injuries can be remembered by '**ATOM CT**':

- **A**irway obstruction
- **T**ension pneumothorax

- **O**pen pneumothorax
- **M**assive haemothorax
- **C**ardiac tamponade
- **T**racheo-bronchial tree injury
- **C**ardiac tamponade.

Potentially life-threatening injuries can be remembered by '**AFOM PD**':

- **A**ortic disruption
- **F**lail chest
- **O**esophageal injury
- **M**yocardial contusion
- **P**ulmonary contusion and **P**neumothorax
- **D**iaphragmatic rupture.

Airway Obstruction

Usually as a result of foreign bodies (e.g. blood, teeth or loss of muscular control of the tongue). More unusual causes include laryngeal trauma and posterior dislocation of the sternoclavicular joint.

Symptoms and Signs. These include tachypnoea, altered level of consciousness (agitated with hypoxia and obtunded with hypercapnia), use of accessory muscles and abnormal sounds such as gurgling, snoring or stridor.

Management. There are a number of airway adjuncts that fall under airway management. These are detailed below:

- Jaw thrust and chin lift – simple first aid may be all that is required to secure a patent airway.
- Nasal airways and Guedel airways – inserted when patients have a reduced conscious level and are obstructing their airway. If the patient's conscious level is not sufficiently reduced, they will not be tolerated.

HINTS AND TIPS

A nasal airway is sized to the patient's little finger, and a safety pin is placed in the end (to stop it going up the nose!). A Guedel airway is sized from the corner of the patient's mouth to the angle of the jaw. It is inserted upside down and rotated to lie over the patient's tongue.

- Intubation – if the techniques below are not successful, the patient will need to be intubated. This is a definitive airway – an ET in the trachea with an inflated cuff and secured with tape.
- Surgical airway – rarely used, but in patients with severe maxillofacial trauma or airway swelling they may be required. They consist of needle cricothyroidotomy (jet insufflation) and surgical cricothyroidotomy. Tracheostomy is NOT a technique for an emergency airway.

PROCEDURE

CRICOTHYROIDOTOMY

Needle cricothyroidotomy – performed by surgically preparing the neck and infiltrating local anaesthetic, then inserting a large-bore cannula through the cricopharyngeal membrane (this can be confirmed by aspirating air into a syringe attached to the cannula once in the correct position). The plastic cannula is then advanced into the trachea, oxygen tubing is attached to the cannula with a side hole and 15 L O_2 is delivered. The side hole is occluded for 1 s and left open for 4 s. This will allow 30–40 min of ventilation before the CO_2 rises to high.

Surgical cricothyroidotomy – performed by preparing the neck and infiltrating local anaesthetic, then making a transverse incision in the cricothyroid membrane. This is then dilated (using the handle of the scalpel or a clip) and a size 5.0–7.0 tracheostomy tube is inserted.

Tension Pneumothorax

Injury results in the formation of a 'one-way' valve – air enters the pleural cavity but is unable to escape, therefore pressure (or tension) in the chest rises, causing distortion of the vena cava and trachea.

Symptoms and Signs. Tachypnoea, use of accessory muscles, cyanosis, hypotension (due to kinking of vena cava and decreased venous return), deviated trachea (away from the affected side), distended neck veins (variable sign), hyper-resonant percussion and absent breath sounds.

Management. This is a clinical diagnosis. Immediate management is the placement of a wide-bore cannula in the second intercostal space in the midclavicular line. A chest drain must then replace this as the tension pneumothorax has been converted to a simple pneumothorax.

HINTS AND TIPS

Remember to insert the cannula along the upper border of the third rib to avoid the intercostal vessels.

Open (Sucking) Pneumothorax

Produced by injuries that cause large defects of the chest wall, i.e. gunshot wounds. The injury leads to intrathoracic and atmospheric pressure equalising. If the defect is greater than two-thirds of the diameter of the trachea, air will preferentially enter the defect and bypass the lungs and thus produce hypoxia.

Symptoms and Signs. Tachypnoea, use of accessory muscles, cyanosis, obvious chest wound.

Management. Immediate management is the placement of a dressing secured on three sides to create a 'flutter-valve' (securing on four sides will produce a tension pneumothorax). A chest drain distant from the injury must then be placed.

Haemothorax and Massive Haemothorax

Most often due to penetrating injury to the hilar or systemic vessels. Can occur with blunt injury with rib fractures and damage to intercostal vessels – a massive haemothorax is defined as immediate evacuation of 1.5L at insertion of a chest drain or >200mL every hour for 2–4h after drain insertion. It produces hypoxia by the pressure effect of the additional volume in the thorax compressing the lung but also by hypovolaemia.

Symptoms and Signs. Signs of shock, tachypnoea, using accessory muscles, cyanosis, dull percussion note and absent breath sounds.

Management. Obtain i.v. access prior to insertion of chest drain, as rapid infusion of fluids may be needed. If blood loss from the chest drain is massive, it should be clamped in an attempt to re-tamponade the bleeding and consider using cell salvage. Thoracotomy if >1.5 L immediately or >200 mL/h (for 2–4 h) is lost.

Cardiac Tamponade

Usually occurs when, as a result of penetrating trauma, blood within the pericardium compresses the heart leading to cardiogenic shock.

Symptoms and Signs. Beck's triad (distended neck veins, hypotension, muffled heart sounds), pulsus paradoxus, Kussmaul's sign (↑JVP with inspiration), small complexes on ECG, EMD and on a FAST scan (see p. 61).

Management. Emergency thoracotomy by a qualified surgeon as soon as possible. If surgical intervention is not possible, needle pericardiocentesis or a pericardial window (performed at laparotomy) can be immediately life-saving, but definitive management requires thoracotomy.

PROCEDURE

NEEDLE PERICARDIOCENTESIS

This is both therapeutic and diagnostic: removal of as little as 20mL of blood can lead to improvement in symptoms. Surgically prepare the chest and infiltrate local anaesthetic, then insert a 16–18G needle 2cm below the xiphisternum and advance upwards towards the tip of the left scapula. The procedure should be performed with ECG monitoring. If the needle is advanced too far, there will be ECG changes such as ST elevation, etc. Once all the blood has been aspirated, a catheter with a three-way tap can be left in case of reaccumulation. Ultrasound guidance can facilitate accurate insertion.

Tracheobronchial Injury

Larynx. Rare, usually due to direct trauma.

Symptoms and Signs. May present late, these include hoarseness, stridor, subcutaneous emphysema and fracture crepitus.

Management. Intubation.

Trachea. Usually injured by penetrating trauma.

Symptoms and Signs. Include noisy breathing and visible bubbles in the neck wound.

Management. Surgical repair.

Bronchi. Rare, usually fatal at the scene, occurs due to severe deceleration injury; it is usually within 2.5 cm of the carina.

Symptoms and Signs. Haemoptysis, subcutaneous emphysema, tension pneumothorax, large air leak after placement of a chest drain.

Investigations. Bronchoscopy is diagnostic.

Management. May require further chest drain if large air leak, intubation of opposite bronchus if acutely hypoxic followed by surgical repair.

Aortic Disruption (TRA)

This is due to deceleration injuries such as in RTAs or a fall from a great height; the body rapidly decelerates, but the organs continue to move. It particularly affects sites where a mobile part of an organ meets a relatively fixed point (i.e. renal pedicle, duodenum at the ligament of Treitz and the aorta). The commonest point of deceleration injury in the aorta is in the ascending aorta just proximal to the innominate artery and at the point of attachment of the ligamentum arteriosum. Tears in the ascending aorta often have associated cardiac damage and rarely reach hospital; tears at the ligamentum arteriosum may be contained by adventitia and allow the patient to reach hospital (typically young males).

Symptoms and Signs. These are variable. The patient may have no signs or be moribund with signs of massive haemothorax. Other signs include upper extremity ↑BP with diminished pulses in the lower limbs, diminished pulses in the upper limbs (due to occlusion of vessels along the aortic arch) and neurological compromise from spinal ischaemia.

Investigations

- CXR (signs include widened mediastinum, fractured first or second rib, obliterated aortic knuckle, pleural cap – small amount of blood in the pleural cavity, deviated trachea to the right, elevation of right bronchus and right deviation of NG tube)
- Arch aortogram
- CT (comparable with aortogram)
- Transoesophageal echo.

Management. Traditional management has been by surgical repair with resection of damaged segment and replacing with a graft. This has been superseded by endovascular repair (TEVAR) and is associated with lower mortality and morbidity.

Flail Chest

Occurs when more than two adjacent ribs are fractured in two or more places. This results in a segment of the chest moving paradoxically with respiration (in with inspiration and out with expiration). Contrary to belief, it is not the paradoxical chest movement that causes respiratory problems but the lung contusion underlying the rib injury.

Symptoms and Signs. Pain, bruising, tachypnoea, paradoxical respiratory movement (often not present acutely due to muscle splinting).

Management. Analgesia, high-flow oxygen, judicious fluid replacement (at risk of pulmonary oedema due to the lung contusion), regular ABGs to identify patients at risk of respiratory failure and the need for artificial ventilation. Rarely, surgical fixation of the rib fractures is needed.

Oesophageal Injury

Can occur with penetrating or blunt injury. Penetrating injury is more common. Cervical oesophageal injuries present in a similar manner to tracheal injuries. With blunt injury, blows to the oesophagus can result in traumatic rupture (similar to Boerhaave's syndrome); this most commonly occurs in the lower left posterolateral oesophagus.

Symptoms and Signs. Haemo/pneumothorax with no rib fractures, pain and shock out of proportion to the apparent injury, particulate matter in the chest drain.

Management. Give i.v. antibiotics, surgical repair (in early diagnosis), with late diagnosed injuries the management is via antibiotics, chest drainage and oesophageal diversion.

Myocardial Contusion

Blunt injury. Difficult to diagnose. May result in a number of ECG abnormalities such as multiple ectopics, sinus tachycardia, atrial fibrillation or raised ST segments (similar to an MI).

Management. Cardiac monitor and treat arrhythmias as and when they arise.

Pulmonary Contusion

Common injury in blunt trauma. Analogous to a soft tissue bruise, with haemorrhage and oedema into the lung parenchyma. This impairs gas exchange and leads to respiratory failure (especially in the elderly and in those with coexistent lung disease).

Management. As for flail chest.

Pneumothorax (→ Ch. 9)

May occur with blunt or penetrating injury. A laceration of the lung parenchyma occurs, and air enters the pleural space; this results in loss of the negative intrapleural pressure, and the lung collapses. The collapsed segment of lung is perfused, but the blood is not oxygenated, leading to hypoxia.

Symptoms and Signs. Tachypnoea, use of accessory muscles, cyanosis, decreased breath sounds, resonant percussion note.

Management. Chest drain.

Diaphragmatic Rupture

Can occur with blunt or penetrating trauma. Blunt trauma usually results in tears of the left posterolateral hemidiaphragm. Penetrating injury may be missed and present many years later with visceral herniation.

Symptoms and Signs. Respiratory compromise, hypoxia and CXR appearance (bowel in chest cavity, 'fluffy' hemidiaphragm, NG tube in chest).

Investigations

- CT
- Thoracoscopy
- Laparoscopy.

Management. Surgical repair.

Miscellaneous Thoracic Injuries

Rib Fractures. Common injury following blunt trauma. Rib fractures can lead to:

- Pneumothorax (rib fragments lacerate lung parenchyma)
- Haemothorax (rib fragments lacerate intercostal vessels)
- Pain: impairs ventilation that may lead to atelectasis and pneumonia.

Rib fractures can indicate other potential injuries:

- Fractures of ribs 1–3: head injury, spinal injury, great vessel injury
- Fractures of ribs 10–12: hepatosplenic injury.

Symptoms and Signs. Pain, crepitus, visible deformity, respiratory compromise, CXR (fractures are not always visible).

Management

1. Analgesia – oral, i.v., intercostal block with local anaesthetic, epidural
2. Chest drain (if associated with pneumo/haemothorax)
3. Chest physiotherapy
4. Frequent ABGs in the elderly or patients with coexistent lung disease to assess impending respiratory failure.

Sternal Fractures

Blunt injury. Usually occurs at the manubriosternal junction. Associated with myocardial and pulmonary contusions.

Management. Cardiac monitoring and analgesia. ABG assessment if pulmonary contusion suspected.

Scapular Fractures

Considerable force is required, therefore suspect associated injuries. Fractures are divided into:

- Body – sling and analgesia
- Neck – may need ORIF if displaced glenoid
- Glenoid – ORIF if loss of joint congruity
- Acromion – ORIF only if gross displacement.

PULMONARY HAEMATOMA. Produced by intraparenchymal bleeding, mechanism of injury is similar to a contusion but respiratory dysfunction is less. A traumatic pneumatocoele (cavity in the pulmonary substance) may develop after resolution of a haematoma.

Symptoms and Signs. May be some respiratory signs, CXR may appear more dramatic with a sharp demarcated edge to the opacity.

Management. Conservative, the haematoma will resolve over 2–3 weeks.

Air Embolism

A rare event that occurs with penetrating trauma when a fistula is formed between the bronchus and a pulmonary vein. When breathing normally, the pressure is higher in the vein than bronchus – this results in haemoptysis. However, if the patient performs a Valsalva-type respiration, i.e. grunts or is intubated, pressure is higher in the bronchus and air will enter the pulmonary vein.

Symptoms and Signs. Haemoptysis. After air has entered the circulation, presentation includes the development of focal neurological signs, sudden cardiovascular collapse after intubation and froth when an ABG is obtained.

Management. Immediate thoracotomy, clamp the hilum of the injured lung and repair the laceration. If air is seen in the coronary vessels, the ascending aorta can be occluded for a few seconds to push out the air.

PROCEDURE

CHEST DRAIN INSERTION

The drain is placed in the fifth intercostal space in the anterior axillary line; this area is sometimes referred to as the 'triangle of safety' – an area bordered by the lateral edge of pectoralis major, the anterior edge of latissimus dorsi, a line from the nipple level (i.e. fifth intercostal) and an apex in the axilla. Surgically prepare and drape the chest; infiltrate local anaesthetic down to the pleura. Make a 2–3 cm horizontal incision and, with blunt dissection, open the wound over the *top* of the rib. Puncture the pleura and then enlarge the hole with your finger and sweep away any organs or adhesions. Then, using a suitable clamp to hold the tip of the drain (either 34 or 36 F), insert the drain through the hole and direct it up and posteriorly. Connect to an underwater seal and suture in place; look for fogging of the tube and 'swinging' of the drain to confirm position. Obtain a CXR.

EMERGENCY THORACOTOMY

Indications for emergency thoracotomy include witnessed arrest and a thoracic injury (especially from penetrating trauma) and severe postinjury hypotension as a result of cardiac tamponade, air embolism or thoracic bleeding. Surgically prepare the chest and fully abduct the patient's arm (if you have time, place a rolled sheet between the scapulae). Make an incision in the fourth intercostal space from the sternal border to the midaxillary line. Once into the pleura, open the full length of the wound with mayo scissors and insert a rib retractor. Objectives at this stage include: releasing cardiac tamponade, controlling intrathoracic bleeding, controlling air embolism, performing open cardiac massage and clamping the descending aorta to control infradiaphragmatic bleeding.

HINTS AND TIPS

Insertion of a chest drain can be very painful. Make sure that the local anaesthetic is infiltrated all the way to the pleura and you have given a strong analgesic (e.g. morphine). If the patient has not had adequate analgesia, the patient may move suddenly, and you will lose the track that you have been dissecting.

Abdominal Trauma

Abdominal trauma may be blunt (direct, deceleration and rotational forces are applied) or penetrating. Injury to an abdominal viscus should be suspected in any blunt injury to the thorax or abdomen or in penetrating injuries anywhere between the nipple and perineum. Obtain information about the injury from the patient, relatives and ambulance personnel.

The abdominal cavity can be divided into peritoneal and retroperitoneal cavities. The peritoneum can be further divided into 'intrathoracic', abdominal and pelvic:

- 'Intrathoracic' abdomen – from the diaphragm to the costal margins; it contains the liver, spleen, stomach and transverse colon (remember that the diaphragm can rise to the fourth intercostal space in expiration).

- Abdominal – small and large bowel, distended bladder, pregnant uterus
- Pelvic – sigmoid colon, rectum, small bowel, bladder, uterus and ovaries.

Organs in the retroperitoneum include:

- Kidneys and ureter
- Duodenum – except the first 2.5 cm (1 inch) of the first part
- Pancreas
- Caecum and ascending colon
- Two-thirds of the descending colon
- Lower rectum
- Aorta and IVC.

Penetrating Trauma

Causes of penetrating trauma include stab wounds and gunshot wounds. The most commonly injured organs are the liver and small bowel. Significant injury is much greater with gunshot wounds (80%) compared with stab wounds (30%).

Management. Initial management is via ATLS protocols; however, note specific points to remember:

1. Look for the wound – wounds on the back are easy to miss.
2. Look for the exit wound in GSWs, which may indicate likely injuries. Remember abdominal GSWs may traverse the thorax, and vice versa.
3. High-velocity GSWs injure widely along their path (cavitation).
4. Low-velocity GSWs injure along their path only.
5. ALL penetrating trauma secondary to GSWs should be explored via a laparotomy due to high risk of injury.
6. Penetrating injury secondary to knife wounds in the absence of haemodynamic instability, signs of peritonism, evisceration or free air under the diaphragm on CXR can be managed expectantly. Alternatively, a diagnostic laparoscopy can be performed to confirm peritoneal breach (the majority of stab wounds do not breach the peritoneum and those that do, do not always injure any organs).

Blunt Trauma

Abdominal injury due to blunt trauma may result from direct injury, deceleration or rotational forces. Blunt trauma is more common in the UK and results from RTAs, falls and pedestrian/vehicle accidents. The most commonly injured organs are the spleen and liver.

Symptoms and Signs. Skin abrasions, bruising, seat belt imprints (particularly with lap belts), fractures of ribs 10–12, abdominal tenderness or rigidity (peritonism), distension, absent bowel sounds, shock and haematuria.

Investigations in Abdominal Trauma.

1. CXR – part of the ATLS protocol, may show free air in a stable patient with penetrating trauma who is able to sit upright
2. Abdominal X-ray (AXR) – not part of the ATLS protocol and unlikely to add a great deal to patients with blunt or penetrating trauma
3. Ultrasound – this can be done in the A&E department and is known as FAST scanning. It simply aims to look for fluid in three areas of the abdomen (perihepatic, perisplenic and pelvic) and for a cardiac tamponade (pericardial).

Detects a minimum of around 200 mL of fluid; must be interpreted with clinical findings. A positive FAST scan is *not* an absolute indication for laparotomy.

4. CT – sensitive and specific for the injured organ; also allows an assessment of severity. Not suitable for unstable patients.
5. DPL – rarely needed with the availability of FAST scans. Basically entails placing a catheter into the abdomen; if frank blood is aspirated, it is a positive test; if not, a litre of fluid is run in and then drained off, which is then sent for analysis. A positive test is indicated by >100,000 RBCs/μL, bile or faecal matter.

Indications for laparotomy include:

- Hypotension refractory to resuscitation
- Peritonitis
- Air under the diaphragm on CXR
- Evisceration
- All GSW
- Positive investigations, i.e. CT.

Specific Organ Injuries

Gastrointestinal Tract. These are shown in Table 4.2.

Pancreas. Secondary to blunt trauma, typically an epigastric blow; the pancreas is compressed against the vertebral column.

Symptoms and Signs. Difficult to diagnose; classically presents with severe abdominal pain that decreases over 1–2h and then increases in severity.

Investigations

- Serum amylase – may be raised in pancreatic injury
- CT.

Management. Distal pancreatectomy; Whipple's procedure in severe injuries with proximal duct injury, injury involving the CBD or ampulla and devascularising injuries.

Complications. Fistula.

Liver. Most commonly injured intra-abdominal organ. Injury does not always need operative intervention. In general, management is based on CT appearances. However, transfusion of >3 units of blood and the patient is still shocked is an indication for laparotomy. Indications for nonoperative management include:

- Haemodynamically stable
- No persistent or increase in abdominal pain
- <4 Units transfusion
- CT – <500 mL blood in the peritoneum, parenchymal laceration or intrahepatic haematoma.

Symptoms and Signs. Few, other than haemodynamic instability in severe injuries; suspect with RUQ bruising/abrasions or broken right 10–12th ribs, right shoulder tip pain.

Management

Nonoperative. With no signs of peritonitis and no haemodynamic instability, the injury can often be managed nonoperatively. CT scan can be a useful guide to the

TABLE 4.2

INJURIES TO THE GASTROINTESTINAL TRACT

Organ	Mode of Trauma	Symptoms and Signs	Management	Complications
Stomach	Usually penetrating	Peritonitis, air under the diaphragm, bloody NG aspirate	Surgical repair, occasionally resection if severe	Fistula, abscess
Duodenum	Usually penetrating. Blunt trauma classically occurs with severe frontal impacts, e.g. hitting handlebars of a motorbike (usually involves the third part of the duodenum)	Bloody NG aspirate, retroperitoneal air, raised amylase (with associated pancreatic injury)	Depends on severity, ranges from simple closure to pancreaticoduodenal resections and complex drainage procedures (duodenal diverticulisation)	Fistula, abscess
Small bowel	Commonly injured in penetrating trauma. Blunt trauma occurs with: • Crushing between abdominal wall and vertebra • Sudden increase in intraluminal pressure, i.e. blast injuries • Deceleration injuries causing tears at fixed points, e.g. ligament of Treitz, ileocaecal area	Peritonitis, air under diaphragm, absent bowel sounds, particulate matter on DPL	Simple repair, resection $\pm$ stoma	Anastomotic leak, obstruction, abscess, fistula
Colorectal	Usually penetrating trauma. <5% are due to blunt trauma (indicates a significant force). Rectal injuries are also rare. They may be associated with pelvic fractures, penetrating trauma in the buttock and perineum – divided into extraperitoneal and intraperitoneal injuries	Peritonitis, absent bowel sounds, faecal matter on DPL, blood on PR	Further assessment can be made intraop via an EUA. Colonic injuries – primary repair, resection and resection and colostomy (Hartmann's procedure). Rectal injuries – primary repair for intraperitoneal injuries and extraperitoneal injuries that can be mobilised intraperitoneally or repaired transrectally. If extensive or delay in presentation, a proximal loop colostomy $\pm$ drainage	Colonic injuries – abscess, anastomotic leak and stoma-related problems. Rectal injuries – abscess, fistulae, incontinence (urinary and faecal), stricture and loss of sexual function

severity of injury, but in the main it is the absence of hypotension or tachycardia that dictates nonoperative management. Other points to consider include persistent or increased abdominal pain or the transfusion of >3 units of blood. Frequent checks of haemoglobin and haematocrit, clinical examination and invasive monitoring (i.e. CVP) will identify patients failing nonoperative management.

Radiological. If CT demonstrates extravasation, indicating arterial bleeding, an option is to perform angiography and embolisation. This can also be performed after operative packing if bleeding continues.

Operative. Operative intervention with liver trauma includes the following alone or in combination:

- Packing the liver with gauze rolls to compress the injured segment (this can be helped by mobilising the injured lobe); the packs can be left for 48h but antibiotics should be given
- Diathermy to superficial bleeding
- Deep liver sutures
- Hepatotomy and vascular ligation (i.e. open laceration more to suture bleeding vessels)
- Resect injured lobe – if a lobe is shattered, it may be better to resect.
- If exsanguinating, Pringle's manoeuvre can be performed – compression of the structures of the free edge of the lesser omentum (can be left for approximately 45min).

Complications. These include rebleeding, bile leaks, jaundice, coagulopathy, hypoglycaemia, ischaemic segments, infection/abscess and haemobilia.

SPLEEN. Most commonly injured in blunt trauma.

Symptoms and Signs. LUQ bruising or abrasions, lower rib fractures, shoulder tip pain (Kehr's sign); LUQ mass (Ballance's sign), displacement of gastric bubble on CXR. Following resuscitation, indications for nonoperative management include:

- Haemodynamically stable
- <2 Units transfused
- Stable serial haemoglobin (Hb) estimation
- No increase in size of splenic haematoma on serial USS
- No deterioration of condition on close observation
- Needs observation for 7–10 days, as there is a risk of delayed rupture of a splenic haematoma.

Management

Nonoperative. The patient must be haemodynamically stable, have <2 units transfused, have no evidence of other intra-abdominal organ injury, no evidence of active bleeding on CT and no evidence of shattered spleen or hilar injury (both mandate operative intervention). The patient should have frequent checks of haemoglobin and haematocrit. Clinical examination and invasive monitoring (i.e. CVP) will identify patients failing nonoperative management.

Radiological. As with liver injury, certain splenic injuries can be managed via angiography and embolisation.

Operative. Operative management depends on the severity of injury but may include the following, either alone or in combination:

- Packing
- Diathermy
- Topical haemostatics, e.g. Surgicel
- Wrapping in a mesh bag to tamponade bleed
- Suture lacerations
- Ligation of splenic vessels – decreased function with arterial ligation but preferred to splenectomy
- Partial splenectomy for polar injuries.

Complications. These include LUQ haematoma (may progress to abscess), pleural effusion, pseudoaneurysm of the splenic artery, arteriovenous fistula between the artery and vein, pancreatic injury/fistula and overwhelming postsplenectomy infection (OPSI →Ch. 15). With splenic haematomas that were treated nonoperatively, there is a small risk of delayed rupture, which can occur days or weeks later. It is prudent to monitor these patients with a repeat USS to identify an enlarging haematoma.

Urinary Trauma

RENAL. The most commonly injured part of the genitourinary tract; the majority of injuries (i.e. contusion) can be treated conservatively. However, more severe injury presenting as haemodynamic instability may require surgical intervention.

Symptoms and Signs. Flank bruising/abrasion, fractured ribs or transverse processes of lumbar spine, haematuria (poor sign: 30% patients with severe trauma have no haematuria and many patients with serious abdominal trauma will have microscopic haematuria with no renal injury).

Investigations. Intravenous urography (IVU), CT.

Management. Depends on whether the patient is stable or unstable. In unstable patients, the choice is immediate surgery. Options include simple suture, partial nephrectomy or nephrectomy. In stable patients following suitable imaging, the majority of injuries can be managed conservatively.

Complications. Urinomas, abscess, bleeding, renal artery thrombosis, hypertension (late).

Other Urinary Tract Injuries

These are shown in Table 4.3.

Limb Trauma

Limb trauma involves injury to: soft tissues, blood vessels (→Ch. 16), nerves, bones (→Ch. 18). It can be life- or limb-threatening.

They can range from minor cuts to extensive deep contaminated wounds and crushed muscle. The types of injuries include:

- Incision – a cleanly cut wound, i.e. surgical
- Avulsion – implies tissue loss
- Degloving – form of laceration in which skin is sheared from the underlying fascia, usually by rotational forces, i.e. car tyre
- Contusion – crushing of the skin to split it
- Haematoma – like a contusion but skin is intact, may devitalise overlying skin if large enough; occasionally they need to be evacuated.
- Abrasion – loss of superficial epithelium caused by friction
- Laceration – tearing of skin, the skin is stretched to its mechanical breaking point.

TABLE 4.3

URINARY TRACT INJURIES AND THEIR MANAGEMENT

Site	Mechanism of Injury	Symptom and Signs	Investigations	Management	Complications
Ureter	Devascularization, deceleration and ureteric avulsion (usually at the pelvi-ureteric junction (PUJ) and more common in children), penetrating trauma (usually affects the upper ureter) and iatrogenic injury	Haematuria is uncommon. If missed may present with ileus, ↑ urea, urinoma, sepsis or urine in an abdominal drain	IVU	Unstable – ureter can be left alone, stented or ligated and repaired later ± percutaneous nephrostomy. Stable patients – depends on the site of injury. PUJ to pelvic brim perform an end-to-end ureteroureterostomy. Below the pelvic brim perform a ureteroneocystostomy. A ureteric stent should be used with all repairs	Stricture, anastomotic leak, urinoma
Bladder	Usually blunt trauma; they may be intraperitoneal (30%) (blunt trauma and full bladder) or extraperitoneal (70%) (pelvic fractures)	Inability to void, haematuria, suprapubic pain, raised urea and creatinine and low sodium (with intraperitoneal injuries)	USS, CT, retrograde cystography	Extraperitoneal – urethral or suprapubic catheter drainage for 2 weeks and then a check cystogram for leaks. Intraperitoneal – repaired and drained with a urethral and/or suprapubic catheter and a check cystogram performed in 2 weeks.	Fistula, abscess and urinary ascites (if undiagnosed)
Urethra	Posterior (membranous) or anterior (bulbar); the majority are due to blunt trauma. Posterior injuries occur above the urogenital diaphragm and are associated with pelvic fractures. Anterior urethral injuries are associated with a 'straddle' type injury	Blood at the urethral meatus; unable to void; high riding prostate on PR (posterior injury); sleeve haematoma of penis (if Buck's fascia intact); butterfly haematoma (if Buck's fascia is torn but Colles' fascia is intact)	Retrograde urethrogram	• Anterior – suprapubic catheter and leave for 2 weeks. If no extravasation at urethrogram, catheter removed; if extravasation, will need end-to-end urethroplasty at approximately 6 weeks. • Posterior – The initial options include suprapubic catheter or urethral re-alignment over a catheter. Following suprapubic catheter, a urethrogram is performed after 2 weeks; around 30% will be able to have the catheter removed. If obstruction is demonstrated, the patient will require a urethroplasty (stretch of the urethra). • Penetrating – immediate surgery, repair and placement of a suprapubic catheter.	Stricture, impotence, incontinence, fistula and abscess

General principles of management:

1. Initial management is by ATLS protocols until immediate life-threatening injuries have been ruled out.
2. The injured limb should be examined for vascular compromise, nerve or tendon damage.
3. The patient should be taken to theatre and have thorough debridement of devitalised or necrotic tissue, cleansing and irrigation, and removal of any foreign bodies (X-rays in two planes may be needed to locate some foreign bodies).
4. If the wound is clean and <6–12h old, primary closure can be undertaken. If the wound is >12h old or grossly contaminated, delayed primary closure should be performed. After 3–4 days if there is no oedema, erythema or pus, the wound can be closed.
5. Antibiotics should be used in contaminated wounds or where dead tissue has been excised.
6. The tetanus status of the patient should be assessed. Some may require a booster dose. In cases of heavy contamination, i.e. farming injuries, they may require human antitetanus immunoglobulin.
7. Larger wounds that cannot be closed primarily may need plastic surgical intervention or regular dressings to heal by secondary intention.

Vascular Trauma

(→Ch. 16)

Skeletal Trauma

(→Ch. 18)

Nerve Injuries

Injuries to nerves can occur due to penetrating trauma or as a result of blunt injuries. Nerve injuries can be classified as follows:

Neuropraxia. A condition of transient physiological block without degeneration. There is continuity of the axons, and the myelin sheaths remain intact. Function returns spontaneously in about 6 weeks.

Axonotmesis. Usually, the result of compression or traction injuries causing disruption of the axons with intact myelin sheaths. The distal axons show degeneration, but since the myelin sheaths are intact, return of function can be anticipated. The axons regenerate at the rate of about 1mm/day. Return of function can be anticipated but may take many months.

Neurotmesis. This is division of the nerve in whole or in part which occurs after incised or lacerated wounds, or may be a complication of a fracture. There is complete disruption of both the axon and the myelin sheath. Surgical repair is required. Residual neurological deficit is likely, and neuroma may occur.

Symptoms and Signs. These depend upon the site of injury to the nerve.

- **Upper trunk lesion of brachial plexus (Erb–Duchenne palsy)** – injured by falls where the head is pulled away from the shoulder on the same side. Causes traction injury to C5–C6 roots. Leads to paralysis of a range of muscles that leads to the classical 'waiters tip' position.
- **Lower trunk lesion of brachial plexus (Klumpke's palsy)** – upward traction of the arm, i.e. fall and grab to save themselves. Damages T1, leads to paralysis of

intrinsic muscles of the hand causing a 'claw' deformity and an area of numbness on the inner forearm.

- **Long thoracic nerve** – can be damaged by blows to the posterior triangle of the neck. Leads to paralysis of serratus anterior and difficulty raising the arm above the head, also causes the classic 'winged scapula' deformity.
- **Axillary nerve** – damaged in fractures of the surgical neck of the humerus and anterior dislocations of the shoulder. Leads to loss of abduction (deltoid) and 'badge' patch loss of sensation over the shoulder.
- **Radial nerve** – damage to the radial nerve can occur at a variety of sites:
  - **Axilla:** secondary to fracture/dislocations of the proximal humerus. The patient will be unable to extend the elbow, wrist (wristdrop) or fingers. There is a variable area of sensory loss of the lateral aspect of the dorsum of the hand.
  - **Spiral groove:** secondary to midshaft fractures of the humerus. The triceps are preserved, but the patient cannot flex the wrist (wristdrop) or fingers.
  - **Radial head:** fractures of the proximal radius and dislocations of the radial head lead to damage to the deep branch of the radial nerve. Supinator and extensor carpi radialis longus are unaffected and allow wrist extension.
  - **Wrist:** penetrating trauma at the wrist leads to damage to the superficial nerve and an area of sensory loss over the lateral aspect of the dorsum of the hand.
- **Ulnar nerve** – damage to the ulnar nerve can occur at the elbow or the wrist:
  - **Elbow:** secondary to fractures of the medial epicondyle or dislocations. Leads to a 'claw hand' deformity and loss of sensation in the medial one and a half fingers.
  - **Wrist:** penetrating trauma is the commonest cause. Results in a similar lesion but with a greater degree of clawing.
- **Median nerve** – damage to the median nerve can occur at the elbow or wrist:
  - **Elbow:** secondary to supracondylar fractures of the humerus, leads to loss of forearm pronation, weakness of wrist flexion and loss of sensation on the lateral palm and the radial three and a half digits.
  - **Wrist:** usually as a result of penetrating trauma, the thenar muscles are paralysed and opposition of the thumb is impossible. Sensory loss is as above.
- **Femoral nerve** – injury is rare, but may be damaged by penetrating groin wounds. The patient cannot extend the knee and there is sensory loss over the anteromedial aspect of the thigh, the medial side of the lower leg and the medial border of the foot as far as the ball of the big toe.
- **Sciatic nerve** – rare to have a complete injury; it may be damaged by penetrating wound fractures of the pelvis and dislocations of the hip. It leads to loss of movement in all muscles below the knee and in the foot: the patient will have 'foot drop'. Sensation is lost below the knee apart from that supplied by the femoral nerve.
- **Common peroneal (fibular) nerve** – injured relatively commonly, particularly by fractures of the neck of the fibula. Leads to foot drop and a loss of sensation to the dorsum of the foot and lower lateral leg.
- **Tibial nerve** – rarely injured due to its deep location. Penetrating trauma may lead to division and results in loss of plantar flexion and loss of sensation over the sole of the foot.
- **Obturator nerve** – occasionally injured by penetrating wounds or with anterior dislocation of the hip. Leads to loss of adductors and a small area of sensory loss over the medial thigh.

Investigations. Clinical. Nerve conduction.

Management

- Peripheral nerve injuries are frequently associated with limb trauma.
- A thorough inspection and examination of the limb should be carried out to establish the presence of a nerve lesion before any treatment is undertaken. This is important for medicolegal reasons.
- Nerve injuries associated with closed trauma do not usually require exploration. Physiotherapy will be needed to prevent contractures and muscle wasting while nerve recovery occurs.
- Penetrating injuries should be explored and nerve repair undertaken. Immediate surgical repair should be undertaken for digital nerves in clean wounds involving sharp lacerations. In contaminated wounds, repair may be delayed. It is wise to mark the nerve at the time of initial exploration with a suture to facilitate later identification. In extensive wounds with contusion and extensive tissue damage, e.g. GSW, nerve grafting may be necessary.

Chapter 5

Preoperative and Postoperative Care

Katherine I. Bridge

CHAPTER OUTLINE

The care of a surgical patient is not limited to their operation alone. Excellent preoperative and postoperative care is vital in achieving the highest level of success of any surgical procedure.

PREOPERATIVE PREPARATION

The purpose of preoperative evaluation is to identify the problems that may increase the operative risk and predispose to postoperative problems. Preoperative evaluation should begin as soon as you first meet a patient, whether that be in the outpatient clinic or in the emergency department.

HINTS AND TIPS

For planned elective surgery, preoperative assessment usually takes place in a preassessment clinic. This may occur at a variety of times after the patient's first visit to the outpatient clinic. A full history and examination should be carried out, with particular emphasis on any changes that may have occurred since the outpatient visit, e.g. has the lump become bigger/smaller, has there been a new diagnosis of a significant comorbidity? If so, a senior colleague should be informed before an operation date is confirmed.

Assessment

1. *Full history*: present illness, past illnesses, bleeding tendencies, medication, allergies
2. *Examination*: directed not only at the presenting complaint but also including a thorough examination of all systems, especially the cardiovascular and respiratory
3. *Laboratory tests*: Haemoglobin (Hb), FBC and U&E for all but the most minor surgery

4. *Radiographs*: Chest X-ray (CXR) should be obtained in all patients with cancer and cardiac, respiratory and renal disease. A routine preoperative CXR is unnecessary in young patients unless there are abnormalities on auscultation.
5. *ECG*: obtain in all patients over the age of 40 and in those with a history of cardiac, respiratory or renal disease.

Principles of Preoperative Preparation

1. Correct any abnormalities that affect surgical risk.
2. Obtain informed consent. Explain all forms of possible treatment available for the condition. Explain the likely outcome without surgery. Explain the nature of the operation and the risks. Obtain the signature of the patient, parent or legal guardian. There is a special consent form for Jehovah's Witnesses.
3. Details of preparation:
    a. Nil by mouth for 4–6 h preoperatively
    b. i.v. fluids
    c. NG aspiration
    d. Bowel preparation
    e. Medication planning, e.g. steroids, insulin, antihypertensives
4. Laboratory investigations, e.g. blood sugar in diabetes, K^+ in renal failure
5. Crossmatch of blood if major operation with expected blood loss
6. Physiotherapy – breathing exercises
7. Deep vein thrombosis (DVT) prophylaxis, e.g. graded compression stockings (TED), subcutaneous low-molecular-weight heparin, e.g. Clexane
8. Anaesthetic premedication
9. Methicillin-resistant *Staphylococcus aureus* (MRSA) screening. All patients should be screened for carriage of MRSA prior to admission (for elective cases) or at admission (for emergency cases). If found to carry MRSA on their skin, patients should be 'decolonised' prior to admission using Octenisan (body wash) and Bactroban (nasal spray) for 5 consecutive days. Emergency admissions seen to be at high risk of MRSA infection (this applies to all surgical patients) should receive this therapy from admission (in advance of their screening results).
10. Mark the surgical site.

HINTS AND TIPS

The surgical site should be clearly marked for all 'unilateral' operations, e.g. a right-sided hernia repair, a left-sided hip replacement. The site should be marked with an arrow, drawn in permanent marker, which will be visible after the drapes are applied, but not so large that it interferes with the area through which the incision will be made. Some surgeons also like to mark the intended operation (e.g. L DHS, when a left dynamic hip screw is planned) next to the arrow. Ensure that the patient agrees that the arrow is on the correct side! In some hospitals, a correct side form is also needed for unilateral operations; this should be completed and signed by the person marking the patient, the nurse before the patient leaves the ward, the anaesthetist before the anaesthetic is given, and the surgeon after the operation has taken place.

For some operations, additional marking is required. For example, in elective bowel resections, it is common practice to mark the site of a planned or potential stoma; for varicose vein surgery, the site of all varicosities should be marked with the patient standing prior to any anaesthetic (as they will disappear once the patient lies down!).

POSTOPERATIVE CARE

Monitor the patient's progress at least daily postoperatively and more frequently if indicated. Record in the notes at least daily.

1. *Detailed operation note* including intraoperative drugs; postoperative instructions should accompany the patient to the ward.
2. *Monitoring of vital signs*. Monitor BP, pulse and respiratory rate every 15 min until the patient is stable (usually done in theatre recovery) and thereafter hourly for 24 h. Monitor central venous pressure (CVP) after major surgery in the elderly and those with cardiac disease. Continuous ECG monitoring is advisable in those with cardiac disease or elderly patients undergoing major surgery.
3. *Early mobilisation*. Patients requiring prolonged bed rest should be turned regularly from side to side to avoid pressure sores. Nurse on airbed. Protect sacrum and heels, especially in diabetic patients.
4. *Diet*. NG tubes are used in a number of abdominal operations. However, increasingly, these are taken out at the earliest opportunity to allow the patient to eat. If the patient is at high risk of ileus, they may be retained for 24–48 h. In operations not involving the gastrointestinal (GI) tract, the patient may drink when fully awake after a GA.
5. *Intravenous fluids*. Administer according to requirements – monitored by clinical examination, urine output and CVP.
6. *Intake/output chart*. Monitor closely to avoid dehydration or fluid overload.
7. *Urinary output*. If the patient is catheterised, monitoring is easy. If the urine output falls below 30 mL/h, action is required. If the patient is not catheterised, inform the surgeon if urine has not been passed within 8 h postoperatively.
8. Medication:
    a. Analgesics: the dose, frequency and route of administration should be clearly indicated.
    b. Antibiotics as indicated
    c. Routine medication as indicated; if the patient is 'nil by mouth', essential medication should be given parenterally.
9. Laboratory tests. After major procedures, the Hb, FBC and U&Es should be checked 24 h postoperatively and thereafter according to indications.
10. Radiographs and ECG. Carry out according to indications and not as routine. CXR may be necessary if pyrexia continues after 24 h postoperatively, if there is sputum production or chest signs.

HINTS AND TIPS

Do not underestimate the importance of urine output in the monitoring of a postoperative patient. The kidneys are very sensitive to small changes in physiological condition. Following major surgery, careful monitoring of urine output in a catheterised patient can help you to identify someone who is volume depleted hours before there will be a change in blood pressure or heart rate.

Progress

The following points should be noted:

- General condition, e.g. well, ill, improving, deteriorating; pain
- Vital signs, e.g. pyrexia, tachycardia
- Mobility
- Chest, e.g. clear, reduced air entry, consolidation
- Abdomen, e.g. distended, bowel sounds, tender
- Legs, e.g. DVT
- Wound, e.g. discharge, infection
- Intake/output
- Diet
- Results of any laboratory tests.

CONDITIONS AFFECTING SURGICAL RISK

General Problems in Surgical Patients

Age

Problems occur at the extremes of life. There are limits to cardiac, respiratory and renal reserves in the elderly. Fluid overload is tolerated poorly. Smaller doses of narcotics, sedatives and analgesics are required.

Obesity

This often results in poor wound healing and a higher incidence of respiratory problems. DVT and pulmonary embolism (PE) are more common. Pressure sores can develop. Delay elective surgery until the patient loses weight.

Compromised Host

There is reduced response to trauma and infection, e.g. immunosuppressive drugs or uraemia. Malnutrition, e.g. vitamin deficiencies or liver disease, can also be a factor.

Allergies

Check for these preoperatively. Unsuspected reactions may occur. In severe cases, anaphylactic shock may result. Sensitivity to surgical dressings (e.g. Elastoplast) may occur.

Drugs

Current drugs, e.g. insulin and steroids, should be monitored carefully. Diabetic patients may require conversion to sliding-scale insulin (see below). Patients on steroids may need to continue their normal dose, but with major surgery, have additional steroid cover. Adjust anticoagulant therapy, e.g. conversion from warfarin to heparin over the perioperative period. Clopidogrel is contraindicated with regional anaesthesia (may cause epidural haematoma). Aspirin does not generally pose a problem in general surgical procedures. ACE inhibitors and ARBs should be stopped 24h before surgery to prevent severe and refractive hypotension.

Medical Problems in Surgical Patients

Cardiovascular

In elderly patients, the following are common: angina, cardiac failure, arrhythmias, valvular heart disease, hypertension, cerebrovascular disease, peripheral vascular disease (PVD). It is necessary to obtain a cardiology opinion, optimise medical treatment and assess operative risk. The decision to operate rests with the surgeon and anaesthetist.

Myocardial Infarction and Angina. Unstable angina and recent myocardial infarction (MI) greatly increase the operative risk. Emergency surgery following recent MI has a mortality of 30%. Delay elective surgery for 6 months.

Cardiac Failure. Treat prior to surgery. Stabilise at least 1 month prior to surgery. Digoxin. Diuretic. Check K^+ prior to surgery. Mild CCF well controlled with digoxin and diuretics carries little risk. CCF with dyspnoea on exertion, orthopnoea and PND carry a significant risk.

Arrhythmias. Uncontrolled atrial fibrillation (AF) may cause perioperative CCF. Digitalise adequately preoperatively. Some degrees of heart block require a prophylactic temporary transvenous pacemaker. Check digoxin levels in patients who have bradycardia. Arrhythmias developing during surgery may be due to hypoxia, hypercapnia or high or low K^+.

Valvular Heart Disease. May result in MI, CCF, arrhythmias, embolism or bacterial endocarditis in the perioperative period. Newly discovered murmurs require a cardiology opinion. Elective cases should be deferred until the murmur has been evaluated. Prophylactic antibiotics are important in the perioperative period and for patients with prosthetic valves. Check if patient is on anticoagulants.

Hypertension. Mild hypertension without renal or cardiac complications does not significantly affect surgical risk. Control BP at or below 160/95 mmHg. Defer and investigate elective cases with newly diagnosed hypertension. Check K^+ in patients on diuretics. Severe and poorly controlled hypertension should be adequately controlled prior to surgery.

Cerebrovascular Disease. High risk of intraoperative CVA. Previous history of TIAs or stroke. Carotid bruits. Aspirin may be protective. Avoid intraoperative hypotension.

Peripheral Vascular Disease (PVD). Patients with peripheral ischaemia may develop arterial thrombosis if hypotensive. Take care to avoid pressure sores, which may not heal and lead to the need for amputation. Patients with PVD should not wear TED stockings.

Respiratory Disease

This is a major cause of postoperative morbidity and mortality in the elderly. COPD, asthma and bronchiectasis are precipitating causes. Smoking, obesity, old age, general debility and cardiac disease are contributory. Preoperative investigations include CXR, lung function tests (e.g. FEV_1, peak expiratory flow rate, spirometry), sputum culture, ABG.

Perioperative Management of Respiratory Disease

- Stop smoking, preferably 4 weeks prior to surgery.
- Preoperative chest physiotherapy and breathing exercises
- Drugs, e.g. bronchodilators, nebulised salbutamol, antibiotics
- Anaesthetic – local or spinal if possible
- Analgesia. Avoid narcotic analgesics that may lead to respiratory depression. Consider epidural pain relief.
- Postoperative physiotherapy
- Early mobilisation.

Renal Disease

This should be managed jointly with a nephrologist. Symptoms of renal failure do not usually become apparent until 80–90% of renal function has been lost and there is little renal reserve.

Mild Impairment of Renal Function. Mildly raised urea or creatinine. Refer to a nephrologist and delay elective surgery until a diagnosis has been reached and appropriate treatment instituted. Deterioration of renal function may occur after major surgery, especially if dehydration is allowed to occur. Adequate preoperative rehydration. Monitor CVP. Caution with nephrotoxic drugs, e.g. gentamicin, computerised tomography (CT) contrast.

Grossly Impaired Renal Function (Nondialysis Dependent). Inadequate management may precipitate end-stage renal failure. Problems include fluid overload, dehydration, hyperkalaemia, metabolic acidosis. Chronic anaemia occurs, but patients are well adapted to this. Uraemia is immunosuppressive, and prophylactic antibiotics are required. Uraemia alters platelet function and bleeding may be a problem.

Dialysis-Dependent Renal Failure

Haemodialysis. Dialysis should take place 24 h prior to surgery to allow the effects of heparin to wear off. Check U&Es, creatinine and HCO_3 postdialysis. CXR to exclude pulmonary oedema. Check K^+ postoperatively, as hyperkalaemia may occur following surgery under GA. If possible, delay postoperative dialysis for 24 h in view of risk of bleeding with heparin.

Continuous Ambulatory Peritoneal Dialysis (CAPD). Check U&Es prior to surgery. If abdominal surgery, CAPD may need to be discontinued and patient instituted on haemodialysis via a central line until intra-abdominal healing has occurred.

Hepatic Disease

There is a high incidence of morbidity and mortality with cirrhosis. Predisposing factors are anaemia, electrolyte disturbances, abnormal clotting, malnutrition, abnormal drug metabolism, ascites, portal hypertension. Defective synthesis of clotting factors in the liver and thrombocytopenia due to hypersplenism may result in excessive bleeding. The Child–Pugh score can be used to assess the 'hepatic reserve': the higher the score, the greater the operative risk (measures albumin, bilirubin, prothrombin time and the presence and severity of ascites and encephalopathy).

Care must be taken to assess a past history of jaundice. This may be due to hepatitis, obstructive jaundice or haemolytic disease.

Hepatitis. Hepatitis A in the past carries little risk; hepatitis B and C may be carried permanently. Check HBsAg.

Obstructive Jaundice. There is usually a clear history. Surgery will usually have been necessary to deal with the problem.

Haemolytic Disease. May cause jaundice.

Perioperative Management of Patients With Liver Disease/Obstructive Jaundice

1. Full clinical examination
2. Hb, FBC, U&Es, Cr, LFTs, PT, glucose
3. Correct hypoglycaemia
4. Correct coagulation defect, e.g. vitamin K parenterally, but in severe disease FFP may be required. Platelet transfusion.
5. Avoid saline infusions (risk of hypernatraemia).
6. Avoid hepatotoxic drugs.
7. Avoid drugs metabolised by liver, e.g. opiates.
8. Correct protein deficiency.
9. Antibiotics.

The main postoperative problems are bleeding, infection and poor wound healing.

Haematological Disease

Anaemia. Mild anaemia, e.g. Hb >10 g/dL, imposes little risk. Anaemia may be related to the condition for which surgery is being undertaken, e.g. GI cancer. Hb <10 g/dL should be treated by preoperative iron therapy or transfusion. Unsuspected anaemia noted prior to elective surgery should be investigated and the operation deferred.

Polycythaemia. Hb >18 g/dL. PCV↑. Risks of arterial and venous thrombosis. Venesect prior to surgery. Myelosuppressive drugs may be required.

Bleeding Disorders

Inherited. Haemophilia is treated with cryoprecipitate preoperatively and until the danger of postoperative haemorrhage is over. Von Willebrand's disease is treated with FFP or cryoprecipitate.

Anticoagulant Therapy. Warfarin – the patient may have a history of thromboembolic disease, valvular heart disease or prosthetic heart valves. Anticoagulation may need to be continued during surgery, albeit at a reduced level. The safest procedure is to discontinue warfarin 3–4 days preoperatively and start heparin i.v. This can be more readily adjusted and is more easily reversed (with i.v. protamine sulphate) if bleeding occurs, and has a much shorter half-life (around 30 min) compared with warfarin. If a patient's INR needs to be reduced for urgent operation, they may be given vitamin K (takes 4 h to work), FFP or, in extreme cases, prothrombin complex concentrate (Beriplex or Octaplex), which will reverse the warfarin in under 30 min.

Disseminated Intravascular Coagulation (DIC). Coagulation and fibrinolysis occur simultaneously. Surgically important causes precipitating the condition include Gram-negative septicaemia, acute pancreatitis, malignancy, major surgery, e.g. ruptured aortic aneurysm. Clinical features include extensive bruising, oozing from drip and venepuncture sites, oozing from the wound, tracheostomy or bowel that occurs in a severely ill patient. Diagnosis is confirmed by PT (prolonged); PTT (prolonged); thrombocytopenia; decreased fibrinogen level; raised FDPs. Treatment is by FFP, platelets and cryoprecipitate. Heparin i.v. may halt the coagulation element. Aggressive treatment of the underlying disease.

Clotting Disorders

Acquired. Antiphospholipid syndrome (associated with SLE; there is a higher risk of venous and arterial thrombosis. However, unless there is a history of thrombosis, no further intervention is required other than normal DVT prophylaxis). Malignant thrombosis associated with advanced malignancy (all patients are considered high risk for a DVT).

Inherited. These include antithrombin deficiency, protein C and protein S deficiency, factor V Leiden and prothrombin 20210A. These patients will require rigorous DVT prophylaxis, particularly if they have had a previous thrombosis.

Sickle Cell Anaemia. These patients are at increased risk of surgical complications. Homozygote patients have 90–100% HbS. Compared with normal adult haemoglobin (HbA), HbS is a long-chain polymer, and its presence results in distortion of the shape of red blood cells, from smooth, doughnut-shapes into spiky, sickle shapes. They may require transfusion if they are anaemic, or to decrease the amount of HbS. Heterozygote patients or those with the sickle cell trait have 20–40% HbS and are generally asymptomatic. Surgery and anaesthesia may lead to dehydration, hypoxia and vascular stasis. These may then lead to a sickle cell crisis with pain and ischaemia (even in trait patients). This can be avoided by adequate hydration, supplemental oxygen and avoiding blood stasis (e.g. pneumatic compression stockings and avoidance of the use of tourniquets).

Endocrine Disease

DIABETES. This poses numerous risks and affects many systems. Complications include:

- Vasculopathy: heart – increased risk of MI; PVD – risk of lower limb ischaemia with ulcers and gangrene; risk of stroke
- Nephropathy – risk of CRF
- Neuropathy – peripheral neuropathy with risk of pressure ulcers on heels and autonomic neuropathy with risk of cardiac arrest and gastric stasis with aspiration
- Retinopathy leading to blindness – problems with management of blind patient in unfamiliar surroundings; anticoagulation, if needed, may make retinal haemorrhage worse
- Increased incidence of infection.

The principles of management of diabetes in the perioperative period depend on whether patients are insulin dependent, on oral hypoglycaemics or controlled by diet.

Insulin Dependent

1. Admit 2 days preoperatively: CXR, ECG, FBC, U&Es, glucose, glycosylated Hb (HBA1c).
2. Establish good diabetic control (glucose 4–10mmol/L).
3. First on morning list. Check glucose.
4. Dextrose/insulin/K^+ infusion
5. Check glucose intraoperatively and U&Es postoperatively.
6. Monitor glucose regularly in early postoperative period.
7. Continue infusion until full oral diet is established and then reinstitute normal insulin regimen.

HINTS AND TIPS

All hospitals should have a standard proforma for perioperative insulin administration for insulin-dependent diabetic patients. These will provide a comprehensive guide as to how to convert a subcutaneous insulin regimen into an i.v. regimen suitable for the perioperative period. Diabetes specialist nurses will be available to see all patients requiring insulin in hospital; if in doubt, ask! Accurate control of blood sugars in the perioperative period will reduce the risk of complications and allow for a smoother transition back to the patients' normal treatment once oral diet can be resumed.

Oral Hypoglycaemics

1. Review control.
2. Major surgery: convert to insulin/glucose/K^+ infusion as above.
3. Minor surgery: omit oral hypoglycaemic agent. Check blood sugar. If greater than 13mmol/L, give small dose of subcutaneous insulin.

Diabetic Patients Controlled by Diet Alone

1. Review control.
2. If preoperative control is adequate, no other measure required other than routine check of blood sugar pre- and postoperatively.

Thyroid Disease.

Hypothyroidism. Patients should be euthyroid prior to elective surgery. Emergency surgery in a patient who is clinically hypothyroid presents a very high risk. Patients are at risk from MI, hypotension, hypothermia, hypoglycaemia and hyponatraemia (may cause convulsions) and coma (hypothyroid coma has a 50% mortality).

Hyperthyroidism. Patients should be euthyroid prior to elective surgery (→Ch. 12). Hyperthyroidism is associated with arrhythmias and hypertension. A thyroid crisis is associated with oversecretion and may be triggered by infection. This presents as hyperthermia, arrhythmias, cardiorespiratory failure and coma.

Adrenal Disease.

Adrenocortical Insufficiency. This may be due to destruction of the adrenal gland by autoimmune disease, tumour, infection, infarction or the sudden withdrawal of steroid therapy. It should be considered in all patients with postoperative hypotension that is refractory to fluid replacement or inotropes with no obvious cause. Patients taking steroids, or who have taken steroids in the last 9 months, should have supplemental steroid cover. A guide to additional hydrocortisone cover is 25mg i.v. hydrocortisone at induction for minor surgery; 25mg i.v. hydrocortisone at induction, followed by 100mg in the postoperative period for moderate surgery; and 100mg hydrocortisone on induction followed by 100mg 6-hourly for 48h or until blood pressure is stable, in major surgery.

Cushing's Syndrome. Patients have excess levels of glucocorticoids and are at risk of hypertension, hypokalaemia, hypernatraemia and diabetes. May be corrected by metyrapone, which inhibits steroid synthesis. These patients are often obese, making surgery more challenging with poor wound healing and increased risk of respiratory complications.

AMERICAN SOCIETY OF ANESTHESIOLOGISTS' CLASSIFICATION OF PHYSICAL STATUS (ASA GRADING)

When an operation is planned, and there are problems concerning the patient's fitness for anaesthetic, the anaesthetist should be involved as soon as possible. The ASA has produced a grading system that attempts to quantify the risks of anaesthetising patients with various clinical conditions.

The ASA grading system for quantifying anaesthetic risk is as follows:

I. A healthy patient with no systemic disease process, e.g. a fit patient with an inguinal hernia.
II. A patient with mild to moderate systemic disease process caused either by the condition to be treated surgically or by other pathological process which does not limit the patient's activity in any way, e.g. mild diabetic, treated hypertensive.
III. A patient with a severe systemic disturbance from any cause and which imposes a definite functional limitation on the patient, e.g. severely limiting organic heart disease, severe diabetes with vascular complications, severe COPD.
IV. A patient with severe systemic disease that is a constant threat to life, e.g. severe unstable angina, advanced liver failure.
V. A moribund patient who is unlikely to survive 24h with or without surgery, e.g. ruptured aortic aneurysm in a patient with severe COPD.

POSTOPERATIVE COMPLICATIONS

All operations carry a risk of complications (a classification is shown in Table 5.1). These should be explained to patients as part of the consent process. Complications may be divided into:

- General complications of any operation, e.g. infection, bleeding, scar; and those associated with the general anaesthetic, e.g. MI, stroke

TABLE 5.1

POSTOPERATIVE COMPLICATIONS

Haemorrhage	Early postoperative Secondary haemorrhage
Wound	Infection Bleeding Haematoma Seroma Suture sinus Breakdown: • Burst abdomen • Incisional hernia • Anastomotic breakdown – peritonitis, abscess, fistula
Cardiovascular	Cardiac arrest MI Pulmonary oedema Arrhythmias DVT
Lung	Atelectasis Aspiration Pneumonia PE Pulmonary oedema Pneumothorax ARDS
Cerebral	Confusion: • Sepsis • Electrolyte/glucose • Hypoxia • Alcohol withdrawal Stroke
Urinary	Acute retention UTI Acute renal failure
Gastrointestinal	Paralytic ileus Mechanical obstruction Acute gastric dilatation Constipation
Other	Pressure sores

- Specific complications of individual operations
- Timing of complication, e.g. immediate, early or late.

Specific complications and timing of complications are discussed in relation to specific operations and conditions in the various chapters in this book.

Haemorrhage

Early Postoperative

Inadequate haemostasis, unrecognised damage to blood vessels, defective vascular anastomosis, slipped ligature, massive blood transfusion without adequate clotting factors, use of intraoperative anticoagulants, e.g. in vascular surgery. Treatment depends on cause. Check clotting screen. Surgical re-exploration is usually required.

Secondary Haemorrhage

Several days postoperatively. Related to infection, which erodes vessels. Treatment of the infection and appropriate surgery to deal with the bleeding.

Wound Problems

Infection

Incidence varies according to type of surgery and potential for contamination (→Ch. 6). Factors leading to increased risk of wound infection include: haematoma, poor nutritional state, diabetes mellitus, reduced immunity, nasal carriage of *Staphylococcus aureus*.

Symptoms and Signs. Painful red incision with discharge. General malaise. Examination reveals pyrexia and a red, hot, tender wound. A purulent discharge may be apparent.

Treatment

1. If pus is present, it should be evacuated.
2. Culture and sensitivity of pus (take samples prior to commencing any antibiotic treatment)
3. Appropriate antibiotic if cellulitis present or compromised patient, e.g. diabetic, taking steroids
4. If cavity present, pack with alginate dressings, e.g. Sorbsan. A larger cavity may require a period of vacuum assisted closure (VAC).

Wound Breakdown

Factors which delay wound healing include: old age, obesity, malnutrition, poor vascularity, sepsis, carcinoma, jaundice, uraemia, steroids, haematomas, raised intra-abdominal pressure and previous radiotherapy.

Burst Abdomen

This is a sudden bursting of the wound to reveal the bowel. This is often preceded by discharge of a salmon pink fluid (pink sign). Usual cause is inadequate suturing of abdominal wall. Coughing, straining at stool may be contributory. Cover the abdominal contents with sterile saline-soaked packs. Return the patient to theatre and repair with large bites of whole thickness of the abdominal wall using deep tension sutures. This complication has a mortality of around 20%.

Incisional Hernia

The overall incidence is about 10%. In addition to factors delaying wound healing, causes include poor suture technique, raised intra-abdominal pressure (e.g. paralytic ileus), coughing, straining (e.g. constipation), prostatism. Rarely a broken suture is responsible. These herniae often have a wide neck, and strangulation is rare.

Treatment. If the patient is unfit, a surgical belt may be worn. If the patient is fit, surgical repair should be carried out.

Anastomotic Breakdown

This is a major cause of postoperative morbidity and mortality after bowel surgery.

CAUSES. These include:

- Poor surgical technique
- Ischaemia at the anastomosis
- Perioperative sepsis
- Distal obstruction
- Residual inflammatory disease, e.g. Crohn's or malignant disease
- General condition, e.g. uraemia, jaundice, malnutrition, steroids.

Anastomotic breakdown may result in generalised peritonitis, paracolic abscess, abscesses between loops of bowel or fistula formation. However, presentation can be surprisingly subtle with mild pyrexia, persistent tachycardia and general failure to progress as the only signs of anastomotic leak (→ Ch 15).

Haematoma

This is a localised collection of blood beneath the wound. May be an obvious tender mass with surrounding bruising. Treatment is by aspiration percutaneously or may require opening of the wound and clot evacuation.

Seroma

This is a localised collection of serous fluid. Often occurs where skin flaps have been raised, e.g. chest wall in mastectomy, or where lymphatics have been divided, e.g. groin or axilla. Examination reveals a nontender fluctuant mass. Small areas may be left and may absorb spontaneously or may be needled percutaneously. Large ones may need formal drainage.

Stitch Sinus

Sutures may act as nidus of infection, especially at the knot. This is becoming less common since absorbable sutures and monofilament nylons replaced silk. Often the suture will extrude through the sinus spontaneously and the sinus will then heal. Occasionally, exploration and removal of the suture are required.

Cardiovascular Problems

Cardiac arrest following surgery is usually due to an underlying cardiac condition aggravated by a precipitating cause, e.g. hypoxia, shock, MI, anaesthetic overdose, hyperkalaemia, hypokalaemia or drug reactions. Cardiac arrest may follow respiratory arrest, e.g. following an obstructed airway (laryngeal oedema or tongue blocking airway) or inhalation of vomit. DVT may follow prolonged bed rest.

Lung Problems

Lung complications are a common postoperative problem. They include atelectasis, aspiration, pneumonia, PE, pulmonary oedema, pneumothorax and acute respiratory distress syndrome (ARDS).

Atelectasis

Mucus is retained in the bronchial tree, blocking the smaller bronchi and resulting in absorption of alveolar air with collapse of an area of lung. Infection may then occur and progress to pneumonia. Minor degrees are common. Smoking and COPD are predisposing factors. Anaesthesia may increase bronchial secretions and depress ciliary action. Postoperative abdominal pain inhibits coughing and allows secretions to accumulate. To prevent atelectasis, pain relief following abdominal surgery should be sufficient to allow a patient to take deep breaths in and out.

Symptoms and Signs. Minor atelectasis may be accompanied by mild pyrexia alone; greater degrees are accompanied by dyspnoea, tachypnoea, rapid pulse and elevated temperature. Major degrees may be accompanied by cyanosis and respiratory collapse. The signs include widespread rales, reduced air entry and dullness to percussion.

Diagnosis. Clinical:

- CXR
- ABG
- Sputum culture.

Treatment. Minor degrees require only chest physiotherapy. Adequate pain relief facilitates mobility and physiotherapy. Nebulised bronchodilators. More severe degrees may require bronchoscopy to remove mucous plugs. The most severe case may require intubation and ventilation.

Aspiration

Aspiration pneumonitis following inhalation of acidic gastric contents is known as Mendelson's syndrome. This tends to affect the right lung more than the left, as the right bronchus is wider and more in line with the trachea. Aspiration may occur during induction, or at the termination, of anaesthesia. It may also occur in patients with bowel obstruction or paralytic ileus who vomit in the early postoperative period. Prevention includes preoperative 'nil by mouth' in elective cases, NG suction in the emergency case and cricoid compression in 'crash' induction. If aspiration occurs, suction, intubation and saline lavage should be carried out. Steroids may help. Antibiotics will prevent super-added infection. Oxygen by mask.

Pneumonia

Predisposing factors include smoking, atelectasis, COPD, aspiration, debilitated patients. A classic cause of pyrexia in a patient who is >48h postoperation.

Symptoms and Signs. Cough, respiratory distress, sputum. Signs include fever, tachypnoea, tachycardia, cyanosis, consolidation and rales.

Diagnosis

- Sputum culture
- CXR
- ABG.

Treatment. Chest physiotherapy. Antibiotics, e.g. amoxicillin or co-amoxiclav until results of culture are known. Oxygen by mask. If no improvement with basic measures, the patient may need to be moved to a critical care facility for positive airway pressure ventilation (e.g. CPAP) or intubation and ventilation.

Pulmonary Oedema

Usually elderly patient with compromised cardiac function or young patient with history of cardiac or renal disease.

Symptoms and Signs. Tachypnoea, tachycardia, orthopnoea, raised JVP, pink frothy sputum, widespread crepitations.

Diagnosis

- CXR
- Raised JVP.

Treatment. Stop i.v. fluids. Sit patient upright. Oxygen by face mask. Give i.v. furosemide. Small doses of opiates. Glyceryl trinitrate (GTN)/i.v. infusion of nitrates.

Pulmonary Embolus (PE)

Complication of silent or overt DVT. Passage of a clot from pelvic or leg veins into the pulmonary artery. Major PE with overt DVT is usually obvious clinically. In some cases, diagnosis relies on a high index of clinical suspicion. Postoperative patients should be examined for any sign of DVT as part of their daily review.

Symptoms and Signs. Usually 4–10 days postoperatively. Sudden dyspnoea and collapse. Hypotension. Pleuritic chest pain. Haemoptysis. Pleural rub.

Diagnosis

- CXR: wedge-shaped collapse
- ECG: right heart strain, S1, Q3, T3 pattern
- ABG: hypoxia
- V/Q scan: mismatch of ventilation/perfusion areas, i.e. ventilation normal but perfusion deficient (rarely performed now)
- CTPA – most commonly used test
- Pulmonary angiography is most accurate – used prior to surgery or thrombolysis.

Treatment

- *Patients without shock.* They may be treated by i.v. heparin sufficient to maintain the APTT at 2.5×normal. Start warfarin after 2 days of heparin and continue for 6–9 months. With recurrent pulmonary emboli it should be continued for life.
- *Profound shock.* Inotropic support. Urgent pulmonary angiography. Thrombolytic therapy or pulmonary embolectomy.
- *Recurrent pulmonary embolus.* This should be treated by insertion of a filter, e.g. Greenfield filter percutaneously via the venous route into the IVC.

Pneumothorax

Rare complication of surgery. Rupture of subpleural bulla or complication of insertion of central line perioperatively.

Symptoms and Signs. Respiratory distress. Reduced breath sounds and hyperresonance to percussion of affected side.

Treatment

- Small: treat expectantly
- Large: chest drain.

ARDS (Shock Lung)

This is acute respiratory failure with tachypnoea, hypoxia, decreased lung compliance and diffuse pulmonary infiltrates on CXR. The exact aetiology is unknown, but there

TABLE 5.2
CAUSES OF ACUTE RESPIRATORY DISTRESS SYNDROME

Infection	Septicaemia
Inhalation	Smoke, vomit, water, high O_2 concentrations, chlorine, ammonia
Embolism	Fat, amniotic fluid, air
Cerebral	Head injury, cerebral haemorrhage
Drugs	Opiates, barbiturates
Others	Pancreatitis, DIC, blood transfusion, cardiopulmonary bypass, major trauma with shock

is interference with the pulmonary epithelial/endothelial cell interface with increased interstitial oedema, vascular congestion and ultimately fibrosis (Table 5.2).

Symptoms and Signs. Present a few days after diagnosis of a serious underlying condition. Breathlessness; deterioration in clinical condition.

Investigations

- CXR shows whiteout with sparing of costophrenic angles
- ABG: hypoxia resistant to oxygen administration
- May be difficult to distinguish from pulmonary oedema in early stages but latter usually shows cardiomegaly on CXR and response to diuretics.

Treatment

1. Treat the underlying disease, e.g. septicaemia.
2. Treat the pulmonary problem:
   a. Mechanical ventilation to maintain PaO_2. PEEP may be necessary.
   b. Monitor fluid balance. CVP to monitor right atrial pressure. Left atrial pressure is monitored as pulmonary wedge pressure with a Swan–Ganz catheter.
   c. Careful monitoring for development of secondary lung infection. Administration of appropriate antibiotics.
   d. Renal failure is a common complication. Early administration of dopamine in renal doses may be appropriate.

The mortality rate for ARDS is 70–90%.

Cerebral Problems

Confusion

Confusion postoperatively is not uncommon, especially at night in the elderly. However, there may be an underlying cause, e.g. sepsis, hypoxia, alcohol withdrawal, electrolyte or glucose imbalance, cerebral bleed, postoperative pancreatitis, opiate analgesia.

Investigations

- Hb
- FBC
- U&Es
- Glucose
- Amylase
- ABGs

- Blood culture
- Urine analysis
- Sputum culture
- CXR
- Brain scan.

Treatment

- Correct electrolyte or glucose disturbance.
- Correct hypoxia – 35% oxygen by mask or nasal cannula.
- Investigate and treat any sepsis.
- Tranquillisers may be required, e.g. chlorpromazine or haloperidol, but these should be used only when the patient's confusion is putting themselves or others at risk.
- For acute alcohol withdrawal, i.v. clomethiazole and parenteral vitamin B may be used. For patients who are known to drink to excess, a reducing dose of chlordiazepoxide should be initiated on admission to prevent acute symptoms.

Stroke

May occur in the elderly postoperatively. Avoid intraoperative hypotension in patients with TIAs or carotid bruits. In some centres, preoperative carotid duplex with subsequent asymptomatic carotid endarterectomy prior to major surgery (e.g. cardiac surgery) is becoming routine practice, to reduce the overall risk of stroke.

Urinary Tract Problems

Acute Retention

Common postoperatively, especially in elderly males.

Symptoms and Signs. Usually suprapubic discomfort, although this may not be apparent if the patient has been given analgesia postoperatively. Usually, nurse reports that patient has not passed urine for several hours postoperatively. Examination reveals a palpable bladder dull to percussion. If the patient has no desire to micturate and the bladder is not palpable, oliguria must be considered and corrected.

Treatment. Conservative. Ensure adequate analgesics. Stand patient up. If no benefit and the patient is fit enough, take to bathroom and leave tap running to encourage micturition. If conservative measures fail, pass a urinary catheter.

Urinary Tract Infection (UTI)

This is common, especially in females. Catheterisation may predispose.

Symptoms and Signs. Dysuria/frequency/dribbling/smelly urine. May be found on investigation of undiagnosed pyrexia postoperatively.

Investigations. MSSU.

Treatment. Appropriate antibiotic.

Acute Renal Failure (ARF)

Oliguria is passage of <30 mL of urine per hour. Anuria is failure to pass any urine.

Causes

Prerenal. Reduced cardiac output, shock, e.g. hypovolaemic, cardiogenic, septic.

Renal. Pre-existing renal disease, e.g. diabetes, glomerulonephritis. Nephrotoxic drugs, e.g. gentamicin. Myoglobinuria in crush syndrome. Haemoglobinuria with haemolysis.

Postrenal. Obstruction, e.g. damage to ureters, benign prostatic hypertrophy.

Treatment of Anuria/Oliguria

1. Check that the catheter is patent. If patient not catheterised, pass catheter.
2. Check BP to exclude hypotension.
3. Fluid challenge, e.g. 1 L normal saline over 1 h. Give sufficient fluid to restore CVP. If elderly patient, a fluid challenge is best done with CVP monitoring.
4. If no improvement in urine output after adequate fluid administration and the BP is low, the patient may require transfer to a critical care/high-dependency facility for inotropic support.
5. Check ABG (for acidosis), K^+ and HCO_3^-. Serum urea and creatinine. ECG (signs of hyperkalaemia)
6. Stop any nephrotoxic drugs.
7. Contact renal physician and manage jointly. In the presence of hyperkalaemia and metabolic acidosis, dialysis will be required until a diuresis ensues. Fluid overload may be treated with CVVH.
8. Furosemide is generally not used to increase a patient's urine output unless they are in CCF.

HINTS AND TIPS

Postoperatively, the vast majority (55–90%) of cases of oliguria/anuria will be prerenal. A quick bladder scan done on the ward can identify a patient in retention and hint towards a blocked catheter (or the need for a catheter!). Once obstruction has been ruled out, prompt and adequate fluid resuscitation is vital, and early review by renal physicians essential if the situation does not improve.

Gastrointestinal Problems

Paralytic Ileus

This is the cessation of GI motility. Aetiological factors include fractures of the spine and pelvis, retroperitoneal haemorrhage, peritonitis, hypokalaemia, drugs, e.g. ganglion blockers and anticholinergic agents, abdominal surgery, immobilisation. Atony of the bowel may be expected for 24–48 h postoperatively. Paralytic ileus continuing after 48 h may have an underlying cause.

Symptoms and Signs. Abdominal distension, vomiting, constipation. Tense tympanitic abdomen. Absent bowel sounds (Table 5.3).

Investigations. Abdominal X-ray (AXR): gaseous distension with fluid levels throughout the large and small bowel.

TABLE 5.3

FACTORS DISTINGUISHING PARALYTIC ILEUS AND MECHANICAL OBSTRUCTION

	Ileus	Obstruction
Time	Usually settles in 3–4 days	May persist longer
Bowel sounds	Absent	High-pitched and tinkling
Pain	Painless	Colicky abdominal pain
AXR	General gaseous dilatation of small and large bowel	Localised small bowel distension with absent gas in colon and rectum

Treatment

1. Pass NG tube, leave on free-drainage and aspirate hourly.
2. Ensure adequate hydration.
3. Correct any potassium imbalance.
4. Paralytic ileus rarely lasts for more than 4 days.
5. If symptoms persist, look for continuing cause and exclude mechanical obstruction with an abdominal CT.

Mechanical Obstruction

Early (Within 2 Weeks of Surgery). May be due to *fibrinous* adhesions. Obstruction may settle with i.v. fluids and NG suction or it may progress and require laparotomy.

Late (After 2 Weeks). May be due to obstruction by adhesions – fibrous bands arising as part of peritoneal healing. Symptoms may settle with i.v. fluids and NG suction ('drip and suck'). If they do not or signs of strangulation appear, laparotomy will be necessary.

Gastric Dilatation

Acute gastric dilatation may occur in the early postoperative period and may be associated with shock. Vomiting with aspiration may occur.

Treatment. NG suction, which may aspirate several litres of brownish/black fluid with altered blood. Fluid and electrolyte losses must be replaced.

Constipation

Uncomfortable for patient. Precipitating factors include starvation, dehydration, inactivity, opiates.

Treatment

1. Check daily if patient has had bowels open. Do not delay treatment.
2. Lactulose should be given as soon as the patient is eating.
3. Glycerine suppositories. PR to exclude faecal impaction.
4. Enemas may be required. With faecal impaction, oil enemas may be necessary.
5. Attention to diet. High-fibre diet or bulking agent.

POSTOPERATIVE PYREXIA

A common problem in the postoperative period is pyrexia. The most likely underlying cause will vary depending on the time from surgery, the type of surgery that the patient has undergone and their clinical presentation. A number of the complications described above may be relevant. Table 5.4 provides a guide as to which complications are more common at different times during the postoperative period. Ultimately, the diagnosis will come by taking careful note of the history and performing a full clinical examination, followed by focused investigations.

TABLE 5.4

CAUSES OF POSTOPERATIVE PYREXIA*

First 24 h	Systemic response to trauma, pre-existing infection
Days 1–3	Atelectasis, chest infection, cannula/line site infection
Days 4–7	Chest infection, wound infection, intra-abdominal sepsis, UTI
Days 7–10	Wound infection, UTI, intra-abdominal, sepsis, DVT/PE

*Drug/transfusion reaction may occur at any time.

HINTS AND TIPS

The following is a recommended routine for the initial assessment of a patient with a postoperative pyrexia:

1. Inspect the wound – infection or haematoma.
2. Inspect cannula/line sites – infected phlebitis.
3. Examine the chest – chest infection, pulmonary collapse, infarct (PE).
4. Examine the abdomen (if postabdominal surgery). Distension, tenderness, mass – peritonitis from an anastomotic leak, intra-abdominal abscess
5. Rectal examination – pelvic abscess
6. Examine the legs – DVT.
7. Send urine for culture – UTI.
8. Send stool for culture – *Clostridium difficile* enterocolitis.

Depending on your findings, institute the investigations detailed under the relevant headings in the section on postoperative complications.

POSTOPERATIVE PAIN RELIEF

Pain must be expected from most surgical procedures but usually subsides gradually over the first few days. Patients respond differently to pain. However, excess pain in the postoperative period may be a symptom of a developing complication.

Methods of Postoperative Pain Control

Full explanation of the operation and postoperative course and an attempt to relieve preoperative anxiety may reduce the severity of postoperative pain.

Oral Analgesia

First-line analgesia for patients who are tolerating diet, usually used for mild to moderate pain, e.g. groin hernia repair or varicose vein surgery. Suitable agents include paracetamol, NSAIDs, nefopam, weak opioids such as codeine and oral morphine (Oramorph).

Parenteral Analgesia

Intermittent Intramuscular Opiates. Commonly used. Usually given p.r.n., 4-hourly. Many patients still complain of pain.

Intravenous Opiates. Given for acute pain. Dose titrated to gain adequate pain relief. Beware respiratory depression in the elderly and patients with renal failure.

Patient-Controlled Analgesia (PCA) Pump. This device allows patients to self-administer a preset dose of analgesic drug by pressing a button connected to a pump. This in turn is connected to an i.v. cannula. There is a preset interval before the infusion will deliver another dose, i.e. the 'lock-out' time. This is a very effective method of pain control but is expensive.

Patient-Controlled Epidural Anaesthesia (PCEA) Pump. This is similar to the above but is administered as an epidural.

Spinal. Local anaesthetic is placed in the intrathecal space. This allows a period of regional anaesthesia for several hours or may be 'topped' up if a catheter is left in situ. Not used for pain relief in the postoperative period.

Epidural. A catheter is placed in the epidural space and local anaesthetic or opioids may be infused. This can be as a continuous infusion or as a patient-controlled pump.

Intercostal Nerve Blocks

These are useful for upper abdominal surgery or in thoracic injuries, e.g. fractured ribs.

Direct Infiltration

Bupivacaine, a long-acting local anaesthetic, can be injected directly into the wound, e.g. for repair of an inguinal hernia. It may be also injected around the nerve supplying the area of the wound, e.g. the ilioinguinal nerve in hernia repair. Infiltration of local anaesthesia may be continuous with catheters placed in between the muscles of the abdominal wall in which the sensory nerves run.

BLOOD TRANSFUSION

Blood transfusion is not without risk. Decision to transfuse blood should have a clear indication, and alternative therapy, e.g. plasma substitutes for hypovolaemia and iron therapy for anaemia, should be considered first. Screening programmes for HIV, hepatitis B and C have made transfusions safer. Unless a patient has severe cardiorespiratory disease (generally need Hb >10g/dL in these patients), there is no change in cardiac output until Hb falls below 7g/dL. In chronic anaemia, even lower levels may be tolerated.

There are numerous different blood types, but the two most common systems are the ABO system and the Rhesus status. ABO is divided into type O (46%), A (42%), B (9%) and AB (3%). Rhesus is divided into positive (85%) and negative (15%). Therefore O Rh positive is the most common and AB Rh negative is the rarest.

Blood Products and Alternatives to Transfusion

Blood products used in clinical practice include:

- *Whole blood*. Rarely used
- *Packed cells*. Used in major haemorrhage or treatment of anaemia. Can be stored at 5°C for approximately 30 days. Increases Hb by 1g/dL per unit transfused.
- *Human albumin* (5% or 20%). Main use is in hypoproteinaemic state, e.g. nephrotic syndrome, ascites in chronic liver disease. Also used as a plasma substitute, e.g. in burns.
- *FFP*. Contains all the clotting factors in plasma. Dose is 10–15mL/kg. Main indications for use include reversal of warfarin, DIC, massive transfusion and liver disease.
- *Cryoprecipitate*. Contains FVIII, FXIII, fibrinogen and von Willebrand's factor. It is pooled from 10–20 adult donors. Used in hypofibrinogenaemia (<1g/dL), massive transfusion, DIC and haemophilia.
- *Platelet concentrates*. Stored at room temperature for 5–7 days. Main indications are for massive transfusions, DIC and thrombocytopaenia with active bleeding or in a thrombocytopaenic patient requiring surgery.

Alternatives to the use of stored blood include:

- *Autologous transfusion*. This includes preoperative autologous donation (blood is donated by the patient prior to surgery for that same patient), acute normovolaemic haemodilution (blood is removed immediately preoperatively; this is replaced with crystalloid) and perioperative red cell salvage (includes blood from drains being re-transfused, e.g. after knee replacements and cell salvage intraoperatively).

- *Pharmacological methods*. These include aprotinin (a serine protease inhibitor that inhibits fibrinolysis and has been shown to reduce blood loss in cardiac surgery), tranexamic acid (inhibits fibrinolysis), desmopressin (increases factor VIII – used in mild haemophilia and von Willebrand's disease) and erythropoietin (can be used to stimulate red blood cell production preoperatively).
- *Blood substitutes*. Largely in the research stage. However, some oxygen-carrying fluids, such as fluorinated organic compounds, have been tested.
- *Plasma substitutes*. Include gelatin solutions (Gelofusine, Haemaccel). They are used to restore circulating volume until blood becomes available.

Clinical Aspects of Blood Transfusion

1. The patient's ABO and Rh groups are established.
2. Each unit of group compatible blood is then crossmatched against the recipient's serum.
3. Minor incompatibilities may occur and require further crossmatching.
4. If blood is required urgently, O negative (universal donor) may be given in an emergency with comparative safety.
5. 'Group and save'. In some operations, transfusion is unlikely but occasionally possible. Blood is taken preoperatively and grouping assessed. The serum is retained in the laboratory, and blood is crossmatched as required.
6. For some operations, blood should be immediately available. Blood is grouped, crossmatched and available on the day of surgery.
7. Mistakes with mismatched transfusions often have serious and occasionally fatal consequences. To avoid mistakes, blood specimens sent to the laboratory must be carefully labelled with the name, date of birth and hospital unit number of the patient.
8. Each unit of blood subsequently transfused must be carefully matched to make sure that the label of the bag of blood corresponds with the name, blood group and hospital number of the patient.

Complications of Blood Transfusion

Acute

Haemolytic Transfusion Reaction. This is secondary to ABO incompatibility and is usually due to human error. Patient may have a temperature, shortness of breath, rigours, loin pain, hypotension and oliguria. Jaundice and haemoglobinuria may occur. If the patient is unconscious, a pyrexia and a drop of BP >10 mmHg should cause concern. Initial management includes ABC, stopping the transfusion, checking the identity of the patient, checking blood group of patient and donor blood group, taking blood for haemolytic screen and clotting. Management involves maintaining a diuresis with fluids and mannitol. ARF may occur and should be treated appropriately. Reaction to other red blood cell antibodies is not as dramatic.

Allergic Reaction. Itching, skin rashes and urticaria may occur. Slow down or discontinue transfusion and administer antihistamine. Rarely anaphylaxis may occur.

Transfusion-Related Acute Lung Injury (TRALI). Similar to ARDS. Due to agglutination of WBCs due to HLA antibodies in the donor plasma (usually occurs in multiparous women).

Nonhaemolytic Febrile Transfusion Reaction (NHFTR). Fever or rigours. Due to prior sensitisation to WBC antigens, e.g. after pregnancy or previous transfusions (possible to get leukocyte depleted blood). Managed by slowing transfusion and giving paracetamol.

Bacterial Sepsis. Uncommon.

Circulatory Overload. Blood should be given slowly in the elderly or those in heart failure. Each unit of blood may be given with a small dose of furosemide.

Hypothermia

Hyperkalaemia

Delayed

Delayed Haemolytic Transfusion Reaction (DHTR). Occurs when a patient has been exposed to red blood cell antigens, e.g. previous transfusion. After 5–10 days an immune response develops and the transfused cells are destroyed. It presents with fever, anaemia, jaundice and haemoglobinuria.

Iron Overload

Graft Versus Host Disease. Rare. Donor lymphocytes engraft into the recipient's marrow. They then recognise the recipient as foreign and cause an immunologic reaction.

Immune Modulation. Increased risk of infection and increased risk of tumour recurrence.

Infections. Rare. All blood is checked for HBV, HCV, HIV and syphilis. Bacterial contamination of blood products can occur.

Post-transfusion Purpura. Rare. Occurs 5–10 days and is due to HLA antibodies in the recipient. Presents with low platelets and bleeding. May be treated with i.v. steroids and immunoglobulins.

Massive Blood Transfusion

This is defined as a transfusion equal to or greater than the whole blood volume in <24h. Specific complications include thrombocytopaenia, decreased coagulation factors, hypothermia, hypocalcaemia due to citrate-binding, hyperkalaemia and acidosis. In major trauma, it has been shown that transfusion of blood, FFP and platelets in a 1:1:1 ratio is associated with improved survival. The majority of hospitals will have a massive transfusion protocol, and requesting this will result in the blood bank providing all of the necessary blood products in the correct ratio for optimum results.

FLUID AND ELECTROLYTE BALANCE

The basic principle of fluid and electrolyte balance is that which is lost must be replaced.

Water loss in a normal individual is approximately 2500mL/day (urine=1–1.5L, faeces=100mL, sweating=600mL and water vapour via breathing=400mL). In the uncomplicated patient, 2.5–3L of fluid replacement is adequate. In the postoperative patient these losses may be much greater. Sources include sweating (10% increase in insensible losses for every 1°C rise in temperature) and GI losses from vomiting, diarrhoea and fistulae. In addition to water replacement, it is important to consider electrolyte replacement, mainly Na^+ and K^+. The loss of Na^+ is around 100mmol/day (mainly from the urine), but 40mmol/day is lost in sweat (therefore it is more in the febrile patient). Some 80mmol/day of K^+ is lost in the urine and a small amount in the faeces (more if diarrhoea). Generally GI losses can be replaced with normal saline. The amount of 'fluid' a patient needs should be based on their size. This can be calculated either from the 4/2/1 (4mL/h for the first 10kg; 2mL/h for the second 10kg and

1 mL/h for every kg thereafter = hourly rate of fluid) or 100/50/20 rule (100 mL/kg for first 10 kg; 50 mL/kg for next 10 kg and 20 mL/kg thereafter = 24 h fluid requirement). In a 70 kg man this is around 2.5 L/day or 110 mL/h. It is also important to replace electrolyte losses. These can be calculated as 1–2 mmol/kg per day for Na^+ and 0.5–1 mmol/kg per day for K^+.

Before understanding the effects that different fluids have on a patient's circulation, it is necessary to understand a few important physiological points:

- In a man weighing 70 kg, the TBW is 42 L.
- Two-thirds or 28 L is intracellular fluid (ICF).
- One-third or 14 L is ECF – two-thirds of this or 10 L is interstitial and one-third or 4 L is plasma.
- A small amount of fluid is termed 'transcellular' and is not exchangeable, e.g. cerebrospinal fluid (CSF), aqueous humour.

Crystalloid and Colloid

Intravenous fluids can be divided into crystalloids and colloids.

Normal Saline. This is 0.9% saline solution with 154 mmol of sodium and chloride. pH5.5. This fluid is isotonic and therefore stays in the ECF (i.e. is distributed over 14 L). Therefore, as the intravascular part is only 3.5 L, only 25–30% of a litre of fluid remains in the intravascular compartment.

Five Percent Dextrose. The added glucose is metabolised (giving 837 kJ/L of energy). This means the fluid is no longer isotonic but hypotonic and thus distributes over the TBW. As plasma only contributes 7–8% of the TBW, only 7–8% of a litre of 5% dextrose remains intravascular.

Dextrose Saline. Contains one-fifth the amount of sodium of normal saline, i.e. 30 mmol/L and 4% dextrose.

Hartmann's Solution. This has a chemical composition closer to plasma. Contains 131 mmol Na^+, 112 mmol Cl^-, 5 mmol K^+, 2 mmol Ca^{2+} and 28 mmol HCO_3^-.

With this in mind, a suitable regimen of postoperative fluids may include:

- 1 L normal saline and 2 L of 5% dextrose with 20 mmol KCl in each of the bags. Each bag is given over 8 h and provides 3 L of fluid, 154 mmol Na^+ and 60 mmol K^+.
- 3 L dextrose saline with 20 mmol KCl in each bag. Each bag is given over 8 h and provides 3 L of fluid, 90 mmol Na^+, 60 mmol K^+. This regimen is better in the first 24 h postoperatively as the adrenal response to surgery/trauma tends to conserve sodium.
- 1 L Hartmann's fluid (no K^+ added) with 2 L of 5% dextrose each with 20 mmol KCl. Each bag is given over 8 h and provides 3 L of fluid, 131 mmol Na^+ and 45 mmol K^+. This is a good regimen after surgery due to lower sodium and lower potassium (K^+ is released with tissue damage during surgery, thus requirements are lower).

Fluid and Electrolyte Depletion

Surgical patients may suffer large losses of fluid and electrolytes as part of the disease process, operation or postoperative complications. In addition to obvious losses, e.g. vomiting and diarrhoea, fluid may be lost into 'new' spaces resulting from the disease process, e.g. the intestine during paralytic ileus, the peritoneum in peritonitis, the retroperitoneum in acute pancreatitis or intracellular shifts in shock. These losses are called 'third space' losses and must be promptly replaced, as the problems they cause are just as important as external losses. These fluids are eventually reabsorbed, and care must be taken that circulatory overload does not occur.

Management of Na^+ and K^+ Imbalance

Hyponatraemia (i.e. Low Na^+). In a surgical patient, this is usually due to water overload and results from administration of inappropriate amounts of 5% dextrose. If the hyponatraemia associated with fluid overload is mild, it is best treated by restricted fluid intake, avoiding the administration of saline and giving furosemide i.v. to force a diuresis. Electrolytes should be checked twice daily. Hyponatraemia is associated with symptoms, e.g. confusion, convulsions, coma, if the Na^+ falls below 120 mmol/L. In hyponatraemia with hypovolaemia, saline should be given.

Hypernatraemia (i.e. High Na^+). This is uncommon in the surgical patient. It may occur during dehydration and in the postoperative period if too much saline is given at a time when aldosterone secretion is high and sodium is being conserved. Rarely it may be caused by Conn's syndrome (→ Ch. 12). If the cause is dehydration (i.e. clinically dry with low CVP and oliguria), the patient will need water replacement, whereas in the postoperative period with normovolaemia, sodium restriction is required.

Hypokalaemia (i.e. Low K^+). Preoperatively, this may be due to diuretic therapy diarrhoea, fistula or excessive mucus loss from a villous adenoma of the rectum. Postoperatively it is usually due to inadequate K^+ replacement. It may occur with pyloric stenosis (with an associated metabolic alkalosis). Symptoms include muscle weakness, cardiac arrhythmias (T wave flattening on ECG) and paralytic ileus. Treatment is by K^+ replacement, but this should not exceed 15 mmol/h, as cardiac arrhythmias may arise with high infusion rates.

Hyperkalaemia (i.e. High K^+). Preoperatively, this may be due to CRF, crush injuries or absorption from massive haematomas. Massive transfusions of stored blood may also cause hyperkalaemia. Postoperatively, it is usually due to excessive administration and is usually asymptomatic. A K^+ above 7 mmol/L is an emergency. Intravenous insulin and glucose should be given and the K^+ checked. ECG changes include elevated T waves. If ECG changes are marked, calcium gluconate should be given i.v. Other methods of reducing the serum K^+ (particularly in the case of chronic hyperkalaemia) include calcium resonium orally or rectally, and if renal function is compromised, dialysis.

Acid–Base Balance

Abnormalities of acid–base balance usually occur in seriously ill patients and include:

Metabolic Acidosis. Severe tissue hypoxia, e.g. septicaemia, hypovolaemia or cardiogenic shock; renal failure; diabetic ketoacidosis; and after aortic surgery when the clamp is removed. The patient compensates by rapid deep respiration to 'blow off' CO_2. Excretes acid urine. ABGs show pH↓, HCO_3↓, $P\text{CO}_2$↓. Management involves treatment of the underlying condition. Bicarbonate infusion may be necessary in severe cases.

Metabolic Alkalosis. This occurs with prolonged vomiting or NG aspiration. Pyloric stenosis. To compensate, the kidney conserves hydrogen ions at the expense of K^+ excretion. ABGs show pH↑, $P\text{CO}_2$↑. Low K^+. Treatment is by rehydration with normal saline, potassium supplements and treatment of the underlying condition.

Respiratory Acidosis. This results from CO_2 retention. After surgery, this is usually due to severe chest complications, e.g. atelectasis from sputum retention or respiratory depression due to narcotics. Respiratory acidosis is compensated for by H^+ being excreted by the renal tubules and HCO_3^- being reabsorbed. ABGs show pH↓, $P\text{CO}_2$↑. Treatment is of the underlying cause.

Respiratory Alkalosis. Hyperventilation due to anxiety. Excessive mechanical ventilation. Compensation occurs by renal excretion of HCO_3^-. ABGs show pH↑, $P\text{CO}_2$↓. Treatment is of the underlying condition.

NUTRITIONAL SUPPORT

Poor nutrition results in increased postoperative morbidity and mortality. Poor wound healing occurs and there is a reduced resistance to infection. General examination of the patient will show evidence of weight loss, e.g. general appearance, loose skin folds. The patient will often be aware of how much weight has been lost and over what time period.

Causes of Malnutrition

- Increased catabolism, e.g. sepsis, major surgery with complications
- Increased losses, e.g. chronic liver disease with loss of albumin, protein-losing enteropathy
- Decreased intake, e.g. dysphagia, vomiting, general debility
- Decreased absorption, e.g. intestinal fistulae, short bowel syndrome
- Other causes, e.g. major trauma, chemotherapy, radiotherapy.

Indications for Nutritional Support

Most patients requiring surgery are well nourished and will stand a few days of starvation. They will recover from surgery sufficiently to resume eating before they become malnourished. Some patients will be clearly malnourished prior to surgery, while others may develop complications that delay resumption of normal diet and require parenteral nutrition. Others may have conditions, e.g. short bowel syndrome, which require long-term or permanent nutritional support.

Indications for nutritional support include:

- Preoperatively in malnourished patients
- Postoperatively in malnourished patients and those who develop malnutrition because of complications
- Patients with sepsis or major postoperative complications
- Patients with fistulae
- Patients with chronic liver disease
- Patients undergoing chemotherapy or radiotherapy for certain tumours
- Patients with short bowel syndrome or malabsorption syndrome.

Evaluation of Nutritional Status

1. History: duration of illness, weight loss, change in appetite, dietary habits
2. Physical examination, general appearance, loose skin folds, loss of skin contours over bony prominences, muscle wasting, peripheral oedema
3. Weight: in relation to height
4. Anthropometric measurements, e.g. triceps skin fold thickness
5. Laboratory tests, e.g. Hb, serum albumin, serum iron.

Administration of Nutritional Support

Oral Nutrition

This is the most efficient, least expensive, most pleasant and safest route for the patient. If the GI tract is available and the patient is able to take oral nutrition, this method is the most appropriate. Liquidised food, Clinifeed or supplements may be given this way. Patients undergoing elective surgery as part of an 'enhanced recovery programme' or 'fast-track surgery' are given oral nutritional supplements preoperatively to maximise their nutritional status prior to surgery.

Enteral Nutrition

This is used for patients with a functioning small bowel unable to take nutrients by mouth, e.g. those who are seriously ill, unable to swallow or have a mouth lesion, e.g. herpes.

Fine-Bore Nasogastric Tubes. Liquidised food, Clinifeed or supplements are given via a tube passed via the nose into the stomach.

Surgically Created Gastrostomy or Jejunostomy. These are appropriate for long-term enteric feeding.

In both of the above methods the feed is dripped slowly into the GI tract. Bolus feeding should be avoided, as it gives marked diarrhoea and, if given via a NG tube in large volumes, may result in regurgitation and aspiration pneumonia.

Complications. Complications of enteral feeding depend on the route of administration and the enteral feed itself. They include:

Nasogastric Feeding. Removal, blockage, aspiration, reflux, vomiting, diarrhoea, hyperglycaemia.

Gastrostomy/Jejunostomy. Pain, bleeding, peritonitis, infection, blockage, diarrhoea, hyperglycaemia.

Parenteral Nutrition

This is used where GI function is inadequate and nutrition is administered via the venous system.

Peripheral Line. Short-term feeding (up to 5 days) may be given via drip in a peripheral vein. Solutions used with this method must be of a special type, which causes little thrombophlebitis. The correct composition of feed for each individual patient is prepared by the pharmacy based on up-to-date blood results. This method may be used preoperatively for patients with malnutrition of moderate degree for which oral nutrition is unsatisfactory, e.g. malignant strictures of the oesophagus.

Central Line. This is the most appropriate route and is used for total parenteral nutrition (TPN). For short-term use, a percutaneous internal jugular line may be used. For longer-term and permanent nutrition, a tunnelled subcutaneous line (Hickman or Broviac) should be used. Hypertonic solutions are infused via the catheter into a large-bore vein with good flow to prevent thrombophlebitis.

Total Parenteral Nutrition (TPN)

This is usually provided in 3L bags either prepared in the hospital pharmacy or bought commercially. This provides all the nutrients required for a 24-h period. Controlled rates of administration are essential and this is achieved either by a special counting device attached to the drip line or via an infusion pump. Any additional fluid and electrolyte to restore losses, or administration of drugs, should be via a separate peripheral line.

Components of TPN

- Calories: these are supplied as a combination of carbohydrate and fat. Most patients require approximately 2000 kcal/day – or more if they have sepsis or burns.
- Protein: this is supplied as amino acids. Nitrogen requirements are about 15 g/day but may be as high as 30 g/day in hypercatabolic states.
- Water
- Vitamins
- Electrolytes, e.g. Na^+, K^+, calcium, phosphate, magnesium
- Trace elements, e.g. zinc, copper, manganese.

Monitoring TPN

Blood sugar, U&Es should be checked daily. Until fluid and nitrogen balance is obtained, the capillary blood glucose should be monitored 6-hourly. LFTs, calcium, phosphate and FBC should be checked twice weekly. If the patient becomes pyrexial, blood cultures should be obtained both peripherally and from the line ('paired cultures'). The site of catheter insertion should be dressed twice weekly under aseptic conditions. If the patient develops a pyrexia and no other cause is found, it may be necessary to remove the catheter and send the tip for culture. The catheter should be used for feeding only. Any other substances, e.g. additional electrolytes or drugs, should be given via a separate peripheral line.

Complications of TPN

Catheter Related. Pneumothorax or arterial puncture may occur during insertion. If the catheter is not correctly positioned in a large vein but is in a chamber of the heart, arrhythmias may occur. Rarely the catheter may erode through a vessel wall and give rise to haemopericardium. Air embolus may occur when manipulating the line, and this should be avoided by keeping the patient supine. Thrombosis of a central vein may occur. Prophylactic heparin 1000 μ/L of the infusion is useful prophylaxis.

Metabolic. Too much or too little of the components of i.v. feeding may be given. Careful monitoring for the following is required:

- Fluid overload
- Hyperglycaemia
- Hypoglycaemia (may occur if infusion of hypertonic glucose is suddenly stopped)
- Electrolyte abnormalities
- Hepatic cholestasis.

Home TPN

Long-term TPN in ambulatory patients is practicable providing it is properly monitored. Patients with short bowel syndrome are the most appropriate. The patient or a partner is taught the technique and backup is provided by a specially trained team able to provide regular biochemical monitoring. A Broviac or Hickman tunnelled central line is used. The feeding solution may be administered overnight and the catheter disconnected to allow activity during the day. Alternatively it may need to be administered throughout 24 h, depending on the patient's requirements.

Chapter 6

Infection and Surgery

Michael Delbridge

CHAPTER OUTLINE

The surgical patient is exposed to potentially harmful microorganisms prior to admission, during admission and after discharge. The outside surfaces of the body, including the aerodigestive tract, are normally colonised with bacteria – a defence mechanism that is disrupted by stress and antibiotic therapy. With the prevalence of hospital-acquired infections, such as *Clostridium difficile* and methicillin-resistant *Staphylococcus aureus* (MRSA), and the potential for blood-borne virus transmission, the practising surgeon needs to be aware of safe antimicrobial techniques and treatments, to protect both the patient and healthcare staff. Effective communication therefore needs to be present between surgeon and microbiologist.

PRINCIPLES OF WOUND MANAGEMENT

Healing by Primary Intention

When appropriate, the wound edges are approximated as soon after the injury as possible, e.g. clean traumatic wounds or surgical incisions. This is known as primary closure and the wound heals by first intention.

Healing by Secondary Intention

The wound edges are not apposed and the wound is left to heal by second intention. Granulation tissue grows up from the base of the wound and the skin grows over in a centripetal manner. This type of healing is appropriate for large, grossly contaminated wounds.

Delayed Primary Closure

The wound is left open and observed for several days. If the wound then appears healthy, it may be closed as for a primary closure. This type of closure is suitable for wounds that have low-grade infection or for surgical incisions where infection may be expected, e.g. abdominal incisions following operations for gross faecal peritonitis.

Factors Affecting Wound Healing

Age. Younger patients heal better than older patients.

Nutritional State. Malnutrition impedes wound healing. Patients who are poorly nourished should be given appropriate feeding, e.g. total parenteral nutrition (TPN) prior to surgery.

Drugs. Steroids delay wound healing.

Tissue Oxygenation and Vascularity. Hypoxaemia and ischaemia delay wound healing. Highly vascular areas, e.g. face, heal quicker than poorly vascularised areas, e.g. shin.

Radiotherapy. Causes endarteritis obliterans of small vessels resulting in local ischaemia and poor healing.

Local Sepsis. This is probably the commonest cause of delayed healing.

Factors Predisposing to Infection in Surgery

Age. Increasing age is a significant independent predictor of risk.

Underlying Illness. Those with an ASA score of III or more have been found to have a significantly higher risk of surgical site infection.

Obesity and Smoking. Are both associated with an increased risk of surgical site infection.

Wound Classification. See below.

Classification of Surgical Wounds

Clean. An incision in which no inflammation is encountered in a surgical procedure, without a break in sterile technique, and during which the respiratory tract, alimentary or genitourinary tracts are not entered, e.g. varicose vein surgery, hernia repair. The risk of postoperative wound infection is about 5%.

Clean Contaminated. An incision through which the respiratory, alimentary or genitourinary tract is entered under controlled conditions but with no contamination encountered, e.g. cholecystectomy, partial gastrectomy. The risk of postoperative wound infection is about 10%.

Contaminated. An incision undertaken during an operation, in which there is a major break in sterile technique or gross spillage from the gastrointestinal tract, or an incision in which acute, nonpurulent inflammation is encountered. Open traumatic wounds >12–24h old. The risk of postoperative wound infection is >50%.

Dirty. An incision undertaken during an operation in which the viscera are perforated or when acute inflammation with pus is encountered (e.g. faecal peritonitis), and for traumatic wounds where treatment is delayed, there is faecal contamination or devitalised tissue is present.

PREVENTION OF SURGICAL SITE INFECTION (INCORPORATING NICE GUIDELINES 2008)

Preoperative Precautions

- Adjust patient lifestyle. Improve diet and body mass index. Advise to stop smoking.
- MRSA screening and subsequent decolonisation if positive (see below)
- Consideration of delay of elective surgery if concurrent infection detected
- Advise patients to take a bath or shower using soap within 24h prior to surgery.
- If hair removal desired, use electric clippers on the day of surgery.

Perioperative Precautions

- Staff to wear specific nonsterile theatre wear in operating suite, sterile gowns in the theatre
- Keep staff movements in and out of theatre to a minimum.
- Operating team to remove hand jewellery, nail polish and artificial nails

- Scrub hands with nail cleaning with a brush or pick prior to the first operation.
- Scrub hands prior to subsequent operations and if hands are soiled.
- Patient skin preparation with povidone-iodine or chlorhexidine prior to incision
- Maintain adequate patient temperature, oxygenation and perfusion throughout.
- Cover surgical wounds with an appropriate dressing at the end.

Postoperative Precautions

- Use an aseptic technique to change dressings.
- Use sterile saline to cleanse wound up to 48h after surgery.
- Patients may shower 48h after surgery.
- Use an appropriate dressing for wounds healing by secondary intention.

ANTIBIOTICS IN SURGERY

Antibiotics are never a substitute for sound surgical technique. Pus, dead tissue and slough need removing. Antibiotics should be used carefully and only with positive indications. Prolonged or inappropriate use of antibiotics may encourage resistant strains of organisms to emerge. Except in straightforward cases, advice of a microbiologist should be sought.

Principles of Antibiotic Therapy

Selection of Antibiotic

The decision to prescribe antibiotics is usually clinical and is based initially on a 'best-guess' policy, i.e. based on experience of that particular condition, what the organism is likely to be, and to what it is most likely to be sensitive. The following sequence of events usually occurs:

1. A decision is made on clinical grounds that an infection exists.
2. Based on signs, symptoms and clinical experience, a guess is made at the likely infecting organism.
3. The appropriate specimens are taken for microbiological examination, i.e. culture and sensitivity testing.
4. The most effective drug against the suspected organism is given in line with individual hospital guidelines. If doubt exists, this is discussed with a microbiologist.
5. The clinical response to treatment is monitored.
6. The antibiotic treatment is altered, if necessary, in response to laboratory reports of culture and sensitivities.

Occasionally the response of the infection to an apparently appropriate antibiotic is poor. Possible causes for this include:

- Failure to drain pus, excise necrotic tissue or remove foreign bodies
- Failure of the drug to reach the tissues in therapeutic concentrations, e.g. ischaemic limbs
- Organism isolated is not the one responsible for the infection.
- After prolonged antibiotic therapy, new organisms develop due to selection pressure.
- Inadequate dosage or inappropriate route of administration.

Route of Administration

Antibiotics should be given i.v. in severe infections in seriously ill patients. Some antibiotics, e.g. gentamicin, can only be given by the parenteral route. When the patient improves and the gastrointestinal (GI) tract is functioning satisfactorily, drugs may be given orally.

> **HINTS AND TIPS**
>
> It is best to avoid the intramuscular route if possible, as it is uncomfortable for the patient, and in shocked patients absorption would be inadequate.

Duration of Therapy

This depends on the individual's response, laboratory tests and the underlying cause of infection. For most infections that show an appropriate response to treatment after 48h, a suitable 'course' should be for 5–7 days. Infections such as osteomyelitis require prolonged courses of antibiotics administered long after symptoms and signs of infection have resolved.

Dosage

The dosage may need to be modified in renal and liver disease.

Complications of Antibiotic Therapy

- Adverse reactions:
  - Side effects, e.g. nephrotoxicity, ototoxicity
  - Hypersensitivity
  - Anaphylaxis
- Development of resistance
- Iatrogenic infection, e.g. C. *difficile* with the use of cephalosporins, clindamycin.

> **HINTS AND TIPS**
>
> The importance of an adequate drug and sensitivity history cannot be overemphasised. Always make sure before giving parenteral antibiotics, especially penicillins, that resuscitation equipment and the appropriate medication to treat anaphylaxis is available. Remember that there is a cross-sensitivity between penicillins and cephalosporins: the incidence may be as high as 10%. If possible, avoid cephalosporins in penicillin-sensitive patients.

Prophylactic Antibiotics

Despite aseptic techniques, some operations carry a high risk of postoperative wound infection, bacteraemia or septicaemia. Administration of antibiotics in the perioperative period will reduce the risks.

Indications for Prophylactic Antibiotics

These include:

- Implantation of foreign bodies, e.g. cardiac prosthetic valves, artificial joints, prosthetic vascular grafts

- Patients with pre-existing cardiac disease who are undergoing surgical procedures, including dental procedures, e.g. patients with mitral valve disease as prophylaxis against infective endocarditis
- Organ transplantation
- Immunosuppressed patients
- Diabetic patients
- Amputations, especially for ischaemia or crush injuries, where there is dead muscle; risk of gas gangrene is high especially in contaminated wounds; penicillin is the antibiotic of choice
- Compound fractures and penetrating wounds
- Surgical incisions, where there is a high risk of bacterial contamination, e.g. (1) clean-contaminated wounds – prophylactic antibiotics are indicated; (2) contaminated – antibiotics are given as therapy not prophylaxis; (3) dirty – antibiotics are given as therapy not prophylaxis.

Most prophylactic antibiotics are given to prevent wound infection. In some cases, they are given prior to instrumental procedures in potentially infected sites, e.g. when performing cystoscopy, when they are given to prevent septicaemia. In most cases, one dose is given preoperatively either orally if under local anaesthetic (1 h preoperatively) or i.v. if under GA. The aim is to achieve therapeutic levels at the time of surgery. Individual hospital policy should be followed with regard to the use of specific agents and their duration as prophylaxis.

Specific Antibiotics (→ Table 6.1)

SURGICAL INFECTIONS

Sepsis

Sepsis is generally related to the body's response to infection. However, sepsis is probably better defined as a group of conditions that include:

- SIRS which is defined as any two from:
  - Pyrexia – >38°C or <36°C
  - Tachycardia – >90 beats/min
  - Tachypnoea – >20 breaths/min
  - WCC – >12 or <4
- Sepsis – SIRS plus a documented infection
- Sepsis syndrome – sepsis plus organ dysfunction and hypoperfusion
- Septic shock – refractory hypotension plus documented infection.

SIRS is seen in many surgical patients and does not always result from an infective process. It is commonly seen in pancreatitis, trauma and burns. SIRS is a normal response to injury and in the early stages is protective. A number of stages in the evolution of SIRS may occur:

- In the region of injury there is local production of inflammatory mediators and cytokines. These lead to vasodilatation, increased vascular permeability and the recruitment of cells that fight infection.

TABLE 6.1

SOME COMMONLY USED ANTIBIOTICS

Class	Antibiotic	Route	Activity	Uses	Side Effects	Cautions
Penicillin	Benzylpenicillin; phenoxymethylpenicillin	Oral, i.v.	*Streptococcus* *Pneumococcus* Clostridia *Neisseria*	Soft tissue and wound infection	Hypersensitivity Urticarial rash Anaphylaxis Cross-sensitivity Convulsions at high doses	Allergy to penicillins Renal failure Cardiac failure (i.v. forms contain K^+ and Na^+ salts)
	Flucloxacillin	Oral, i.m., i.v.	*Staphylococcus*	Soft tissue and wound infections		
	Amoxicillin; ampicillin	Oral, i.m., i.v.	*Strep. faecalis* *Haemophilus influenzae*	Urinary tract infection Chest infection		
	Co-amoxiclav	Oral, i.v.	Coliforms *Staphylococcus* Bacteroides	Soft tissue infection Chest infection (hospital acquired pneumonia/aspiration pneumonia) Intra-abdominal infection		
	Meropenem; imipenem	i.v.	Broad spectrum Anaerobes, aerobes	Life-threatening sepsis (including neutropenic sepsis)		
	Piperacillin	i.m., i.v.	Bacteroides Coliforms *Klebsiella* *Pseudomonas*	Used with tazobactam for severe sepsis – chest, soft tissue, biliary tree		

Continued

TABLE 6.1

SOME COMMONLY USED ANTIBIOTICS—cont'd

Class	Antibiotic	Route	Activity	Uses	Side Effects	Cautions
Cephalosporin	Cefuroxime	Oral, i.m., i.v.	Broad spectrum	Second line in UTI, chest infection (for mild penicillin allergy)	Use is often restricted in hospitals due to the risk of *Clostridium difficile* pseudomembranous colitis 10% cross-sensitivity with penicillin allergy Rashes Pyrexia Transient elevation in LFTs	Dose reduction in renal failure
	Cefotaxime/ceftazidime	i.m., i.v.	Broad spectrum *Pseudomonas*	Orbital cellulitis Sepsis due to Gram-negative bacilli		
Sulphonamide and trimethoprim	Co-trimoxazole (sulfamethoxazole and trimethoprim)	Oral, i.m., i.v.	Broad spectrum	PCP pneumonia	Nausea Vomiting Rash Mouth ulcers Marrow suppression Hyperkalaemia	Avoid in pregnancy Potentiates the action of warfarin and ciclosporin
	Trimethoprim	Oral, i.v.	Broad spectrum	Simple UTI		
Macrolide	Erythromycin	Oral, i.v.	Broad spectrum *Streptococcus* Clostridia *Staphylococcus* *Campylobacter*	Used as a second line agent in patients sensitive to penicillins Skin and soft tissue infections Chest infection Legionnaires' disease *Campylobacter* enteritis	Diarrhoea (oral) Phlebitis (i.v.)	Potentiates action of warfarin and ciclosporin

Aminoglycoside	Gentamicin	i.m., i.v.	Gram-negative Coliforms *Pseudomonas* *Staphylococcus*	Surgical prophylaxis (has largely replaced cefuroxime for intra-abdominal surgical procedures)	Ototoxicity (vertigo, deafness) Nephrotoxicity	Monitor serum levels Caution in renal failure
Quinolone	Ciprofloxacin	Oral, i.v	Broad spectrum *Pseudomonas* *Staphylococcus*	Simple UTI (oral) Acute prostatitis Acute pyelonephritis	i.v. use is often restricted in hospitals due to the risk of *C. difficile* pseudomembranous colitis Nausea Diarrhoea Vomiting Anxiety Insomnia Nervousness Convulsions	Potentiates action of warfarin
Glycopeptide	Vancomycin	Oral (does not cross the gut lining), i.v.	*Staphylococcus* MRSA *Streptococcus* Clostridia	Severe infections Oral for pseudomembranous colitis MRSA +ve skin and soft tissue infections	Phlebitis (i.v.) Ototoxicity Nephrotoxicity	Monitor serum levels to control dosage Renal failure Hepatic failure
	Teicoplanin	i.v., i.m.	*Staphylococcus* *Streptococcus* *Enterococcus* *Listeria* anaerobes	Prophylaxis in orthopaedic surgery		

Continued

TABLE 6.1

SOME COMMONLY USED ANTIBIOTICS

Class	Antibiotic	Route	Activity	Uses	Side Effects	Cautions
Tetracylcine	Doxycycline	Oral	*H. influenzae* Coliforms *Mycoplasma* pneumonia *Streptococcus*	Used as a second line agent in patients sensitive to penicillins Skin and soft tissue infections Chest infections GU infections (Chlamydia)	Hypersensitivity to sunlight Rash	Caution in liver impairment
Other	Metronidazole	Oral, i.v., topical, p.r.	Anaerobic bacteria Protozoa	Prophylaxis in colorectal surgery Intraperitoneal sepsis Gynaecological sepsis Giardiasis Amoebiasis Amoebic liver abscess In combination with penicillins for diabetic foot sepsis	Anorexia Sore tongue Metallic taste Disulfiram-like reaction if taken with alcohol	Potentiates action of warfarin
	Clindamycin	Oral, i.v.	*Staphylococcus* *Streptococcus* *Bacteroides*	Inhibits toxin synthesis therefore used in necrotising fasciitis, skin and soft tissue infections	Pseudomembranous colitis (*C. difficile*) Diarrhoea Nausea Vomiting	Not to be used with macrolides
	Fusidic acid	Oral, i.v.	*Staphylococcus* *Corynebacterium*	Osteomyelitis	Jaundice	Pregnancy

- In more severe injury the cytokine release has a systemic effect; this includes the production of acute phase proteins, pyrexia and an increase in peripheral leukocytes. This response is regulated by a group of counter-regulatory cytokines.
- In patients with SIRS there is an exaggerated response and the production of cytokines exceeds the counter-regulatory mechanisms. Cytokines such as IL-1 and TNF-α produce vasodilatation leading to hypotension, increased vascular permeability leading to oedema and third space fluid loss. There is also widespread activation of leukocytes that can cause damage in organs distant from the site of injury, e.g. lungs.

Management of SIRS

- Resuscitation
- Identify source of sepsis. Likely possible sources include: the wound; intravascular access (arterial, central venous, cannulas); urinary catheters/urinary tract infection; prosthetic implants; chest infection.
- Administration of appropriate antibiotics – empirically initially and then changed after antibiotic sensitivities are known
- Definitive management of the course of sepsis, i.e. surgical or radiological guided drainage of abscess.

Cellulitis

A spreading inflammation of connective tissue. It is usually subcutaneous and caused by β-haemolytic streptococci or *Staphylococcus aureus*.

Symptoms and SIRS. Redness, oedema and localised tenderness. A scratch, insect bite, ulcer or surgical wound may be apparent. There is usually fever and malaise. Lymphangitis or lymphadenitis may be present. Lymphangitis produces red tender streaks in the line of lymphatics extending from the area of cellulitis towards the regional lymph nodes. Lymphadenitis is represented by enlarged tender regional lymph nodes. Occasionally the overlying skin is red and the glands may be fluctuant.

Investigations

- WBC
- Blood cultures
- CRP
- Blood glucose.

Drawing a line around the erythema with permanent marker pen enables observation of progression/regression of the leading edge and can be used to gauge response to treatment.

Treatment. *Streptococcus* and *Staphylococcus* are usually sensitive to flucloxacillin. Elevation of a limb may be required. Occasionally an abscess with thin watery pus forms and requires drainage.

Erysipelas is an uncommon skin infection caused by a streptococcus (group A). The condition is usually encountered on the scalp, face and neck. Pain and redness of the skin are apparent, the margin being well demarcated and raised above the normal skin. Pyrexia and malaise usually accompany the local signs. Treatment is with penicillin.

Necrotising Fasciitis

This is a rapidly progressive and potentially fatal bacterial infection that spreads along fascial planes and causes vascular thrombosis resulting in necrosis of the tissues involved. If present in a limb distal to the elbow or knee, organisms often involved include β-haemolytic streptococci and staphylococci. Coliforms and Gram-negative anaerobes may be synergistically involved elsewhere such as the scrotum (Fournier's gangrene). Necrotising fasciitis may result from a small puncture wound, surgical incision or penetrating trauma of a hollow viscus.

Symptoms and Signs. Pain and tenderness at the leading edge of the infection can be agonising. Redness, oedema, necrotic insensate skin patches, haemorrhagic bullae, crepitus and discharge. The patient is febrile and exhibiting signs of systemic sepsis. A test incision either at the bedside or in an operating theatre producing a grey/brown 'dishwater' exudate aids diagnosis, as does a 'sweep test' where a finger placed into the test incision and turned into the soft tissues easily separates the tissue planes digested by bacterial enzymes.

Investigations

- WBC
- Blood culture
- Swabs – culture and sensitivity
- Radiograph may show gas in tissues.

Treatment. Patients should be resuscitated and transferred urgently to the operating theatre for surgical debridement of all infected and dead tissue. A critical care bed should be requested for postoperative recovery. The tissue is usually oedematous, grey and odorous. The subcutaneous fat and fascia are involved. Muscle is often viable but may also be necrotic. The microbiologist should be informed if a diagnosis of necrotising fasciitis is suspected. Fresh specimens of tissue should be sent for urgent Gram stain and microscopy. Antimicrobial treatment is with Tazocin, clindamycin and one dose of gentamicin. In patients who are penicillin allergic the combination would be vancomycin, clindamycin (inhibits the Streptococcal toxin) and a dose of gentamicin. Antibiotics are changed according to culture and sensitivities. The patient's systemic state is observed carefully postoperatively and the wound is inspected regularly, often with a planned second look under general anaesthetic at 24 or 48h, and any further necrotic tissue excised. When the infection has been controlled, large skin defects can be reconstructed with skin grafts. Mortality rate is about 25% in extensive cases.

HINTS AND TIPS

Although necrotising fasciitis is rare, it is important to know about it. Necrotising fasciitis is difficult to diagnose in its initial stages, as it mimics cellulitis. A high index of suspicion is necessary. Early features include pain, tenderness and systemic illness out of proportion to the local physical signs. Urgent surgical referral and prompt surgical debridement are essential.

Gas Gangrene

Myositis and cellulitis caused by *C. perfringens*, an anaerobic, spore-forming and gas-producing organism. The organism is found in soil and faeces. It is an infection associated with deep, penetrating, contaminated wounds usually involving an extremity, and rarely is seen as a complication of amputation of an ischaemic limb. Intravenous drug users may inadvertently inject *C. perfringens or C. tetani* into the soft tissues. It may involve the abdominal wall following penetrating trauma of, or surgery to, the GI tract. Clostridial myonecrosis is also associated with *C. septicum*, which has an association with previous or occult bowel malignancy. If *C. septicum* is cultured, the patient should be investigated for a possible occult or recurrent malignancy following acute management.

Symptoms and Signs. Acute onset 6h to 3 days after injury. Severe pain at site of injury. The tissues are swollen; brownish, serous, malodorous fluid may drain from the wound. Patchy necrosis and crepitus occur. The patient is toxic and may be confused or delirious. The temperature is not always elevated.

Investigations

- WBC
- Bilirubin raised because of haemolysis
- Gram stain of discharge shows Gram-positive bacilli
- Radiograph shows gas in tissues.

Treatment

Prophylactic. Adequate debridement of wound at time of initial injury. All contused and dead tissue should be removed and the wound thoroughly irrigated and left open. Prophylactic penicillin should be given to all patients with contaminated wounds and to patients with ischaemic limbs undergoing amputations.

Therapeutic. Radical debridement of all necrotic tissue is mandatory. If the muscle of a limb is involved, amputation will be necessary. This should be done at a level where the muscle bleeds and contracts when cut. Large doses of penicillin should be given intravenously. Anti-gas gangrene serum either prophylactically or therapeutically is of unproven value.

HINTS AND TIPS

Gas gangrene is a surgical emergency. Delaying treatment can lead to shock, renal failure and coma. Death can occur within 48h of onset of symptoms. Prompt treatment is therefore essential.

Tetanus

This is a rare condition in the UK owing to widespread immunisation. It is caused by *C. tetani*, an anaerobic Gram-positive bacillus that produces a neurotoxin. It is found in soil and faeces. The neurotoxin enters peripheral nerves and travels to the spinal cord where it blocks inhibitory activity of spinal reflexes resulting in the characteristic features of the disease. The disease follows the implantation of spores into deep, devitalised tissues.

Symptoms and Signs

History of Injury. This may be as minor as the prick of a rose thorn. The incubation period is 1–30 days. Muscle spasm usually occurs first at the site of inoculation and is followed by trismus resulting in the typical risus sardonicus (lock-jaw).

Stiffness in the neck, back and abdomen follow together with generalised spasms which may cause asphyxia. The muscles remain in spasm between convulsions. Opisthotonos (arching of the back and neck due to spasm) may occur. This stage is followed by convulsions which are extremely painful and during which the patient is conscious. Death may occur from asphyxia due to involvement of respiratory muscles or from inhalation of vomit with aspiration pneumonia.

Differential Diagnosis

- Strychnine poisoning: the muscles are flaccid between convulsions
- Tetany: usually carpopedal spasm and does not affect the trunk
- Epilepsy
- Meningitis: there is usually only neck stiffness but convulsions may occur
- Hysteria.

Treatment

Prophylactic

- Active immunisation with tetanus toxoid. All children should be immunised, and this is repeated at 6 weeks and 6 months after the initial dose. Booster doses should be given at 5-year intervals. All patients attending an A&E department with new trauma, however mild, should have a booster, unless one has been given within the previous 5 years.
- Contaminated and penetrating wounds should be debrided and prophylactic penicillin administered. A tetanus toxoid booster dose should be given to the previously immunised patient. Those not previously immunised should be given human antitetanus immunoglobulin.

Therapeutic

1. Involve the critical care team. Discuss with microbiology.
2. Isolate the patient in a quiet darkened room. Give diazepam or chlorpromazine. In severe cases, the patient will need to be paralysed and ventilated. Feeding should be given via a fine-bore nasogastric tube. Ventilation may need to be continued for up to 4 weeks. A trial period of weaning off relaxants without recurrence of spasm will indicate when ventilation is no longer required. Tracheostomy may be required.
3. Administer penicillin, tetanus toxoid and human antitetanus immunoglobulin.
4. Excise and drain any contaminated wound.
5. Regular physiotherapy will be required during the recovery period.

Prognosis. The mortality rate is inversely proportional to the length of the incubation period. If spasm occurs within 5 days of the time of injury, the prognosis is poor. The mortality rate is also directly proportional to the severity of the symptoms.

METHICILLIN-RESISTANT *STAPHYLOCOCCUS AUREUS* (MRSA)

MRSA is a major nosocomial pathogen. It may cause severe morbidity and mortality. Up to 40% of nosocomial *S. aureus* infections may be methicillin resistant. They are also resistant to flucloxacillin, amoxicillin, co-amoxiclav, cephalosporins and Tazocin. Many inpatients are colonised or infected, and up to 25% of hospital personnel may be carriers. The organism may be carried in the anterior nares, inguinal, perineal and axillary areas. Spread often occurs by the hands, usually of nursing or medical staff.

Risk Factors for Colonisation. These include advanced age, previous hospitalisation, length of hospitalisation, stay in ITU, chronic illness, prior and prolonged antibiotic therapy, presence of a wound, exposure to colonised or infected patients, presence of invasive indwelling devices, nursing home residency.

Clinical Presentation. These principally include line sepsis, surgical site infection and pneumonia.

Infection Control. This includes screening of patients and staff. If MRSA is suspected, swabs should be taken from the hairline, nose, axilla, groin, perineum. Important factors in infection control include hand washing, use of gowns and gloves, isolation of infected or colonised patients (barrier nursing) and environmental cleaning.

Management

Carriers. Carriers may be treated by application of antiseptics, e.g. mupirocin to nose; use of antiseptic soaps and shampoos for 5 days. Check swabs should be taken at 2, 9 and 16 days after use of antiseptics.

Patients With MRSA Infection. These patients should be nursed using special precautions. Vancomycin is the antibiotic of choice. Linezolid and daptomycin are alternative treatments.

INFECTION AND THE SURGEON

The surgeon – as indeed are any medical, nursing or paramedical personnel – is at risk from three main blood-borne viral infections: HIV, hepatitis B, hepatitis C.

HIV

Infection with HIV is permanent, and it is likely that all carriers will eventually develop AIDS. Surgical personnel are at high risk. Infection with HIV results from the passage of infected body fluid (usually blood) from one person to another. Needlestick injuries and scalpel injuries are possible sources of infection. In the general population, HIV may be transmitted by unprotected anal, vaginal and oral intercourse, sharing needles in drug abuse and infected blood products (e.g. as has happened in the past with haemophiliacs).

Risk Categories

The following are at risk of becoming HIV-positive: homosexual or bisexual males; prostitutes (male and female); intravenous drug abusers; haemophiliacs who were treated before routine testing became available, i.e. October 1995; sexual partners of the above and children of infected mothers.

Prevention of HIV

Care at operation needs to be exercised with patients who are known to have AIDS or be HIV-positive. Patients with anorectal disease related to homosexuality, haemophiliacs and sexual partners and children of the above should be treated with appropriate caution.

Counselling is required and consent must be obtained for HIV testing. If a patient refuses and is suspected of being HIV-positive, then precautions must be taken with nursing care and any invasive procedures from simple venepuncture to major surgery.

The chance of seroconversion from a needlestick injury is approximately 0.3%.

Hepatitis B

Infection is largely blood-borne. It may be transmitted by blood transfusion; inoculation via sharp injuries from blood or blood products; droplet transmission; syringe and needle sharing in drug addicts; sexual intercourse with an infected partner; homosexual practices; tattooing or ear piercing, etc. with unsterile equipment. Antigen carriage is a risk for hospital staff, especially those in 'high-risk' areas, e.g. theatre staff. Dialysis units are often quoted as being a 'high-risk' area, but following outbreaks many years ago, all staff and patients are tested for HBsAg.

Hepatitis B vaccine is offered to all high-risk staff. These categories include: surgeons; theatre nurses; other operating department personnel; pathology department staff; A&E unit staff; liver transplant unit staff; gastrointestinal unit staff; workers in residential units for the mentally handicapped; staff of infectious and communicable diseases units.

The chance of seroconversion from a needlestick injury in unvaccinated individuals is approximately 30%.

Hepatitis C

HCV is present in blood and spreads in the same way as HBV, by blood transfusion; syringe and needle sharing in drug addicts; mother-to-baby transmission; sharps injuries; tattooing, ear piercing, etc. with unsterile equipment; sharing toothbrushes and razors. Sexual transmission occurs but is uncommon. The incubation period is 6 weeks to 2 months. About 0.7% of the population are chronically infected with HCV.

The disease is often asymptomatic; only about 25% becoming symptomatic and jaundiced. Around 20% of those infected will clear the virus in the acute stage. Of those that do not, some will never develop liver damage; many will develop only moderate liver damage, with or without symptoms; 20% will progress to cirrhosis during 20 years or so, and of that 20%, some will progress to liver failure and some will develop hepatocellular carcinoma. Carriers are a source of infection and include drug addicts; recipients of blood and blood products before September 1991; children of infected mothers; and healthcare workers from occupational injuries.

The chance of seroconversion from a needlestick injury is approximately 3%.

Precautions for the Care of Known and Suspected HIV, HBV and HCV Carriers

Sources of infection are:

- Contact – blood, urine, faeces, saliva, tears, cerebrospinal fluid (CSF)
- Air-borne – use of power tools
- Inoculation – sharps injuries, e.g. needlestick, scalpels.

Universal Precautions

This refers to those precautions taken to protect theatre staff from infection in all cases. They include:

- Gowns
- Masks
- Surgical gloves
- 'No touch' technique.

Special Precautions

These are used for all high-risk patients, e.g. hepatitis, HIV or patients suspected of having these conditions:

- All personnel involved in patient care should be aware of the risk.
- Any patient considered as a risk should be indicated as belonging to a high-risk category on the operating list (*under no circumstances should the actual disease causing the risk be placed on the operating list, for reasons of patient confidentiality*).
- Arrangements should be made for contaminated fluid, dressings, etc. to be handled and disposed of correctly.
- Appropriate theatre techniques should be adopted:
  - Minimise theatre staff; only essential personnel – no spectators.
  - Remove all but essential equipment.
  - Disposable drapes and gowns
  - Double-gloving and use of 'indicator' glove systems
  - Visors to prevent splashing in eyes
  - Blunt suture needles
  - Stapling devices rather than needles where possible
  - Pass instruments in kidney dish.
  - 'No touch' technique
  - All disposable equipment should be removed in specifically marked containers.
  - The theatre should be thoroughly cleansed with dilute bleach solution at the end of the procedure.
  - Recovery staff must also be aware of the risk.

Management of Sharps Injuries

- Let the site of injury bleed.
- Wash area with soap and water.
- Immediately report the incident to supervisor/senior officer/occupational health.
- Visit the occupational health department or nearest emergency department as soon as possible.

Procedure at Occupational Health or Emergency Department

- Take detailed information – details of injury; how long ago it occurred; was the skin penetrated; did it bleed; was the sharp visibly contaminated with blood; was the source patient known to be infected and with what; any first aid measures used.
- Explain that transmission risk is small.
- Offer blood test but only after appropriate counselling.
- If the source patient is known (i.e. the original user of the needle in needlestick injuries), they should be asked to consent for testing for HIV, HBV or HCV. They should be counselled before the tests are done.
- The person sustaining the sharps injury should be advised about the risks of transmission until such time as test results are received. They should practise safe sex and not donate blood.

Postexposure Prophylaxis

Hepatitis B

- If the source patient tests positive for HBV, the healthcare worker should have been vaccinated and serum antibody positive.

- If antibody levels are low, a dose of hyperimmune anti-hepatitis B IgG plus one dose of vaccine should be given.
- In the unvaccinated, one dose of hyperimmune anti-hepatitis B IgG should be given and a course of vaccination commenced.
- Similar procedures should be followed when the source patient cannot be identified or refuses to be treated.

Hepatitis C

- After 6 weeks and 12 weeks, serum analysis with polymerase chain reaction. If positive, can give interferon and ribavirin.

HIV

- Carry out tests after counselling at 3 months and 6 months.
- No vaccine is available.
- Postexposure prophylaxis should be given within 1 h of exposure in cases involving high-risk or known HIV carriers.

Triple agent prophylaxis with drugs from two classes should be used – an example is Tenofovir disoproxil and Emtricitabine (these are Nucleoside reverse transcriptase inhibitors) and Raltegravir (an Integrase inhibitor) – this is from the BASH PEP guidelines.

Chapter 7

Management of Malignant Disease

Marcus J.D. Wagstaff • Katherine I. Bridge

CHAPTER OUTLINE

Patients with malignant disease form a major part of the workload of a surgical unit. The total number of patients with malignant disease is rising owing to increased life expectancy; as many as one in three people in the Western world will be diagnosed with cancer in their lifetime. Due to the complex and often aggressive management of cancer, these patients are assessed and managed by a multidisciplinary team consisting of surgeons, oncologists, radiologists, pathologists and nurses. Where possible, the aim should be to prevent malignancy, e.g. cessation of smoking in the prevention of lung cancer, avoidance of excessive ultraviolet light in the prevention of skin cancer and vaccination against HPV in the prevention of cervical cancer. Screening programmes aim to make earlier diagnoses of common, treatable forms of cancer and hopefully maximise the cure rate. This chapter aims to introduce the reader to the concepts regarding cancer screening, assessment, management and palliative care.

SCREENING

This is the examination of an asymptomatic population at risk of a particular condition, with a view to early diagnosis and consequent increase in cure rate. The basis for screening a normal population is to diagnose cancer at an asymptomatic stage, treatment at which point results in greater survival than with cancers diagnosed at a symptomatic stage. For a screening programme to be successful it must adhere to certain principles:

- The cancer being detected must be common enough to represent an important health problem.
- The natural history of the cancer should be established, i.e. its development from a latent phase to symptomatic disease.
- A test should be available to detect the latent stage; the test should be sensitive and specific to the cancer and be acceptable and safe to the patient.
- Early detection of the cancer should lead to a benefit in terms of cost of treatment and survival of the patient.

- Examples of screening programmes being carried out at present are:
  - Cervical smears for cervical carcinoma
  - Mammography for carcinoma of the breast
  - Faecal occult bloods for carcinoma of the colon.

PREMALIGNANT CONDITIONS

A symptom, collection of symptoms or disease that if left untreated has the potential to develop into a malignant condition. It is therefore important that these conditions are recognised and appropriate action taken. Examples of premalignant conditions include:

- *Skin*: actinic keratoses, Bowen's disease, erythroplasia of Queyrat (penis)
- *Gastrointestinal (GI) tract*: leukoplakia (mouth and tongue), Plummer–Vinson syndrome, Barrett's oesophagus, villous adenoma, familial polyposis coli, ulcerative colitis, Crohn's disease, Ménétrier's syndrome
- *GU tract*: leukoplakia of the bladder, bilharzia.

GENERAL SYMPTOMS AND SIGNS OF MALIGNANT DISEASE

These may relate to the primary tumour, metastases or generalised systemic manifestations.

They may be broadly classified as follows:

Primary Tumour

Palpable Swelling. This is usually painless unless invading other structures. Common examples include the palpable masses of the primary tumour in carcinoma of the breast, carcinoma of the thyroid, carcinoma of the caecum.

Obstruction. Examples include dysphagia in carcinoma of the oesophagus, obstructive jaundice in carcinoma of the head of the pancreas, large bowel obstruction in carcinoma of the colon, vomiting in gastric outlet obstruction from carcinoma of the gastric antrum.

Bleeding

- Overt: haemoptysis, haematemesis, haematuria, rectal bleeding
- Occult: carcinoma of the stomach or carcinoma of the caecum. Microcytic anaemia occurs.

Symptoms Due to Compression or Invasion of Local Structures. SVC obstruction with bronchial carcinoma (an oncological emergency); back pain with retroperitoneal invasion with pancreatic cancer; invasion of nerves, e.g., facial paralysis with carcinoma of the parotid gland, recurrent laryngeal nerve palsy with anaplastic carcinoma of the thyroid or lung carcinoma.

Metastases

- Enlarged lymph nodes: may be discrete or hard, irregular and matted
- Hepatomegaly: primary in stomach, colon, bronchus or breast
- Jaundice: from nodes in the porta hepatis, with primary in the stomach, pancreas or colon
- Ascites: ovarian or any GI malignancy
- Abdominal mass due to omental secondaries – often in association with ascites
- Pathological fractures from bony metastases, e.g. breast, bronchus, thyroid, prostate, kidney

- Pleural effusion, e.g. from breast cancer
- Fits, confusion, personality change from cerebral metastases, e.g. breast, bronchus, malignant melanoma.

HINTS AND TIPS

'Paired and midline organs' may help you to remember the most common causes of bone metastases – breast, bronchus, thyroid, prostate and kidney. This is important in the patient who presents with incidental bony metastasis or pathological fracture; it will help in focusing examination and investigations to locate the primary tumour.

Generalised Manifestations. Examples include cachexia, PUO (lymphoma, hypernephroma), hypertrophic pulmonary osteoarthropathy (carcinoma of the bronchus), thrombophlebitis migrans (carcinoma of the pancreas), neuropathies and myopathies (carcinoma of the bronchus), endocrine manifestations, e.g. ADH or ACTH production in bronchial carcinoma and clubbing (lung carcinoma, mesothelioma and neurogenic tumours).

Asymptomatic Incidental Findings. Axillary lymphadenopathy on routine examination, e.g. with small impalpable carcinoma of the breast. Silent pulmonary primary or metastases on routine chest X-ray (CXR).

HINTS AND TIPS

A diagnosis of advanced malignancy will often be obvious. However, early, and even late, malignant disease can present with fairly nonspecific symptoms and be the cause of illness in the patient who you think is 'just not quite right'. A high index of suspicion is required.

STAGING AND GRADING OF CANCER

The extent, or stage (i.e. the size of a tumour and how far it has spread from its origin), of a malignant tumour is established to provide an indication of the prognosis and to act as a guide for the type of treatment. It is also necessary for comparing the efficacies of different treatments in clinical trials. Two methods may be used – clinical and pathological. A tumour's apparent growth rate may be graded according to its histological appearance, and its resemblance to mature cells of its lineage (degree of differentiation) can be commented on to indicate aggression.

Clinical and Pathological Staging

The TNM classification was developed by the Union of International Cancer Control (UICC). This method uses both clinical and laboratory results to grade the tumour. The clinician assesses three factors:

- Extent of the tumour (T)
- Node status (N)
- Presence of metastases (M).

(→ Ch. 11 – Breast, Ch. 20 – Melanoma).

A method that is based on pathological staging only is Dukes' classification for colorectal carcinoma (→Ch. 15).

The FIGO staging for gynaecological malignancies divides disease into five stages: 0 – carcinoma in situ, I – confined to the organ of origin, II – invasion of surrounding organs, III – spread to nodes within the pelvis and IV – distant metastasis.

Grading of Tumours

The histological appearance of specimens is graded according to various criteria such as the proportions of cells undergoing mitosis, the degree of differentiation, the degree of nuclear pleomorphism, etc. This represents the 'aggressive' nature of the cancer. Examples include Broder's grading of squamous cell carcinoma or the Bloom–Richardson grading of breast carcinoma.

DIAGNOSTIC PROCEDURES

Biopsy. This is mandatory and may be carried out in a variety of ways:

- Fine-needle aspiration using a 22G needle: smear produced on slide; read by experienced cytologist. Can be used for solid lesions or for cytology from a malignant effusion
- Core biopsy, e.g. Tru-Cut: core of tissue removed for histological examination
- Incisional biopsy: removes a small accessible piece of the lesion for histological examination
- Excisional biopsy: the complete removal of a discrete lesion without a wide margin and without it being considered curative of the malignancy
- Evaluation under anaesthetic: to assess presence or extent of disease, e.g. staging laparotomy (largely superseded by computerised tomography (CT) scanning), panendoscopy, mediastinoscopy, bronchoscopy, thoracoscopy with biopsy of suspicious or high-risk areas.

Imaging (e.g. Ultrasound, CT or Magnetic Resonance Imaging (MRI)). This is used for confirming a suspected diagnosis, assessing spread and quantifying response to treatment. A negative study does not exclude microscopic disease.

Positron Emission Tomography (PET). This is described in detail in Chapter 3.

TUMOUR MARKERS

These are substances present in the body in a concentration related to the presence of a tumour. They are rarely sufficiently specific to be of diagnostic value. The tumour marker may be a substance secreted into the blood or other body fluid or expressed at the cell's surface by malignant cells in larger quantities than that of their normal counterparts. Detection is by measuring the concentration of the marker in the body fluids, usually by immunoassay, although some markers may be detected in histological sections by immunohistochemistry. The main value of tumour markers is in following the course of a malignant disease and monitoring the response to treatment and hence determining the prognosis. They may also be used for tumour localisation and antibody-directed therapy. The following are examples of tumour markers in common use.

α-Fetoprotein (AFP). Normally synthesised in the foetal yolk sac and liver. It is increased in hepatocellular cancer and germ cell tumours, i.e. testicular teratoma.

It can be useful in monitoring the presence of metastases and response to treatment. Non-neoplastic causes of a raised AFP include cirrhosis, hepatitis and pregnancy.

Carcinoembryonic Antigen (CEA). Normally produced by the foetal gut, liver and pancreas. It is raised in tumours of the colon, pancreas and stomach. In colonic malignancy, CEA is raised in 3% of Dukes' A, 25% of Dukes' B, 45% of Dukes' C and 65% of metastatic cancer. It can be useful in assessing response to treatment and diagnosing recurrence before clinical detection. Non-neoplastic causes of raised CEA include ulcerative colitis, Crohn's and cirrhosis.

Human Chorionic Gonadotrophin (HCG). This was one of the first tumour markers to be recognised. It is raised in choriocarcinoma and hydatidiform moles. β-HCG is a valuable tumour marker for testicular cancers.

Prostate-Specific Antigen (PSA). PSA is a serine protease. Its normal function is to liquefy gel around spermatozoa. It is a very useful marker in prostatic cancer – it is organ-specific. In patients with a PSA of 4–10 ng/mL, 20–30% will have prostate cancer. With a PSA <20 ng/mL, bony metastases are rare. Non-neoplastic causes of a raised PSA include benign prostatic hypertrophy and prostatitis.

CA19-9. A tumour antigen elevated in GI malignancy. It is not diagnostic but has been used commonly in association with pancreatic malignancy. It has a sensitivity and specificity of 80–90% for pancreatic cancer and is used to monitor the success of chemotherapy. It can also be elevated in pancreatitis, gallstones, cholecystitis and cirrhosis.

CA125. Most commonly used tumour marker in ovarian malignancy. It is associated with nonmucinous tumours. An elevated level is not diagnostic of ovarian malignancy – fewer than 50% of patients with stage I have a raised CA125. In addition, raised levels are also seen in pregnancy, endometriosis and cirrhosis. CA125 is also elevated in advanced nonovarian malignancies.

CA15-3. This is a mucin marker used in the assessment of breast cancer. Patients with stage I disease may only show raised CA15-3 in approximately 10–20% of cases. In advanced cancer, the number of patients with increased levels is 50–100%. Benign breast disease may lead to elevated levels. However, CA15-3 has been used in assessing recurrence and has been shown to be prognostic – initially elevated levels are associated with a poorer prognosis. CA15-3 levels may also be raised in benign breast or ovarian disease or endometriosis.

THE MULTIDISCIPLINARY TEAM (MDT) MEETING

Patients' case histories are presented at regular MDT meetings, e.g. for breast, head and neck or skin cancer. These are attended by professionals with a specialist interest e.g. surgeons, oncologists, radiologists, pathologists and nurses. The clinical findings are correlated with the radiological and pathological investigations, including staging and grading where known, and if the findings are concordant with a diagnosis, a course of action is decided. This may be, for example, surgery with curative or palliative intent, primary radiotherapy or chemotherapy, neoadjuvant therapy or further investigation prior to treatment.

HINTS AND TIPS

PROPER PREPARATION FOR AN MDT DISCUSSION IS CRUCIAL

A patient presents to clinic with a history and/or examination findings suggestive of malignancy. Regional nodal groups and common metastatic sites should be examined.

The patient should be informed of your suspicion and the need to exclude malignancy by further investigation.

For referral to the MDT the patient needs the following to form the basis for planning management:

- Clinical presentation of findings including social and past medical history
- Tissue diagnosis with grade
- Clinical stage.

Therefore, there need to be appropriate plans for imaging the affected region (CT, MRI, endoscopic retrograde cholangiopancreatography (ERCP), magnetic resonance cholangiopancreatography (MRCP), etc.), to examine the size of the tumour and extent of invasion into the surrounding structures (T stage).

Also imaging of the common metastatic areas (regional nodal groups and distant metastatic spread), to suggest an N and M stage.

A biopsy may be performed at the time of imaging. Discuss this with your MDT radiologist, as some images are best interpreted without the changes that occur after a biopsy.

Discuss your diagnostic suspicions with the MDT pathologist to ensure you send any biopsy specimen in an optimum media (fresh, formalin, etc.). They will also give you an estimated time for diagnosis given specialist stains and/or techniques may be required.

Prepare your clinical findings, including social circumstances and comorbidities, for presentation and your investigation results for discussion. WHO performance status can be useful for decisions on operative fitness – 0 is fully active, I is restricted in strenuous activity. II is ambulatory but unable to carry out work activities, III is capable of limited self-care but in bed/chair >50% of day, IV is totally confined to bed and V is dead.

TREATMENT OF CANCER

Major treatments are surgical excision, radiotherapy, chemotherapy and hormonal manipulation. Cancers vary in their indications for treatment modalities, and different tumours vary in their response to these modalities.

Surgery

Curative

The ideal operation for cancer is the one that completely extirpates the tumour. This may require wide excision of the tumour together with removal of the lymph nodes in continuity with the tumour. Premalignant conditions may also be treated by surgery. Other modes of management such as curettage and cautery, cryotherapy or photodynamic therapy (the ablation of pharmacologically photosensitised cells using a laser, e.g. in Bowen's disease or Barrett's oesophagus) are also available.

Palliative

When operating on a tumour, it may be discovered that it is impossible to remove the primary lesion. However, a palliative operation may be carried out. The aim of palliative surgery is to alleviate symptoms and improve function and/or quality of life in the patient, e.g. bypassing an obstructing tumour in the GI tract to prevent the symptoms of intestinal obstruction.

Occasionally, operations are planned purely for palliative reasons when it is known that it will be impossible to remove the primary tumour, e.g. for bleeding, pain, obstruction. Occasionally, surgery is used to 'debulk' a tumour. This can be the case in extensive ovarian malignancy where removal of the greater mass of tumour will improve the efficacy of subsequent chemotherapy. Solitary (e.g. lung, liver, brain) metastasis or multiple metastases (subcutaneous) may be amenable to surgery, and other modalities such as radiofrequency ablation may be possible for liver metastases.

Radiotherapy

Delivery of Radiotherapy

Radiotherapy can be delivered to the site of a tumour in four ways:

- External beam radiation
- Proton beam therapy
- Implantation radiotherapy
- Systemic irradiation.

Radiation damages cells by inducing DNA damage. Cancer cells are affected more than normal cells because their DNA repair mechanisms are impaired. As a general rule, the higher the mitotic rate of a tumour, the greater the response to radiotherapy.

The absorbed dose of radiotherapy is quantified as the SI unit, the Gray (Gy) where $1\,Gy = 1\,J/kg^{-1}$. The total dose (typically around 50 Gy in solid tumours) is often divided into multiple exposures or fractions, to enable normal cells to recover and to ensure more cancer cells are exposed during radiosensitive points in the cell cycle.

External Beam Radiation. This method is the most commonly used form of radiotherapy for deeper tumours. The doses from beams from several angles can summate deep to the skin, thus avoiding the severe skin lesions that previously were a side effect of radiotherapy. Three-dimensional conformational mapping using a planning CT scan and intensity-modulated radiotherapy (IMRT) enables accurate dosing of radiotherapy fractions of photons through computer-controlled X-ray accelerators for deep asymmetric tumours, while minimising collateral damage.

Proton Beam Therapy. This uses a beam of protons to irradiate diseased tissue. The chief advantage of proton beam therapy is a steep fall-off in dose, sparing normal tissues. Therapy is the ability to precisely localise the radiation dose compared with other types of external beam radiotherapy. It is useful in treating hard-to-reach cancers, such as spinal tumours (chordomas), with a lower risk of damaging surrounding tissues and causing side effects. It has been used successfully to treat paediatric neoplasms such as medulloblastoma. Indeed, its ability to precisely target the tumour and spare surrounding tissues is particularly beneficial in children where traditional radiotherapy may affect the surrounding tissue, causing stunting of growth.

Proton beam therapy is not available in the UK at present, although its introduction at two centres is being planned Figure 7.1. Its use is controversial and expensive. It is now available at the Christie and UCHL.

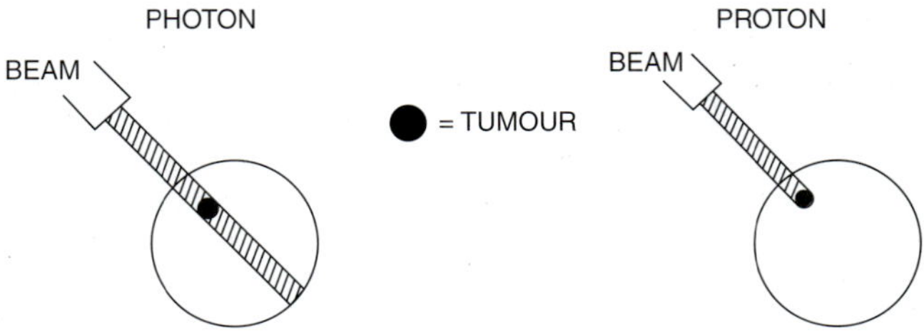

FIGURE 7.1

Comparison of photon beam and proton beam. The proton beam is more accurately aimed at the tumour and does not pass through limiting damage to surrounding tissues.

Implantation Radiotherapy (e.g. Intracavitary or Intralesional) – Brachytherapy. The source of irradiation may be placed within a cavity, e.g. in the vagina for irradiation of the cervix or directly into the lesion, e.g. iridium-192 (^{192}Ir) wires in carcinoma of the tongue. A common use is in prostate cancer with permanent seed brachytherapy in which radioactive seeds are left in the prostate and deliver radioactivity over months.

Systemic Irradiation. ^{131}I can be administered orally for follicular and papillary carcinoma of the thyroid gland. Experimentally, radioisotopes can be directed at cancer cells by attaching them to tumour-specific antibodies.

Use of Radiotherapy

Radiotherapy can be used in four ways:

- Primary treatment (radical radiotherapy)
- Neoadjuvant prior to surgery and adjuvant after surgery
- Palliation
- Systemic treatment.

Primary Treatment. Radiotherapy is used as the primary treatment with a view to a cure. Certain tumours, e.g. laryngeal, have a cure rate equal to surgery. Examples of tumours treated by radiotherapy include:

- Basal cell and squamous cell carcinoma of the skin
- Some head and neck tumours and laryngeal tumours
- Treatment of cervical cancer with chemoradiotherapy.

Hodgkin's Disease (Adjuvant and Neoadjuvant Treatment). Neoadjuvant treatment is used preoperatively to down-stage tumours, i.e. decrease size and potentially convert an inoperable tumour into an operable one. Adjuvant radiotherapy aims to control microscopic tumour deposits that have spread beyond the resection margins or are spilt during surgery. An example is radiotherapy to the scar, axillary nodes, supraclavicular and internal mammary nodes in breast cancer.

Palliative Radiotherapy

- Bony metastases – pain relief is often dramatic
- Cerebral metastases

TABLE 7.1

COMPLICATIONS OF RADIOTHERAPY

General	Tiredness, malaise
Skin	Rashes, moist desquamation
Blood vessels	Endarteritis obliterans. Impairs blood supply. Progresses for many years after treatment. Many of the effects on other systems may have endarteritis obliterans as a precipitating cause
Healing	This is delayed, e.g. failure of skin grafts, anastomotic breakdown, intestinal fistulae
Renal tract	Frequency, cystitis
GI tract	Nausea, vomiting, anorexia. Radiation proctitis (after irradiation of the cervix or prostate), causes rectal bleeding and tenesmus. Small bowel irradiation may give rise to intestinal fistulae and strictures
Head and neck	Xerostomia (dry mouth). Epiphora (red-watery eye) due to damage to tear duct. Osteoradionecrosis of the mandible

- Ulcerating or fungating breast cancer – controls oozing and bleeding and allows skin healing
- Lung cancer – to prevent cough and haemoptysis.

The complications of radiotherapy are shown in Table 7.1.

Systemic. Two types of systemic radiotherapy are used:

Total Body Irradiation. Leads to bone marrow failure and thus necessitates a bone marrow transplant; it is used in the treatment of leukaemia.

Radioactive Isotopes. This form of radiotherapy uses radioisotopes that are concentrated in the tumour and lead to local irradiation of the tumour. Examples include ^{131}I in thyroid cancer and strontium-89 in prostatic metastatic disease. Radium 223 also is used for bone metastasis in prostate cancer.

Chemotherapy

Chemotherapeutic agents destroy tumour cells in a variety of different ways. Most tumours are treated by a combination of cytotoxic drugs, the combinations being chosen so that their toxic effects on any particular organ are minimised. The most appropriate combinations have usually been established by clinical trials based on initial empiricism. Drugs are usually given in short courses with a period of rest between courses to allow recovery of the normal tissues (chemotherapy 'cycles'). The total number of cycles is varied depending upon the extent of disease, the sensitivity of the cancer to chemotherapy and the number of side effects experienced by the patient. Chemotherapy can be given in isolation, with either curative or palliative intent, or in combination with other treatments. As with radiotherapy, chemotherapy given before surgery is referred to as neoadjuvant chemotherapy (NACT) and attempts to down-grade the tumour and increase the likelihood of curative surgery. Chemotherapy following surgery to treat micrometastasis and reduce the risk of recurrence is 'adjuvant chemotherapy'.

The response of tumours to chemotherapy is very variable. Some are highly sensitive, whereas others are insensitive.

Highly sensitive tumours in which there are prospects of a cure include Hodgkin's disease, testicular teratoma, childhood leukaemias, osteogenic sarcoma (lung secondaries).

Moderately sensitive tumours where palliation is the aim include ovarian tumours, breast cancer and bronchial carcinoma.

Apart from oral and intravenous administration, cytotoxic agents may be directly administered into a tumour, e.g. 5-fluorouracil for liver metastases and close intra-arterial injection in malignant melanoma; instillation into the bladder for superficial bladder tumours.

Side Effects

Chemotherapy is toxic not only to malignant cells but also to normal body cells, especially those with a high turnover rate, e.g. bone marrow and GI epithelium. Many side effects are extremely unpleasant and should be carefully explained to and discussed with the patient prior to starting the course (→Table 7.2).

Chemoradiotherapy

The use of chemotherapy can make cancer cells more sensitive to radiation. This synergistic effect in combination has led to effective chemoradiation regimens for local/regional treatment in head and neck, anal, cervical and oesophageal cancer. This treatment can be used in the neoadjuvant setting or instead of surgery.

Hormonal Manipulation

This is applicable to carcinoma of the breast and carcinoma of the prostate. Removal of the source of hormones or blocking their effect may inhibit tumour growth.

Breast

The options available for hormonal treatment in breast cancer include:

- Inhibition of ovarian function

TABLE 7.2

SIDE EFFECTS OF CHEMOTHERAPY

Nonspecific	Nausea, vomiting, metallic taste, general malaise
GI tract	Oral ulceration, diarrhoea
Reproductive system	Loss of libido, sterility, mutagenesis
Bone marrow	Bone marrow suppression with anaemia, thrombocytopaenia, (bleeding), leukopaenia (infection)
Immune system	Immunosuppression. Opportunistic infections, e.g. candidiasis and *Pneumocystis jiroveci*
Skin	Rashes, ulceration, hair loss (regrows after course is stopped)
Urinary tract	Cystitis (cyclophosphamide), gout due to massive tumour destruction, leads to hyperuricaemia, which may lead to renal failure – prevented with allopurinol
Oncogenesis	Twenty-fold increase in incidence of other malignancies

- Blocking the binding of oestrogen to cancer cells
- Blocking peripheral oestrogen production.

Inhibition of Ovarian Function. There are three methods available to decrease oestrogen production by the ovaries:

- Surgery – oophorectomy
- Pelvic irradiation – radiotherapy
- Luteinising hormone releasing hormone (LHRH) agonists, i.e. goserelin.

Inhibition of ovarian function is important in the management of breast cancer in premenopausal women. Meta-analysis of various trials of ovarian ablation in women <50 years old demonstrated a 26% reduction in annual recurrence and 25% reduction in the annual death rate.

Blocking the Binding of Oestrogen to Cancer Cells. The anti-oestrogen tamoxifen is effective in pre- and postmenopausal women with oestrogen receptor–positive breast cancer. Tamoxifen is a nonsteroidal drug that competes with oestrogen to bind the oestrogen receptor. Meta-analysis of trials demonstrated a 25% reduction in annual recurrence and a 17% reduction in annual death rate. Tamoxifen is also a first-line drug in metastatic disease. Long-term use may be associated with an increased risk of endometrial cancer. Fulvestrant is a new anti-oestrogen that causes down-regulation of the oestrogen receptor. It can be used in tamoxifen-resistant metastatic disease.

Blocking Peripheral Oestrogen Production. Following the menopause, the main source of oestrogen production is by the peripheral conversion of adrenal androgens in liver, muscle, breast and fat – which is mediated by the aromatase enzymes. The aromatase inhibitors, e.g. anastrozole, are useful in first-line treatment and in patients who have tamoxifen-resistant metastatic disease.

Prostate

The main aetiological factor in prostate cancer is dependence on testosterone. A number of modalities are available to reduce androgen exposure.

Surgical Orchidectomy. The gold standard; has become less popular with the advent of medical alternatives.

Luteinising Hormone Releasing Hormone (LHRH) Analogues, e.g. Goserelin. This results in chemical castration by the down-regulation of receptors in the pituitary gland. It must be remembered that initial use will stimulate androgen production before inhibition (androgen flare). This may result in an exacerbation of symptoms and thus should always be given with an antiandrogen.

Oestrogen, e.g. Diethylstilboestrol. Rarely used due to considerable side effects. Results in castration levels of androgens in 1–2 weeks.

Antiandrogens. These may be steroidal or nonsteroidal. Steroidal antiandrogens, e.g. cyproterone acetate, inhibit LH release from the pituitary and decrease the binding of dihydrotestosterone to androgen receptors. Nonsteroidal antiandrogens, e.g. flutamide, block dihydrotestosterone binding but not LH production.

Biological Therapies

Human-made agents targeting specific cellular processes, rather than the DNA itself, have been developed and are used in certain cancers. Examples include tyrosine kinase inhibitors (e.g. imatinib for GI stromal tumours), immunotherapy (e.g. local administration of BCG in carcinoma of the bladder) and MAb. The use of MAb is a leading area of research, and these are increasingly being used in the first-line treatment of a number of cancers.

Examples of MAb agents currently in use include:

- Trastuzumab (Herceptin) in HER2 receptor–positive breast cancer
- Rituximab targeting the CD20 antigen overexpressed in non-Hodgkin's lymphoma
- Ipilimumab, which prevents the action of CTLA-4, an antigen that is usually responsible for inhibiting the action of T cells. Ipilimumab blocks the action of CTLA-4, and thus allows cytotoxic T cells to recognise and destroy cancer cells. Used in malignant melanoma.
- Bevacizumab (Avastin) targeting vascular endothelial growth factor (VEGF) to inhibit angiogenesis in bowel cancer.

HINTS AND TIPS

PUTTING IT TOGETHER – TO 'GET YOUR HEAD AROUND' CANCER MANAGEMENT

Think of a cancer in terms of three areas:

- Local (T stage)
- Regional (draining lymph node groups) (N stage)
- Metastasis (M stage).

The primary should be adequately treated (often by surgical excision with adequate margins, to prevent local recurrence). Excision may be easier after pretreatment (neoadjuvant therapy) with chemotherapy and/or radiotherapy, which can shrink the tumour. Some cancers are best treated by chemotherapy, radiotherapy or chemoradiation alone. Local treatment may be performed early enough to prevent regional or systemic spread. This spread may already have occurred without being clinically or radiologically detectable at the time.

Regional lymph nodes may be sampled at the time of excision of the primary (e.g. sentinel node biopsy for breast cancer or melanoma) to stage the disease better with a view to planning management. Positive nodes on biopsy would indicate treatment of the area (see below). Regional lymphadenectomy or radiotherapy/chemoradiation in the absence of lymphadenopathy can be undertaken (elective lymphadenectomy). This may be recommended if there is a high (e.g. >20%) chance of existing subclinical metastases at a given T stage of a tumour and is weighed against the risks.

Biopsy-proven regional disease is treated with surgical lymssphadenectomy (axilla, groin, neck) or with radiotherapy ± chemotherapy. In the absence of regional control, the nodes will grow with significant morbidity (ulceration, bleeding, pain), which may prove fatal (carotid artery or femoral artery erosion). It does not prevent metastasis, which may already be present.

Subclinical systemic metastases are treated by systemic treatment e.g. adjuvant chemotherapy. The probability of presence or absence of metastases is calculated using a variety of methods, normally from the pathological T and N stage, and the evidence of the benefits of systemic therapy is balanced against the side effects.

Clinically or radiologically apparent metastases may be treated by surgery if isolated (e.g. brain/lung/liver metastases) or subcutaneous; with chemotherapy if multiple; with radiotherapy to prevent degradation/restore function to a particular area, e.g. painful bone metastases; or with other modalities such as radiofrequency ablation for liver metastases. Solitary oligometastases can now sometimes be treated with sterotactic ablative radiotherapy (SABR), which delivers a very high dose of radiotherapy to a small area of disease.

PALLIATIVE CARE

Most patients with disseminated malignancy deteriorate until they reach a terminal phase. This phase is often accompanied by many unpleasant symptoms that are difficult to control. Support should be not only medical but also emotional, psychological and spiritual. Patients with a complex need in any of these areas should be referred to a specialist palliative care team, which is available in the community as well as in hospitals. Initially, it may be possible to manage the patient at home with the support of family, friends, palliative care nurse (Macmillan nurse in the UK) and family doctor. Death should be met with privacy and dignity. Eventually, hospitalisation may be required for terminal care. Patients may be best managed in a hospice where all expertise is available to support the patients and their relatives.

Most hospitals in the UK now employ an end-of-life care pathway that can be tailored to the needs of the individual patient. Patients in the UK have previously been treated using the Liverpool Care Pathway (LCP). The chief principle of the LCP was to provide gold-standard hospice-style care for those who were dying, regardless of where they were. The LCP was heavily criticised in the UK national press in 2013, and as a result, the Department of Health released a statement indicating that the LCP should be phased out over the following 6–12 months and replaced with individually designed care pathways to suit the needs of each individual patient. It is important to remember that a care pathway is not a substitute for clinical judgement which should be applied if and when the case arises.

Principles of Palliative Care

1. Assess prognosis.
2. Discuss prognosis with patient and relatives.
3. Inform the family doctor of the situation and encourage regular visits. Maintain continuity out-of-hours.
4. Ensure all support that the patient may need to remain at home as long as possible, e.g. commodes, home help, district nurse, Macmillan nurse.
5. Provide support for carers.
6. Anticipate symptoms and try to prevent them, e.g. nausea, constipation, pain.
7. Regular review of medication to make sure pain relief is adequate and nausea and vomiting are well controlled.
8. Arrange appropriate hospital or preferably hospice accommodation when/if required.

Treatment of Symptoms

Pain

Regular opiates are needed to prevent 'breakthrough' pain. Suitable analgesics include morphine sulphate tablets (MSTs), fentanyl patches, morphine elixir, subcutaneous morphine, PCA via pump and spinal opioids; local blocks may help. In addition, steroids and chlorpromazine may be helpful. The correct dose of analgesic is that which relieves the pain. Opiate dependency and respiratory depression are irrelevant in the dying patient.

Nausea and Vomiting

Antiemetics should be given, e.g. metoclopramide, domperidone, prochlorperazine. Ondansetron is a very effective antiemetic. Levomepromazine can be used for intractable nausea and vomiting in palliative care. In addition, haloperidol is increasingly used to help with nausea in the dying patient. If there is a mechanical reason for the nausea and vomiting, it may be difficult to control. If possible, a tube gastrostomy carried out under local anaesthetic may help. It allows the patient to swallow a suitable liquidised diet, which will then drain through the gastrostomy tube without subsequent vomiting.

Constipation

Regular laxatives and enemas may be required.

Dysphagia

A stent may be already in situ. Tasty liquidised food is helpful.

Mouth Care

Careful attention to oral hygiene may prevent problems. 'Swish and swallow' nystatin may prevent candidiasis. If ulcers develop, they may be treated with local anaesthetic gel and metronidazole gel.

Cough

This may be treated with morphine or codeine. Antisecretory medications (e.g. hyoscine butylbromide) should be used to reduce respiratory secretions.

Insomnia and Agitation

Treat with chlorpromazine or benzodiazepines (midazolam).

HINTS AND TIPS

Most hospitals have an end-of-life care pathway, which contains a list of anticipatory medications that should be prescribed PRN for all of those who are in the terminal phase of their illness. In hospital, these medications can then be administered as soon as they are needed without having to wait for a doctor to sign the prescription. Similarly, any patient discharged home should be given a prescription for a limited supply of each of these medications so that they can be given by district nurses or Macmillan nurses as soon as they are needed.

Chapter 8

Head, Neck and Otorhinolaryngology

Mr Neil Baillie

CHAPTER OUTLINE

The head and neck region is complex and accounts for a diverse range of benign and malignant conditions in both the paediatric and adult population. Lumps in the head and neck are relatively common, and patients may present to the ENT, general, dental or maxillofacial surgery clinics.

SCALP AND FACIAL SWELLINGS

These largely are lesions of the skin, adnexa and subcutaneous tissue and include epidermoid cysts, boils and abscesses, lipomas, papillomas, squamous cell carcinomas, basal cell carcinomas and malignant melanomas (→Ch. 20). In addition, an ivory osteoma may occur as a smooth, hard swelling of the outer table of the skull. The skin moves freely over it. Confirmation is by X-ray. It is asymptomatic and should only be excised if it enlarges.

NECK SWELLINGS

The neck is divided topographically into an anterior and posterior triangle by the sternocleidomastoid muscle. The anterior triangle is bounded by the midline anteriorly, the anterior border of sternocleidomastoid posteriorly and the lower border of the mandible superiorly. The posterior triangle is bounded anteriorly by the posterior border of sternocleidomastoid, posteriorly by the anterior border of trapezius and inferiorly by the middle third of the scapula. A convenient classification for lumps in the neck includes superficial swellings, lymph nodes and deep swellings (→Table 8.1).

The key to assessment and diagnosis of soft tissue neck swellings is careful history taking and examination of the site, size and nature of the swelling (soft or firm, mobile or fixed, transilluminates, presence of a bruit). In adults, the gold-standard initial investigation for a lump in the neck is USg FNAC. Computerised tomography (CT), positron emission tomography-CT (PET-CT) or magnetic resonance imaging (MRI) are also useful imaging modalities and may be combined with other investigations such as Mantoux skin testing or blood tests for FBC, ESR, CRP or HIV, depending on the differential diagnosis.

TABLE 8.1

SWELLINGS IN THE NECK

Superficial	Sebaceous cyst Lipoma Dermoid cyst Abscess
Lymph Nodes	
Deep	
Anterior triangle	Move on swallowing: • Thyroid nodule • Thyroglossal cyst Do not move on swallowing: • Salivary glands • Branchial cyst • Peripheral nerve tumours • Carotid body tumour • Carotid aneurysm • Sternocleidomastoid 'tumour'
Posterior triangle	Cervical rib Peripheral nerve tumours Cystic hygroma

HINTS AND TIPS

Assume all patients over 40 years of age with a new-onset neck lump to have malignant disease until proven otherwise.

Superficial

Superficial lumps can occur in either the anterior or posterior triangle of the neck, and they arise within the skin or subcutaneous tissues; these include epidermoid cysts, lipomas, dermoids and infective lesions, e.g. boils and abscesses (→Ch. 20).

Lymph Nodes

There are over 300 lymph nodes in the neck arranged in a superficial and deep lymphatic drainage system. Superficial lymph nodes predominantly lie along the course of the external and anterior jugular veins, while deep lymph nodes are distributed in a horizontal and vertical arrangement. The horizontal chain of deep cervical lymph nodes consists of the submental, submandibular, preauricular and occipital nodes, whilst the vertical group contains a lateral chain of lymph nodes in the anterior triangle of the neck closely related to the IJV and a central neck compartment of lymph nodes surrounding the trachea and thyroid gland. There are also lymph nodes in the posterior triangle of the neck. On the left side of the neck, lymph drains into the terminal portion of the left thoracic duct and into the right lymphatic duct on the right side. The causes of cervical lymphadenopathy are shown in Table 8.2.

TABLE 8.2

CAUSES OF CERVICAL LYMPHADENOPATHY

Infection	Local lesions on head and neck Upper respiratory tract infection Tonsillitis Glandular fever Toxoplasmosis Tuberculosis HIV Cat-scratch disease
Malignancy	Primary: • Lymphoma • Leukaemia Secondary: • Upper aerodigestive tract carcinoma • From solid tumours almost anywhere in the body, e.g. breast, lung, renal, prostate
Inflammatory	Sarcoidosis Kawasaki's disease Rosai–Dorfman disease

Investigation of Cervical Lymphadenopathy

1. A full ENT clinical examination is required, including flexible nasopharyngolaryngoscopy. Look for skin lesions on the face, neck or scalp, and pay attention to the oral cavity, nasal cavity, postnasal space, oropharynx (tonsil and tongue base), hypopharynx, larynx and thyroid gland.
2. A full general examination of the chest, breast, abdomen, testes and lower limb is required. Check for axillary and inguinal lymphadenopathy. Check for hepatosplenomegaly.
3. Hb, FBC, ESR, EBV, *Toxoplasma* screen, viral antibodies, HIV
4. FNAC (under ultrasound guidance if available)
5. Chest X-ray (CXR) for hilar nodes or primary lung tumour
6. MRI or CT of the head and neck to examine nodes, and look for possible primary site if malignancy suspected
7. Endoscopic examination under anaesthesia with of the nasopharynx, oropharynx, hypopharynx, larynx, trachea, upper bronchi and upper oesophagus ± stomach, and biopsy of suspicious areas or possible primary sites, i.e. nasopharynx, tongue base, tonsil and pyriform fossae
8. Excision biopsy of lymph node – only if diagnosis is uncertain and after a UADT malignancy has been excluded, or lymphoma is suspected and tissue is required for histological subtyping.

Deep Swellings of the Anterior Triangle

These can be classified into lumps that move on swallowing and those that do not.

Swellings That Move on Swallowing

THYROID. Swellings of the thyroid gland are dealt with in Chapter 12.

THYROGLOSSAL DUCT CYST. This is an embryological remnant of the thyroid duct and may present as a fluctuant swelling in the midline of the neck. It is the most common midline neck cyst, affecting 1–7% of the population, with an equal male-to-female preponderance. Thyroglossal duct cysts may occur anywhere along the line of the thyroid gland descent but is most common just above the body of hyoid bone (in over 75% of cases).

Symptoms and Signs. Painless cystic swelling in midline of the neck that moves on swallowing or tongue protrusion. Occasionally (in approximately 5% of cases) it may become infected, with associated pain, tenderness, erythema and increased swelling.

Treatment. Cyst and tract excision including middle third of the hyoid bone (Sistrunk's procedure). Ultrasonography should be performed preoperatively confirming the thyroid gland is in its normal anatomical position, as the thyroglossal duct cyst may occasionally contain the only thyroid tissue present.

Swellings That Do Not Move on Swallowing

SALIVARY GLANDS: INFLAMMATORY. Causes of salivary gland swellings are shown in Table 8.3. Although the parotid gland lies mainly over the ramus of the mandible, lesions of the parotid tail often present in the upper neck.

ACUTE SIALADENITIS. Acute inflammation of the salivary glands may arise due to bacterial or viral pathogens. Worldwide, the most common cause of viral sialadenitis in childhood and teenagers is mumps, which causes bilateral parotid swelling.

Acute bacterial sialadenitis is more commonly unilateral from *Staphylococcus aureus* infection. The parotid gland is usually involved in elderly, dehydrated and debilitated patients, whilst other secondary causes include radiation therapy or immunosuppression. The submandibular gland is affected from duct obstruction due to sialolithiasis (over 80% of the time) or, less frequently, from odontogenic infection.

Symptoms and Signs. Pain and swelling over the salivary glands, made worse by eating, associated with general malaise. Examination reveals erythema, tenderness and swelling in the region of the gland, plus or minus purulent discharge from the involved salivary duct.

Treatment. Viral parotitis – supportive treatment with analgesia, rehydration and sialogogues. Acute bacterial sialadenitis is treated with analgesia, antibiotics, rehydration, sialogogues and good oral hygiene. Calculi, if present, should be removed by

TABLE 8.3

SWELLINGS OF THE SALIVARY GLANDS

Inflammatory and infective	Acute sialadenitis, e.g. mumps parotitis Chronic sialadenitis, e.g. calculus, duct stenosis
Neoplastic	Benign: • Pleomorphic adenoma • Warthin's tumour Malignant: • Mucoepidermoid carcinoma • Adenoid Cystic Carcinoma • Metastasis
Autoimmune	Sjögren's syndrome

surgical removal or basket retrieval. If an abscess forms, surgical drainage may be required, paying attention to protect the facial nerve, if the parotid gland is involved. Recurrent parotitis should be investigated by USS or sialography to exclude sialectasis and areas of duct stricture.

CHRONIC SIALADENITIS. In the submandibular gland, this is usually due to a calculus in Wharton's duct. Salivary calculi involve the submandibular gland in over 80% of cases, are composed of calcium phosphate and carbonate and are usually radio-opaque. Sialolithiasis tends to affect adults in the third and fourth decades of life, with males more commonly affected than females. Chronic parotitis from recurrent bacterial infection may occur secondary to duct ectasia or strictures, but the exact pathogenesis is poorly understood.

Symptoms and Signs. Pain and swelling of the affected gland occur on eating and drinking, which is reproducible in clinic by oral administration of sialogogues such as lemon juice. Infection and abscess formation may ensue. Inspect the duct orifice. In the case of submandibular gland calculi, the swelling may be observed in Wharton's duct. Feel along the duct in the floor of mouth with a gloved finger whilst also externally palpating the gland. The calculus may be felt.

Investigations

- USS is the investigation of choice, as it permits assessment of the gland, duct system and calculus which usually has an acoustic shadow.
- 'Floor of mouth' radiographic view for submandibular calculi in Wharton's duct where ultrasound findings are equivocal or unavailable
- If no stone is seen, consider sialography.
- Sialoendoscopy is increasingly used in the diagnosis and treatment of salivary gland outflow obstructive conditions.

Treatment

- Submandibular duct stones that are easily palpable in the floor of the mouth may be removed by incising directly over the stone into the duct. Beware of potential injury to the closely related lingual nerve. The stone is extracted, and the duct may be closed or marsupialised. Smaller stones under 7mm in size may be removed using wire basket retrievers inserted into the duct under endoscopic or sialographic guidance in specialist centres.
- With duct stenosis, a ductoplasty (widening of the duct orifice) or endoscopic balloon dilatation of strictures is performed.
- For intraglandular stones, total (submandibular) or partial (parotid) gland excision is indicated for recurrent symptoms.

SALIVARY GLANDS: AUTOIMMUNE. This is a slow painless enlargement of salivary glands. Two syndromes are described.

Mikulicz's Syndrome. This causes symmetrical enlargement of the salivary glands, both parotid and submandibular. There is involvement of lacrimal glands and a dry mouth (xerostomia). IgG4 levels are elevated whilst anti-Ro (SSA) and Anti-La (SSB) tests are negative. Females are more commonly affected.

Sjögren's Syndrome. Similar symptoms to Mikulicz's syndrome but with keratoconjunctivitis sicca (dry eyes). Positive antibodies to Ro (SSA) and La (SSB), Schirmer's and

Rose Bengal tests, and minor salivary gland biopsy showing lymphocytic foci can aid diagnosis.

Treatment. No treatment may be required, but steroids may help. Dry eyes may be treated with hypromellose drops (artificial tears). Artificial saliva and oral moisturisers can help xerostomia.

SALIVARY GLANDS: TUMOURS. Salivary gland tumours are uncommon, accounting for less than 4% of head and neck neoplasms, with the majority benign. Over 70% of salivary gland tumours arise in the parotid gland, of which over 75% are benign pleomorphic adenomas, whilst the remaining 11% of tumours occur in the submandibular gland and 14% in minor salivary glands. The minor salivary glands are numerous (between 500 and 1000) and situated throughout the submucosa of the upper aerodigestive tract, with the highest concentration in the hard palate. In general, the smaller the salivary gland, the more likely a neoplasm will be malignant.

BENIGN SALIVARY GLAND TUMOURS: PLEOMORPHIC ADENOMA. Some 75% occur in the parotid. The old name of 'mixed parotid' tumour arose from the histological appearance of mixed elements, i.e. epithelial, myoepithelial and stromal components. They are slow growing and may enlarge over many years. The tumour may possess 'pseudopodia' or satellite nodules in up to 25% of cases, hence shelling out (enucleation) of these lesions may leave residual disease, with a high rate of recurrence. The risk of malignant transformation for pleomorphic adenomas is low, at less than 10% in patients observed for a period of over 15 years.

Symptoms and Signs. Affects adults in the third to sixth decades, occurring more frequently in females than males. It presents as a painless slow-growing swelling. Examination reveals a nontender, firm or nodular, mobile swelling, usually behind the angle of the mandible. Always test the integrity of the facial nerve. Diagnosis is made on history, examination and FNAC. MRI findings of a well-defined parotid mass with postcontrast enhancement and high T2 signal may be diagnostic.

Differential Diagnosis. Parotitis, sebaceous cyst, lipoma, preauricular lymph node, tumour of the mandibular ramus.

Treatment. Partial parotidectomy, i.e. removal of the tumour with a surrounding cuff of normal salivary gland tissue, whilst preserving the facial nerve. Over 90% of parotid gland pleomorphic adenomas reside in the superficial lobe and are lateral to the facial nerve; hence the majority of patients will undergo a superficial parotidectomy. Enucleation, or extracapsular dissection, may be associated with a higher incidence of recurrence and hence discouraged.

Complications. These include wound infection, bleeding and haematoma formation, facial nerve palsy (either temporary or permanent), salivary fistula (usually dries up spontaneously) and Frey's syndrome (gustatory sweating due to facial sweat fibres undergoing neoinnervation from parasympathetic secretomotor fibres). The patient should be warned of all these complications, especially the risk of facial nerve palsy, prior to informed consent being obtained.

BENIGN SALIVARY GLAND TUMOURS: ADENOLYMPHOMA (WARTHIN'S TUMOUR). Also known as adenolymphoma or papillary cystadenoma lymphomatosum, this is a mixed cystic and solid tumour containing epithelial and lymphoid elements. It is benign, arising almost exclusively in the parotid gland, accounting for 10% or parotid tumours, and 10% are bilateral. Warthin's tumour affects males more than females in the fifth to seventh decades of life, and there is an association with cigarette smoking.

Symptoms and Signs. Slow-growing painless swelling in tail of the parotid region. It is usually soft and well defined. Uncommonly, there may be pain and increased swelling secondary to an immunological response in the lymphoid component.

Treatment. Surgical excision. If patient is elderly and diagnosis certain, they can be managed conservatively. Recurrence after surgery is uncommon.

MALIGNANT SALIVARY GLAND TUMOURS. Malignant salivary gland lesions are uncommon, with diverse histology and may be primary or secondary, with an estimated incidence of 0.9 per 100,000 in the USA. The parotid gland is involved in 20% of tumours, submandibular gland in 50% of malignant neoplasms, whilst over 70% and 50% of sublingual gland and minor gland tumours, respectively, are malignant.

Mucoepidermoid carcinoma is the most common primary salivary gland malignancy, occurring more frequently in adult females and is also the most common salivary gland carcinoma in children. Adenoid cystic carcinoma (ACC) is another common salivary gland malignancy and occurs in over 50% of submandibular gland carcinomas. Both mucoepidermoid and ACCs can present with tumours of variable grade that determine their pathological behaviour. A predominant histological feature of ACC is perineural invasion, which confers a worse prognosis.

HINTS AND TIPS

In parts of the world with high rates of skin cancer (such as Australia, Europe, etc.), always consider that a malignant parotid mass may be due to metastasis from a cutaneous malignancy, such as squamous cell carcinoma or melanoma.

Other malignant tumours of the parotid include acinic cell carcinoma, carcinoma ex-pleomorphic adenoma, squamous cell carcinoma and salivary duct carcinoma. The parotid gland contains 10 to 20 intraglandular nodes, and as it drains lymph from the scalp, face and ear canal, it is susceptible to metastasis from primary cancers in these regions. Additionally, primary lymphoma of the major salivary glands accounts for 5% of extranodal lymphomas.

Symptoms and Signs. Patients present with a slow-growing, painless, firm, irregular salivary gland mass. Occasionally there may be associated pain or facial nerve palsy.

Treatment. Surgery ± adjuvant radiotherapy. Surgery consists of total parotidectomy with preservation of the facial nerve if it is functioning preoperatively and there is no gross involvement with cancer. An ipsilateral neck dissection may be required depending on the tumour subtype and grade. Lymphomas may require incisional tissue biopsy for diagnosis prior to definitive nonsurgical oncological therapy.

Branchial Cyst

Anomalies of the second branchial arch account for over 95% of branchial cleft disorders.

Symptoms and Signs. The peak age of presentation is in the third decade of life, and it is more common in females. The most common presenting symptom is a lateral neck mass of variable consistency below the angle of the mandible, at the anterior aspect of the sternocleidomastoid muscle. There may be an associated sinus or fistulous tract that opens over the anterior border of sternocleidomastoid. The sinus may extend up between the internal and external carotid arteries and open as a fistula into the tonsillar fossa. Branchial cleft cysts may become inflamed and enlarge following an upper respiratory tract infection.

Differential Diagnosis of a Branchial Cyst. This includes a benign or malignant lymphadenopathy, haemangioma and carotid body tumours. A cystic lateral neck mass arising in an older patient should raise suspicion of a cystic lymph node metastasis from a squamous carcinoma of the upper aerodigestive tract. Diagnosis may be confirmed on FNAC, correlated with radiological findings (on USS, CT or MRI) of a fluid-filled cyst.

Treatment. Surgical excision of cyst, sinus or fistula tract. Infected branchial cysts should have an initial course of antibiotic treatment, prior to surgery once the inflammation has settled.

Carotid Body Tumour

Also known as paraganglioma or chemodectoma, these benign tumours are the most common head and neck paraganglioma and originate from extra-adrenal paraganglionic cells derived from the neural crest. They are slow growing and arise from the carotid body at the carotid bifurcation. Paragangliomas account for 1 in 30,000 head and neck tumours. Rarely do these tumours become malignant.

Symptoms and Signs. Presents at age 40–60 years. Painless, slow-growing lump with transmitted pulsation, that is mobile laterally, but not vertically (Fontaine's sign). With continued enlargement, patients may complain of progressive hoarseness, cough or dysphagia. There may be associated fainting episodes from pressure on the carotid sinus.

Investigations

- MRI with gadolinium demonstrates characteristic diagnostic features. CT scanning with intravenous contrast is a useful alternative.
- Angiography: has been superseded by MRI, but is useful for preoperative embolisation. It shows a vascular blush with splaying of the carotid bifurcation (Lyre sign).

Treatment. Predominantly surgical excision. Large tumours may require carotid bypass grafting. Radiation therapy may be considered in patients not suitable for surgery.

Carotid Aneurysm

A true aneurysm is extremely rare. A false aneurysm may arise following penetrating trauma of the neck. A tortuous carotid artery appearing from under the anterior border of sternocleidomastoid may give the impression of an aneurysm. Careful examination will reveal the tortuosity and lack of an expansile area.

Deep Swellings of the Posterior Triangle

The most common cause of a deep posterior triangle neck swelling is cervical lymphadenopathy. Less common causes are cystic hygroma and cervical rib.

Cervical Rib

This is a supernumerary rib arising from the seventh cervical vertebra. It occurs in 0.2–0.5% of the population, is often asymptomatic and is usually discovered incidentally on radiological imaging. It is occasionally palpable and may cause neurological or vascular symptoms in the arm (→Ch. 16).

Symptoms and Signs. Vascular symptoms, e.g. Raynaud's phenomenon or venous thrombosis in the arm, ± neurological symptoms, such as wasting of the small muscles of the hand (T1 myotome) and paraesthesia on the inner upper aspect of the arm in the dermatomal distribution of T1. There may be a palpable lump in the supraclavicular fossa.

Diagnosis

- CXR to include thoracic inlet
- Count the ribs on the CXR – if there are 13, there is a cervical rib.

Treatment. Surgical excision of rib if symptomatic.

Subclavian Artery Aneurysm

This is often just a poststenotic dilatation distal to a cervical rib. True aneurysms are rare. Treatment is by excision if symptomatic.

Pharyngeal Pouch

See under Voice and Swallowing Disorders, p. 141.

Cystic Hygroma

Also known as lymphangioma, this is a collection of dilated lymphatic sacs that fail to connect with the rest of the lymphatic system.

Symptoms and Signs. Swelling in the lower part of the posterior triangle present at birth or occurring in the first few years of life. The mass is soft, smooth, compressible, transilluminable and nontender. There may be associated difficulty feeding or respiratory compromise depending on the size and location.

Treatment. Surgical excision. Cyst walls are thin and rupture easily. They can be difficult to excise completely. Macrocytic lesions may be successfully treated with sclerotherapy.

ORAL DISORDERS

Stomatitis

Stomatitis is a general term used to describe inflammation of the lining of part or the whole of the mouth (→Table 8.4).

General Principles of Management

Examination. Check dentures, check for sharp teeth, check oral hygiene. Examine clinically for signs of vitamin deficiency, malignancy or haematological disease.

Investigations

- Hb
- FBC
- ESR
- Blood sugar
- CXR
- VDRL
- Mouth swab with film for fungus, and culture and sensitivity for bacteria.

Treatment. Treatment is that of the underlying disease.

TABLE 8.4
CAUSES OF STOMATITIS

Local	Ill-fitting dentures Sharp teeth Smoking Local ulceration Infections, e.g. herpes simplex, candida, Vincent's angina Trauma, e.g. chemical, thermal, irradiation
General	Haematological: • Leukaemia • Agranulocytosis • Anaemia • Vitamin deficiency; B and C Debilitating illness: • Cancer • Tuberculosis • Following major surgery

Ulcers

Oral cavity ulcers may occur due to a variety of benign and malignant conditions. The main causes are the result of local trauma from teeth or thermal injury, recurrent aphthous ulcers, malignancy, drugs (NSAIDs, nicorandil), infective organisms such as the herpes simplex virus, syphilis or TB, as well as a diverse range of systemic conditions such as haematinic deficiencies and rheumatic diseases.

HINTS AND TIPS

A persistent solitary oral cavity ulcer of more than 2 weeks, duration, with no signs of obvious healing, must be considered a malignant ulcer and referred to a head and neck surgeon for urgent assessment and management.

Traumatic. Caused by a sharp tooth, ill-fitting dentures or accidental trauma. They heal rapidly once the causative agent is removed.

Aphthous. These are usually recurrent and affect at least 10% of the population, with a slight female preponderance. They may be minor, major or herpetiform and are usually multiple, painful, ovoid, small ulcers (2–4 mm in diameter, or up to 1 cm for major ulcers) surrounded by an erythematous halo. They may also be solitary. Aphthous ulcers usually heal spontaneously within 10 days. A local anaesthetic gel may relieve pain.

Herpes Simplex. Multiple small painful ulcers of the mouth or lips, and they may occur in debilitated or immunosuppressed patients. Treat with topical acyclovir cream, oral or intravenous acyclovir.

Syphilitic. These are rarely seen. Chancre in primary, 'snail track' in secondary and gumma in tertiary syphilis.

TUBERCULOUS. These are rare and usually found on the tongue. They are painful ulcers with undermined edges and are associated with advanced pulmonary tuberculosis.

MALIGNANT. See below.

Leukoplakia

Leukoplakia may occur anywhere within the mouth but is common on the tongue. Affected areas appear thickened, white and may show cracks and fissures. It is a clinical term with no defined histological definition. Unlike *Candida*, it cannot be rubbed off. The exact aetiology of leukoplakia is poorly understood. Oral leukoplakia carries a 25% risk of progressing to invasive carcinoma.

Erythroplakia

This is a red mucosal plaque with no obvious predisposing mechanical or inflammatory cause. The risk of malignancy is over 30%.

Cystic Lesions of the Lips and Mouth

Mucous Retention Cyst

These occur on the inner surface of the lips and anywhere in the mouth where there are mucus-secreting glands. Obstruction to the duct causes the cyst.

Symptoms and Signs. Painless cystic lesion. Pinkish grey. Transilluminates.

Treatment. Excision or may burst spontaneously.

Ranula

A large mucus extravasation cyst of the floor of the mouth, which resembles a frog's belly (*ranula* is Latin for frog). It occurs in children and young adults, due to obstruction of the sublingual salivary gland, most commonly secondary to trauma. A plunging ranula extends through or behind the mylohyoid muscle and may present as a lump in the neck.

Symptoms and Signs. Soft, fluctuant swelling in the floor of mouth that often transilluminates.

Treatment. Surgical excision of cyst and affected sublingual gland.

Sublingual Dermoid

Dermoid cysts form along lines of embryological fusion. In the oral cavity they are usually midline, arising from inclusion of ectoderm during fusion of the mandibular processes, and account for less than 0.01% of all oral cavity cysts. Although congenital, dermoid cysts are rarely noticed before the age of 10 years.

Symptoms and Signs. Swelling in floor of mouth. Usually painless. May present as 'double chin' if below mylohyoid. In the latter case it may be mistaken for a thyroglossal cyst.

Treatment. Excision or leave alone if diagnosis confirmed and patient is asymptomatic.

Tonsillitis

Acute tonsillitis is a common ENT condition. The most common bacterial organisms are group A β-haemolytic *Streptococcus*. The tonsils are MALT lying in the space bounded by the anterior and posterior faucial pillars formed by the palatoglossus and palatopharyngeus muscles, respectively.

Symptoms and Signs. The patient complains of a sore throat, difficulty swallowing, earache and general malaise. Patients may be pyrexial, with associated cervical lymphadenopathy. Bacterial tonsillitis (β-haemolytic *Streptococcus, Staphylococcus, Haemophilus influenzae*) may present with pus on the tonsils (follicular tonsillitis) and is an indication for broad-spectrum antibiotic therapy.

Investigations

- Diagnosis is clinical. Inflammatory markers such as CRP and white cell count may be elevated.
- Monospot test for infectious mononucleosis (glandular fever).

Treatment. Broad-spectrum antibiotics for bacterial tonsillitis, analgesia and rehydration. Avoid amoxicillin if infectious mononucleosis is suspected, as it may be complicated by a rash.

Lymphoproliferative disorders such as lymphoma should form part of the differential diagnosis of persistent or unilateral tonsillar enlargement, especially in adults.

Tonsillectomy

Tonsillectomy is not usually indicated for infrequent episodes of tonsillitis. Recurrent bacterial tonsillitis, multiple quinsy or respiratory obstruction may warrant surgery. This is performed under general anaesthetic. An incision is made in the mucosa of the anterior faucial pillar and the tonsil dissected from its fossa. Bleeding may be prevalent from its inferior aspect where it is closely related to the tongue base; hence, the lower pole is often ligated to avoid haemorrhage. Recognised complications of tonsillectomy include infection and primary, reactionary or secondary bleeding. Secondary haemorrhage is the most common complication, with rates between 2% and 10% (depending on the institution or tonsillectomy technique), and the majority of these patients only require conservative treatment.

VOICE AND SWALLOWING DISORDERS

Hoarseness

Hoarseness is a very common symptom, and in the majority of cases these disorders are due to benign pathology. However, hoarseness is also a presenting symptom for laryngeal cancer. Careful history and examination will help discriminate between benign and malignant causes of hoarseness. Key points in the history include: occupation (i.e. professional voice user, e.g. musician, teacher, doctor, etc.), smoking and alcohol history, and associated ENT/general symptoms. Flexible laryngoscopy is an essential component of the ENT/head and neck examination.

Hoarseness of less than 2 weeks, duration associated with pyrexia, sore throat and an upper respiratory tract infection is usually due to acute laryngitis that settles with conservative measures. Where the voice change is intermittent and of variable duration with a history of high vocal load ± gastro-oesophageal reflux and normal vocal cord examination, muscle tension dysphonia is the presumptive diagnosis, and these patients may benefit from a voice clinic assessment for speech therapy and further management. Persistent, painless, progressive hoarseness (especially in a smoker) should arouse suspicion for laryngeal cancer, particularly if a unilateral laryngeal lesion is evident on flexible laryngoscopy. Other (benign) causes of constant progressive hoarseness include vocal cord nodules, polyps, cysts, granuloma, papillomas, Reinke's oedema and vocal cord paralysis.

HINTS AND TIPS

Progressive hoarseness in a smoker of more than 2 weeks, duration warrants urgent referral to an ENT surgeon to exclude laryngeal carcinoma.

Vocal Cord Paralysis

Immobility of the vocal cord occurs due to disruption of laryngeal motor innervation. If unilateral, patients may be asymptomatic, or complain of a weak breathy voice, ineffective cough and/or aspiration. Bilateral vocal cord paralysis may result in upper airway obstruction requiring a tracheostomy.

In adults, over 30% of cases have no known cause, 30% are secondary to recurrent laryngeal nerve injury during surgery (e.g. thyroid surgery), whilst the remaining 30% are due to neoplasia (e.g. hypopharyngeal carcinoma, thyroid tumours, paragangliomas). In childhood, unilateral vocal cord paralysis is most commonly due to birth trauma or surgery for other congenital abnormalities. In cases with no history of recent surgery, a CT scan from skull base to diaphragm is a necessary investigation to exclude pathology along the entire course of the vagus and recurrent laryngeal nerves. Most cases of idiopathic vocal cord paralysis recover (can take up to 12 months). Voice rehabilitation may include speech therapy, injection laryngoplasty or permanent vocal cord medialisation in those cases unlikely to recover neural function.

Swallowing Disorders

Swallowing is a complex, highly coordinated physiological process with a number of phases that are mostly under involuntary control. Difficulty swallowing, or dysphagia, is a common symptom for a variety of acute and chronic throat disorders.

Acute dysphagia, with associated pyrexia, sore throat and cervical lymphadenitis, is indicative of a UADT infection and usually settles with supportive therapy. In the absence of systemic symptoms, acute dysphagia may be due to food bolus or foreign body (e.g. coin, denture) impaction, and a history of foreign body or food bolus ingestion is usually forthcoming, but this may be lacking from a child or an elderly patient with dementia.

Constant progressive dysphagia for solids and weight loss should arouse suspicion of an UADT carcinoma, especially with risk factors for head and neck cancer, such as heavy alcohol and tobacco consumption and other ENT symptoms such as otalgia and hoarseness. Progressive dysphagia may develop secondary to CN palsies or other neurological causes (e.g. multiple sclerosis, CVA).

Pharyngeal pouch, or Zenker's diverticulum, is another cause of constant, progressive dysphagia and is usually associated with regurgitation of undigested food and halitosis. This is a pulsion diverticulum of the pharynx occurring between the thyropharyngeus and cricopharyngeus muscles of the inferior constrictor, i.e. through Killian's dehiscence. The peak age of onset is in the seventh decade. A barium swallow reveals the pouch in most cases. Never perform 'blind' endoscopy – the pouch may be perforated if the endoscope passes into it. Treatment is usually by endoscopic pouch stapling for those greater than 2 cm. Cricopharyngeal myotomy and external pouch excision are other treatment options.

The management of dysphagia is directed at the underlying cause. General measures such as dietician assessment, rehydration and nutritional supplementation, with close monitoring for refeeding syndrome, are also important.

CARCINOMA OF THE UPPER AERODIGESTIVE TRACT

Head and neck cancer is the seventh most common cancer worldwide. The management is complex and best done in centres with high-volume, subspecialist experience, as part of a multidisciplinary head and neck oncology team.

All patients with suspected head and neck cancer require a thorough history and general ENT examination, including flexible nasopharyngolaryngoscopy. Investigations are directed at confirming the diagnosis, assessing the extent of primary tumour and status of regional lymph nodes, as well as distant metastasis, in addition to post-treatment surveillance.

Curative treatment involves management of the primary site and neck nodes and is dependent on patient factors (i.e. age, comorbidities), disease factors (TNM stage) and institution factors (i.e. local surgical or radiation oncology expertise). The main aims of therapy are to (1) achieve the best locoregional control and survival rates, (2) maintain form and function of the UADT and (3) minimise associated toxicity from the various treatment modalities.

The Oral Cavity

Squamous cell carcinoma accounts for 90% of oral cancers and may present as a lump or ulcer in any of the oral cavity subsites (i.e. lip, alveolar ridge, oral tongue, floor of mouth, retromolar trigone, buccal region or hard palate). It spreads via lymphatics to cervical lymph nodes, in up to 50% of patients at initial presentation, conferring a worse prognosis. There are over 300,000 new cases of oral cancer per year worldwide, with significant geographical variation. It has predominance for elderly males, but the incidence is increasing in younger adults.

Predisposing Factors. Tobacco and alcohol are the most common preventable risk factors and have a synergistic effect on predisposition. Carcinogenic agents may predispose to epithelial dysplasia that progresses to invasive carcinoma. Betel nut derivatives, which are regularly consumed in large parts of India and Southeast Asia, increase the risk of developing oral cancer. Ill-fitting dentures and sharp teeth have been postulated as risk factors for oral cancer, but this remains controversial. Exposure to sunlight may predispose to carcinoma of the lip.

Investigations

- Imaging: Orthopantogram (OPG), MRI or CT scan of the head and neck, CXR, ± CT chest depending on stage
- FNAC of any suspicious neck nodes
- Intraoral biopsy, incisional or excisional depending on size of tumour
- Panendoscopy and biopsy to exclude synchronous lesions (up to 6% of patients)

Treatment. Surgery ± adjuvant radiotherapy and chemotherapy is the mainstay of treatment, and the extent of surgery or intensification of adjuvant therapy is determined by disease stage.

- Small tumours less than 2 cm can be treated by wide local excision ± neck dissection or sentinel lymph node biopsy, without the need for tissue reconstruction.
- Larger lesions may require more extensive surgery, e.g. subtotal glossectomy, modified radical neck dissection and free flap reconstruction. Occasionally part of the mandible may have to be resected with the tumour.

Prognosis. The 5-year survival is over 75% for stage I and II tumours and under 50% for stage III and IV disease.

Squamous Cell Carcinoma of the Pharynx and Larynx

The upper aerodigestive tract can be further subdivided into the nasopharynx (region posterior to the nasal choana, extending from skull base superiorly to the level of the soft palate inferiorly), oropharynx (from palatoglossus anteriorly, including posterior third of tongue and soft palate, to upper border of epiglottis), larynx and hypopharynx (from upper border of epiglottis superiorly to cricoid cartilage inferiorly, with the larynx anteriorly).

Nasopharyngeal Carcinoma (NPC)

Uncommon in Western populations but endemic in parts of Southern China, Hong Kong and Southeast Asia, with age-adjusted incidence rates of 20 to 30 per 100,000. There is a significant male preponderance. Predisposing factors include nitrosamine-containing foods and the Epstein–Barr virus, with no contribution from cigarette smoking for endemic types of NPC. Local invasion can occur into the sphenoid sinus, oropharynx, orbit or skull base.

Symptoms and Signs. Patients often present late with enlarged nodes in the neck (often bilateral). Other symptoms include epistaxis, nasal obstruction, blood in saliva, conductive hearing loss, tinnitus, sore throat or CN palsies (CN V, VI, IX, X, XII).

Investigations

- MRI or CT scan of head and neck
- CT chest ± abdomen
- FNAC
- USg core biopsy of lymph node if FNAC nondiagnostic
- Panendoscopy of the UADT and biopsy.

Treatment. Radiation therapy for early-stage tumours, or chemoradiation for advanced disease, is the treatment of choice. Salvage surgery to the primary site or neck is reserved for treatment failures.

Prognosis. Stage I and II NPC treated with radiation alone have 5-year survival rates of over 80%, whilst patients with advanced (stage III and IV) disease have a 70% overall 5-year survival.

> **HINTS AND TIPS**
>
> An adult male of Chinese origin presenting with a neck lump, unilateral deafness and epistaxis or blood-stained saliva should be considered to have a nasopharyngeal carcinoma until proven otherwise.
>
> Likewise, an adult male of Chinese origin with a neck lump should be investigated for nasopharyngeal carcinoma.

Oropharyngeal Carcinoma

The oropharynx is further subdivided into the tonsils, tongue base, soft palate and posterior pharyngeal wall (caudal to the nasopharynx and superior to the epiglottis). Most tumours are squamous in origin; however, the high density of lymphoid tissue within the oropharynx means that higher proportions of lymphoma are found in this region. Traditional risk factors for head and neck cancer, such as tobacco and alcohol consumption, are implicated in the pathogenesis of oropharyngeal carcinoma. However, there is increasing incidence of oropharyngeal carcinoma associated with high-risk HPV (subtype 16 and 18) in nonsmoking, nondrinking younger adults. In some parts of the world (e.g. Europe, USA, Australia), HPV-associated oropharyngeal carcinoma currently accounts for 60–80% of new oropharyngeal tumours and is the predominant site for head and neck squamous cell carcinoma.

Symptoms and Signs. Patients often present at an advanced stage with cervical lymphadenopathy ± sore throat, referred otalgia (CN IX or X involvement), oral bleeding or dysphagia. The tonsil fossa is the most frequent location for oropharyngeal tumours (in over 70% of cases), and patients may present with an exophytic mass, fullness or ulceration in the tonsil.

Investigations

- MRI or CT scan of head and neck
- CT Chest
- FNAC
- USg core biopsy of lymph node if FNAC nondiagnostic
- Panendoscopy of the UADT and biopsy.

Treatment. Early-stage oropharyngeal squamous cell carcinoma may be treated with either surgery or radiation therapy. Transoral robotic surgery is increasingly being used as the surgical technique of choice. Advanced primary lesions with extensive tongue base or mandibular involvement may experience significant functional impairment from surgical resection, which often involves a lip split mandibulotomy or lateral pharyngotomy, and/or free flap reconstruction; hence, these patients will be offered primary chemoradiation treatment in most centres.

Most oropharyngeal lymphoproliferative malignancies are usually non-Hodgkin's lymphomas, predominantly B-cell in origin. These are treated with radiation therapy and/or chemotherapy depending on the histological type and stage.

Prognosis. The survival rate for nonsmokers/nondrinkers with HPV-associated oropharyngeal carcinoma is good, with around 85–90% still alive 5 years post-treatment, even for stage III and IV disease. Conversely, smokers with HPV-negative tumours have a poorer outcome, with a 5-year overall survival of 40%.

Carcinoma of the Hypopharynx and Cervical Oesophagus

The hypopharynx is further subdivided into the pyriform sinuses, postcricoid region and posterior pharyngeal wall. The cervical oesophagus comprises the part of the upper oesophagus situated above the thoracic inlet and is contiguous with the postcricoid region superiorly. Hypopharyngeal squamous cell carcinoma is less common compared with other head and neck subsites, with an annual incidence of 1 per 100,000 in the USA, most frequently involving the pyriform sinuses. Aetiological factors include excessive alcohol consumption and cigarette smoking, and less commonly Paterson–Brown–Kelly (Plummer–Vinson) syndrome.

Symptoms and Signs. Presenting complaints include progressive dysphagia, odynophagia, hoarseness, cervical lymphadenopathy and/or referred otalgia. Clinical examination will demonstrate a palpable neck mass in 50% of cases, and the primary lesion may be evident on flexible laryngoscopy.

Investigations

- Barium swallow
- MRI or CT scan of head and neck

- CT chest
- PET-CT
- FNAC of cervical nodes
- Panendoscopy of the UADT and biopsy.

Treatment. Primary conservation surgery and/or radiotherapy are treatment choices for early-stage (I and II) disease. Larger primary lesions may require more extensive resections that will compromise swallowing function; hence, primary chemoradiation with surgical salvage is becoming the standard care in most Western institutions. Total laryngopharyngectomy ± total oesophagectomy, neck dissection and free/pedicled flap reconstruction or gastric pull up may be required when there is disease outside the pharynx/larynx, or for extensive cervical oesophageal involvement.

Prognosis. Advanced stage hypopharyngeal and cervical oesophageal carcinoma are associated with poor prognosis. Less than 30% of patients remain alive at 5 years following curative treatment. Most of these patients succumb either to complications of treatment, second primary tumours or distant metastasis.

Laryngeal Carcinoma

Reflecting its embryonal structure, the larynx is subdivided into three anatomical subsites: supraglottis (above the vocal cords), glottis (vocal cords) and subglottis (below the vocal cords). As per other head and neck subsites, laryngeal cancers are predominantly squamous cell carcinomas and are also the second commonest UADT malignancy, with an annual incidence of over 11,000 cases in the USA. There is a male preponderance, whilst the glottis is the most frequent laryngeal subsite involved with carcinoma, followed by the supraglottis and rarely the subglottis. Risk factors include tobacco use (glottic cancer) and alcohol excess (supraglottic cancer).

Symptoms and Signs. Depends to a degree on subsite, but most patients report voice change or hoarseness. Cervical lymphadenopathy is uncommon with glottic cancer but is frequent with supraglottic cancer and often bilateral. Dyspnoea is a late presenting symptom. Flexible laryngoscopy usually reveals a laryngeal lesion.

Investigations

- MRI or CT scan of head and neck
- CT chest
- FNAC of cervical nodes
- Panendoscopy of the UADT and biopsy.

Treatment. Dependent on site and disease stage. Early-stage I and II tumours may have single-modality surgical or radiation therapy. Advanced-stage III and IV disease is treated with combined-modality therapy, either chemoradiation ± surgical salvage or surgery (partial/total laryngectomy and neck dissection) ± adjuvant radiotherapy.

Prognosis. Early (stage I and II) glottic cancer has a 5-year survival rate of over 80–95%, whilst patients with advanced disease have a 60% 5-year overall survival.

Neck Dissection

This is the removal of lymph nodes and surrounding fibrofatty tissue from between the superficial and/or visceral/deep layers of the deep cervical fascia, in various compartments of the neck.

Cervical lymph nodes are arranged according to a system (levels I–VI) developed by the Memorial Sloan Kettering group:

I. Submental/submandibular nodes. The submental triangle (Ia) lies between the anterior belly of the digastric muscles and the hyoid bone. The submandibular triangle (Ib) is bounded superiorly by the body of the mandible and inferiorly by the anterior and posterior bellies of the digastric muscle.
II. Upper jugular nodes from skull base to level of hyoid bone
III. Middle jugular nodes situated from hyoid bone to lower aspect of cricoid cartilage
IV. Lower jugular nodes located between cricoid cartilage and clavicle
V. Posterior triangle lymph nodes
VI. Anterior compartment neck nodes, extending from level of hyoid bone to the suprasternal notch.

Indications. A therapeutic neck dissection is performed when there is clinical or radiological evidence of metastatic cervical lymphadenopathy in head and neck cancer, and surgery is being used as a treatment modality. When there is no evidence of positive neck nodes (cN0), a prophylactic neck dissection may be performed if the probability of occult cervical metastases is high (arbitrarily >20%), or when access to branches of the external carotid artery/IJV is required for microsurgical anastomosis in free flap reconstruction.

Classification. Traditionally, a radical neck dissection removes all lymph node–containing tissue from levels I–V, whilst sacrificing three nonlymphatic structures, i.e. the spinal accessory nerve, IJV and sternocleidomastoid muscle.

Modified radical neck dissection, similar to a radical neck dissection but with preservation of one or more of the nonlymphatic structures.

A selective neck dissection preserves one or more lymph node levels in addition to the three nonlymphatic structures and is usually performed in the context of the cN0 neck.

Extended neck dissection: any of the procedures described above may become an extended neck dissection when lymph node groups, neural, vascular or musculocutaneous structures not normally removed in a neck dissection are resected.

Complications. Bleeding; infection; marginal mandibular (CN VII); CN X, XI, XII; phrenic or lingual nerve injury; chyle leak; pneumothorax; air embolus; carotid artery injury; cerebrovascular accident; skin flap necrosis.

DISORDERS OF THE EAR

Otitis Externa

Acute or chronic inflammation of the external auditory canal skin. The lifetime general population risk of developing otitis externa is 10%.

Acute otitis externa is the most common form, with an annual incidence of 1%. Risk factors include swimming, warm humid climates, trauma from foreign bodies (e.g. cotton buds and hearing aids), dermatological conditions (e.g. eczema, psoriasis) and diabetes. Most cases are caused by bacteria, particularly *Pseudomonas aeruginosa* and *S. aureus*. Fungal infection, predominantly with *Aspergillus or Candida species, is more frequent in humid climates and in otitis externa previously treated with antibiotics*. Furunculosis can occur around an infected hair follicle and is usually excruciatingly painful.

Necrotising (or malignant) otitis externa is a rare non-neoplastic infection of the external ear canal that progressively spreads along the soft tissues and bones of the lateral skull base, with ultimate involvement of intracranial structures. It predominantly occurs in elderly, diabetic or immunocompromised patients and may be fatal without prompt recognition and treatment. Most cases are caused by *P. aeruginosa*.

HINTS AND TIPS

Adult patients with persistent otitis externa (i.e. over 4 weeks) unresponsive to appropriate antibiotic or antifungal therapy should be referred to an ENT surgeon for urgent biopsy of the ear canal skin to exclude malignancy, most commonly squamous cell carcinoma.

Symptoms and Signs. Pain, swelling, itching and scanty discharge from the ear canal are typical. A conductive hearing loss may be present. Classically, there is tenderness on moving the pinna or tragus, and the ear canal is swollen and contains scanty moist debris. Patients with necrotising otitis externa complain of persisting severe otalgia, *worse at night*, and often have granulation tissue visible on the floor of the ear canal at the bony cartilaginous junction on otoscopy. Lower CN palsies, usually starting with facial palsy, indicates a poor prognosis, and death is usually from intracranial complications, including internal carotid artery or sigmoid sinus thrombosis.

Treatment. Aural toilet and topical antibiotic–steroid eardrops (with pseudomonas cover) are essential components of treatment and usually lead to resolution of symptoms. An ear wick may be required if the external auditory canal is too swollen to admit eardrops. Ear swabs for microbiological analysis should be performed when there is no response to initial topical therapy or where infection has spread beyond the ear canal, which is also an indication for oral or systemic antibiotics.

Necrotising otitis externa is investigated with CT scan/MRI of the skull base/brain to assess the extent of disease and technetium ± gallium scans for bony involvement. Treatment consists of strict diabetes control, regular aural toilet and topical antipseudomonal therapy, with the mainstay of treatment being long-term (6–12 weeks) systemic antibiotics. Interval gallium scanning can help assess response to treatment and determine the duration of antibiotic therapy. Surgery has a limited role and is reserved for debridement of abscesses or sequestra, or when tissue specimens are required for histological or microbiological analysis. More extensive surgery risks facilitating the spread of infection by breaking down natural barriers and exposing uninfected tissue.

Acute Otitis Media (AOM)

This is a suppurative infection of the midde ear mucosa and is one of the commonest infections of childhood, affecting 45–60% of children under the age of 5 years. The incidence in adults is estimated at 1.5–2.3%. AOM is usually a bacterial complication of a viral upper respiratory tract infection. The most frequent causative organisms are *S. pneumoniae, H. influenzae* and *Moraxella catarrhalis*. Eustachian tube dysfunction is the most important contributing factor in the development of AOM and immune dysfunction may also contribute. Children have a shorter, narrower Eustachian tube and a relatively immature immune system, explaining the frequency of AOM in this age group. Pressure from the mucopurlent secretion in the middle ear can compromise the tympanic membrane vasculature, causing painful ischaemia and may cause a perforation.

Symptoms and Signs. Pain, fever, malaise, vomiting. A red/purple and bulging tympanic membrane and mucopurulent aural discharge if the tympanic membrane perforates. A conductive hearing loss is present and may last for weeks to months after the acute infection due to a persisting sterile middle ear effusion (otitis media with effusion or 'glue ear'). Rarely, patients may develop complications such as mastoiditis (recognisable by a red boggy post-aural swelling displacing the pinna), meningitis, facial nerve palsy or labyrinthitis.

Treatment. Most cases resolve spontaneously within 3 days and require only supportive therapy with analgesia, antipyretics and topical anaesthetic drops. Oral antibiotics make little impact on the number of children whose symptoms improve, or the incidence of recurrent infection, short-term hearing loss or tympanic membrane perforation, and should not be offered routinely. Antibiotics should be considered if there is no improvement after 3 days, in children under the age of 2 years and in cases with otorrhoea. Antibiotics should be prescribed immediately on presentation in children and young people who are systemically unwell, have symptoms and signs of a more serious condition, or are at high risk of complications. Amoxicillin is the first-choice antibiotic, with clarithromycin and co-amoxiclav among second-line options. Mastoiditis is rare, with or without antibiotic therapy, but if present requires incision and drainage of the abscess, mastoidectomy, tympanostomy tube insertion and systemic antibiotic therapy.

Recurrent AOM requiring antibiotics (> three episodes in 6 months or four episodes in 12 months) may benefit from myringotomy and tympanostomy tube insertion. OME lasting longer than 3 months with associated hearing loss on audiometry may be offered tympanostomy tube insertion or hearing aids.

Chronic Suppurative Otitis Media (CSOM)

CSOM may be subdivided into two distinct clinical entities depending on the absence or presence of cholesteatoma. A cholesteatoma is an epithelioid cyst caused by ingrowth of squamous epithelium into the normally mucosa-lined middle ear and mastoid air cell system. CSOM without cholesteatoma is due to chronic bacterial inflammation of the middle ear mucosa associated with a tympanic membrane perforation. The tympanic membrane perforation is most commonly a sequela of AOM. It affects 0.9% of children and 0.5% of adults.

Cholesteatomas may be congenital (abnormal focus of squamous epithelium in the middle ear cleft during development) or, much more commonly, acquired as a result of perforation or thinning and retraction of the tympanic membrane due to chronic Eustachian tube dysfunction and previous AOM. In acquired CSOM with cholesteatoma, there is ingrowth of squamous epithelium and trapping of keratin debris within the middle ear air system. The trapped keratin debris becomes infected, most commonly with waterborne pseudomonas, with associated chronic inflammation. Cholesteatoma is a destructive disease process, estimated to affect 5 per 100,000 population in the Western world, with higher incidence in developing countries.

Symptoms and Signs. Persistent or recurrent, usually painless, purulent or clear otorrhoea, hearing loss (usually conductive), swollen auditory canal, tympanic membrane perforation with erythematous, oedematous middle ear mucosa. Otorrhoea associated with cholesteatoma is usually foul-smelling. CSOM with cholesteatoma may also be complicated by ossicular damage (causing conductive hearing loss), labyrinthitis (causing sensorineural hearing loss and vertigo), facial paralysis, cerebral venous sinus thrombosis, meningitis or intracerebral abscess. Untreated, it is often eventually fatal.

Investigations

- Audiometry – most commonly shows conductive hearing loss
- High-resolution CT scan of the temporal bone to determine extent of cholesteatoma and for operative planning

- In cases where doubt exists about the diagnosis or extent of the disease, a diffusion weighted MRI imaging can help distinguish cholesteatoma from other forms of inflammatory tissue.
- Examination of the ear under anaesthesia is sometimes necessary in children who are uncooperative with examination in clinic.

HINTS AND TIPS

A cholesteatoma should be suspected where there is recurring or persisting foul-smelling otorrhoea and hearing loss failing to settle with antibiotic therapy. The diagnosis is essentially a clinical one, based on findings at otoscopic or microscopic examination, with the presence of a tympanic membrane defect and squamous epithelium within the middle ear cleft being the classic observation.

Treatment. Perform regular aural toilet. Topical antibiotic/steroid therapy to control infection and granulation tissue. A tympanoplasty is often curative in CSOM without cholesteatoma but can be complicated with recurrence of AOM if Eustachian tube dysfunction persists. Tympanomastoidectomy surgery to remove all squamous epithelium from the middle ear and mastoid air cells and repair the tympanic membrane is the cornerstone of CSOM with cholesteatoma management. Hearing rehabilitation may be achieved using ossiculoplasty, hearing aids or cochlear implants upon eradication of disease.

FACIAL PARALYSIS. The facial nerve is a derivative of the second branchial arch and contains sensory, parasympathetic as well as motor fibres. The facial nerve has a complex intracranial, temporal and extratemporal course prior to innervating the muscles of facial expression, hence pathology in any of these areas may present with facial weakness.

Bell's palsy is the commonest (idiopathic) cause of facial paralysis, affecting 20–30 people per 100,000 population. It presents with a rapid onset of unilateral facial paralysis occurring within 72h. A diagnosis of Bell's palsy should only be made after a thorough ENT and CN examination ± investigations, following which other causes of facial palsy have been excluded. The exact aetiology of Bell's palsy is unknown, but it is postulated to arise secondary to a viral infection (herpes virus). Other notable causes of facial paralysis include temporal bone fractures, penetrating facial trauma, infections (e.g. Ramsay Hunt syndrome, AOM, necrotising otitis externa, Lyme disease), cholesteatoma, neoplasms (e.g. malignant parotid tumours, facial neuroma, vestibular schwannoma), systemic disease (e.g. sarcoidosis, HIV, multiple sclerosis) or congenital conditions (e.g. Möbius syndrome).

The management of facial paralysis is determined by the underlying cause. General measures include an ophthalmology review to exclude ocular damage and the use of eye protection ± lubricants when eye closure is affected. Physiotherapy with facial massage and exercise may be helpful. For Bell's palsy a reducing dose of oral steroids over a 10–14-day period (1mg/kg up to 60mg/day) is recommended, ideally commenced within 72h of onset of symptoms. The use of oral antivirals (e.g. acyclovir) for Bell's palsy is controversial but may be offered in combination with steroid therapy in severe to complete paralysis (e.g. valciclovir 1g TID for 1 week). Over 85% of patients with Bell's palsy make a full recovery.

HINTS AND TIPS

Progressive facial paralysis is uncharacteristic of Bell's palsy and is more indicative of neoplasia. Such patients, or those previously diagnosed with Bell's palsy, whose facial weakness has not significantly improved within 2–4 weeks of initial onset, require urgent referral to an ENT surgeon for further assessment and management.

DISORDERS OF THE NOSE AND PARANASAL SINUSES

The external nose and nasal cavity can be examined using a headlight or head mirror and nasal speculum. A rigid or flexible nasendoscope allows for a more comprehensive examination of the nasal cavity and postnasal space.

Nasal Obstruction

In the paediatric population, this may be congenital or acquired. More prevalent congenital causes in neonates include choanal atresia or a meningoencephalocele. Neonates are obligate nasal breathers up to 3 months of age; hence, bilateral nasal obstruction in neonates may result in an airway emergency at birth. Common acquired causes of nasal obstruction in childhood include adenoidal hypertrophy, allergic rhinitis and nasal foreign bodies. Foreign bodies are associated with unilateral foul-smelling purulent discharge and may require removal under a general anaesthetic. Consider cystic fibrosis as a cause of childhood nasal obstruction in regions where the disease is more prevalent.

In adults, unilateral nasal obstruction may arise secondary to a deviated nasal septum or a nasal mass, which may be benign (polyp, papilloma) or malignant (tumour). Consider carcinoma in patients with more recent onset of nasal obstruction and associated symptoms of epistaxis, pain or a neck lump.

Bilateral nasal obstruction commonly caused by rhinosinusitis (inflammation of the nasal mucosa) due to allergy, infections (viral, bacterial, fungal, TB) or systemic conditions (sarcoidosis, granulomatosis with polyangiitis (GPA)). A thorough history with particular attention to onset, duration and associated symptoms together with a full ENT examination including nasoendoscopy usually determines the diagnosis in most cases.

NASAL POLYPS. Polyps are pedunculated masses of oedematous mucosa that arise from the sinuses or the lateral nasal wall. They are associated with conditions that cause chronic nasal inflammation, most commonly CRS, but may also arise in asthma, aspirin-exacerbated respiratory disease, cystic fibrosis and autoimmune disease. Treatment is with topical ± systemic steroid therapy with surgical removal for incomplete response. More recently, biologic agents that target type 2 inflammation have shown promise in poorly controlled polyposis. Unilateral polypoid swelling within the nasal cavity should raise suspicion of neoplasia and should be referred urgently to an ENT surgeon for evaluation.

RHINOSINUSITIS. This may be acute (< 4 weeks), recurrent acute (> four acute episodes/year), subacute (4–12 weeks) or chronic (>12 weeks). ARS is a very common disorder and is characterised by inflammation of the nasal and sinus mucosa lasting less than 4 weeks in duration. It is commonly associated with a viral (rhinovirus, influenza, parainfluenza) upper respiratory tract infection followed by secondary bacterial infection (*H. influenzae, Sc. pneumoniae, Staph. aureus*). In the USA, ARS accounts for 25 million physician visits annually.

ARS patients present with nasal obstruction, facial pain and mucopurulent nasal discharge or rhinorrhoea. Nasoendoscopy shows inflamed nasal mucosa, oedematous middle meati ± mucopus. Investigations are not usually required, as the condition is self-limiting. Most patients with a viral ARS recover within 5–7 days without medical intervention, although nasal decongestants can be helpful for symptom relief. Acute bacterial rhinosinusitis is suggested by symptoms including purulent drainage that worsens after 5 days or persists beyond 10 days and/or symptoms that are out of proportion to those typically associated with a viral upper respiratory process. Acute, recurrent acute and subacute bacterial rhinosinusitis should be treated with 7–10 days of broad-spectrum antibiotics, intranasal steroids and decongestants. Acute rhinosinusitis may be complicated by spread of infection and inflammation to the orbit, facial skeleton or intracranial regions. Surgical treatment in the form of endoscopic sinus surgery may be required for resistant cases of ARS, or in the presence of complications.

CRS is persistent inflammation of the nasal and sinus mucosa for more than 12 weeks, duration. It may occur with or without nasal polyps. It can be precipitated by ARS. Overall prevalence is reported as 5–28%. Numerous host (e.g. allergy, mucociliary dysfunction), local (e.g. sinus anatomy) and environmental factors (e.g. smoking, micro-organisms) contribute to the development of CRS, but the exact aetiology remains poorly understood. CRS is associated with asthma, which shows a prevalence of 25% in CRS compared to 5% of the general population.

The diagnosis is based on the presence of at least two of the following: nasal obstruction/congestion, rhinorrhoea, postnasal drip, facial pain and altered smell (hyposmia) lasting 12 weeks or longer. Nasal examination may show rhinitis, polyps, oedematous middle meati and mucopus. Investigations such as skin prick test or RAST may reveal allergic causes, whilst blood tests to exclude chronic granulomatous diseases such as granulomatosis with polyangiitis (antineutrophil cytoplasmic antibodies, ANCA) or sarcoidosis (serum ACE) may be necessary. CT scans of the paranasal sinuses are not necessary for diagnosis but highlight the extent of disease and help plan surgical treatment if required.

The mainstay of CRS treatment is medical, using allergen avoidance, regular saline nasal douching, intranasal steroids ± oral antihistamines and infrequent short periods of rescue oral steroids (prednisolone 1mg/kg). Surgery is reserved for failure of medical therapy and usually involves functional endoscopic sinus surgery (FESS) ± septoplasty.

Fungal Rhinosinusitis (FRS). FRS may be invasive or noninvasive, and disease progression is determined in some cases by the patient's immune status. Noninvasive types of FRS such as fungal balls or eosinophilic fungal disease occur in immunocompetent patients. AIFRS almost always occurs in immunosuppressed individuals (e.g. neutropenia, post-transplant patients) and is invariably fatal if not diagnosed promptly and treated aggressively. It is an ENT emergency. The most common organism in AIFRS is *Aspergillus* sp. (*A. fumigatus*) or mucormycosis.

Unlike AIFRS, chronic invasive fungal sinusitis occurs in patients with little or no immunocompromise. It is a rare disease and is more prevalent in parts of Africa and India. Surgical treatment is usually curative.

TUMOURS. Tumours of the paranasal sinuses are uncommon. Benign tumours include inverted papillomas, juvenile angiofibromas and osteomas. The commonest malignancies are squamous cell carcinomas, minor salivary gland tumours, melanoma and sarcomas.

Patients may be asymptomatic or present with unilateral nasal obstruction. Associated recurrent epistaxis, facial pain or neuralgia, or a lump in the neck should raise the index of suspicion for malignancy.

MRI and CT scans will help identify the extent of the tumour and help plan surgical resection after discussion in the head and neck cancer or skull base MDT. Adjuvant radiotherapy ± chemotherapy may be indicated. Depending on the site and stage of disease, a variety of endoscopic or open surgical techniques may be employed ± free flap reconstruction.

ENT EMERGENCIES

Epistaxis

Acquired causes of nosebleeds include local trauma, anticoagulants, benign and malignant tumours, allergic rhinitis, liver and renal failure and blood dyscrasias, such as primary and secondary thromobocytopaenia, lymphoma, leukaemia and aplastic anaemia. Congenital causes include hereditary haemorrhagic telangiectasia, haemophilia and von Willebrand's disease.

Little's area (on the anterior nasal septum) is the most common site of bleeding, accounting for over 90% of epistaxis. Minor bleeds may cease with local pressure, topical application of adrenaline or silver nitrate cautery.

Heavier bleeds, which do not settle with conservative measures, will require nasal packing using proprietary nasal balloons or tampons or impregnated ribbon gauze (e.g. BIPP) layered within the nasal cavity. Posterior nasal bleeding may be controlled by passage of a Foley catheter into the nasopharynx and inflation of the balloon to tamponade the nasal cavity. Stop and/or reverse anticoagulant therapy as indicated by the underlying medical condition and severity of epistaxis.

Uncontrollable bleeding after cautery and appropriate nasal packing requires examination of the nasal cavity and postnasal space under anaesthesia ± ligation of the sphenopalatine, internal maxillary, anterior ethmoidal or external carotid arteries, following appropriate resuscitation with fluids or blood products. Poor surgical candidates or those failing surgical treatment should be referred to an interventional radiologist for arterial embolisation.

All patients with significant epistaxis should have a full blood count to assess the haemoglobin and platelet count in addition to clotting studies.

Nasal Trauma

A simple 'broken nose' may be reducible by manipulation if managed within 2h of injury, after which swelling may obscure the deformity. However, manipulation can be attempted at 7–14 days postinjury, once swelling has resolved and before significant callous formation prevents fracture mobilisation.

Submucosal nasal septal haematomas require urgent incision and drainage with nasal packing and broad-spectrum antibiotic therapy to prevent cartilage necrosis and a resultant 'saddle-nose' deformity.

Any nasal trauma associated with high-energy trauma and other deformity (e.g. malocclusion, trismus, diplopia) should be investigated with a CT scan.

Swallowed Foreign Body

Chicken or fish bones can become entrapped in the upper aerodigestive tract. The most common site is the vallecula (in the oropharynx), but other subsites such as the palatine tonsils, tongue base or pyriform sinus may be involved. The patient presents with drooling and a feeling of irritation at the back of the throat. Oropharyngeal foreign bodies may be removed under local anaesthetic using forceps.

Foreign bodies in the pyriform sinus or postcricoid region may cause dysphagia, dysphonia or odynophagia. Cervical surgical emphysema suggests pharyngeal perforation. If suspected, this may be confirmed on an urgent water-soluble contrast swallow, prior to rigid endoscopy, which will permit removal of the offending foreign body. In cases of perforation, there is a risk of mediastinitis, and a fine-bore nasogastric feeding tube should be passed under direct vision to bypass the site of perforation. The patient should receive broad-spectrum intravenous antibiotics and be closely observed whilst nil by mouth for 5–7 days. Larger foreign bodies (such as marbles, coins or batteries) swallowed by children become trapped at the level of cricopharyngeus, and in extreme cases may present with stridor and respiratory compromise. Urgent pharyngo-oesophagoscopy and removal is required. Lodged button batteries are of particular concern, as, in contact with mucosa, they rapidly induce an alkaline environment causing tissue necrosis and perforation. They should be removed within 2h.

Peritonsillar Abscess (Quinsy)

The peritonsillar (or quinsy) abscess is an acute suppurative infection in the peritonsillar space that may occur following an episode of acute tonsillitis. Peritonsillar abscesses can arise in patients without a prior history of tonsillitis, leading to suggestions that it may be due to infection and abscess formation within the minor Weber's salivary glands that reside in the submucosa of the soft palate. Patients usually present with odynophagia, 'hot potato' voice, drooling, foul-smelling breath and trismus. If untreated, infection can easily spread to the parapharyngeal space with resultant sequelae. Quinsy is treated by incision and drainage under local or, occasionally, general anaesthetic, after appropriate intravenous rehydration, analgesia and broad-spectrum antibiotic therapy.

Deep Neck Space Infections

These may arise from a myriad of causes such as odontogenic or pharyngeal infections, UADT foreign bodies, penetrating cervicofacial trauma, intravenous drug use or immunodeficiency. In children, ARS is the most common cause of retropharyngeal lymphadenitis, with subsequent retropharyngeal abscess formation in a minority of cases.

The fascial layers and structures of the neck together form a number of real and potential spaces in which infection and abscesses may develop. These include, amongst others, the parapharyngeal, retropharyngeal and masticator spaces. The presenting symptoms and severity of deep neck space infections may depend on which compartments are involved.

Patients may be asymptomatic but usually present with inflammatory symptoms and signs such as pain, fever, neck swelling or erythema, in addition to ENT symptoms such as dysphagia, odynophagia, referred otalgia, trismus, hoarseness or dyspnoea. A full ENT examination including flexible pharyngolaryngoscopy is mandatory and may reveal the underlying source of infection, such as poor dentition. Where available, a contrast CT scan of the head and neck (± chest) is the imaging investigation of choice.

Treatment is directed at urgently securing the airway, then fluid resuscitation, broad-spectrum intravenous antibiotic therapy ± surgical exploration and abscess drainage.

Acute Epiglottitis

Caused by *H. influenza* type B, acute epiglottis is a potentially fatal infection presenting in children of 2–7 years of age. Symptoms include stridor and dyspnoea – worse on lying supine, dysphagia and excessive drooling. The child sits upright (tripod position) and is distressed. Widespread vaccination has reduced the incidence of this, and it responds to amoxicillin therapy. On presentation, humidified oxygen should be administered. Direct laryngoscopy may cause life-threatening obstruction and should only be performed by clinical staff with the means to secure the airway. A tracheostomy may be necessary if orotracheal intubation is difficult.

Acute Sensorineural Hearing Loss (SNHL)

Sudden SNHL may be instantaneous or occur over a period of hours. It is an ENT emergency that requires prompt investigation and treatment. Sudden SNHL is rarely bilateral, affects 5–20 per 100,000 people per year and is usually idiopathic. Peak incidence is in the sixth decade, affecting males and females equally. Infection (e.g. meningitis, Lyme disease, mumps, measles), head trauma, ototoxic drugs, neoplasms (e.g. vestibular schwannoma, meningioma), neurological (e.g. multiple sclerosis) and autoimmune disorders (e.g. SLE, GPA) are other causes. Examination of the ear to exclude wax, tympanic membrane perforation or middle ear effusion is required, in addition to tuning fork test, CN and a full ENT examination. Initial investigations include pure tone and speech audiometry to assess the degree of hearing loss, whilst other tests such as MRI brain or autoimmune screen are directed at excluding other causes of sudden SNHL. Management is determined by the cause and is usually empirical for the majority, consisting of prompt administration of oral steroids (e.g. Prednisolone 60 mg/day for 7 days). Salvage treatment with intra-tympanic steroid injections ± hyperbaric oxygen therapy may be offered for those not responding to oral steroids.

PROCEDURE

SURGICAL TRACHEOSTOMY

This is a surgical procedure to create an opening in the trachea. It may be performed under local anaesthesia (emergency tracheostomy) or general anaesthesia, and the indications include (1) emergent or expectant upper airway obstruction, (2) prolonged orotracheal intubation and requirement for assisted ventilation weaning, (3) bronchial toileting and (4) lower airway protection from aspiration. Early complications include tube dislodgement or mucous plug obstruction, wound infection, bleeding, recurrent laryngeal nerve injury, tracheo-oesophageal fistula, surgical emphysema or pneumothorax. Late side effects include tracheal stenosis, tracheomalacia, tracheocutaneous fistula and, in rare cases, tracheal innominate artery fistula.

PROCEDURE

OPEN TRACHEOSTOMY

- An elective tracheostomy is performed in the operating theatre under general anaesthesia, with the patient in a supine position, neck flexed and head extended.
- The intended tracheostomy tube is selected and the cuff checked for leaks.
- A 4 cm transverse skin incision is made halfway between the cricoid cartilage and sternal notch. The anterior jugular veins may be encountered and can be appropriately ligated if necessary.
- Dissection through the superficial fascia proceeds in a longitudinal direction and the strap muscles (sternohyoid and sternothyroid) retracted in the midline.
- The thyroid isthmus is divided between haemostats and ligated using transfixion sutures. Langenbeck retractors are used to aid tracheal access.
- The pretracheal fascia is gently dissected to expose underlying tracheal rings.
- The anaesthetist is informed that the trachea is about to be opened, and they will need to advance the orotracheal tube caudally, moving the cuff away from the planned incision.
- The stoma is incised below the first tracheal ring, either as a longitudinal split or excised window through the second and third rings.
- The introducer is made ready inside the tracheostomy tube with the cuff deflated, whilst the anaesthetist deflates the orotracheal tube cuff and withdraws the tube in a cephalic direction until the tube is clear of the tracheal opening. The introducer and tracheostomy tube are passed into the tracheal stoma, the introducer removed and the cuff inflated. Depending on the type of tracheostomy tube used, an inner tube is inserted and the whole assembly connected to the anaesthetic circuit.
- Before closing, confirm that a CO_2 trace is observed on the attached capnograph, that breath sounds and chest expansion are present bilaterally, and that there is no obvious leak in the ventilator circuit. If a leak is present, the tracheostomy tube cuff may be damaged or a larger tube may be required.
- The wound is partially closed with skin sutures around the tube, and the tube secured in place with the supplied neck tape, or with sutures.
- Regular warm humidified air and inspection of the wound for signs of infection are essential components of postoperative tracheostomy care.

Percutaneous tracheostomy is being used more commonly. It has gained increasing acceptance as an alternative to conventional surgical tracheostomy. In experienced hands with appropriate patient selection, it is safe, easy and quick. Two important criteria for percutaneous tracheostomy are:

- Ability to hyperextend the neck
- Presence of at least 1 cm between cricoid cartilage and suprasternal notch ensuring that the patient will be able to be reintubated in the case of accidental extubation.

Exclusions include children under the age of 12 years, obesity and patients with clotting defects. The technique used is a Seldinger technique with dilatation under bronchoscopic visualisation.

PROCEDURE

PERCUTANEOUS TRACHEOSTOMY

- With the patient's neck extended, and under local anaesthetic (with adrenalin), a 1.5–2.0cm vertical incision is made through the skin approximately 2cm below the cricoid cartilage.
- Blunt dissection is used to reach the pretracheal plane avoiding the thyroid isthmus.
- Finger dissection is used to palpate the cricoid cartilage and tracheal rings.
- Endoscopist/anaesthetist passes a bronchoscope attached to a video camera down the endotracheal tube.
- The endotracheal tube and bronchoscope are withdrawn to a subglottic level, being careful not to withdraw the tube from the larynx.
- The operator enters the tracheal lumen with an introducer needle under direct bronchoscopic visualisation. The puncture should be made between the second and third tracheal rings.
- A guidewire is inserted, the track dilated over a guidewire and the tracheostomy tube inserted over an introducer which is then withdrawn.
- The tube is secured to the skin with sutures and further secured with a tracheostomy tape.

Chapter 9

Thorax

Yusuf Bayrak

CHAPTER OUTLINE

PLEURA AND LUNGS

Pneumothorax

This is the abnormal presence of air in the pleural cavity (→Figure 9.1). Types of pneumothorax include the following.

Primary Spontaneous Pneumothorax. This usually occurs in young, tall, thin males. There is usually no known underlying lung disease, but it is caused by rupture of blebs/bulla in the apices of upper or lower lobes. Atmospheric pressure changes and smoking are also risk factors.

Secondary Spontaneous Pneumothorax. This occurs due to underlying respiratory pathology, e.g. COPD, primary or metastatic tumours of the lung especially during chemotherapy, lung abscess, cystic fibrosis, ILD or asthma.

Traumatic. (See Ch. 4, p. 56.)

Catamenial Pneumothorax. Pneumothorax that occurs in reproductive-age women without concomitant respiratory diseases. It usually happens within 72h before or after onset of menstruation.

Pleural Effusion

This is abnormal collection of fluid in the pleural space between parietal and visceral pleura and is categorised mainly according to Lights criteria:

Exudative if any of the following three criteria met:

- Pleural total protein/serum total protein ratio >0.5
- Pleural lactate dehydrogenase/serum lactate dehydrogenase ratio >0.6
- Pleural lactate dehydrogenase level >2/3 upper limit of the laboratory's reference range of serum lactate dehydrogenase.

Transudative if the same three criteria simultaneously are not met, but if the clinical appearance is suggestive of a transudative effusion, Dr. Light recommends a serum albumin – pleural albumin <1.2mg/dL, to confirm the effusion is exudative. However, do not use the albumin gradient alone to distinguish transudates from exudates, as it will misidentify ~13% of exudates as transudates.

- Transudative effusions are mainly related to renal, hepatic or cardiac failure and are straw coloured. Congestive heart failure, nephrotic syndrome, cirrhosis, malnutrition should be investigated.

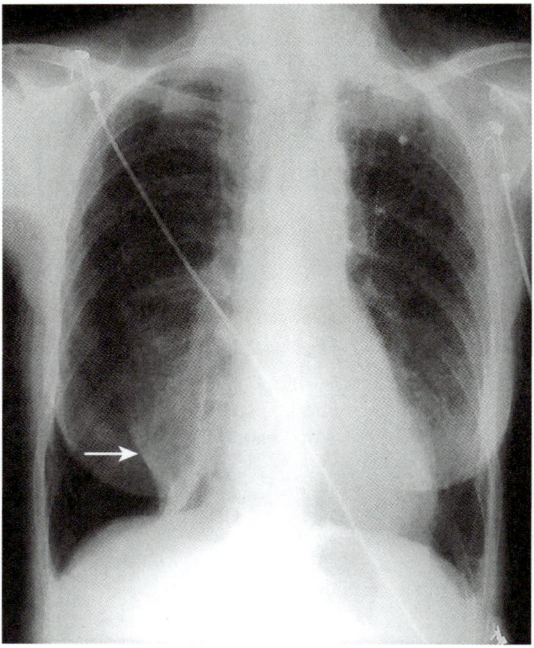

FIGURE 9.1
A pneumothorax is visible on the right side. Note the absence of lung marking at the periphery. The lung edge is visible *(arrow)*.

- Exudative effusions are caused most commonly by infections (empyema, pneumonia, viral infection, tuberculosis) and malignancies (primary lung or metastatic from breast, gastrointestinal (GI) system).
- Special considerations:
  - Chylothorax contains lipids and cholesterol, looks like creamy milk.
  - Haemothorax contains blood, hence it is red coloured and might be associated with trauma, malignancy or parapneumonia.
  - Empyema is turbid and purulent that indicates pus.
- (For causes→Table 9.1).

Symptoms and Signs. Pleuritic chest pain, shortness of breath, signs of congestive heart failure, peripheral oedema. Ipsilateral reduced expansion, dullness to percussion, absent breath sounds.

Investigations

- Chest X-ray (CXR): dense shadow over a lung field with concave upper limit (→Figure 9.2). If the upper border is horizontal, remember the air fluid level in the intestine (ileus) and describe this pathology as hydropneumothorax.
- Diagnostic aspiration – assess protein and LDH content as well as pH, glucose and albumin

TABLE 9.1

CAUSES OF PLEURAL EFFUSIONS

Transudate	Congestive heart failure Renal failure (nephrotic syndrome) Hepatic failure (hypoproteinaemia)
Exudate	Infection: • Pneumonia • Tuberculosis • Empyema • Subphrenic abscess
Malignancy	Primary (adenocarcinoma/mesothelioma) Secondary
Other	Pulmonary embolus (with infarction) Pancreatitis Haemothorax Connective tissue disease

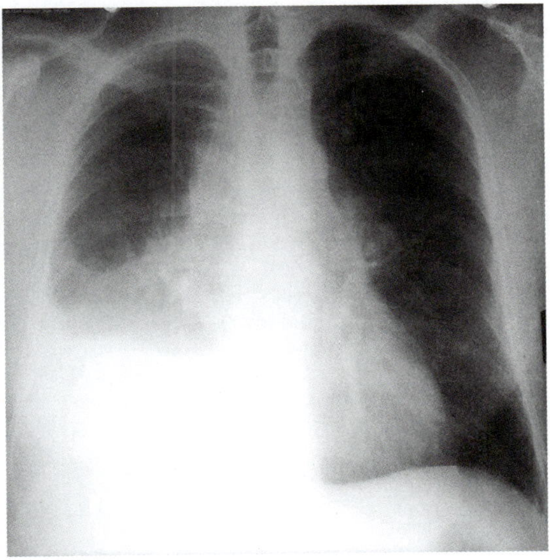

FIGURE 9.2

A right-sided pleural effusion. Note the dense shadow and the concave upper limit of the effusion.

- Culture and antibiotic sensitivity
- TB culture and adenosine deaminase (ADA) level
- Cytology for malignant cells
- Open or video-assisted thoracoscopic surgical pleural biopsy.

Treatment. It is of the underlying cause. Large and symptomatic effusions need drainage. In malignant effusions, aim to achieve chemical pleurodesis by instilling chemicals (sterile talc, bleomycin, doxycycline, tetracycline, poviioidine) into the pleural cavity after drainage. Indwelling tunnelled catheters (Pleurx) might be required in chronic malignant effusions with trapped lungs to palliate symptoms. Decortication of the pleura is effective in the control of effusions and expansion of the lung.

HINTS AND TIPS

Indications for thoracocentesis include diagnostic, symptom control and respiratory distress.

The site for puncture is guided by ultrasound, correlation with CXR, chest computerised tomography (CT) and clinical findings. In a sterile prepared and draped area between the spine and posterior axillary line, a needle is used to perform intercostal nerve block with local anaesthetic. The needle is advanced whilst aspirating and placed over the upper edge of the rib to avoid injury to the neurovascular bundle. Typically, fluid that is aspirated is sent for microbiological, cytological and biochemical analysis. For symptomatic relief up to 1–2 L of the effusions can be evacuated. To avoid re-expansion pulmonary oedema, 1 litre should not be exceeded in the initial process and gradual drainage is essential.

Tumours of the Pleura

Primary tumours of the pleura are not as common as primary lung tumours. The commonest pleural neoplasm is mesothelioma. Mesothelioma occurs in people with a previous history of exposure to asbestos. The disease is exceptionally rare in those who have not been exposed. It is most common in males between 40 and 50 years of age. Symptoms include malaise, weakness, chest pain, cough, dyspnoea, weight loss and fever. Radiograph shows pleural fluid and thickening. Diagnosis is mainly established by VATS pleural biopsy and rarely by fluid analysis. Radiotherapy or chemotherapy is palliative. Some patients might benefit from symptom control with pleurectomy decortication in early disease. Surgery does not alter the prognosis, although extrapleural pneumonectomy and intrapleural hyperthermic chemotherapy offer promising outcomes. Neoplasms of the pleura may also be due to secondary spread from other tumours, e.g., bronchus, breast.

Pulmonary Infections

Bronchiectasis

This is a complication of repeated pulmonary infection where the respiratory pathways are permanently damaged and dilated. It usually affects the lower lobes. The dilated bronchi harbour infected sputum, which is expectorated, often in large amounts. Common pathogens include *Haemophilus* and *Pseudomonas*. Causes of bronchiectasis include whooping cough, measles, tuberculosis, inhalation of foreign bodies, pneumonia, common variable immune deficiency (CVID); exaggerated immune response, e.g. allergic bronchopulmonary aspergillosis (ABPA) and inflammatory bowel disease; or rarely congenital causes, e.g. cystic fibrosis, Kartagener's syndrome (bronchiectasis, sinusitis, dextrocardia), Mounier–Kuhn syndrome and pulmonary sequestration.

Symptoms and Signs. Repeated chest infections, chronic cough, copious purulent sputum. Haemoptysis, malaise, clubbing. Rhonchi, coarse crepitations.

Investigations

- CXR: cystic shadows (possibly with fluid levels), areas of fibrosis, 'tram lines' due to bronchial oedema
- High-resolution CT (gold standard)
- Sputum culture
- Lung function tests
- Sweat test and cystic fibrosis transmembrane conductance regulator (*CFTR*) gene testing
- Ventilation/perfusion scan – Nuclear medicine study to define nonfunctioning lung tissue.

Treatment. Physiotherapy with postural drainage. Antibiotics. Bronchodilators. Surgery for localised disease.

Complications. Recurrent chest infections, haemoptysis (massive haemoptysis may occur), metastatic cerebral abscess. Rarely, pneumothorax may occur.

Lung Abscess

The causes are bronchial obstruction due to carcinoma, inhalation pneumonitis, inhaled foreign body (especially lung abscess in a child), septic embolus, infected pulmonary infarct, transdiaphragmatic extension of subphrenic abscess. Other causes include: infected cyst; secondary to pneumonia, bronchiectasis or TB; immunosuppression; blood-borne, e.g. staphylococcal septicaemia, fungal.

Symptoms and Signs. Obviously ill. Purulent sputum. Haemoptysis. Fever. Rigours. Pleuritic pain. Pyrexial. Clubbing. Reduced breath sounds, dullness to percussion, bronchial breathing, signs of pleural effusion, metastatic abscesses, e.g., cerebral.

Investigations

- Fibreoptic bronchoscopy to exclude endobronchial lesion like foreign body or tumours
- CXR: consolidation early in disease; later, cavitation and fluid level
- Sputum culture and sensitivity, AAFB (alcohol and acid-fast bacilli), fungal stains and cultures.

Treatment. This is of the underlying cause. Postural drainage and antibiotics for no less than 4 weeks. A great majority of cases resolve on medical treatment. Surgery is only required where medical treatment fails or there is a need for treatment of an underlying cause, e.g., removal of bronchial carcinoma.

Tuberculosis

The reader is referred to a textbook of medicine. Surgery is rarely required in this condition at the present time, since antituberculosis therapy is effective in most cases. However, the incidence of multidrug-resistant TB is increasing, and new cases are being seen associated with AIDS. Surgery is required for some of the complications of TB, e.g., bronchopleural fistula, persistent open cavities with positive sputum, bronchiectasis, haemorrhage and destroyed lung. Of historical interest are the operations of thoracoplasty, plombage and phrenic nerve crush. Patients who have had these procedures are occasionally encountered (usually in examinations!). The procedures are designed to collapse the chest wall and the diaphragm onto the lungs, deflating and 'resting' the lungs while healing occurs.

Lung Tumours

Bronchial Carcinoma

This is the leading cause of cancer deaths in males in the UK accounting for approximately 50,000 per year. It is the second commonest in females. Cigarette smoking is attributable for up to 75–80% of all lung cancers. Other aetiological factors include chronic exposure to asbestos, nickel, arsenic, petroleum products and radioactive materials.

Cytologically divided under

Non–small cell lung cancer:

(1) Adenocarcinoma (30–45%)
(2) Squamous cell carcinoma (25–40%)
(3) Undifferentiated large cell carcinoma (rarest)

Carcinoids (typical/ atypical)
Small cell lung cancer (15–25%).

Symptoms and Signs

Primary. The tumour may be asymptomatic and seen on routine CXR. Cough, haemoptysis, dyspnoea, chest pain, wheeze, hoarseness, recurrent chest infections, dysphagia, weight loss, fatigue and fever.

Complications

- Thoracic: pleural effusion, recurrent laryngeal nerve palsy (hoarseness), SVC obstruction, Horner's syndrome (ptosis, myosis, enophthalmia, anhidrosis), especially with Pancoast's tumour (invasive cancer of apex of lung)
- Metastatic: cachexia, malaise; brain (headaches, fits, personality change); bone (pathological fractures); liver (jaundice); adrenal (Addison's disease); electrolyte disturbances especially hyponatraemia and hypercalcaemia
- Nonmetastatic, extrapulmonary: endocrine (syndrome of inappropriate antidiuretic hormone secretion (SIADH), ACTH secretion, hypercalcaemia, gynaecomastia, hypercalcitonaemia, elevated follicle stimulating hormone (FSH)/ LH, hypoglycaemia, hyperthyroidism, carcinoid); neurological syndrome (subacute sensory neuropathy, myasthenic neuropathy, mononeuritis multiplex, Lambert–Eaton myasthenic syndrome, encephalomyelitis, opsoclonus-myoclonus); skeletal (hypertrophic pulmonary osteoarthropathy, clubbing); collagen/vascular (thrombophlebitis migrans, vasculitis, SLE, dermatomyositis and polymyositis); renal (glomerulonephritis, nephrotic syndrome); coagulopathies (thromboembolism, disseminated intravascular coagulation (DIC)); haematogenic (anaemia, raised WCC, eosinophils, thrombocytosis, thrombocytopenic purpura); cutaneous (erythema multiforme, erythema gyratum repens, acanthosis nigricans).

Investigations

- FBC
- ESR
- LFTs
- Calcium

- CXR: PA and lateral (→Figure 9.3), mass, raised diaphragm with involvement of phrenic nerve, pleural effusion
- Sputum cytology for malignant cells
- Chest CT with i.v. contrast
- Bronchoscopic biopsy is best for central lesions, percutaneous biopsy for peripheral lesions – biopsy will confirm histological type.
- Endobronchial ultrasound (EBUS) to biopsy lesions and lymph node stations to allow staging
- Pleural tap if effusion present, cytological examination for malignant cells
- Positron emission tomography (PET)-CT scan: local/distant spread and invasion and assess lesion and mediastinal hot spots to determine likely cancer spread (FDG 18)
- Brain magnetic resonance imaging (MRI) with i.v. contrast for metastases
- Mediastinoscopy (rarely performed now due to EBUS).

Treatment. Depends on histological type and clinical staging. Non–small cell tumours, regardless of size and localisation, may be resected if not locally advanced to mediastinal lymph nodes and patient has enough cardiopulmonary reserves. Other local treatments such as radiotherapy exist for patients with lymph node involvement and not fit for surgery conditions. Small cell tumours are aggressive and are usually

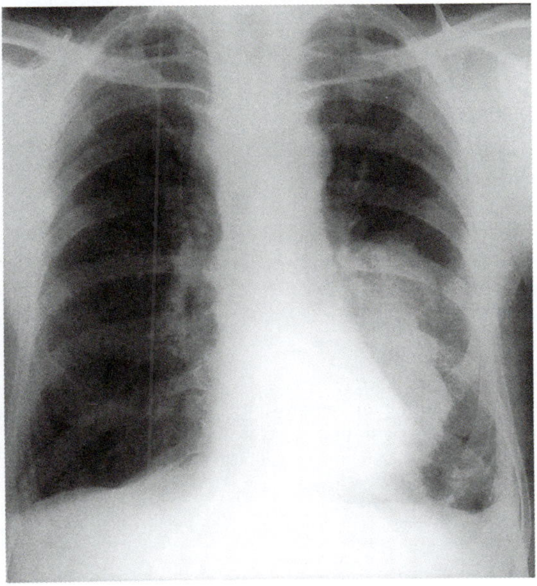

FIGURE 9.3
A large bronchial carcinoma in the left lung.

beyond surgery, having disseminated at the time of presentation. Combination chemotherapy and radiotherapy prolong survival in small cell tumours. Most patients are incurable at presentation. Symptomatic relief is the aim. Radiotherapy is appropriate for a bronchial obstruction with lung collapse, SVC obstruction, bone pain and haemoptysis. Endobronchial and SVC stenting procedures may be carried out. SVC obstruction treated by stenting has a success rate of 90% with insertion of a stent via the right femoral vein. Extensive endoluminal tumour debulking can be carried out using a cryoprobe/laser and endoluminal brachytherapy.

Surgical treatment involves lobectomy, sleeve lobectomy or pneumonectomy and is the only potential cure. Careful selection of patients is required, and operability should be assessed by bronchoscopy, EBUS, PET-CT scan and cardiopulmonary fitness test, e.g. exercise testing (CPEX). Contraindications to surgery include multiple distant metastases, SVC obstruction, malignant pleural effusion, recurrent laryngeal nerve and phrenic nerve involvement.

Prognosis. About 50% survive 5 years after lobectomy and 25% after pneumonectomy. Since 75% are not candidates for surgery, the overall survival for 5 years is about 5–10%. Prognosis ultimately depends on the cell type and stage of the disease at the time of diagnosis. Small cell carcinoma has the worst prognosis.

Metastatic Lung Tumours

Metastatic tumours are common in the lung, which in some cases may be the only site of metastases. Secondaries may be from adenocarcinoma (breast, kidney, colorectal), sarcoma (bone) or malignant melanoma. Rarely, single or multiple metastatic lung tumours may be removed as part of the treatment. The primary tumour must be controlled, and no metastases should be present elsewhere. The best results are obtained with tumours for which there is effective chemotherapy. The best example is the surgical treatment of pulmonary metastases in patients with osteogenic sarcoma. The presence of metastatic colonic tumour in the lung is an indication for 'metastasectomy'. Results are improving.

Solitary Pulmonary Nodules (Coin Lesions)

These are well-circumscribed peripheral nodules seen on routine CXRs of patients who are usually asymptomatic. The lesions may be infective, granulomatous or neoplastic. About 10% are malignant.

Symptoms and Signs. Tends to be asymptomatic. Smokers. Cough, haemoptysis, weight loss, hypertrophic osteoarthropathy. Beware of the overlying skin lesions seen on radiograph.

Investigations

- Picked up on CXR: concentric or heavy calcification suggests benign lesion; documented absence of growth over 1 year suggests benign lesion
- Sputum cytology and culture (mostly not helpful to exclude malignancy)
- CT scan to exclude multiple lesions.

Treatment. Surgical excision if malignancy cannot be excluded or the patient chooses surgery.

HINTS AND TIPS

Any smoker with haemoptysis should have a low dose chest CT, particularly if there are other sinister features such as persistent cough, shortness of breath and weight loss. Screening by low-dose chest CT in adults aged 50–80 who have a 20-pack-year smoking history and currently smoke or have quit within the past 15 years is recommended currently and showed survival advantage. When examining such patients, check for clubbing/hypertrophic pulmonary osteoarthropathy. The symptoms of TB often mimic those of malignancy. Consider this possibility in the elderly, patients on immunosuppression and in the presence of family history.

MEDIASTINUM

Mediastinal masses may be found incidentally on routine CXR or may be symptomatic. CT scan and MRI may be required to localise the mass, indicate its aetiology and determine the invasion to surrounding structures.

Certain lesions are more likely to occur in characteristic mediastinal sites:

- Superior mediastinum: retrosternal goitre
- Anterior mediastinum: teratoma, pericardial cysts, bronchogenic cysts, diaphragmatic hernia (foramen of Morgagni), thymoma
- Posterior mediastinum: neurogenic tumours, e.g., dumbbell tumours, paravertebral mass, TB abscess, phaeochromocytoma, diaphragmatic hernia, hiatus hernia.

In addition to the above, aneurysms and lymph nodes may be apparent in any site. Causes of lymph node enlargement include secondary deposits, sarcoid, lymphoma and TB.

Symptoms and Signs. Asymptomatic, cervical lymphadenopathy, SVC obstruction, hoarseness (left recurrent laryngeal nerve palsy), Horner's syndrome.

Investigations

- α-FP, beta-human chorionic gonadotrophin (β-HCG) and LDH, chest CT ± MRI
- Percutaneous core biopsy (avoid fine needle aspiration which have low diagnostic yield)
- PET scan for staging
- Bronchoscopy and EBUS/EMN
- Upper GI endoscopy and EUS
- Angiography (vascular lesions)
- Mediastinoscopy
- Testis ultrasound in young males.

Treatment. Surgery may be required. Minimally invasive techniques are preferred to confirm the diagnosis and for appropriate treatment.

Thoracic Trauma

This is dealt with in Chapter 4.

Chapter 10

The Heart and Thoracic Great Vessels

Laszlo Göbölös • Gopal Bhatnagar

CHAPTER OUTLINE

HEART AND GREAT VESSELS

The Evolvement of Cardiac Surgery

Cardiosurgical procedures have evolved significantly in the past century from a hardly accepted operative approach to an everyday medical necessity with low risk for standard, elective surgeries and excellent long-term outcomes. Patient assessment for operative suitability and risk stratification applying one of the major scoring systems (Society of Thoracic Surgeons (STS), EUROScore) became sophisticated and relies on several instrumental diagnostic techniques, including echocardiography, angiography, computed tomography (CT), magnetic resonance imaging (MRI), positron emission tomography, in contrast to obtaining medical history with physical examination, and accompanied by a chest radiograph only in the 1950s. Improved operative and perfusion techniques, novel anaesthetics, intensive care, and minimally invasive approaches have revolutionised heart surgery, resulting in enhanced outcomes, effectively reducing complications and markedly decreasing mortality.

Indications for Surgery

- Failed medical treatment or advanced disease not suitable for medical monotherapy
- Where the surgical procedural risk is perceived to be lower than that of the underlying natural pathology orinterventional cardiology procedure and the long-term outcome is more beneficial.

Relative and Absolute Contraindications for Surgery

- Surgical risk/benefit calculation is unfavourable (see scoring systems).
- Irreparable myocardial damage; transplantation still might be an option
- Irreversible organ failure (single or multiple), e.g. extensive stroke, liver, kidney and lung damage
- Unsuitable patient where the post-procedural recovery potential is low (advanced age, advanced malignant disease, bed-bound patient).

Preoperative Assessment

- Established diagnosis and operative plan according to multidisciplinary evaluation. This includes not only a complete physical examination but blood tests (CBC, CMP, ABG, type-and-screen), a variety of instrumental imaging, such

as ECG, chest X-ray (CXR), echocardiography (transthoracic or transoesophageal), carotid- and vein-mapping Doppler, coronary angiography (gradients, FFR), MRI (morphology, contractility, myocardial viability), cardiac CT/CT angiography (re-do, aortic surgery), radionuclide imaging (myocardial perfusion), positron emission tomography (PET)-CT (tumour, infection), 4D CT (3D volume helical data rendered into a cine-image), pulmonary function test, etc. 3D printing is a powerful tool in paediatric cardiac cases for planning complex procedures, visualising the most optimal operative access of the pathology and, as a result, saving valuable myocardial ischaemic time.
- Emotional support, informed consent
- Medical optimisation of heart failure status
- Correction of anaemia, electrolyte imbalance, and nutritional deficiencies
- Chest physiotherapy, optimisation of COPD, smoking cessation (minimum 6 weeks prior to elective surgery).

Surgery

Conventional open-heart surgery is performed via a mid-sternal incision. Minimally invasive approaches, such as a limited sternotomy (L or T shaped) for aortic valve/ascending aorta replacement, right anterolateral mini-thoracotomy for aortic, mitral, and tricuspid valve procedures, are common nowadays. Left anterolateral mini-thoracotomy is utilised for MIDCAB and limited access LVAD placement. A left posterolateral thoracotomy approach is for the ligation of a patent ductus arteriosus in paediatric patients. Robotic surgery has taken minimally invasive methods to a different level due to ergonomics and precision surgery with a 10x power-of-magnification operative images. The ultimate port access surgery is total endoscopic coronary artery bypass grafting (TECAB) at the moment.

Cardiopulmonary Bypass. On cardiopulmonary bypass, the heart and lung functions are replaced by a pump (roller or rotor) and a membrane oxygenator. The venous return to the heart, specifically from the right atrium/venae cavae, is redirected by inserted cannulas and connected lines to the oxygenator and heat exchanger. Next, the pump component forwards oxygenated blood to the body via the arterial cannula placed in the ascending aorta or aortic arch above the cross-clamp level, which later provides a blood-free operative field by the exclusion of the heart from circulation. A small amount of blood draining from the bronchial circulation to the left atrium is returned to the venous reservoir by the aortic vent placed under the cross-clamp, and additional pump suckers clear the collection of fully heparinised blood from the pericardium, after passage through appropriate filters. When the aorta is clamped without any further cardioprotection, the heart quickly becomes ischaemic. However, there are various methods available to preserve myocardial integrity:

- Intermittent or continuous coronary perfusion
- Intermittent cross-clamping
- Reduction of myocardial metabolism (cardioplegia and cooling).

With maintained coronary perfusion, either the heart is operated off-pump or as a 'beating heart' on-pump where coronary perfusion is present throughout the procedure, and the moving organ is positioned for bypass grafting without any haemodynamic compromise. With intermittent cross-clamp fibrillation, the heart is electrically fibrillated between limited durations of ischaemia and periods of normal perfusion, followed by complete reperfusion after each bottom-end coronary anastomosis. Antegrade cardioplegia is provided either via the combined perfusion vent of the aortic root distal to the cross-clamp or via direct cannulation of the coronary ostia, utilising infusion of cold (4–5°C) or warm blood or cold crystalloid solution, arresting the heart in diastole. In case of severe aortic regurgitation or multiple occluded or stenotic coronary arteries, retrograde cardioplegia is delivered through the coronary sinus. The constructed distal anastomosis also allows a selective cardioplegia of the bypassed territory, with the advantage of testing the new bottom-end simultaneously. The primary goal of cardiac arrest with intermittent cardioplegic coronary perfusion is to couple myocardial oxygenation and nourishment with simultaneous reduction of myocardial metabolism. Aortic occlusion is generally well tolerated for 1–2h applying cold blood cardioplegia, but a total ischaemic period over 4h is often critical. After finalising all required cardiac repairs, the heart is allowed to fill up with blood, then de-aired. This is followed by removal of the aortic cross-clamp. The re-established natural coronary perfusion washes out the cardioplegia, and the heart often restarts spontaneously. Once stable haemodynamics is maintained, the cardiopulmonary bypass is weaned

Cannulation Options. Central cannulation is the standard of routine cardiac procedures, with cannulation of the ascending aorta or aortic arch and a two-stage venous return from the right atrium or via bicaval cannulation. Peripheral cannulations might be used for minimally invasive procedures, emergencies, and re-do operations, most commonly utilising the femoral vessels. However, the arterial cannulation spots might be limited in type A aortic dissections due to the pathological process. Various approaches are described in the literature besides the classical femoral arterial target and subclavian cannulation, including innominate artery, right upper pulmonary vein, transapical, cut-down direct lumen cannulation, etc. Recently, the ultrasound-guided direct Seldinger cannulation of the true lumen on the ascending aorta or arch became a guideline recommendation; hence it provides quick perfusion access, rapid re-expansion of the true lumen and antegrade perfusion (Figure 10.1).

Hypothermic Circulatory Arrest, Core Temperature Monitoring. Hypothermic circulatory arrest remains a crucial element of complex aortic and cardiac repairs. The central nervous system is the most prone organ for ischaemia; by lowering the core temperature usually to 20–25°C, the decreased metabolic rate allows a safe circulatory of 20–45min. This period can be further extended by ante- or retrograde cerebral perfusion during the circulatory arrest. Meticulous core temperature monitoring is crucial not only for safe hypothermic arrest but also in the rewarming phase. Extended hypothermia results in coagulopathy, seizures or dysrhythmias. Excessive rewarming can lead to severe neurological damage. Tympanic or pulmonary artery core temperature monitoring is the most reliable; additional measurement points, such as bladder, nasopharyngeal, and rectal sites, warrant the follow-up on the delayed whole body rewarming process. Additionally, brain protection is reassured by near-infrared spectroscopy, monitoring regional cerebral oxygen saturation.

Minimal Extracorporeal Circulation. This closed-loop, tip-to-tip heparin-coated cardiopulmonary bypass system significantly reduces the prime volume, the blood-to-air contact and contains no venous reservoir. It reduces haemodilution and improves tissue perfusion. The system can be run at a significantly lower ACT in comparison to a standard CPB, and the post-bypass systemic inflammatory response is diminished. An airtight system run is mandatory, as no venous reservoir is present (Figure 10.2).

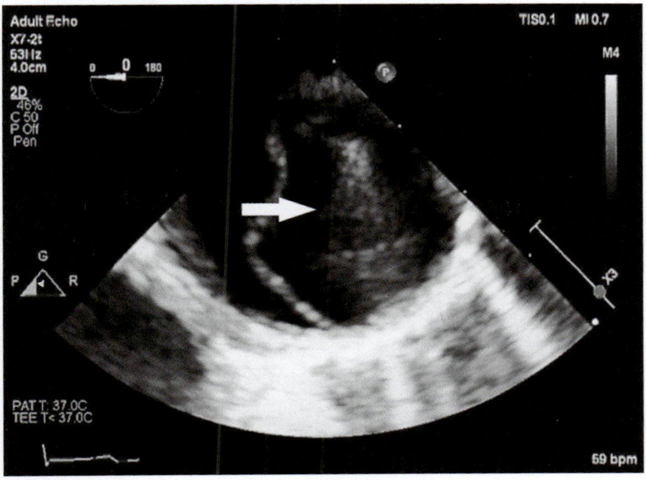

Figure 10.1

Direct cannulation of TAAD true lumen applying the Seldinger method. The arrow marks the inserted cannula on the TOE image. *The photo is from the authors' collection.*

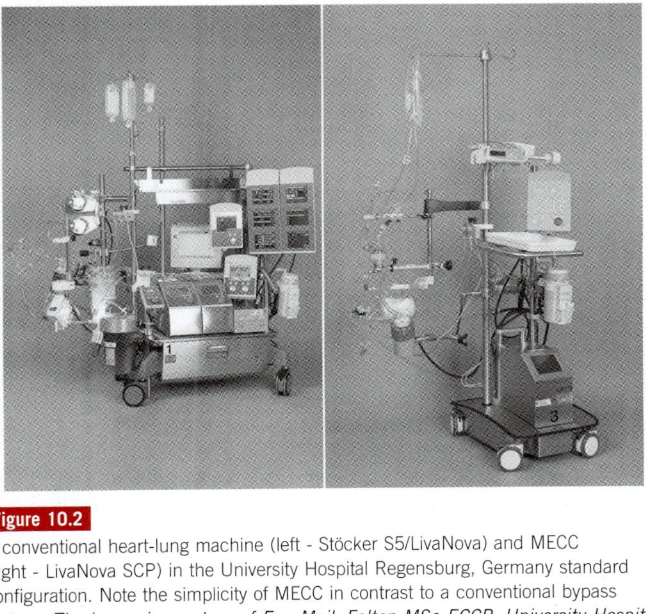

Figure 10.2

A conventional heart-lung machine (left - Stöcker S5/LivaNova) and MECC (right - LivaNova SCP) in the University Hospital Regensburg, Germany standard configuration. Note the simplicity of MECC in contrast to a conventional bypass system. *The image is courtesy of Eng Maik Foltan MSc ECCP; University Hospital Regensburg, Germany.*

Extracorporeal Membrane Oxygenation (ECMO). ECMO is the solution for critical respiratory (veno-venous –; VV-ECMO) or cardiopulmonary failure (veno-arterial-; VA-ECMO). The perfusion system is identical to the MECC system but provides long-term pump runs. The cannulation is usually peripheral; central cannulation is used in post-cardiotomy cases only. They can be used as bridge-to-recovery or bridge-to-final procedure (e.g. PCI, transplantation).

Postoperative Management

> **HINTS AND TIPS**
>
> Post-procedural emergency chest reopening indications:
>
> - Increased chest drain output despite correction of coagulopathy, indicating ongoing surgical bleeding
> - Clinical signs of pericardial tamponade
> - Cardiopulmonary resuscitation, unresponsive to short conservative rescue attempts.
>
> **PROCEDURE**
>
> - After rapid preparing and draping of the operative field, the median sternotomy wound is deeply incised down to the sternal surface.
> - Sternal wires are divided and removed with wire twisters.
> - Sternal edges are retracted, and the pericardial effusion/clot is removed.
> - The heart surface and chest wall are meticulously inspected for a potential source of bleeding, and all residual clots are removed. In case of insufficient cardiac output, direct cardiac massage can be applied, and defibrillation may be delivered.

Common Postoperative Complications

Low Cardiac Output. It may result from cardiac failure, acute blood loss, pericardial tamponade, arrhythmias or pulmonary hypertension.

Myocardial Ischaemia. Another relatively common but potentially devastating complication. It may result from incomplete revascularisation, early graft failure, coronary embolisation or dissection.

Respiratory Tract Infection. It ranges from a common lower respiratory tract infection resulting from insufficient postoperative physiotherapy to extensive pneumonia or life-threatening acute respiratory distress syndrome (ARDS) in usually incompletely prepared emergency cases.

Respiratory Failure. It may result from extensive atelectasis, pulmonary oedema or analgesic overdosage (opioids), leading to definite hypoxia. However, pain from the surgical incision reducing respiratory efforts can also be contributory.

Renal Failure. Renal hypoperfusion from any cause can lead to acute tubular necrosis. Postrenal origin, even unresolved urine retention after urinary catheter removal, may result in kidney failure. Haemofiltration/haemodialysis may be required intermittently or permanently in postoperative renal failure.

Jaundice. Usually, it emerges from polytransfusion or haemolysis, resulting from CPB or a high-velocity paravalvular leak. Rarely, liver failure may originate from the low cardiac output. Seldom, CPB leads to pancreatitis, and concomitant obstruction of the gall passage.

Cerebral Damage. The most common cause is embolism (air or solid particle) or hypoperfusion. The latter can be a consequence of low CPB flow, cerebrovascular disease, or vessel dissection. Cerebral oedema may complicate the process, resulting in brain stem herniation in the worst-case scenario.

Atrial Fibrillation (AF). Postoperative AF occurs in one-third of patients. A sudden drop in cardiac output, especially in heart failure patients or in case of rapid ventricular response or consequent thromboembolic events, can result in life-threatening perioperative situations.

Postoperative Treatment.

Cardiac Output Support. Keeping up satisfactory preload requires adequate filling pressure of chambers, and a sufficient central venous pressure (CVP) is a reliable basic indicator to follow. The myocardial contractility is supported by inotropes, sometimes in combination. Heart rate is maintained around at 90/min in the early postoperative period, and sequential pacing might be required to achieve this goal. Afterload (peripheral resistance) adjustment commences with the aid of vasoconstrictors or vasodilators. Metabolic acidosis and lower mixed venous saturations are valuable indicators of poor peripheral tissue perfusion. Intra-aortic balloon pump insertion improves diastolic coronary perfusion and reduces cardiac afterload. Low cardiac output state necessitating external chest compressions requires urgent re-exploration. Pulmonary hypertension can be sufficiently addressed by milrinone. Dysrhythmias require antiarrhythmic drugs, electric cardioversion or pacing.

Prevention of Respiratory Complications. Optimise haemodynamics, apply adequately targeted positive pressure ventilation and aim for early extubation. Additional supportive therapy consists of analgesics, nebulisers, physiotherapy and diuretics.

Maintenance of Urine Output. Maintain cardiac output by sufficient fluid load and inotropes, e.g. dobutamine. Correcting haemoglobin levels and administering diuretics, e.g. furosemide, may facilitate urine production, ideally ≥1 mL/kg/h.

Avoiding Cerebral Complications. Target BP close to normal range. Eliminate CO_2 overload by positive pressure ventilation, avoid hyperpyrexia, and administer corticosteroids, e.g. dexamethasone, in case of cerebral oedema.

Prevention and Treatment of Postoperative AF. Optimisation of electrolyte balance and early titration of beta-blockers may prevent atrial dysrhythmias. In AF without haemodynamic compromise, chemical cardioversion with amiodarone ± beta-blocker is the therapy of choice. Electric direct current cardioversion is indicated in haemodynamically affected patients or failed chemical cardioversion after 6–12 weeks. All patients require therapeutic anticoagulation whilst in AF. After 24 h of AF, thrombus presence must be echocardiographically excluded in the atria prior to electric cardioversion.

Congenital Heart Disease

The incidence measures 1.2–1.4% of live births. Aetiological factors include genetic traits (familial burden, Down's syndrome, etc.), maternal rubella, diabetes, medications (e.g. warfarin, phenytoin, lithium, isotretinoin and topical retinoids), high alcohol intake and smoking.

The following lesions are most commonly encountered, in order of decreasing frequency: ventricular septal defect (VSD), patent ductus arteriosus (PDA), atrial septal defect (ASD) (secundum type), partial anomalous pulmonary venous connection, AVSD (primum ASD, endocardial cushion defect), pulmonary stenosis, aortic stenosis, bicuspid aortic valve, coarctation of the aorta, mitral cleft, tetralogy of Fallot and transposition of the great vessels. Congenital heart disease can be classified as acyanotic (L-R or no shunt) or cyanotic (dominant R-L shunt).

Common Signs and Symptoms. Arrhythmias, cyanosis (blue lips, fingernails, skin), finger clubbing, shortness of breath, fatigue, oedema, ascites, renal failure and hepatic failure.

Investigations. Physical examination, ECG, CXR, pulse-oximetry, stress test (ECG, echo), echocardiogram (TTE, TOE), CT angiography, MRI scan, left and right heart catheterisation, coronarography, ventriculography, genetic testing.

The reader is referred to a textbook of Paediatric cardiology for the detailed symptoms, signs and investigations of the specific conditions. The treatment and prognosis are discussed below.

Acyanotic Lesions

VENTRICULAR SEPTAL DEFECT (VSD). Of these defects, 90% close spontaneously by 1 year of age; the majority of those that remain patent are amenable to percutaneous closure. Surgery is indicated for extensive or complex lesions, heart failure, pulmonary hypertension or a pulmonary blood flow 1.5 times greater than systemic flow (Q_p:Q_s>1.5). The defect is closed with a prosthetic patch on CPB. Perioperative morbidity and mortality depend on the preoperative patient condition and degree of pulmonary vascular resistance. An uncomplicated VSD is associated with an operative mortality of <1% in high-volume centres.

PATENT DUCTUS ARTERIOSUS (PDA). The pulmonary vascular resistance markedly drops at birth as the lungs inflate, and the ductus arteriosus closes within a few days. Failure of closure mainly occurs in premature babies, albeit maternal rubella in the first trimester or hypoxia can also be causative. Nevertheless, a subset of associated cardiac malformations – i.e. duct-dependent anomalies – are survivable only via a patent PDA to maintain systemic circulation. In these cases, early closure of the ductus without simultaneous repair of the associated lesions is usually fatal (transposition of the great vessels, preductal aortic coarctation, pulmonary artery hypoplasia/atresia, aortic-, mitral-, tricuspid valve atresia, hypoplastic left heart syndrome, etc). Therefore, the ductal flow is maintained with prostaglandin E_1 infusion until a definitive repair is undertaken or a palliative shunt is constructed. In premature babies with isolated PDA, a prostaglandin synthetase inhibitor, e.g. indomethacin, can induce duct closure. All persistent ducts should be closed to prevent infective endocarditis. The ductus is ligated or clipped via left posterior thoracotomy; pedal oximetry/NIRS is mandatory during the procedure to monitor accidental aortic flow limitation. Endovascular occlusion techniques are commonly applied. Procedural mortality measures <0.5%.

ATRIAL SEPTAL DEFECT (ASD). Surgery is indicated at Q_p:Q_s>1.5. The defect is closed with a patch at secundum ASD. Partial AVSD (primum defect) requires mitral cleft closure and ASD patch repair. In complete AVSD, complex AV valvular repair(s) and septal patching (both atrial and ventricular) commence. Ideally, the operation should be undertaken prior to primary school admission. Mortality measures <1% but increases in case of significant pulmonary hypertension. Percutaneous device obliteration is the first therapy of choice for secundum defects.

COARCTATION OF THE AORTA. The above is a luminal narrowing in any location between the arch and bifurcation, most commonly situated at the isthmus. Coarctation can be isolated but often associated with lesions that limit blood flow early in foetal life, i.e.: congenital aortic stenosis, aortic atresia, mitral stenosis, hypoplastic LV, tetralogy of Fallot, pulmonary and tricuspid atresia. VSD may also be present with coarctation. There are two appearances; the common postductal in usually juxtaductal ("next to" ductus arteriosus) position or the rare preductal involving the aortic arch. The ring- or tube-shaped proliferation of the media can cause pinhole lesions to 50% luminal reduction of the aortic cross-section and may extend to the entire aorta and its branches. This results in the development of collaterals to supply the lower body (between internal mammary, vertebral, thyro- or costocervical branches and the descending aorta distal to the occlusion). The presentation is with symptoms emerging after PDA involution, featured by upper body hypertension, LV overload, and lower body hypotension.

A systolic murmur is typical at the left sternal edge (2R2) and posteriorly with absent or reduced femoral pulses. The repair should be performed in stable children before 6 months of age. Operative procedures include resection with end-to-end anastomosis, subclavian flap aortoplasty, and synthetic patch aortoplasty (cave: aneurysm formation). If the gap is too large, an interposition graft is inserted (cave: no growth potential). Complications include recurrent coarctation (ductal tissue remnant), spinal cord ischaemia, recurrent laryngeal nerve palsy, chylothorax and mesenteric "arteritis" resulting from increased pulse pressure. Without surgery, the majority of patients are lost before the age of 40 years. Death occurs from an aortic dissection, rupture, infective endocarditis, heart failure or cerebral haemorrhage. The operative mortality is <2% but can increase to 10% in neonates. Recently, a large proportion of coarctations have been commonly treated by angioplasty in small children. Recurrent coarctations mostly undergo balloon dilatation. Coarctation is associated with bicuspid aortic valve and ascending aortopathy; it is also essential to follow-up on repaired coarctation patients in adulthood.

CONGENITAL VALVE DISEASE IN CHILDREN. Stenosis may occur on a variable spectrum regarding all valves, including atresia and hypoplastic corresponding chamber at the endpoint. Treatment varies between balloon dilatation during cardiac catheterisation and open repair for complex lesions. Valvular regurgitation can be caused by clefts, rudimentary cusps or complex lesions, i.e. Ebstein anomaly.

ANOMALOUS PULMONARY VENOUS CONNECTION. The pulmonary veins connect partially (usually the right-sided ones) or entirely to the systemic venous return and create a large L-R shunt. Survival and the degree of cyanosis depend on the presence of a R-L shunt (ASD, VSD, PDA) in a total anomalous malformation. Partial cases are usually treated by a baffle redirecting blood from the aberrant pulmonary orifice through a present or created ASD to the LA. The total anomalous infra- and supracardiac types are repaired by connecting the pulmonary venous confluence to the posterior wall of the LA. The cardiac type requires coronary sinus unroofing and baffling into the LA. The procedure is performed as soon as the diagnosis is established, and the perioperative mortality was significantly reduced in the past two decades to <5%.

Cyanotic Lesions

Congenital cyanotic heart disease is uncommon. The two common pathologies are the tetralogy of Fallot and transposition of the great vessels. Cyanosis also develops where a L-R shunt reverses owing to pulmonary hypertension (Eisenmenger complex), e.g. ASD, VSD; this stage represents a contraindication for surgical correction.

Tetralogy of Fallot. It consists of pulmonary outflow stenosis accompanied by RV hypertrophy and VSD with overriding aorta. Correction includes reconstruction of the RV outflow tract, usually with a monocusp valve after extensive muscle bundle resection, outflow augmentation by a patch, and closure of the VSD. Nearly all children are corrected in a single combined procedure – early correction in infancy is the therapy of choice. Seldom in small, underdeveloped babies, an aortopulmonary shunt must be used for palliative purposes to increase pulmonary blood flow as a first stage. A classical Blalock–Taussig (BT) shunt is not constructed anymore, but similar interposition graft analogues are utilised. At a second stage, the modified BT shunt is then closed, and all defects are corrected between the ages of 3 and 5 years. There should be a negligible mortality risk associated with the shunt procedure and a low risk for complete correction. These patients often require pulmonary valve replacement as a re-do procedure in their fourth decade of life.

Transposition of the Great Vessels. Here, the aorta arises from the RV and the pulmonary artery from the LV. Survival depends on coexisting malformations, e.g. PDA, VSD, ASD, allowing the mixing of the two separate circulations. Concomitant abnormal coronary anatomy is common. Surgical correction requires an 'arterial switch', where the supracoronary ascending aorta and PA are transected, repositioned over each other's proximal stump and re-anastomosed, i.e. the aorta to the LV and the PA to the RV (LeCompte manoeuvre). The coronary orifices are also mobilised and relocated to the neo-aortic root prior to completing the aortic anastomosis line. The procedure must be undertaken within the first 2 weeks of life before the LV decreases in size and adapts to the lower-pressure pulmonary circulation. Alternatively, a classical interatrial repair can be undertaken at 6 months. Here, a 'baffle' made of pericardium is created in the atrium to direct caval blood behind the baffle to the mitral valve and anatomical LV and PA, with the pulmonary venous return channelled in front of the baffle to the tricuspid valve, anatomical RV and aorta. Operative mortality measures approximately 10%.

Acquired Valvular Heart Disease

Valvular disease is limited mainly to the aortic, mitral and occasionally tricuspid valves. The pulmonary valve is seldom affected. A valve may be narrowed (stenosis) or rendered incompetent (regurgitation), or a combination of both can develop. Surgical treatment of acquired valvular disease consists of either valve repair (common for mitral regurgitation) or replacement. Transcatheter aortic or mitral valve procedures (clip or band) are often undertaken for high-risk surgical patients, although recent studies permit more in the direction of lower-risk transcatheter aortic valve implantation. An increasing number of percutaneous approaches for tricuspid valve repair is emerging.

Valve Replacement Options

Mechanical Valves. All mechanical valves require life-long anticoagulation to mitigate embolisation and valve thrombosis risks. Despite their material being erosion resistant, pannus formation may hinder the impeccable long-term leaflet function, and infective endocarditis can also negatively influence their longevity.

Mechanical valves include:

- *Ball-cage valve.* The Starr–Edwards valve is a metal cage incorporating a silastic ball. Due to the design and weight of the ball, haemolysis is relatively common. They are not implanted nowadays.
- *Tilting disc valve (monoleaflet).* This valve is composed of a single rotating disc on a central metal strut. Medtronic Hall, Björk–Shiley and Omnocarbon valves are the most common, although rarely used recently. They all have a higher gradient than a bileaflet valve due to considerable resistance resulting from a more limited leaflet opening angle and heavier leaflet.
- *Bileaflet valve,* e.g. St Jude (pyrolytic carbon), Sulzer-CarboMedics (carbon discs on a titanium ring), Sorin Bicarbon (carbon discs in titanium housing), On-X (carbon coated graphite and tungsten leaflets, polytetrafluoroethylene sawing cuff). Some are featured by nearly right-angle orifice openings with reduced resistance and cavitation. The hydrodynamically optimised hinges are less thrombogenic; therefore, a lower INR is compatible long-term, following a short initial standard anticoagulation.

Tissue Valves. Biological implants are mainly bovine pericardium or porcine xenografts. Their structure is either stented or stentless. Stented valves are mounted on a woven material-covered metal frame, including a sewing ring. Stentless prostheses do not have a structural frame but are mounted on a woven sewing ring and are typically sutured inside the aortic root. Some of the stentless valves are actually a complete, immunodepleted porcine aortic root. Regarding all tissue valves, the embolic rate is meagre; therefore, anticoagulants are unnecessary. They lack long-term durability, with up to 75% failure rate at 15 years. However, larger-size complete xenograft aortic roots are featured by significantly improved durability. Late failure often results from long-term mechanical damages and concomitant calcification on the valve components. The valve failure emerges gradually with developing heart failure symptoms.

Special purpose tissue valve:

- *Rapid deployment valves.* These tissue valves (e.g. Perceval; Corcym) are usually guided or anchored by three single-bite sutures but deployed within an expanding frame in an effort to reduce myocardial ischaemic and CPB time significantly.
- *Transcatheter valves* are either self-expanding (e.g. CoreValve Evolut Pro plus; Medtronic – external porcine pericardial wrap over the lower cage cells. *Advantage:* lower profile delivery system, greater sizing range. *Disadvantage:* paravalvular leak rates), balloon expandable (e.g. Sapien 3 Ultra/XT; Edwards Lifesciences – bovine pericardial leaflets in a cobalt-chromium frame. *Advantage:* increased outer skirt height, lower profile. *Disadvantage:* heart block, especially left bundle branch rates) or mechanically expanding devices (e.g. Lotus; Boston Scientific – bovine pericardium/multilayer and multipolymer external wrap over lower cells. *Advantage:* easily repositionable. *Disadvantage:* higher postprocedural pacemaker implantation rates. Recently, Boston Scientific announced the discontinuation of the latter valve due to complexities associated with the product delivery system, but the implanted valve durability is not affected).
- *Free aortic homograft* is utilised for aortic root or ascending aortic replacement.

- *Antibiotic-preserved fresh homografts* may also be implanted, although not commonly available nowadays.
- *Human cryopreserved allograft valves* are usually implanted in aortic valve position.

Complications of Artificial Valves

- Thrombosis with valve dysfunction or embolism
- Failure – valve failure mechanisms include leaflet tear or calcification, fracture of a stent post, stent creep and suture line disruption, and embolisation of a complete valve at progressed endocarditis, accompanied by acute heart failure.
- Bacterial or fungal endocarditis
- Pannus formation/obstruction – tissue growth onto valve ring
- Paravalvular leakage – interventional occlusion is often possible
- Haemolysis, although rarely experienced at modern valves.

Valve Reconstruction. Valve reconstructions aim to preserve the own valves, which are less prone to deterioration and infections due to the maintained own blood supply and immune defence, and require no long-term anticoagulation. Indeed, a well-repaired own valve is better than a perfect artificial one.

- *Aortic valve/root repair – e.g.* David repair (the mobilised own aortic root is repositioned inside a tube graft), Yacoub repair (the mobilised own aortic root is reconnected to a proximally aortic annulus-shaped interposition graft; the suture line runs 4–5 mm parallel to the aortic annulus. At this repair, the aortic root support is less.), Ozaki repair (a custom-tailored valve cusp replacement with autologous pericardium) and aortic valve annuloplasty rings (Schäfers, HAART 300 – BioStable Science)
- *Mitral and tricuspid valve repairs* – Excessive leaflet segment resection, plication, neochord implantation, cleft closure, perforation closure by a pericardial patch, etc. Two distinctive mitral repair philosophies present; resect or respect (keep structures, just modify configuration). Nevertheless, most adult AV leaflet repairs require annular stabilisation by a ring (complete – Edwards Physio II, Duran AnCore, etc.; partial – Colvin-Galloway Future Band; seldom used) or band (Cosgrove Edwards Annuloplasty System). The classical DeVega running suture tricuspid annular repair is rarely applied due to inferior long-term outcomes.

Ischaemic Heart Disease

The most common cause of death in Europe. Coronary artery disease affects more and younger men than women, although the incidence in women is increasing. It accounts for one-third of all male deaths and one-quarter of all female deaths.

Aetiology. Male sex, positive family history (first-degree relative – male <55 years/female <65 years), smoking, hypertension, hyperlipidaemia, diabetes, obesity.

Symptoms and Signs. Angina, shortness of breath, dysrhythmias, syncope, myocardial infarction (MI), CCF, sudden death. Often negative noninvasive examination at rest; at any suspicion, a stress test or invasive investigation is indicated. Diabetic signs. Occasionally xanthelasma. Cholesterol nodules. Arcus senilis. Symptoms and signs of concomitant peripheral vascular disease.

Investigations

- Biochemical assessment: Haematology and clinical chemistry (lipid profile and cardiac markers are crucial)

- CXR – cardiomegaly, fluid overload, pleural effusion
- ECG: resting test is negative in up to 75% of patients; ST changes with angina, Q waves, suddenly developing blocks, AF – exercise ECG usually confirms the diagnosis
- Echocardiogram: LV hypertrophy, reduced ejection fraction, regional wall motion abnormalities, thinned-out myocardium, aneurysm formation, acute mitral regurgitation, acute VSD development. Chemical (dobutamine) stress echocardiography might be required in asymptomatic patients who are unable to exercise.
- Cardiac catheterisation and coronary angiography – contrast medium is injected into each major coronary artery, and multiple projections are recorded by video cinematography; the disease extension is assessed. Fractional flow reserve measures pressure differences across coronary stenosis to determine the likelihood that the stenosis impedes oxygen delivery to the myocardium. Also, intravascular ultrasound (IVUS) can assess the significance of the stenosis. LV ventriculogram allows gross estimation of left ventricular ejection fraction (LVEF).
- ECG gated cardiac CT
- ECG gated cardiac computer tomography – a high-resolution CT scan is acquired gated with ECG triggering to eliminate movement artefact, and iodinated intravascular contrast reveals coronary anatomy.
- Cardiac magnetic resonance – this technique allows assessment of global ventricular function/geometry, muscle mass and myocardial perfusion.

Treatment

Conservative. Smoking cessation. Diet optimisation. Adjustment of hyperlipidaemia, anaemia, diabetes, and hypertension. Lifestyle counselling, tailored exercise programme. Vasodilators, e.g. nitroglycerine or calcium antagonist spray; β-blockers, e.g.: bisoprolol; calcium antagonists, e.g. diltiazem; potassium channel activators, e.g. nicorandil; antiplatelets, e.g. aspirin, clopidogrel; lipid-lowering agents, e.g. statins, fibrates, PCSK9 inhibitors; ACE inhibitors, e.g. ramipril; ARB, e.g. valsartan; selective I_f inhibitor, e.g. ivabradine.

Percutaneous Transluminal Coronary Angioplasty (PTCA). The procedure is undertaken to eliminate localised symptomatic coronary narrowing, i.e. causing angina unresponsive to medical treatment. A balloon, usually drug-coated, is inserted into the stenotic area under radiographic control and expanded. Low risk of infarction and mortality is associated with the standard procedure. Bare metal or drug-eluting stents prevent plaque collapse as a scaffold. Chronic occlusions are also recanalised with increasing success. Intracoronary rotablation can open up heavily calcified lesions.

Coronary Artery Bypass Graft (CAB). Surgery is indicated when there is intractable or unstable angina with haemodynamic compromise, triple vessel disease with depressed ventricular function, and left main stem stenosis or in diabetic patients. A concomitant valvular lesion with significant coronary disease requires surgical correction, although catheter-based valvular procedures in combination with PTCA are also emerging. As a standard bypass, a reverse segment of saphenous vein is anastomosed between the aorta and the coronary artery distal to the obstruction. Total arterial revascularisation is increasingly common. Both right and left internal mammary or radial arteries are used, as an arterial replacement. The gastroepiploic artery is rarely utilised for the distal right system.

The long-term postoperative outcomes are excellent when left ventricular function is in normal range, with a mortality of approximately 1%.

Surgery for Complications of Myocardial Infarction (MI)

Ventricular Aneurysm. The prognosis without surgery is moderately compromised: 45–50% of patients survive 5 years on medical treatment, and 75–80% with surgical resection, usually in combination with CAB. Death is due to LVF, MI and stroke caused by embolisation; rupture is rare but fatal.

Mitral Regurgitation. Infarct affects the papillary muscles, which may even rupture, resulting in a haemodynamic disaster. Treatment is by valve replacement with CAB if appropriate. Valve repair is increasingly popular, although outcomes are still variable due to challenges caused by the tethered subvalvular apparatus and remodelled LV geometry.

Ruptured Interventricular Septum. The defect is repaired with a Dacron patch, although associated with a high perioperative mortality rate (30–50%). The necrotic tissues are challenging to be sutured and not stable; it is an advantage if the patient's condition allows an operative delay of 1 week so that more robust fibrotic transformation may start on the lesion rims. VA-ECMO treatment may bridge the patient through the critical initial period. Limited, beneficially located defects might be amenable by percutaneous closure.

Pericarditis

This is inflammation of the parietal and visceral layers of the pericardium. It may occur as an isolated lesion or as part of a systemic disease. It is often idiopathic (probably viral), but it can be tuberculotic or tumour-related (direct invasion or metastatic), bacterial (*Staphylococcus*, *Streptococcus* or *Haemophilus* septicaemia), rheumatic fever, collagen diseases, uraemia, traumatic, postpericardiotomy syndrome, MI (Dressler's syndrome) may also cause it.

Symptoms and Signs. Sharp precordial pain radiating to shoulders and neck, often accompanied by malaise, fever, and pericardial friction rub. Heart sounds are diminished in case of an effusion that may evolve to tamponade, with concomitant tachycardia, hypotension, raised JVP, and pulsus paradoxus.

Investigations

- FBC – WCC elevated
- ESR/CRP raised
- U&Es – uraemia
- Blood culture
- CXR: globular heart if effusion
- ECG: ST elevation, R wave reduction due to pericardial fluid causing impedance
- Echocardiogram: exudates may show bright echoes on pericardium – pericardial effusion; in chronic cases, the pericardium might be thickened and calcified
- Diagnostic aspiration
- Biopsy

Treatment. As of the underlying cause or consequent pathologies.

Complications of Pericarditis

Cardiac Tamponade. A pericardial effusion as small as 100–150 mL may induce symptomatic tamponade if it develops rapidly, while gradual accumulation may render much larger amounts well tolerated. A compressing effusion interferes with diastolic filling and leads to limited cardiac output. The fluid may consist of blood (postoperative collection, ruptured ventricular aneurysm, type A aortic dissection, trauma) or inflammatory exudate (any pericarditis). Surprisingly, even air can lead to tamponade if an organ-pericardial connection has a valve-like element (e.g. oesophageal or gastric fistula) and a pressurised pericardium builds up.

Symptoms and Signs. Tachycardia, hypotension, raised JVP with systolic descent, pulsus paradoxus, reduced heart sounds, distended heart silhouette on CXR. The Earth-Heart sign on CXR is a feature of tension pneumomediastinum.

Treatment. Urgent when there are signs of cardiogenic shock. Tamponade is treated by pericardiocentesis with a wide-bore needle or pigtail catheter inserted under the xiphoid process. Samples are sent for microbiological and cytological examination in case of an exudate. Persistence or recurrence of symptoms is an indication for surgery to create a pericardial window for internal drainage. The pericardium is opened via an anterior mini-thoracotomy, or a VATS procedure is undertaken. If the cause is traumatic, a coexistent heart injury may require treatment.

Constrictive Pericarditis. The thickened, rigid pericardial sac limits the ventricular filling. Often idiopathic, while aetiological factors include postoperative status, irradiation, TB, renal failure and autoimmune process.

Symptoms and Signs. Dyspnoea, fatigue, oedema, ascites, renal and hepatic failure. Raised JVP, often accompanied by Kussmaul's sign, tachycardia, pulsus parvus, ascites, hepato-splenomegaly.

Investigations

- ECG: low voltage, T inversion
- CXR: calcified pericardium might be visible
- Echocardiogram: thickened and calcified pericardium, reduced cavity motions, especially in the filling phase.

Treatment. Surgical resection of the thickened pericardium.

Thoracic Aorta

Aneurysms

Aneurysms of the thoracic aorta are true (fusiform, saccular) or false (thrombus covers a perforation and gradually grows under pressure). Aortic aneurysms carry the risk of rupture or aortic dissection above a specific diameter. Risk factors for aneurysm development are male sex, hypertension, hypercholesterolemia, smoking, age and genetic predisposition (familial, Caucasian race). Certain monogenetic conditions such as Marfan's, Ehlers–Danlos, Loeys–Dietz and other connective tissue diseases predispose to early aneurysms. In addition, familial polygenetic conditions account for up to 20–25% of aneurysms, with the remainder of 'degenerative' aneurysms emerging typically over 60 years of age. Other essential associations include a bicuspid aortic valve (and aortic coarctation), post-trauma, inflammatory conditions (e.g. Takayasu's arteritis), drug abuse (cocaine) and historically, syphilis.

Symptoms and Signs

Asymptomatic. Incidental discovery on imaging. Ascending aortic involvement might be associated with valvular incompetence (dilated aortic root), hoarseness can be caused by pressure on the recurrent laryngeal nerve, back pain by vertebral erosion, dysphagia by pressure on the oesophagus and dyspnoea by phrenic nerve involvement. Rarely pain results from erosion of the sternum.

Investigations

- VDRL: syphilis
- CXR: mediastinal widening
- CT/CT angio scan. 3D reconstruction assisted operative planning
- Echocardiogram (especially regarding valvular lesions)
- MRA
- Genetic testing.

Treatment. Indications for surgery include size criteria, conservative treatment-resistant symptomatic aneurysms irrespective of size, dissection, rupture, documented rapid enlargement and significant aortic valve incompetence. Aneurysms of the ascending aorta and arch require a prosthetic graft replacement on CPB with or without circulatory arrest; in hypothermia/cerebral perfusion. In addition, replacement of the aortic valve/root and reimplantation of coronary orifices may be necessary. Aneurysm of the descending thoracic aorta is classically replaced by an interposition tube graft on partial left heart bypass. Nowadays, TEVAR of the descending aorta and increasingly in the arch region after debranching the supraaortic vessels is the therapy of choice. The most severe complication of repair of descending thoracic aortic aneurysms is paraplegia, occurring in about 5% of patients. Controlling the cerebrospinal pressures in all cases and selective perfusion of the Adamkiewicz artery during open repair may prevent this devastating complication.

Aortic Dissection

Aortic dissection is a discontinuation in the intimal lining of the aorta, resulting in conduction of blood flow in a false passage through the media. The latter may re-fenestrate into the true lumen creating a double lumen aorta between the entry and re-entry, and the patient may survive. In other cases, rupture, most commonly into the left hemithorax with exsanguination, or occlusion of the true lumen obstructing the blood flow via the major branches occur. As dissection advances, occlusion of aortic side branches may emerge with distinctive symptoms, e.g. coronaries (MI), carotids (stroke), spinal branches (paraplegia), renal arteries (anuria and renal failure) and visceral arteries (ischaemic bowel). The aortic dissection can also rupture into the pericardium, resulting in pericardial tamponade. Aetiological factors include hypertension, genetic predisposition and cystic medial necrosis. Most commonly classified according to Stanford criteria (clinical approach), where type A dissection involves the ascending aorta (corresponding to DeBakey I and II) and type B does not (DeBakey III). The arch area is a grey zone regarding the treatment, although isolated arch dissection is rare. European guidelines view it as non-A non-B dissections, the latest US criteria as type B dissection with a preference for supraaortic vessel debranching and TEVAR treatment. The DeBakey classification is an anatomical approach: type I: ascending and descending aorta; type II: ascending aorta only; and type III: descending aorta only. Although the Stanford classification is useful for everyday clinical decision-making, as type A dissection requires surgical and type B medical management, new classifications emerge to refine the therapeutic pathways. The Penn classification distinguishes type A dissection patients as non-ischaemic (Aa), branch ischaemic (Ab), generalised (Ac) or combined ischaemic (Abc) groups. The TEM (*T*ype, *E*ntry, *M*alperfusion) classification further divides the Stanford criteria into subcategories (Type A, B, non-A non-B; E0 – nondetectable, E1 – ascending aortic, E2 – aortic arch, E3 – descending aortic entry; M1 – coronary, M2 – supraaortic, M3 – descending aortic branch malperfusion) (Figure 10.3).

Symptoms and Signs. Sudden excruciating chest pain radiating to the back, sometimes challenging to distinguish from acute coronary syndrome. Shock. Signs of cardiac tamponade. MI may occur if the disease extends proximally. Sudden shortness of breath at acute aortic regurgitation. Hypotension. Claudication. Disparity of pulses or BP in extremities. Acute peripheral arterial occlusion. Neurological symptoms, coma. Acute abdomen.

Investigations

- ECG may exclude MI
- CXR: mediastinal widening, left pleural effusion if rupture
- CT angiography is the key investigation for diagnosis and planning treatment
- Echocardiogram (aortic flap, RWMA, pericardial effusion, aortic regurgitation).

Treatment

Medical. Control hypertension, e.g. labetalol infusion (decreases shear stress by controlling the heart rate), followed by nitrates such as sodium nitroprusside (cave: reflex tachycardia) or calcium channel blockers. Negative inotropic therapy (β-blockade) is essential to narrow the gap between the systolic and diastolic pressures, which may prevent the progression of dissection. Obtain CT

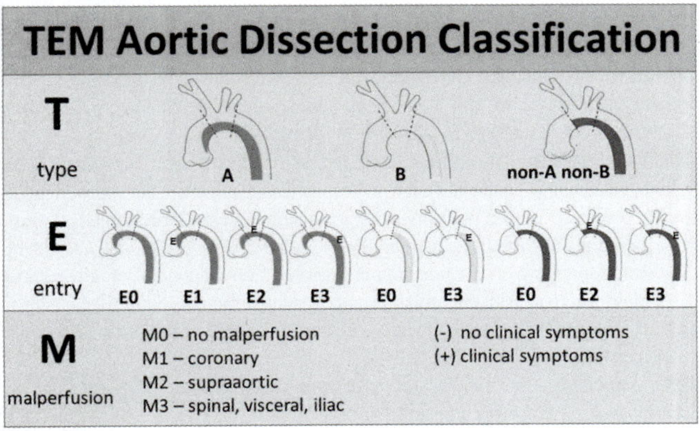

Figure 10.3

Type, Entry site, Malperfusion (TEM) classification of acute aortic dissections. Details are present in the text. *Sievers HH, Rylski B, Czerny M et al. Aortic dissection reconsidered: type, entry site, malperfusion classification adding clarity and enabling outcome prediction. Interact Cardiovasc Thorac Surg. 2020;30(3):451-457. The image is courtesy of Prof Bartosz Rylski MD PhD, Heart Centre Freiburg University, Germany, with permission of Oxford University Press.*

angiogram and echocardiogram (to detect pericardial effusion/tamponade, assess aortic valve function and coronary ostial anatomy). Long-term medical treatment includes long-acting β-blockers (e.g. nebivolol) and angiotensin II receptor blockers (e.g. losartan). The latter controls the blood pressure and the neutrophil-macrophage activation cascade, which is crucial in chronic vasculitis progression.

Surgical. In type A aortic dissection, urgent surgery is mandatory due to the high risk of fatal complications. The ascending aorta is replaced with a tube graft with or without aortic valve/root replacement. The procedure aims to remove the aortic dissection entry and reapproximate the layers of the aorta at the distal suture line; technically, we convert a type A dissection into a type B. Blood now enters the true lumen, decompressing the false channel and restoring blood flow through the branches. At type B dissection, primary medical therapy is indicated; if insufficient, endovascular or surgical treatment may be undertaken. Intervention, usually TEVAR, is indicated for intractable pain or hypertension, progressive malperfusion and rupture. Paraplegia may emerge resulting from compromised spinal cord blood flow.

Prognosis. Thirty-day perioperative mortality measures 10–15% in specialised aortic centres, which might be doubled in low-volume hospitals. Therefore, the latest guidelines suggest transferring aortic dissection patients to a specialised centre if reasonably possible. Postoperatively or in case of type B dissection, patients require regular follow-up with adequate BP control and imaging to monitor disease progression and to intervene by a lower-risk procedure (e.g. TEVAR) in a timely fashion if necessary.

Heart transplantation

Heart transplantation aims to enhance the quality of life and extend survival. Although transplant numbers are constantly increasing worldwide, there is still a considerable discrepancy between donor organ availability and potential recipient numbers. In this regard, bridge-to-transplant VAD therapy is crucial for transplant candidates. A heart transplant is indicated in end-stage heart failure refractory to maximal optimised medical treatment (usually LVEF<20%, VO_2<12 mL/kg/min).

Candidate Selection. The above-mentioned heart failure criteria. No systemic illness with less than 2 years of expected survival despite transplantation. No recent neoplasm in the last 5 years. No fixed pulmonary hypertension (PVR>6 Wood units, pulmonary systolic pressure >60 mmHg, transpulmonary gradient >15 mmHg). The age cut-off is 60–70 years, depending on the transplanting geolocation. In general, an advanced age which would interfere with the ability to recover from the procedure is the selection limitation. The psychiatric aspect is also relevant in that the patient will be compliant with the complex, life-long therapy.

Donor Selection. After the declaration of brain death, blood typing, serology, ECG, echocardiogram, ± coronary angiography of older donors or those with potential risk for coronary disease. Coronary disease is often accelerated in the graft after transplantation. Contraindications for donor suitability are ongoing sepsis, malignancy, excessive inotropic support requirements, and persistent LVEF reduction under 40% despite medical optimisation of therapy. Adequate donor procurement is essential for transplant success.

Surgical Technique. The biatrial orthotopic transplant technique was the first used, but the bicaval method is getting more common in the last two decades. Sinus node dysfunction, atrial arrhythmias, tricuspid regurgitation, and inferior atrial haemodynamics are higher with the biatrial approach. Total orthotopic or heterotopic techniques are seldom applied nowadays.

Immunosuppression. There is significant institutional variability present in immunosuppressive protocols. IL-2 antagonists and polyclonal antilymphotic antibodies are commonly used in the early postoperative period. In the long-term treatment, a combination of calcineurin inhibitors (tacrolimus, cyclosporin) or mTOR inhibitors (sirolimus, everolimus) with antiproliferative agents (mycophenolate, azathioprine) and corticosteroids is utilised.

Survival. The median survival measures approximately 50% at 10-year post-transplantation. Acute rejection or severe infections on immunosuppressive therapy are the leading cause of death. Cytomegalovirus infection is common with multiorgan involvement, its role is known in rejections and lymphoproliferative disorders, but direct mortality from the virus is low due to antiviral treatment. Emerging malignancies may join the picture resulting from chronic immunosuppression at later stages.

Rejection. ECG, echocardiography and endomyocardial biopsy are the routine follow-up for rejection; gene expression profiling from biopsies completes the rejection surveillance. Antithymocyte globulin (ATG) and high dose of intravenous corticosteroids are the treatment of choice in acute rejection. In addition, plasmapheresis or immune apheresis can be added for antibody-mediated rejection.

Cardiac Allograft Vasculopathy. Long-term complications and mortality are significantly associated with allograft vasculopathy, which diffusely affects the coronary arteries, in contrast to atherosclerotic coronary disease. Higher donor age is a risk for allograft vasculopathy. Therefore, follow-up including coronary angiography in combination with IVUS is recommended.

Chapter 11

Breast

Bahar Mirshekar • Lisa Caldon

CHAPTER OUTLINE

The majority of patients (90–95%) presenting with breast symptoms have benign disease, although at presentation most will fear they have cancer. Therefore a rapid, efficient, sympathetic approach to assessment and diagnosis is required. As such, breast assessment clinics are designed to permit the vast majority of women to be assessed, diagnosed and receive a management plan in one visit (one-stop clinics).

THE ASSESSMENT OF BREAST DISEASE – TRIPLE ASSESSMENT

Patients with breast disorders are assessed using a triple assessment (Fig. 11.1), namely clinical (history and examination), imaging (ultrasound and mammography) and pathology (FNAC and core biopsy). The three modalities are then viewed together to minimise the risk of inaccurate diagnosis. The accuracy of clinical and imaging assessment vary with the patient's age, being least accurate in the young but increasing with age as the breast involutes (and density reduces), resulting in abnormalities being easier to differentiate from normal breast tissue.

Patients with a mass or indeterminate findings on clinical or imaging assessment must have a biopsy, unless the diagnosis is clearly benign.

Clinical Assessment

History

- Symptoms: breast lump or thickening, skin tethering, nipple change or discharge, change in colour or size of the breast or breast pain. Take note of the description of symptoms, their duration, pattern and any precipitating or alleviating factors (including relation to the menstrual cycle).
- Assess the risk factors for breast cancer (see Table 11.1).
- Note any factors that might influence triple assessment, e.g. possible pregnancy (concern about radiation exposure), lactation, previous breast surgery, drugs or conditions that increase the risk of bleeding with biopsy (i.e. warfarin).

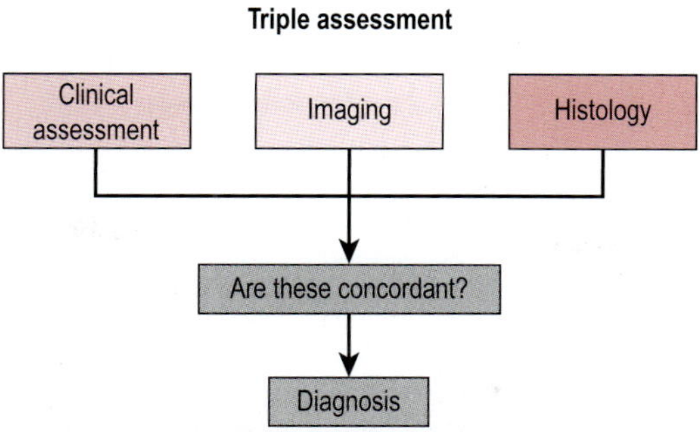

	1	2	3	4	5
P (Palpation)	Normal	Benign	Indeterminate	Suspicious	Cancer
U (Ultrasound)					
M (Mammogram)					
B (Biopsy)					

FIGURE 11.1
Triple assessment.

HINTS AND TIPS

Breast pain alone or pain with lumpiness are very common presenting complaints (18% and 33% of all patients respectively). It is almost always (95%) benign in nature. The pain may originate from the breast (cyclical) or chest wall (noncyclical, more common). However, pain that is severe, unilateral, focal, persistent (>3 months) and associated with focal discrete tenderness should be regarded as suspicious for cancer.

Examination

Look (Observation)

- The patient should be upright, with the arms down by their sides and breasts fully exposed. Observe for symmetry, colour, masses, skin tethering (dimpling), *peau d'orange*, nipple changes (inversion, rashes, etc.) and previous scars.
- Then observe with hands raised above head, to exaggerate any skin tethering.

Feel (Palpation)

- Lie the patient at about 30°, with the hands behind the head. This stretches the breast over the chest wall optimally for palpation.
- Palpate each quadrant of the breast and the axillary tail using a flat hand, feeling with the sensitive skin over the finger pulps and distal interphalangeal joints.
- Examine the nipples. If inversion is present, is it central (duct ectasia) or eccentric (cancer or scarring after periductal mastitis)? Are you able to evert the inverted nipple? Is there discharge? Note the colour of any discharge and whether it is unilateral or bilateral, and emerges from single or multiple ducts.
- Palpate for axillary and supraclavicular fossa lymph nodes. Are nodes palpable, soft or firm, mobile or fixed?

TABLE 11.1
RISK FACTORS FOR BREAST CANCER

Sex	99% of breast cancer occurs in women
Increasing age	Rare under 30 years 80% are > age 50 years 35% are > age 70 years
Endogenous oestrogen exposure	Early menarche
	Few/no pregnancies
	Age at first pregnancy >35 years
	Late menopause
	Breastfeeding history (risk is 4% lower for every year of breastfeeding)
	Chronic liver disease
	Postmenopausal obesity (BMI >28)
Exogenous oestrogen exposure	Contraceptives (increased risk during use, lowers to baseline at 10 years after discontinuation)
	HRT for >5 years > age 50 years
Genetics	Ancestry; founder genetic mutations, i.e. Ashkenazi Jews, Icelanders, Norwegians, etc.
Family history of breast and/or ovarian or other cancers	
High-risk gene mutations	*BRCA1*, *BRCA2* and *PALB2* mutations (most common); family history of breast and/or ovarian cancer, especially under age 40 years
Moderate risk gene mutations	Li–Fraumeni syndrome, Cowden's disease, Peutz–Jeghers syndrome, *CHEK2* mutations. Kleinfelter's syndrome in men
History of previous breast cancer	Invasive breast cancer or DCIS
Increased breast density	
Specific forms of benign breast change	Florid proliferative breast change; usual type hyperplasia, sclerosing adenosis, multiple papillomas, ADH, LCIS
Exposure to chest wall ionising radiation	Mantle radiotherapy as a child or teenager. Risk of cancer starts 10 years after the treatment
Lifestyle factors	Obesity, higher socioeconomic status, smoking, alcohol, inactivity

HINTS AND TIPS

Examining for axillary nodes can be a difficult technique to perform correctly, unless shown. Examine with the patient in the 30° lying position. It is easier to palpate the right axilla with the left hand and the left axilla with the right hand. With your fingertips directed into the axilla, get the patient to flex their elbow to 90° and rest it on your other hand. Push upwards and medially in the direction of the sternal notch. Palpate posteriorly to anterior on the curve of the chest wall high in the axilla and continue to do this while gradually retracting your hand.

Move. Is the mass fixed or mobile? If you are unsure, repeat your examination with the pectoralis major tensed (this is achieved by asking the patient to sit with their hands pressed on their hips).

General Examination Findings. BMI. Breast ptosis and symmetry. If relevant, examine for distant metastases.

Investigations

- *Breast USS*: universal imaging modality in breast assessment. It is more accurate than mammography in young patients, those with dense breasts and those with lobular cancers.
- *Staging axillary USS*: performed if the other investigations are suspicious for cancer, to look for any enlarged nodes with increased cortical thickness. If these are noted, an FNA or core biopsy is taken for diagnosis.
- *Mammography*: accuracy increases with increasing age and more radiolucent breasts (due to involution with fatty replacement). Mammograms are generally unreliable under 40 years because of the density of glandular breast tissue, so are only used in those over 40 years or when other investigations are suspicious for cancer. Mammograms look for the lesion in question and features suggestive of other foci of in situ or invasive breast cancer. Two-view mammography is performed, craniocaudal (CC) and medial lateral oblique (MLO). More recently, contrast enhance mammography is being used to improve accuracy and for local staging of breast cancers as a more cost-effective alternative to breast MRI. Mammograms are performed after the administration of i.v. iodinated contrast.
- *Breast MRI:* detects subtle morphological changes but differentiates poorly between benign and malignant lesions. Specific indications include lobular cancers undergoing breast conservation surgery (as the extent can be occult on mammogram and, less commonly, on USS) and patients with dense breast tissue. It is also used for family history surveillance in moderate- and high-risk women under 40 years (dense breasts) and among those with known *P53* gene mutations (risk of radiation-induced cancers with mammograms). Other indications include patients with implants if good mammographic Eklund views are not achievable, or if ruptured implants are suspected (linguine sign).

Pathology

- *Core biopsy*: three to five 1.6mm diameter cylinders of tissue (14G needle) are removed under local anaesthetic.
- *Vacuum-assisted biopsy (VAB or Mammotome)*: a larger biopsy, reserved for cases of diagnostic difficulty or microcalcification. Vacuum-assisted excision (VAE) can be used for therapeutic purposes (excision of radial scars, fibroadenomas <3cm in diameter).
- *FNAC*: reserved for very small and/or superficial lesions that would be difficult to biopsy via other techniques (including axillary nodes).
- Where possible, core and VAB are performed under ultrasound or mammographic guidance to optimise accuracy of sampling.
- A small radiolucent clip is placed at the time of biopsy in nonpalpable lesions and after diagnosis in patients having neoadjuvant chemotherapy (where the tumour can shrink or disappear) to help with intraoperative localisation.

The Multidisciplinary Team (MDT)

In the UK, all available information on patients undergoing full triple assessment are reviewed and discussed at an MDT meeting. Core members of the MDT comprise breast surgeons, breast clinicians, clinical nurse specialists, radiologists, pathologists and oncologists. The aim of the MDT is to minimise the risk of missed and delayed breast cancer diagnosis and ensure all relevant information for optimal treatment planning is available, correct and taken into consideration. Cases are re-discussed in the MDT whenever new information is available, e.g. postoperatively for adjuvant therapy planning.

CARCINOMA OF THE BREAST

This is the most common malignancy in females. The baseline risk of breast cancer in the UK is 10–12%, or 1 in 8 women, and the incidence is rising. Incidence increases with age. Survival has improved significantly over time, with 5-year survival rates for all breast cancer at 85%.

Risk Factors for Breast Cancer

Breast cancer has a multifactorial aetiology, with a combination of oestrogen exposure, environmental, genetic and behavioural factors (obesity, alcohol-induced liver disease) being implicated. Recognised genetic mutations account for only 5–10%. The risk factors are outlined in Table 11.1.

Presentation

- Symptomatic local/regional disease: painless breast lump or thickening; skin dimpling; breast asymmetry; skin erythema; nipple inversion or discharge (blood-stained or serosanguinous). The majority of breast cancers (50%) are located in the upper outer quadrant, as the majority of the breast's terminal ductolobular units are located at this site. On examination: a hard irregular mass, which can be mobile, fixed to skin or fixed deeply to the chest wall; a discrete asymmetric thickening; skin erythema; *peau d'orange*; Paget's disease of nipple; enlarged, mobile, fixed or matted axillary or supraclavicular lymph nodes
- Symptomatic metastatic disease: bone pain, breathlessness, increased abdominal girth, jaundice, headache, fits, personality change. Signs may include: liver (jaundice, hepatomegaly, ascites), lung or pleural (pleural effusion, consolidation), bone (bone tenderness or pathological fractures), brain (papilloedema)
- Asymptomatic detected via screening
- Incidental finding, e.g. on chest CT.

Investigations

- Triple assessment. A mammogram of a patient with breast cancer is shown in Figure 11.2.
- If indicated (large cancer, locally advanced disease, multiple lymph node metastases), staging for distant metastases; FBC, LFTs and calcium; and either CT chest/abdomen and pelvis plus isotope bone scan (current standard in the UK) or PET-CT. CT of the brain is not routinely performed unless indicated by symptoms.

Types of Primary Breast Cancer

These can be subdivided into in situ and invasive breast cancers. The types, classic features and frequency are shown in Table 11.2.

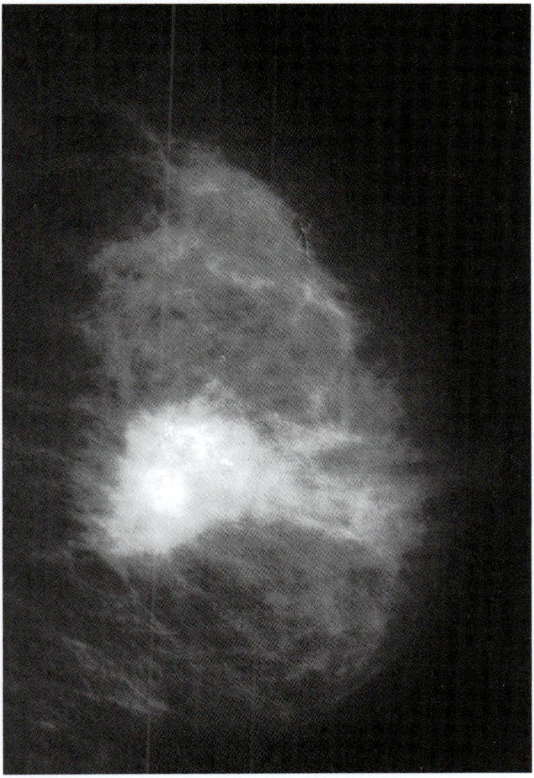

FIGURE 11.2

A mammogram showing a carcinoma of the breast.There is a dense mass with microcalcification. Malignant microcalcification requires careful examination of the film with magnification: it does not reproduce well in photographs.

Clinical Staging

Two forms are in wide use (Tables 11.3, 11.4). Table 11.4 and 11.5 show the prognosis associated with the different stages of breast cancer.

Treatment of Breast Cancer

The treatment of breast cancer is multimodal, involving local (surgery, radiotherapy) and systemic (chemotherapy, biological, endocrine and bisphosphonate) treatments. Treatment is planned by the MDT and takes into account cancer type, biology and stage, plus patients' comorbidities. Traditionally, surgery was done first, and was followed by adjuvant chemo or radiotherapy; however, neoadjuvant chemotherapy is now being used more frequently, particularly in triple-negative or HER2-positive tumours greater than 2 cm or associated with axillary metastases. This reduces the

TABLE 11.2

TYPES OF PRIMARY BREAST CANCER

Invasive Breast Cancer	Features	% of Invasive Breast Cancer
Ductal	Classical firm lump	78%
Lobular	Can present as a less well-defined thickening. Tend to be grade 2, ER+ HER2−. Less responsive to chemotherapy	10%
Mucinous	Dispersed cancers cells in lakes of mucin. Can masquerade as a complex cyst	5%
Tubular	A ductal subtype. Tend to be grade 1, ER+, HER2− good prognosis cancers	
Medullary	A rare ductal subtype. Soft to palpation. High grade in appearance but low grade in behaviour. Usually lymph node negative	<5%
Papillary	Usually in postmenopausal women, often grade 2 and associated with DCIS	1–2%
In Situ Breast Cancer		**% of In Situ Breast Cancer**
DCIS	Usually impalpable and screen detected as linear branching microcalcification. The disease and, therefore, treatments are local	90%
LCIS	Usually impalpable and screen detected. Pleomorphic LCIS is treated as per DCIS. The classical variety is regarded as risk lesion for breast cancer, and monitored	10%

TABLE 11.3

AMERICAN JOINT COMMITTEE ON CANCER (AJCC) STAGING BASED ON TNM CLASSIFICATION

Primary (T)	Tis – carcinoma in situ T0 – no primary tumour located T1 – tumour <2 cm T2 – tumour 2–5 cm T3 – tumour >5 cm T4 a – extension to chest wall (excluding pectoralis major muscle) b – ulceration, ipsilateral satellite nodules, *peau d'orange* c – both T4a and T4b d – inflammatory carcinoma
Nodes (N)	N0 – no nodal involvement N0i+ – isolated tumour cells N1a – 1-3 ipsilateral axillary nodes involved N1mi+ – micrometastases N2a – 4-9 ipsilateral axillary nodes involved N3a – ≥10 ipsilateral axillary nodes involved
Metastases (M)	M0 – no metastases M1 – distant metastases

TABLE 11.4

UNION FOR INTERNATIONAL CANCER CONTROL CLASSIFICATION OF BREAST CANCER

		TNM	5-Year Survival	10-Year Survival
Stage 0		Tis, N0, M0	99%	98%
Stage I	A	T1, N0/N1mi, M0	90–94%	85%
	B	T0/T1, N1, M0		
Stage II	A	T0, N1, M0 T1, N1, M0 T2, N0, M0	70%	60%
	B	T2, N1, M0 T3, N0, M0		
Stage III	A	T0, N2, M0 T1, N2, M0 T2, N2, M0 T3, N1, M0 T3, N2, M0	50–55%	40%
	B	T4, any N, M0	42–48%	
	C	Any T, N3, M0		
Stage IV		Any T, any N, M1	13%	10%

TABLE 11.5

NOTTINGHAM PROGNOSTIC INDEX*

		Predicted 10-Year Survival (%)	
Score	*Prognostic Group*	*No Adjuvant Chemo.*	*Tamoxifen if ER+*
<2.4	Excellent	95	–
2.41–3.4	Good	85	89
3.41–4.4	Moderate I	70	78
4.41–5.4	Moderate II	50	63
>5.4	Poor	20	41

*0.2 × diameter (cm) + LN (lymph node) status (0 = 0, 1–4 = 2, >4 = 3) + grade (1 = 1, 2 = 2, 3 = 3).

chance of delays to systemic therapy (e.g. due to surgical complications). Neoadjuvant chemotherapy can also be used to make surgery possible (large, locally advanced, inoperable cancers) or less cosmetically disruptive (downsize to make excision less extensive), or to guide adjuvant chemotherapy by using the pathological tumour response as a biomarker for the effectiveness of neoadjuvant therapy. In patients who require genetic testing, it also allows time for this, which can affect surgical management (e.g. bilateral mastectomy instead of breast-conserving surgery in patients with a breast cancer-specific gene mutation). Neoadjuvant endocrine therapy is also sometimes used in ER-positive HER2-negative tumours where surgery may be delayed. Primary endocrine therapy can be used as the sole therapy in ER-positive HER2-negative tumours in patients who are unsuitable for surgery.

Local Treatments (Surgery and Radiotherapy)

The aim is to achieve local control of the disease.

Surgery

There are a number of surgical options, from simple mastectomy to breast conservation surgery (BCS) / wide local excision (WLE), where the disease is removed with a sufficient margin to ensure all of the disease has been removed. Recent trends are to more BCS, and mastectomy rates are reducing internationally. Over recent years the surgical approach to breast cancer has been refined further as plastic surgical approaches and techniques have been integrated into the specialty. This new approach is called oncoplastic breast surgery.

Breast Conservation Surgery (BCS). BCS options involve simple WLE, which can be performed alone or with either volume replacement (such as perforator artery flaps), or volume displacement (such as therapeutic mammoplasty) techniques. Surgery is now performed with a view to fully excising the disease while also minimising the cosmetic impact of the surgery (preserving the volume and contour of the breast), i.e. the oncoplastic approach.

WLE is removal of the lesion with a margin of normal breast tissue, to minimise the risk of local recurrence. If the lesion is impalpable (such as those detected by screening), it is localised under radiological guidance prior to the surgery. Wires used to be the mainstay of localisation, but a variety of techniques are now available including radioactive radioisotope injection (ROLL), insertion of radioactive markers (I^{125}seeds), magnetic seeds, radiofrequency identification tags and radar localisers. Marker seeds allow the lesion to be localised prior to the day of surgery, and in some cases before neoadjuvant chemotherapy instead of a marker clip.

Mastectomy. Mastectomy is required for multifocal cancers (more than one tumour in a breast quadrant), multicentric cancers (tumours in more than one breast quadrant), large cancers in smaller breasts, or may be chosen by patients who have cancers technically suitable for BCS. The most common version of mastectomy is a simple mastectomy, where pectoralis major and minor are preserved. Mastectomy can be performed alone or with immediate reconstruction. When combined with an immediate reconstruction, the skin and/or NAC can be preserved. If radiotherapy after mastectomy is likely, most surgeons defer definitive reconstruction due to increased complications and worse cosmetic outcomes.

Staging and Management of the Axilla. Whichever excision technique is used, the axilla should be formally staged and treated. Axillary staging can be performed by SNB, axillary node sampling or ALND (previously referred to as axillary node clearance). In the UK patients with a normal axilla on preoperative staging USS have a SNB to improve accuracy of axillary staging. The sentinel lymph node is the first in the chain of lymph nodes draining a region (see Fig. 11.3). Radioisotope (Tc^{99}) and/or blue dye (Patent Bleu) or magnetic tracer (Magtrace) are used to identify the node. Traditionally patients with positive nodes would proceed to ALND or radiotherapy.

Complications of Surgery

- Surgery to the breast: infection, bleeding, seroma, pain/numbness, poor cosmesis

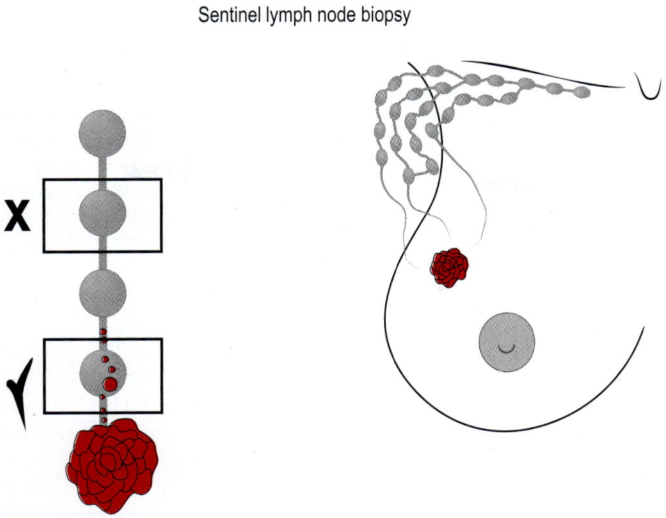

FIGURE 11.3
The sentinel lymph node is the first in the chain of lymph nodes draining an anatomical region. The assessment of this specific node provides the most accurate axillary staging information, with minimised risk of the complication of lymphoedema.

- Surgery to the axilla: numbness of the upper inner arm (intercostobrachial nerve distribution), shoulder stiffness, lymphoedema of the arm (1–2% risk with SNB, 10–25% risk with ALND)
- Psychological: associated with the impact of the cancer diagnosis and surgery.

Radiotherapy

Radiotherapy is used to reduce the risk of local recurrence, both after BCS and also among those who are most at risk after mastectomy (larger grade 3 cancers, inflammatory cancers, cancers close to the chest wall and those with high-volume axillary lymph node metastases). Radiotherapy is also given as a targeted local treatment to bony metastases, and can be used to gain control in locally advanced breast cancer.

Complications of Radiotherapy. Common early complications are fatigue, skin soreness and erythema. Later side effects include fibrosis of local structures including breast, lung (pneumonitis) and coronary arteries (increased risk of cardiac disease), and osteoradionecrosis (rib fractures). Poor healing should be expected when operating on tissue that has previously been exposed to radiotherapy.

Systemic Therapies (Chemotherapy, Endocrine Therapy and Biological Therapies, Plus Bisphosphonates)

Chemotherapy

The decision to give chemotherapy is based on the presence of overt metastases or the statistical probability that metastases are present. The probability of metastases being present is estimated using one of a number of tools such as the Nottingham Prognostic Index (Table 11.5) or an online tool such as PREDICT, which incorporates receptor status, biological features, tumour turnover markers, in addition to size, grade and nodal status, to allow more accurate individualised prediction of prognosis with and without chemotherapy. Because chemotherapy works most effectively on rapidly dividing cells, the greatest and most rapid response is seen among the more aggressive breast cancers (ER-, HER2+, triple-negative, and grade 3 invasive ductal cancers). For ER+ HER2- tumours with an intermediate risk of distant recurrence, tumour gene profiling assays (e.g. Prosigna, Oncotype DX) can be used to provide extra information about the risk of distant recurrence and therefore the recommendation for chemotherapy.

Biological Therapies

These include monoclonal antibody targeted against HER2 protein, e.g. trastuzumab (Herceptin). Twenty percent of patients' cancers are HER2+. Most of these are grade 3 cancers. As with endocrine therapy, these treatments only work in the presence of the appropriate receptor. Before the provision of adjuvant therapy against HER2, the presence of these receptors was associated with worse prognosis. They are now equivalent as long as optimal therapy is received.

Complications of Chemotherapy and Biological Therapies. Short-term side effects include gingivitis, nausea, vomiting, diarrhoea, bone marrow suppression (anaemia, thrombocytopenia and neutropenia), mild cognitive impairment, early menopause, peripheral neuropathy, cardiotoxicity and osteoporosis.

Bisphosphonates

Bisphosphonates were used in breast cancer treatment to counteract the osteopenic side effects of aromatase inhibitors (AIs). They are now recognised to independently reduce metastases and improve survival.

Endocrine Therapy

Endocrine therapy is only given to patients whose cancers have oestrogen receptors on their surface (ER+ cancers). Endocrine therapy is divided into selective oestrogen receptor modulators (SERMs) like tamoxifen and raloxifene, and AIs such as anastrozole, letrozole and exemestane. SERMs block oestrogen receptors. AIs inhibit the conversion of circulating steroids to oestrogen. Endocrine therapy reduces the risk of local recurrence, contralateral ER+ invasive breast cancer and increases survival. There is evidence that AIs are more effective than SERMs in postmenopausal women. Premenopausal women need the total oestrogen receptor blockade provided by SERMs, as their primary source of oestrogen is ovarian. Ovarian oestrogen production can also be stopped with oophorectomy or a synthetic luteinising hormone releasing hormone (LHRH) analogue (goserelin). Endocrine therapy is given as both adjuvant and primary treatment. Primary endocrine therapy can be offered as an alternative to surgery in patients who refuse surgery or have a poor life expectancy (<5 years), either due to advanced age or higher risk of mortality from another cause. Neoadjuvant endocrine therapy can also be used to downstage and downsize breast cancers prior to surgery.

Complications of Endocrine Therapies. These include menopausal symptoms, weight gain, bone/joint pain, fatigue, dry skin, hair thinning, loss of libido, insomnia and depression. Osteoporosis is a specific side effect of AIs, and thromboembolic events and endometrial cancer are side effects of tamoxifen.

A summary of the various treatment modalities is shown in Table 11.6.

TABLE 11.6

SUMMARY OF TREATMENT MODALITIES

Treatment Modality	Indication
Surgery	
BCS (WLE +/- therapeutic mammoplasty or local flap reconstruction)	• Cancer resectable with clear margins, leaving sufficient residual breast volume • Patient choice • Able to undergo radiotherapy
Mastectomy	• Multifocal cancer • Cancer too large for breast-conserving surgery • Unsuitable for radiotherapy/history of previous radiotherapy to same breast • Patient choice e.g. breast cancer gene mutation carrier
Salvage mastectomy	• Locally advanced cancer ± chest wall resurfacing with skin graft or flap
Sentinel lymph node biopsy	• Invasive cancer with no evidence of axillary metastases on preoperative imaging • DCIS with high risk of invasion (e.g. mass-forming) or if patient undergoing mastectomy

Axillary lymph node dissection	• At least one biopsy-proven axillary metastasis on preoperative imaging
	• Patients who have positive lymph nodes on sentinel lymph node biopsy. However:
	  ◦ postmenopausal patients with T1 tumour, grade 1-2, ER+, HER2- undergoing whole breast radiotherapy and endocrine therapy can avoid further axillary treatment
	  ◦ patients with 1–2 positive sentinel lymph nodes can have axillary radiotherapy instead of ALND (reduced risk of lymphoedema)
	• Inflammatory breast cancer

Radiotherapy	
Whole breast	• To reduce local recurrence risk • Invasive cancer; all having BCS • Most DCIS unless low risk
Tumour bed boost	• Given with or after whole breast radiotherapy to reduce risk of local recurrence • For patients with high risk of local recurrence e.g. age under 50 years
Partial breast	• Radiotherapy targeted to tumour bed • For patients with low risk of local recurrence
Chest wall ± supraclavicular fossa radiotherapy	• Mastectomy with high local recurrence risk, i.e. grade 3, high-volume lymph node disease • Local disease control in palliation
Electron boost	• Local disease control in palliation
Targeted local	• Bone metastases
Chemotherapy	
Neoadjuvant	• Downstage locally advanced cancer prior to surgery • Downsize to increase potential for BCS • Use tumour as a bioassay to assess response to neoadjuvant therapy and therefore guide adjuvant treatment

Continued

TABLE 11.6
SUMMARY OF TREATMENT MODALITIES

Treatment Modality	Indication
Primary	• Palliation for local disease control
Adjuvant	• For proven or predicted systemic metastases • Palliation for local disease control
Biological Therapies	
	• Targeted neoadjuvant or adjuvant treatment for HER2+ and triple-negative breast cancer
Endocrine Therapy	
	Targeted neoadjuvant or adjuvant treatment for ER+ breast cancer that reduce or block the effects of circulating oestrogen. These include: • AIs in postmenopausal women • SERMs, oophorectomy, or LHRH analogues + AIs in premenopausal women
Electrochemotherapy	
	• Local disease control for cutaneous metastases

Follow-up

- Routine breast self-examination
- Clinical follow-up is in accordance with local protocols
- Mammography is traditionally performed annually for 5 years.

LOCALLY RECURRENT DISEASE. May be treated by:

- Surgery if operable
- Radiotherapy if this has not been given to the area before
- Endocrine therapy or chemotherapy and/or biological therapy.

Palliation

Multimodality treatments are used to palliate locally advanced and stage IV disease. Psychological support and best supportive care should be viewed as an essential part of the management of advancing disease.

Palliation of locally advanced breast cancer

- Local control of extensive or fungating lesions: salvage surgery or radiotherapy are options but may result in large chest wall defects requiring closure by skin graft or myocutaneous flap.

Palliation of metastatic breast cancer

- Reduce tumour burden: endocrine therapy or palliative chemotherapy and/or biological therapy
- Bony metastases: localised radiotherapy, bisphosphonates, ± prophylactic fixation of areas at risk of pathological fracture
- Spinal metastases at risk of cord compression: decompression and stabilisation
- Pleural effusion: aspiration of and instillation of cytotoxic agents
- Skin metastases: electrochemotherapy shows promising results for local control.

Breast Reconstruction

Following mastectomy, patients are provided with an external prosthesis that fits into their bra, which provides a 'normal' appearance when clothed. It is now increasingly common for patients to undergo breast reconstructive surgery, either at the time of resection (immediate reconstruction) or after the completeness of excision is confirmed and/or adjuvant treatments complete (delayed reconstruction). Reconstruction can be achieved using breast implants or autologous tissue according to patient preference, size of breast, availability of donor-site material, fitness for surgery and risk of complications. Autologous reconstruction is achieved using a pedicled or microsurgical free tissue transfer. The techniques used are described in Chapter 20.

Breast Screening

Screening is intended to facilitate the early detection of breast cancer, to improve the prognosis. As a result, the 1-year survival rate of screen-detected malignancies is very high (96%). Currently, all women aged 50–70 years in the UK are invited to have two-view mammography every 3 years. In 2012, there was a trial (AgeX) extending this to women aged 47–73 years – the results are awaited. Suspicious lesions on mammography require further imaging with further mammography (magnified paddle views or tomography) ± USS and image-guided core biopsy or VAB, and then appropriate treatment is undertaken.

Ductal Carcinoma In Situ (DCIS)

DCIS represents an area of dysplasia within the breast ducts between atypia and malignancy. The dysplastic cells reach but do not invade the basement membrane. It is therefore a localised disease that cannot metastasise. It can be low, intermediate or high nuclear grade and has a variety of histological subtypes. The majority (90%) are asymptomatic and are therefore detected by breast screening programmes, where they appear as linear branching microcalcification (see Fig. 11.2). DCIS represents 25–30% of screen-detected breast cancers. It can also present with symptoms such as a lump, blood/serosanguinous nipple discharge or Paget's disease. As the size of DCIS increases, the likelihood of it containing focal areas of invasion rises.

TREATMENT. Treatment is local, as it is a localised disease.

- Surgery: WLE with 2mm margins +/- oncoplastic techniques or mastectomy (± immediate breast reconstruction) if DCIS is widespread or multifocal
- Radiotherapy: required in those who have WLE unless they have very low risk of local recurrence (ALL of: age over 50 years, size less than 2.5cm, low/intermediate grade and clear margins)
- Endocrine therapy: some centres now test DCIS for ER status and offer endocrine therapy accordingly.

If histology confirms invasion, management is as for invasive breast cancer.

STAGING.

- Axillary USS staging is routine.
- Surgical axillary staging with SNB is performed within some centres routinely when a patient has BCS for a large area of DCIS (typically >4–5cm) and in those having mastectomy.

Lobular Carcinoma In Situ (LCIS)

LCIS is subdivided into classical and pleomorphic LCIS. The classical variety is now regarded as a risk lesion for breast cancer rather than preinvasive disease and is monitored with increased surveillance, rather than excised. Pleomorphic LCIS is treated like DCIS.

Paget's Disease of the Nipple

This is associated with DCIS, with the abnormal cells spreading within the epithelium on to the nipple.

Symptoms and Signs. Red, eczematous-like lesion that starts on the nipple, eventually eroding the nipple, then spreads outwards onto the areola. There may be a palpable mass.

Differential Diagnosis. Eczema of the nipple (usually bilateral, itchy and not erosive).

Investigations. Triple assessment, usually including a punch biopsy of the nipple.

Treatment. The treatment is as for DCIS.

Prognosis. In the absence of any invasive component, the prognosis is excellent.

Inflammatory Carcinoma of the Breast

This rare form of breast cancer (1–4%) is the most aggressive. It develops rapidly (can progress visibly in days) and metastasises early and widely. It is more common in younger patients and can present in pregnancy or lactation. The Black population is at slightly increased risk. The diagnosis should be considered in postmenopausal women presenting with features suggestive of bacterial mastitis; this is very uncommon in women who do not smoke, or are not pregnant or breastfeeding.

Symptoms and Signs. Warm/hot, enlarged, heavy, red/pink breast, which remains unchanged despite receiving antibiotics for presumed bacterial mastitis. Generalised breast enlargement with extensive skin changes (thickening, oedema, erythema and *peau d'orange*). Pathological axillary nodes are often palpable at presentation.

Diagnosis

- USS
- Mammogram may not be possible due to lack of tissue compliance and tenderness
- Core biopsy of USS-detected lesions or punch biopsy of the skin
- Staging for distant metastases: CT chest/abdomen and pelvis plus isotope bone scan, or PET-CT.

Treatment. Combination of primary chemotherapy, followed by mastectomy and ALND, and chest wall radiotherapy.

Prognosis. Prognosis is poor compared with other forms of breast cancer, but has improved dramatically (from <5% to 50% at 5 years provided that there are no distant metastases) since the adoption of comprehensive multimodal treatment.

Special Contexts for Breast Cancer

Pregnancy

This is uncommon (1 in 3000 to 10,000 pregnancies and comprises 1–3% of breast cancers). These are typically ER-, PR-, HER2+ invasive ductal cancers. One to four percent are inflammatory cancers.

Investigations

- US with core biopsy is the investigation of choice.
- Digital mammography with abdominal shielding.
- MRI: is probably safe, but adequate human data is not available.
- Chest X-ray (with abdominal shielding) and liver US for further staging if required.

Treatment. Specific treatment is tailored to the cancer biology, trimester and whether the patient wishes to proceed with the pregnancy or undergo a termination. An obstetrician specialising in high-risk pregnancies should be involved. Specific differences in the management of this group include:

- Surgery can be undertaken in any trimester but there is an increased risk of spontaneous abortion. Immediate breast reconstruction should be avoided to reduce length of general anaesthetic and asymmetry.
- SNB using isotope only, as blue dye cannot be used due to possible teratogenicity.
- Chemotherapy can be given after the first trimester. Tamoxifen and trastuzumab (Herceptin) are contraindicated in pregnancy.
- Radiotherapy should be delayed until after delivery, therefore avoid breast-conserving surgery in first trimester as there will be a prolonged delay before radiotherapy.

Prognosis. Stage for stage, the prognosis for breast cancer in pregnancy is the same as that diagnosed in nonpregnant women. However, patients typically present at a later stage (60% with regional lymph node metastases) as symptoms and signs are often masked by pregnancy-related breast changes.

Male Breast Carcinoma

This is rare and predominantly occurs in older men (mean age 61–70 years). It presents with a unilateral, hard, painless mass. Most are ER+.

Investigation

- Triple assessment
- USS for axillary node staging
- Staging for distant metastases: CT chest/abdomen and pelvis plus isotope bone scan, or PET-CT.

Treatment

Local treatment

- Mastectomy
- Axillary management; depends on axillary staging
- Radiotherapy: often given to reduce the risk of local recurrence (increased compared with female patients due to more locally advanced disease with closer proximity of cancer to skin and chest wall – 40% stage III or IV at diagnosis).

Systemic treatment

- If ER+ tamoxifen; tolerance due to side effects is a problem. AIs have been used, but are associated with reduced efficacy. Other options are orchidectomy and LHRH analogues.
- Chemotherapy; adjuvant or neoadjuvant depending on stage and indication.

Prognosis. The prognosis of male breast cancer is thought to be identical to that of the female type when compared stage for stage. However, males tend to present at a later stage with more locally advanced disease, therefore overall prognosis tends to be worse.

Pseudolipoma

This is a soft lobulated swelling of the breast resembling a lipoma. It is caused by an underlying carcinoma causing retraction of the suspensory ligaments of the breast resulting in bunching of the fat between the skin, septae of the breast, and the carcinoma. Beware the diagnosis of lipoma of the breast, especially in the older patient. Mammography is advised.

Risk Reduction in Women With Moderate and High Risk

NICE guidelines published in 2013 clarified risk reduction strategies among women of greater than baseline population risk of breast cancer.

- All groups are offered lifestyle modification and breast self-examination/awareness information.
- Moderate and high-risk women are offered additional enhanced breast screening and chemoprophylaxis with tamoxifen or raloxifene if premenopausal and AI if postmenopausal.
- High-risk women and those with a ≥10% risk of breast cancer-associated gene mutation are offered genetic testing (for BRCA1, BRCA2 and PALB2) and risk reducing surgery. Mastectomy ± reconstruction reduces risk by about 90%; and salpingo-oophorectomy around age 40 years offers risk reduction of approximately 50% for breast cancer and 90% for tubo-ovarian cancer in BRCA1 and BRCA2 patients.

CONGENITAL DISORDERS OF THE BREAST

This includes duplication, absence and hypoplasia of breast structures.

Duplication

Accessory nipples (polythelia, affects 1–6% of women) or breasts (polymastia, affects 1–2% of women) can occur anywhere along the mammalian ('milk') line, which extends from the axilla to groin. The most common site for an accessory breast is the axilla, and the most common site for accessory nipples is just below the inframammary fold.

Treatment

- No treatment required unless symptomatic.

Absence and Hypoplasia

The absence of breast tissue (amasia) can occur in isolation or associated with absence of the NAC (athelia) and/or the pectoralis muscles.

Breast hypoplasia can be congenital or iatrogenic, uni- or bilateral. It often becomes evident at puberty. Iatrogenic hypoplasia can result from exposure of the developing breast to surgery or ionising radiation in childhood (i.e. radiotherapy for lung metastases from Wilms' tumour, mantle radiotherapy for non-Hodgkin's lymphoma). Individuals exposed to radiotherapy are at increased risk of breast cancer, and should be placed on high-risk breast surveillance programmes.

Treatment

- Treatment is aimed at improving cosmesis and symmetry. In women this involves breast augmentation with prostheses or lipofilling (also called fat transfer).

HINTS AND TIPS

Surgery on the developing breast should be avoided, as any damage to the breast bud can cause significant long-term deformity.

ABERRATIONS OF NORMAL DEVELOPMENT AND INVOLUTION

Many breast conditions which used to be labelled benign breast diseases are now considered physiological aberrations (very common and occur at a consistent time point), and are classified under the encompassing term aberrations of normal development and involution (ANDI).

The breast has three phases in its lifecycle: development (<25years), mature reproductive life (25–40 years) and involution (35–55 years). Aberrations can occur in the stroma and lobular components in any of these phases.

Aberrations of Development (<25 Years of Age)

Major duct structures are present behind the nipple in both sexes and remain identical until puberty, when oestrogen levels rise and stimulate duct proliferation. This is greater in females, and lobules develop at their termination. Externally the breast bud develops under the NAC, then the breast enlarges. Lobules do not develop in males; for this reason males do not develop lobular cancer.

Juvenile Hypertrophy. Initially breast development is normal, but then the adolescent girl experiences uncontrolled excessive growth due to an aberration of stromal development. Patients complain of discomfort and self-consciousness due to the breast volume.

Treatment. Breast reduction.

Fibroadenoma

Fibroadenomas are common, comprising 60% of all palpable lumps in women under 20 years and 13% of all breast lumps in the UK. They develop from the excessive division of a single lobule. This results in a densely whorled mass, which compresses surrounding normal tissue creating a pseudocapsule. They sometimes go unnoticed by the patient until the breast softens with involution, or they may be an incidental finding noticed on the first screening mammogram, where they are seen as a rounded or lobulated radiopaque density.

Giant fibroadenomas are an uncommon variant (0.5% of all fibroadenomas) and are over 5 cm in diameter.

Symptoms and Signs. The classic history is of a mobile, nontender breast lump, which usually does not vary in size with the menstrual cycle. On examination there is a discrete, smooth, rubbery swelling which is very mobile (commonly termed a breast 'mouse'). There is no evidence fibroadenomas undergo malignant transformation.

Investigation. Triple assessment to exclude carcinoma. Core biopsy can be omitted if the patient is under 25 years, there is no history of rapid growth, and US appearances are classic of a fibroadenoma.

Treatment

- Reassurance only: if the diagnosis is certain and the lump not symptomatic.
- Regular monthly breast self-examination; and seek reassessment if the lump starts to enlarge rapidly or become painful. Over time 10% will enlarge, a third will shrink, and the rest will remain unchanged. Phyllodes tumour can masquerade as a fibroadenoma; and the two cannot necessarily be differentiated on clinical, imaging or pathological assessment (unless the entire lesion is removed). For this reason, some surgeons advocate excision of all fibroadenomas over 3 cm.
- Excision should be performed if there is any uncertainty about the diagnosis.

Phyllodes Tumours

Phyllodes tumours are rare. Microscopically, there is a leaf-like structure, with a higher mitotic count than seen with fibroadenomas. There is a spectrum of benign (70%), to borderline (20%), to malignant (10%) phyllodes tumours. In contrast to fibroadenomas (which arise from the lobular elements of the breast), they arise from the breast stroma. Malignant phyllodes are classified as soft tissue sarcomas, and metastasise (very rare) with a similar pattern (lungs). The history tends to differ from that of the fibroadenoma; they tend to occur in an older age group (40–50 years), and there is often a history of rapid growth of the discrete, rubbery breast lump, sometimes with accompanying pain from compression of normal surrounding breast tissue.

Investigation. Triple assessment.

Treatment. Excision: with a 5 mm rim of normal breast tissue to minimise local recurrence (10–20% risk with the benign variety). There is no indication for SLNB in Phyllodes tumours.

Aberrations of Mature Reproductive Life (25–40 Years of Age)

The fully developed breast undergoes cyclical changes associated with the menstrual cycle in mature reproductive life. In the premenstrual phase, cyclical breast pain is common and regarded as physiological. It is only regarded as an aberration if pain is particularly severe or protracted.

BENIGN BREAST CHANGE. This is the pathological term given to focal breast nodularity associated with cyclical breast activity. It is the most common cause of a breast 'lump' among women in this age group and accounts for about 38% of all UK breast referrals. This is often associated with exaggerated cyclical breast pain. Terms like 'fibrocystic disease', 'fibroadenosis' and 'cyclical mastitis' were used to describe this condition before it was recognised as an aberration of normal physiology.

Symptoms and Signs. Premenstrual breast lumps/lumpiness/thickening, which can be tender. Examination reveals tender lumpy or nodular breasts with thickened areas, most commonly in the upper outer quadrant.

Investigations. Triple assessment to exclude carcinoma if a dominant mass or asymmetric thickening is present. USS will confidently confirm the presence of benign breast change. Mammography is indicated if the patient is ≥40 years. Core biopsy is performed if clinical or imaging assessments are indeterminate.

Treatment. Keeping a breast pain diary documenting severity and symptoms in relation to menstrual cycle can help differentiate between cyclical and noncyclical breast pain. Ninety percent of patients only require:

- A clear, sympathetic explanation and reassurance regarding their diagnosis. Normal imaging can facilitate full reassurance.
- Simple analgesia
- Firm supporting bra: worn day and night while symptomatic, to minimise movement and counteract the pull of the breast on the chest wall via the supporting ligaments.

Rarely, other management strategies are required for particularly severe symptoms:

- Pain team assessment and management; the condition occasionally responds to hypnotherapy and acupuncture.
- Danazol: is occasionally given in the luteal phase of the cycle. Although it works well, the androgenic side effects put most patients off a trial of treatment and only 50% of patients prescribed danazol tolerate it.
- Antioestrogen therapy (tamoxifen and goserelin): not licensed for breast pain, but is effective. They can be prescribed off licence by a specialist and should be closely monitored. Only a short, low-dose course of tamoxifen should be given and treatment limited to the luteal (premenstrual) phase of the cycle.

Aberrations of Involution (35–55 Years of Age)

During involution the stroma undergoes fatty replacement. As a result the breasts become less radiodense, softer and ptotic (droopy). As lobules undergo involution, areas of fibrosis and microcysts develop, and the number of glandular elements increase.

MACROCYSTS. Palpable (macro) cysts are distended involuted lobules. They are very common (15% of all symptomatic breast lumps), and affect 7% of women. Breast cancer has been reported to be two to three times higher in patients with cysts, but evidence suggests this is merely coexistence in the ageing population.

Symptoms and Signs. Breast lump that appears rapidly (sometimes overnight). Patients may have a history of previous breast cyst. On examination a rounded, smooth, possibly fluctuant lump is palpated. They are sometimes tender. Cysts can be asymptomatic (noted on mammogram).

Investigation. Triple assessment:

- USS: cysts have a classic rounded or oval shape and halo appearance, with a black centre and discrete white wall. If blood is aspirated or a cyst wall mass is noted, intracystic papillary carcinoma should be excluded (this is a rare).
- Mammogram: cysts appear as a rounded opacity or opacities and may be bilateral.

Treatment

- Aspiration: for symptomatic cysts.
- Excision: considered in recurrent complex cysts normal on biopsy (to exclude carcinoma).
- Patients with cysts should be warned further cysts may occur and new lumps require assessment.

SCLEROSING LESIONS. Fibrosis is an involutionary change, but if excessive, it is classified as an aberration. Sclerosing adenosis is excessive fibrosis of the lobule. If associated with atypia (atypical ductal hyperplasia), it is recognised to be a 'risk lesion' for the development of DCIS or invasive cancer. Therefore, this group should undergo increased (annual) surveillance mammography for 5 years.

Localised, excessive stromal fibrosis produces radial scars (<1 cm) and complex sclerosing lesions (>1 cm). They appear as asymmetric spiculated densities on screening mammography, are common (incidence 1 in 500 women screened) and should be biopsied to differentiate from breast cancer. Once diagnosed, resection is indicated, as 10% of complex sclerosing lesions contain foci of DCIS or grade 1 invasive ductal cancer.

Duct Ectasia. During involution, the major ducts up to 2–3 cm deep to the nipple undergo fibrosis, leading to dilatation and shortening. The nipple flattens and undergoes slit-like central inversion. The findings are often bilateral, in contrast to the unilateral, more eccentric inversion seen with breast cancer.

Symptoms and Signs. Patients present with central (often bilateral) nipple inversion or cream, yellow, green or brown nipple discharge, from multiple duct openings. Patients commonly complain discharge is provoked by squeezing the nipple, or is spontaneous after a warm shower or bath.

Differential Diagnosis

- DCIS or intraductal papilloma if discharge is dark brown.
- Breast cancer with nipple inversion.

Investigations

- USS: reveals dilated ducts containing material.
- Mammogram: can reveal an opaque mass of fusiform dilated ducts. Skin indentation may be apparent.
- Nipple fluid cytology: can be performed to confirm or refute the presence of blood within nipple discharge if it is dark brown or serosanguinous. The presence of blood may indicate an underlying papilloma or DCIS.

Treatment

- Reassurance
- Total duct excision (Hadfield" procedure) if there is diagnostic uncertainty, or if discharge is of large volume, marking their clothes and causing embarrassment
- Cosmetic eversion of nipple if requested.

Intraductal Papilloma. Papillomas are common (2–3% of women), can be solitary or multiple, and are classified as aberrances rather than neoplasms. Most are small and located in a solitary duct near the nipple. If multiple or large (>2 cm in diameter), there is a reported increased risk of intralesional papillary cancer.

Symptoms and Signs. Persistent spontaneous blood-stained or serosanguinous single duct nipple discharge, with at least two episodes a week, in a patient older than 50 years. A small mass may be palpable, or pressure over a particular region of the areola may precipitate the discharge.

Investigations

- Triple assessment
- USS: may reveal a lump within a dilated duct. If seen, a core biopsy is taken.
- Mammography: to exclude DCIS and carcinoma. Core biopsy is performed if microcalcification is identified.

Treatment

- Excision: of confirmed papilloma.
- Those with persistent spontaneous symptoms should undergo diagnostic surgery. Options include microdochectomy (single duct excision if the duct orifice in question can be identified and cannulated at surgery) or total excision of the major nipple ducts (Hadfield" procedure).

> **HINTS AND TIPS**
>
> Only 10% of those with blood-stained discharge will be found to have a papilloma or DCIS. The majority have duct ectasia.
>
> It can be difficult to distinguish serosanguinous discharge from a pale cream discharge associated with the more common duct ectasia. The 'tissue test' can be used to differentiate between them: serosanguinous discharge wicks rapidly on a tissue, while the other type remains as a sticky blob.

OTHER BENIGN CONDITIONS OF THE BREAST

The breast can be affected by infections, trauma and inflammation.

Bacterial Mastitis and Breast Abscess

Bacterial breast abscess most commonly occurs following suppuration of acute mastitis in the lactating breast (incidence 3% of lactating women, 80% occur in the first month postpartum). The infecting organism is usually *Staphylococcus aureus*. Occasionally abscesses occur in the glands of Montgomery. These present as a boil-like lesion on the areola and should be treated as for a boil.

Symptoms and Signs

- Lactating breast. Patient generally unwell with painful, tender, red and warm swelling of breast. The swelling may become fluctuant and eventually the abscess points and discharges.

Investigation

- USS to identify collections and their extent
- Culture of aspirated or drained fluid.

Treatment

- Antibiotics may settle the early phase of acute mastitis.
- Aspiration of purulent collections is required and may need to be repeated. Ultrasound-guided drainage of deeper collections may be necessary.
- Incision and drainage is avoided if possible to minimise the risk of milk fistula and poor cosmesis. However, it can be necessary for large loculated abscesses or those with very thick pus that cannot be aspirated.

Periductal Mastitis

This is a common, poorly understood condition that occurs primarily in the 35–55 years age group. It is more common among smokers. It is characterised by periductal inflammation rich in plasma cells. Microbiology cultures are often sterile but may grow *S. aureus, Enterococcus or anaerobes*. Periductal mastitis is sometimes used interchangeably with duct ectasia, but there is a growing body of evidence that it is a separate entity.

Symptoms and Signs. Pain and periareolar erythema many be accompanied by creamy, purulent or sometimes blood-stained discharge from the nipple or a periareolar fistula. There may be a tender periareolar mass that can become fluctuant. Chronic inflammation can occur with the presence of granulation tissue and chronic fistulae. Over time, healing occurs by fibrosis, with shortening and dilatation of the major ducts, and eccentric nipple inversion.

Differential Diagnosis. Carcinoma of the breast with nipple inversion.

Investigations

- Triple assessment; ultrasound is used to differentiate inflammation from abscess formation. Mammogram shows an opaque mass of dilated ducts and skin indentation.
- Microbiology on any discharge or fluid aspirate.

Treatment

- Antibiotics if infection is present; guided by history of smoking and culture results – often need broader-spectrum than flucloxacillin e.g. co-amoxiclav.
- Aspiration if an abscess is present. Repeat aspiration is often required.
- Surgical drainage is reserved for those not settling with repeated ultrasound-guided aspirations or patients with multiloculated abscesses not amenable to aspiration.
- Chronic mammillary fistulae can be treated by fistulectomy. This comprises laying open of the fistula and excision of all granulation tissue; however, this is not advised if the patient continues to smoke, as there are often problems with wound healing.

Fat Necrosis

This is due to trauma with rupture of fat cells resulting in an inflammatory reaction, which may become calcified with time. Fat necrosis accounts for 2–3% of all benign breast lesions.

Symptoms and Signs. There is usually a history of trauma, often minor (fall, RTA, seat belt injury) followed by the appearance of a lump. Teeth bites may be an aetiological factor, and the patient may be embarrassed to explain this. The lump may have decreased in size before the patient is seen in clinic. Fat necrosis (especially during the inflammatory phase and later fibrotic phase) can mimic cancer, being firm, irregular and sometimes associated with skin tethering.

Investigations. Triple assessment to exclude carcinoma.

Treatment. Conservative. Ultimately, fat necrosis may evolve into an oil-filled cyst that can be aspirated if symptomatic.

Hamartoma

This is a disorganised overgrowth of normal breast constituents, where one constituent dominates. They present as a lump. Triple assessment should be performed and excision offered if the patient is symptomatic or if there is diagnostic uncertainty.

Gynaecomastia

Gynaecomastia is benign hypertrophy of duct and connective tissue elements of the male breast, usually caused by an increased ratio of oestrogens to androgens. It may occur in the following instances:

- At birth (maternal oestrogens crossing placenta)
- At puberty, where it may be unilateral or bilateral (embarrassing to the patient; it may resolve or may need surgery)
- In older age (senile gynaecomastia – due to reduced endogenous testosterone)
- Drug induced (cimetidine, spironolactone, digoxin, methyldopa, oestrogens, cyproterone acetate)
- Use of alcohol, anabolic steroids, cannabis
- Secondary to liver failure
- In association with testicular tumours.

Investigation. Triple assessment is required if any suspicious features are present or if the finding is unilateral.

Blood tests to identify the cause of gynaecomastia: 9 am testosterone, thyroid function tests, liver function tests, beta-human chorionic gonadotrophin, alfa-fetoprotein

Treatment. Reassurance. Removal of precipitating cause if possible. A short course of tamoxifen can be used off licence for painful gynaecomastia. Surgical excision or liposuction is performed by some centres.

Other Related Conditions

These conditions are not of breast origin, but occur in the skin or chest wall in the region of the breast, e.g. Tietze's disease, Mondor's disease, lipoma, epidermoid cysts.

Patients may occasionally present with apparent pain in the breast, where the condition responsible for the pain is not within the breast.

TIETZE'S DISEASE. This is costochondritis and usually involves the second, third and fourth costal cartilages. The cause is unknown, and radiographs are unhelpful. The condition is self-limiting, although NSAIDs and a well-fitting bra can help. If the pain is severe, infiltration with local anaesthetic and steroids may be helpful.

MONDOR'S DISEASE. This is superficial thrombophlebitis of the subcutaneous veins of the chest (and/or abdominal) wall. The cause is uncertain, but it can be associated with trauma, infection and (rarely with) underlying breast cancer. The vein becomes a red, tender cord which often extends onto the anterior axillary fold. As the inflammatory reaction settles the patient is left with a linear depression over the vein. Triple assessment should be conducted. The condition is self-limiting (2 weeks to 6 months), and the active inflammatory stage usually settles in 10 days. NSAIDs and good bra support can provide symptomatic relief.

Chapter 12

Endocrine Surgery

Simon Pain • Mark Rochester • Peter Truran • Barney J. Harrison

CHAPTER OUTLINE

THYROID

Congenital

The embryological line of descent of the thyroid gland is from the foramen caecum at the base of the tongue to its normal position in the neck. Occasionally, it may descend lower to the superior mediastinum.

Lingual Thyroid

This is undescended thyroid tissue found at the foramen caecum at the base of the tongue. It is often asymptomatic but may interfere with speech or swallowing. A radioiodine scan should be performed to confirm the presence of functioning thyroid tissue elsewhere in the neck. Treatment is by suppression of TSH with thyroxine to prevent gland enlargement. Surgical excision should be considered if hormonal therapy is ineffective or the patient has obstructive symptoms.

Thyroglossal Cyst

(→Ch. 8)

Thyroglossal Fistula

This is not congenital but follows rupture or inadequate excision of a thyroglossal cyst or fine-needle aspiration. Recurrent inflammation occurs. Treatment is by excision of the fistula and may require dissection as far as the foramen caecum of the tongue and removal of the middle third of the hyoid bone (Sistrunks procedure).

Examination of the Thyroid Gland

> **HINTS AND TIPS**
>
> Palpate the thyroid gland from behind the patient and remember to examine the lymph nodes, position of the trachea and thyroid status.

Inspection should be carried out initially from the front. Give the patient a glass of water to swallow and check that the mass moves up on swallowing. Confirm that there is a mass in the neck in the area of the thyroid gland. Gently place a finger in the suprasternal notch and check that the trachea is central. Examine the thyroid from behind. Place the thumbs on the vertebra prominens and the fingers on the anterior part of the neck on either side. Palpate up and down in the area of the thyroid. Applying gentle pressure to one side of the neck over the thyroid facilitates palpation of the contralateral lobe. Decide whether there is a single nodule, many nodules or whether there is diffuse enlargement of the thyroid gland. Palpate up and down the deep cervical chain of lymph nodes to check for lymphadenopathy. Try to get below the lower limit of the thyroid swelling to exclude retrosternal extension. Percussion over the sternum to check for retrosternal extension is inaccurate and outdated. In patients with Graves' disease, auscultate over the gland. Very vascular toxic glands may have a systolic bruit. Look for signs of thyroid eye disease in patients with Graves' disease.

Symptoms of Thyroid Disease

Swelling in the Neck

- A goitre is an enlargement of the thyroid gland (for classification→Table 12.1). It may be smooth or nodular. Patients may be hyperthyroid, hypothyroid or euthyroid.
- A solitary nodule in the thyroid may be a cyst, benign nodule or cancer. They should all be investigated.
- Enlarged lymph nodes may be palpable in papillary or medullary thyroid cancer (MTC) and are sometimes the presenting feature.

Hoarse Voice. This is due to pressure on and/or malignant infiltration of one or both recurrent laryngeal nerves.

Dysphagia. This may occur with very large goitres.

Dyspnoea. It is due to tracheal deviation or compression. Stridor may be apparent.

Pain. This may occur with haemorrhage into a nodule, locally advanced carcinoma, subacute thyroiditis or, occasionally, Hashimoto's disease.

Eye Symptoms. Staring or protruding eyes (exophthalmos) in patients with Graves' disease, double vision, dry 'gritty' eyes, difficulty closing eyes. The latter may lead to pain due to corneal ulceration.

TABLE 12.1

CLASSIFICATION OF THYROID SWELLINGS

Diffuse	Simple hyperplastic goitre: • Puberty • Pregnancy • Iodine deficiency Graves' disease
Nodular (dominant/multiple)	Multinodular goitre Toxic multinodular goitre Thyroid cancer
Solitary thyroid nodule	Thyroid cyst Colloid nodule Follicular nodule Thyroid cancer
Inflammatory	De Quervain's thyroiditis Riedel's thyroiditis
Autoimmune	Hashimoto's thyroiditis

Hyperthyroidism. Palpitations, dyspnoea, nervousness, irritability, tremor of hands, sweating. Increased appetite with weight loss, diarrhoea. Preference for cold weather. Amenorrhoea. Pretibial myxoedema may be found in Graves' disease.

Hypothyroidism. Slowness of thought, speech and movement. Weight gain. Cold intolerance, tiredness, lethargy, constipation. Loss of hair. Change of voice (hoarseness). Carpal tunnel syndrome.

Incidental Finding on Imaging for Another Problem. The increased use of ultrasound / computerised tomography (CT) / magnetic resonance imaging (MRI) / positron emission tomography (PET) frequently identifies asymptomatic abnormalities in the thyroid. Most nodules are benign but should be investigated if a nodule is over 1 cm and/or has radiological features of concern. A PET-CT avid nodule has an approximately 40% risk of malignancy.

HINTS AND TIPS

Benign and malignant thyroid disorders are associated with genetic/environmental factors. Ask all patients about family history of thyroid disease and exposure to ionising radiation.

Investigation of Thyroid Dysfunction/Swellings

HINTS AND TIPS

Patients with a new thyroid mass need clinical examination, thyroid function tests and usually neck ultrasound. A fine-needle aspiration for cytology should be taken if a solitary or dominant nodule is present.

Laboratory Tests. TSH is the initial test for assessment of thyroid function. If abnormal levels are identified, free T4 is measured. TSH is elevated in hypothyroidism, low or suppressed in thyrotoxicosis. Raised titre of thyroid autoantibodies suggest immune aetiology of disease. Thyroid receptor antibodies (TRAB) are elevated in Graves' disease. Thyroid peroxidase antibodies are elevated in autoimmune hypothyroidism.

Fine-Needle Aspiration. Carried out under ultrasound guidance, this will distinguish between a solid lesion and a cyst and is used to discriminate benign from malignant disease. Cytology cannot distinguish between benign and malignant follicular lesions.

Plain Radiograph of Chest (to Include Thoracic Inlet). May show tracheal displacement or compression, retrosternal extension.

Ultrasound Scan. It establishes the size and shape of the gland, indicates if nodules are single or multiple, and their size in addition to lymph node abnormalities. It will also distinguish cystic from solid nodules. An experienced radiologist should comment on features that indicate increased risk of malignancy (hypoechogenicity, irregular margins, intranodular vascularity, microcalcification).

Radioisotope Scan. Rarely indicated except in some patients with thyrotoxicosis. In Graves' disease the uptake is increased and diffuse. In toxic nodular goitre the uptake is patchy and multiple or unifocal depending on the pathology.

CT/MRI (→ Fig. 12.1). Performed to assess airway narrowing and displacement, retrosternal extension, extent of lymph node involvement and local invasion in thyroid cancer.

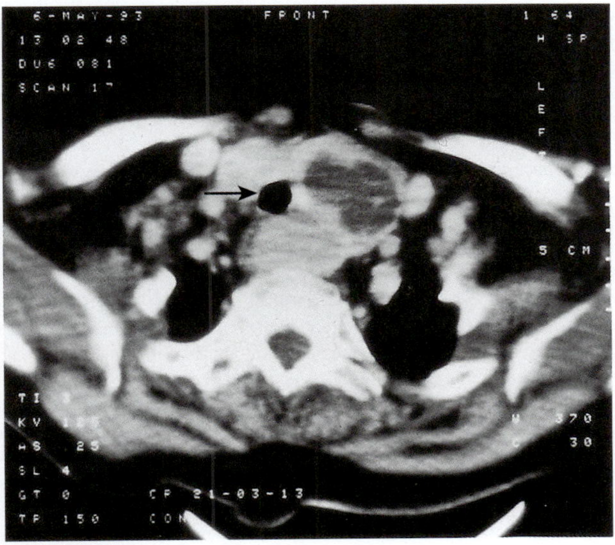

FIGURE 12.1
A CT scan of the neck showing a goitre (large mass in the left lobe of the thyroid gland). The trachea (arrow) is slightly deviated to the right.

The Patient With a Thyroid Swelling (Goitre)

HINTS AND TIPS

Thyroid enlargement is a common topic in undergraduate and postgraduate exams.

Goitre – a descriptive term for the enlargement of the thyroid gland. It does not indicate the underlying pathology. Palpation of the neck may reveal diffuse or nodular thyroid enlargement. A classification of goitres is shown in Table 12.1.

Diffuse Enlargement

Simple Goitre. Worldwide, iodine deficiency is the most common pathological cause. In the UK it is rare, as iodide is added to table salt. Physiological enlargement is seen during puberty and pregnancy.

Symptoms and Signs. The patient is usually euthyroid with a smooth goitre that may be minimally or markedly enlarged.

Treatment. Addition of iodised salt to diet in areas where iodine deficiency occurs to prevent goitre development. Thyroidectomy is indicated only if the gland is very large and/or causing pressure effects.

Graves' Disease

Symptoms and Signs. Tachycardia, palpitations, atrial fibrillation, tremor, sweating, weight loss, diarrhoea and increased tendon reflexes. Symptoms of thyroid eye disease include grittiness of the eyes and double vision. The signs to be assessed are exophthalmos, lid retraction and lid lag. Occasionally in thyrotoxic patients a bruit is heard over the gland.

Investigations

- Low TSH; free T4 (↑); free T3 (↑)
- High titres of TPO and stimulating TRAB.

Treatment

Antithyroid Drugs (Carbimazole, Propylthiouracil). Carbimazole inhibits the action of thyroid peroxidase with a consequent reduction in thyroid hormone synthesis. Side effects of carbimazole include rashes and neutropenia – patients must be warned to report any sore throat or mouth ulcers occurring. Fifty percent of patients with Graves' disease remain euthyroid when the drug is discontinued after 1 year. Patients who relapse are offered definitive treatment with radioiodine or surgery.

Radioiodine. ^{131}I is administered orally. It usually takes 8–12 weeks before the patient becomes euthyroid. It is appropriate treatment for most patients with thyrotoxicosis, but is not used in children and patients with moderate or severe eye disease. Radiation protection legislation/safety may limit its use in patients with young families. Hypothyroidism will occur in most patients.

Surgery. This is the treatment of choice for younger patients, children and patients with thyroid eye disease or large goitres. The patient must be rendered euthyroid prior to surgery. Total thyroidectomy or subtotal thyroidectomy is performed.

Nodular Enlargement

Clinically will be a solitary nodule, multiple nodules or dominant nodule in multinodular goitre. A clinically solitary nodule will often be part of multinodular change on thyroid ultrasound. Thyroid cancer may present as any form of nodular enlargement of the thyroid.

Multinodular Goitre. This is the most common cause of goitre in the UK and more common in women. With large glands, tracheal deviation and/or compression may occur. Some patients will develop hyperthyroidism due to the size of the gland and/or autonomous function.

Symptoms and Signs. In endemic areas, nodular goitre appears at 15–30 years, while sporadic goitre occurs later at 25–40 years. Dyspnoea, dysphagia may occur if the gland is very large. Pain is not usually a symptom of benign nodular disease.

Investigations

- TSH, free T4
- CXR/CT if retrosternal extension is suspected. The interpretation of thoracic inlet views is difficult and generally unhelpful.
- Fine-needle aspiration cytology of an enlarging or dominant nodule is advised.

Treatment. If the patient is clinically euthyroid and the goitre is small/asymptomatic, no treatment is required. Patients with thyrotoxicosis should be rendered euthyroid with antithyroid drugs but require definitive treatment with radioiodine or surgery. If an enlarged gland, symptoms/signs of airway/oesophageal compression thyroidectomy may be indicated.

Retrosternal Goitre

The thyroid may enlarge into the mediastinum. A retrosternal goitre is not an absolute indication for surgery, but patients may require surgery based on compressive symptoms, thyrotoxicosis or malignancy concerns (see below). Occasionally a sternotomy is required to remove the thyroid.

Solitary Thyroid Nodule

CYST. Present as thyroid swelling, sometimes painful. Needle aspiration confirms the nature of the swelling and provides fluid for cytology. Recurrent cyst is an indication for surgery.

COLLOID NODULE. Presents as thyroid swelling and may cause airway/oesophageal compression. Benign nature of the nodule is confirmed by ultrasound and/or cytology. Indications for surgery are:

- compressive symptoms
- enlargement
- uncertain diagnosis
- patient concern.

FOLLICULAR NODULE (AS DESCRIBED ON CYTOLOGY). Present as a thyroid swelling of varying size. The diagnosis of a follicular lesion on ultrasound and/or cytology mandates further assessment. Cytology does not distinguish follicular adenoma from follicular carcinoma. The finding of a follicular lesion in a euthyroid patient has a 20–30% risk of malignancy. Diagnostic hemithyroidectomy should be performed. Functioning adenomas may cause hyperthyroidism (toxic adenoma), and an iodine uptake scan will show high uptake in the nodule with low uptake in the surrounding gland.

Thyroid Cancer

HINTS AND TIPS

Differentiated thyroid cancer (papillary or follicular) accounts for 90% of thyroid malignancy. It has a generally good prognosis. Treatment for most patients is surgery, radioiodine and TSH suppression.

Papillary cancer spreads to the lymph nodes whereas follicular cancer spreads via the blood to the bone and lungs.

MTC does not respond to radioiodine because it arises from parafollicular C-cells. It is familial in 25% of cases (MEN type 2 syndrome). Treatment is surgery.

Thyroid cancer is rare and accounts for 1% of all malignancies, and the large majority are primary tumours. Metastatic carcinoma to the thyroid is rare. The main types of thyroid cancer are described below.

Symptoms and Signs. Clinical presentation of benign and malignant disease may be similar – a thyroid swelling. Features of concern include a rapidly enlarging nodule or new nodules in young patients (less than 20 years) or patients over 50. Patients present with a thyroid mass and/or lymph node mass and are usually euthyroid. Stridor, dysphagia, pain and hoarseness due to involvement of the recurrent laryngeal nerve may occur in locally advanced disease. Advanced medullary carcinoma may present with diarrhoea. Anaplastic carcinoma occurs in the elderly and presents with rapidly growing locally advanced disease causing airway and/or oesophageal compromise.

Differentiated Thyroid Cancer

PAPILLARY (70%). Papillary carcinoma occurs at any age with a peak incidence in the 30–40 years age group. Usually a slow-growing nodule, which may metastasise early to regional lymph nodes. It is often multifocal within the thyroid gland. The tumour is TSH dependent.

FOLLICULAR (20%). Follicular carcinoma has a peak incidence in the 40–60 years age group. It spreads via the blood stream. Distant metastasis is normally to lung and bone. Occasionally, the disease presents with bony secondaries. The tumour is TSH dependent.

Treatment. Surgery for differentiated thyroid cancer includes hemithyroidectomy or total thyroidectomy (± cervical lymph node dissection in papillary thyroid cancer). Many patients will undergo radioiodine remnant ablation and subsequent lifelong thyroxine treatment. Thyroxine at a higher dose is prescribed in many patients to achieve low-normal or suppressed TSH depending on their risk of recurrent disease. Serum thyroglobulin is measured as a marker of recurrent disease. Recurrent thyroid cancer is diagnosed by symptomatic presentation, cross-sectional imaging, radioiodine scans or elevated thyroglobulin. Surgery, ^{131}I therapy or external beam irradiation may be indicated to treat recurrent disease.

Prognosis. In general prognosis is excellent for most patients, and there is a move for less intensity in treatment in view of the excellent prognosis. The overall 10-year survival rate is 80–90%. Adverse prognostic factors include increasing age (over 45 years) at first presentation, male sex, incomplete resection, extrathyroidal invasion and distant metastatic spread.

Anaplastic Carcinoma (5%)

Rare aggressive tumour that occurs in older patients. Usually rapidly growing and locally invasive, with early spread via the lymphatics and bloodstream to lungs, bone and brain. Stridor, dysphagia, recurrent laryngeal nerve palsy may occur. Treatment (surgery or radiotherapy) is usually palliative to relieve airway compromise. Prognosis is very poor.

Medullary Carcinoma (5%)

Arises from parafollicular C-cells, secretes calcitonin/CEA. It may be familial (25%) and associated with MEN type 2 syndromes/FMTC (see MEN section). Onset in familial disease can occur in the first year of life (MEN type 2B), in the first decade (MEN type 2A) or the second decade (FMTC). Family history and genetic screening (rearranged during transfection (*RET*) mutation analysis) should be performed in all patients with medullary cancer. Phaeochromocytoma must be excluded in all MTC patients prior to treatment. MTC presents with a thyroid nodule or diffuse mass and spreads early to cervical nodes. Preoperative diagnosis can be made with FNAC and/or calcitonin levels. Treatment is total thyroidectomy and cervical node dissection. Prognosis can be determined by post-treatment calcitonin levels and calcitonin/CEA doubling times. Prophylactic thyroidectomy is performed for known MEN type 2/FMTC gene carriers at 6 months to 20 years depending on the specific gene mutation.

Lymphoma (1%)

Presents with a history of rapidly enlarging thyroid mass and airway compromise. Patients often have a history of hypothyroidism / Hashimoto's thyroiditis. May be diagnosed on FNAC or core biopsy. In the acute setting after biopsy, airway compromise responds quickly to steroid therapy. Definitive treatment (chemotherapy–radiotherapy) by the lymphoma team depends upon the subtype and disease stage.

Inflammatory Conditions of the Thyroid

Subacute Thyroiditis (De Quervain's)

This is a self-limiting condition. Symptoms include pain, swelling, enlarged tender thyroid, malaise, myalgia. The ESR is raised. Aspirin and steroids give symptomatic relief. The acute symptoms last 10–14 days. Surgery is not required.

Riedel's Thyroiditis

This is a woody hard goitre that infiltrates into the adjacent muscle. It may compress the trachea and may be associated with retroperitoneal fibrosis and other similar conditions. The differential diagnosis includes anaplastic carcinoma, so incision biopsy may be required for an accurate diagnosis. Treatment with tamoxifen is associated with reduction in the size of the goitre; surgery is sometimes required if there is airway compromise.

Hashimoto's Disease

An autoimmune disorder that occurs almost exclusively in females characterised by thyroid enlargement, varying degrees of hypothyroidism and diffuse lymphocytic infiltration of the thyroid gland. There is destruction of functioning thyroid tissue. TPO antibody titres are raised. Hypothyroidism is treated with thyroxine. Surgery is very rarely performed and is reserved for patients with severe pressure symptoms.

Thyroidectomy

Indications

Possible (clinical/radiological/cytological concern) or proven malignancy, thyrotoxicosis. Symptoms/signs of tracheal/oesophageal compression, cosmetic concerns.

Preoperative Preparation

Thyrotoxic patients should be rendered euthyroid preoperatively with antithyroid medication. Patients with a malignant thyroid mass or a history of previous thyroid/parathyroid surgery or any changes to voice should undergo laryngoscopy to assess vocal cord mobility, as the recurrent laryngeal nerves are at risk during thyroidectomy. Informed consent should be obtained and include a discussion about potential complications of surgery – see below.

Operations

- Hemithyroidectomy is performed for unilateral benign disease or diagnostic uncertainty.
- Total thyroidectomy is performed for the treatment of bilateral benign disease and for most patients with papillary/MTC. Patients with good-prognosis follicular

cancer are often treated with hemithyroidectomy alone. In some countries patients with benign bilateral disease may be treated with less than total thyroidectomy to preserve normal thyroid function and avoid the need for thyroxine replacement.

- New techniques. Thyroidectomy is usually performed under general anaesthetic with a transverse cervical incision. Video-assisted thyroidectomy is a new development.

PROCEDURE

PRINCIPLES OF HEMITHYROIDECTOMY

- General anaesthesia with endotracheal intubation
- Support (e.g. litre bag i.v. fluid/sandbag) under shoulders and head positioned on a ring. Neck extended
- Skin crease incision about two fingers breadth above the sternal notch. The incision should reach the sternocleidomastoid on each side
- Raise skin flaps (including subcutaneous fat and platysma) to the thyroid cartilage superiorly and the sternal notch inferiorly
- Make a vertical incision through the deep fascia between the strap muscles and retract the strap muscles. If the goitre is large, the strap muscles are divided at their upper extremity because their nerve supply enters the lower part of the muscles
- Divide the middle thyroid veins
- Draw down the upper pole and identify the superior thyroid vessels
- Ligate/clip the superior thyroid vessels close to the upper pole of the thyroid to avoid the external branch of the superior laryngeal nerve
- Draw the lobe of the thyroid gland medially and dissect the lateral connective tissue and identify the inferior thyroid artery and the parathyroid glands
- Identify and preserve the recurrent laryngeal nerve throughout its course
- Ligate/clip individual branches of the inferior thyroid artery at the capsule of the thyroid
- Ligate/clip the inferior thyroid veins
- The lobe is now free and may be removed by dividing the isthmus
- Meticulous haemostasis
- Close the wound in layers.

Complications

HINTS AND TIPS

The main complications of first time thyroidectomy are neck haematoma requiring urgent intervention (1:100), permanent vocal cord palsy (1:100). After bilateral surgery hypocalcaemia occurs in 1:4 temporary, 1:20 permanent.

HAEMORRHAGE. Wound haematoma (1:100 cases) is rare but serious, as it may cause airway obstruction due to subglottic oedema. It is potentially fatal. Emergency crico-thyroidoctomy may be required. Treatment is by opening the wound, evacuating the haematoma and securing haemostasis. This may need to be done on the ward. Instruments to remove clips or stitches must be within ready reach in the postoperative period.

Vocal Cord Palsy Due to Recurrent Laryngeal Nerve Injury. This may be unilateral, bilateral (2–4 per 1000 thyroidectomies), temporary (<12 months) or permanent. Unilateral injury causes voice change with varying degrees of loss of power and a breathy voice. In bilateral cord palsy, airway obstruction due to vocal cord adduction or failure of airway protection on swallowing occurs (abducted cords) – tracheostomy is required.

Superior Laryngeal Nerve (External Branch) Injury. Singers, actors and others who rely on their voice professionally should be warned of this possible complication.

Thyroid Storm (Thyrotoxic Crisis). Hypercatabolic state due to circulating thyroid hormone excess – when an inadequately prepared patient has undergone surgery for thyrotoxicosis. Seen rarely nowadays because of better preoperative preparation. Symptoms include hyperpyrexia, confusion, restlessness, sweating, tachycardia and cardiac arrhythmias. Treatment includes cardioselective beta-blocker, hydrocortisone, sedation, cooling.

Hypocalcaemia. This results from ischaemia or inadvertent removal of the parathyroid glands after bilateral surgery. The lowest calcium value may occur up to 72h postoperation. Symptoms include circumoral paraesthesia with tingling of the extremities. Chvostek's sign (tap the facial nerve in front of the external auditory meatus – contraction of facial expression muscles occurs in hypocalcaemia), Trousseau's sign – inflation of blood pressure cuff on the arm results in carpal spasm. Hypocalcaemia in most cases responds to oral calcium and vitamin D supplementation. Treatment with intravenous calcium is sometimes necessary.

Hypothyroidism. All patients will require thyroxine after total thyroidectomy. One in three patients require lifelong thyroxine supplements after hemithyroidectomy.

Other Complications. Wound infection, recurrent thyrotoxicosis and the possibility of keloid scarring should also be discussed preoperatively with the patient.

PARATHYROID

Hyperparathyroidism

Primary Hyperparathyroidism

HINTS AND TIPS

Primary hyperparathyroidism is not uncommon: 0.5–1% prevalence. Careful biochemical investigation is needed to confirm the diagnosis. Surgery is the only curative treatment for primary hyperparathyroidism with a cure rate of 98% in experienced hands.

Primary hyperparathyroidism has a prevalence of 0.5–1%. This may result from a parathyroid adenoma (85%), parathyroid hyperplasia (15%) and, rarely, carcinoma. Hyperparathyroidism is the most frequent component of MEN type 1 syndrome.

Symptoms and Signs. These are classically 'stones, bones, abdominal groans and psychic moans'.

Stones. Renal calculi occur in 5% of patients with hyperparathyroidism. All patients with renal calculi should have their serum calcium and phosphate checked.

Bones. Bone pain, fractures, osteoporosis.

Abdominal Groans. Peptic ulcer disease, constipation, pancreatitis.

Moans. Psychiatric manifestations may occur, e.g. confusion, depression, psychosis. However, many patients have nonspecific symptoms, e.g. weakness, fatigue, lethargy, arthralgia, anorexia.

Other. Many patients are identified with hypercalcaemia as an incidental finding on routine blood tests.

Investigations

- Adjusted Ca↑- raised calcium with increased or inappropriate level of parathyroid hormone is primary hyperparathyoroidism (once familial hypocalciuric hypercalcaemia (FHH) is excluded).
- Phosphate sometimes↓
- PTH↑
- 24h urine collection and blood samples for calcium/creatinine ratio
- SPECT-CT – radioactive uptake with Sestamibi – uptake is superimposed on CT.

Differential Diagnosis. Need to exclude other causes of hypercalcaemia, e.g. malignancy (bone metastases, parathyroid related protein (PTHrP)), vitamin D excess, myeloma, sarcoidosis, milk-alkali syndrome. PTH is low in these conditions. FHH.

Treatment. Surgery is the only curative treatment. Preoperative single-gland localisation with ultrasound and methoxyisobutylisonitrile (MIBI) scans allow a targeted neck exploration to identify and remove only the abnormal gland. If localisation studies are not performed or are negative/nonconcordant, bilateral neck exploration is required to assess all four parathyroid glands. Enlarged parathyroid glands are removed.

Failure to cure hypercalcaemia at neck exploration (<5% of cases when surgery is performed by an experienced surgeon) may result from surgeon inexperience, or supernumerary or ectopic (including mediastinal) parathyroid glands. Complications of parathyroidectomy include hypocalcaemia, recurrent laryngeal nerve injury and neck haematoma.

Secondary Hyperparathyroidism

High levels of PTH in response to dietary calcium deficiency, vitamin D deficiency, renal failure. Patients in chronic renal failure are unable to synthesise active vitamin D and develop hypocalcaemia, hyperphosphataemia and impaired calcium absorption.

Symptoms and Signs. Bone pain, pruritus, extravascular calcification.

Investigations. Serum calcium is normal. Hyperphosphataemia. PTH very high.

Treatment. Patients with chronic renal failure receive phosphate binders to reduce serum phosphate levels. Activated vitamin D, calcium supplements and high-calcium dialysate are given to treat hypocalcaemia. Surgery is required in patients refractory to medical treatment (total parathyroidectomy).

Tertiary Hyperparathyroidism

Hyperparathyroidism that persists in patients who have had a successful renal transplant. This reflects the autonomous production of PTH after a long period of secondary hyperparathyroidism. Treatment is by total parathyroidectomy.

ADRENAL GLAND

HINTS AND TIPS

Two questions related to adrenal masses: Is it functioning? Is it malignant?
An adrenal mass should never be biopsied or operated upon without biochemical proof that it is not a phaeochromocytoma.

Adrenal Cortex

Cushing's Syndrome

Increased circulating cortisol of any origin, the causes include: adrenal adenoma, adrenal carcinoma, macronodular adrenal hyperplasia, administration of exogenous corticosteroids, Cushing's disease (overproduction of ACTH by the anterior pituitary), ectopic ACTH secretion, e.g. small cell bronchial carcinoma.

Symptoms and Signs. The presentation is variable. Any or all of the following may occur: truncal obesity, buffalo hump, moon face, proximal myopathy of the limbs, skin striae, acne, hirsutism, capillary fragility with bruising, oedema, hypertension, osteoporosis, psychiatric disturbances, diabetes, peptic ulceration, pancreatitis, cataracts, skin pigmentation, avascular necrosis of bone.

Investigations

- U&Es: hypokalaemia
- Blood sugar ↑
- Plasma cortisol at midnight and morning: the diurnal variation is lost in cortisol excess
- Urinary free cortisol is elevated in Cushing's – beware of false positives
- Overnight low-dose dexamethasone suppression test – failure to suppress cortisol levels below 50 nmol/L suggests cortisol excess. Forty-eight-hour dexamethasone suppression test required
- ACTH levels: high in pituitary-dependent cases, low or undetectable with adrenal tumour, may be very high with ectopic ACTH secretion
- CT or MRI of adrenals or pituitary fossa or chest depending upon abnormal biochemistry.

Treatment

ACTH-Independent Hypercortisolism. If an adenoma or carcinoma, the abnormal adrenal gland is removed.

ACTH-Dependent Hypercortisolism. For pituitary tumours, surgery is required via trans-sphenoidal resection. For ectopic ACTH secretion, the source should be excised if possible, e.g. lung surgery for small cell lung cancer.

Patients who have undergone surgery for endogenous cortisol excess will require peri-operative steroid replacement therapy, lifelong after bilateral adrenalectomy. After unilateral adrenal surgery, recovery of the hypothalamic–pituitary–adrenal axis should be proven (Synacthen test) before discontinuing oral steroid replacement.

Primary Hyperaldosteronism

There is excess secretion of aldosterone and suppression of plasma renin. The production of excess aldosterone by the adrenal glands is bilateral or unilateral. The primary type must be distinguished from secondary hyperaldosteronism where there is an increased plasma renin due to increased activity of the renin–angiotensin mechanism in renal artery stenosis, cirrhosis, CCF or nephrotic syndrome. Conn's syndrome is an aldosterone-producing adenoma and a cause of primary hyperaldosteronism.

Symptoms and Signs. Hypertension, lethargy, fatigue, muscle weakness (due to hypokalaemia), polyuria, polydipsia.

Investigations

- U&Es (hypokalaemia, alkalosis)
- Plasma aldosterone raised (antihypertensive drugs/diuretics may influence results)
- Plasma renin levels low.

When the biochemical diagnosis is confirmed, CT scan/MRI of the adrenal glands is required to identify abnormal morphology.

Treatment. Unilateral hypersecretion of aldosterone can be treated by surgery or spironolactone; bilateral hypersecretion is treated medically. Selective adrenal vein catheterisation to measure aldosterone levels is sometimes required to distinguish unilateral from bilateral disease.

Adrenal Medulla

Phaeochromocytoma

A catecholamine-producing tumour that arises from the chromaffin cells of the adrenal medulla. Functioning paraganglioma are ectopic phaeochromocytomas that arise from sympathetic nervous tissue. Phaeochromocytoma/paraganglioma may be multiple, bilateral, malignant, familial (associated with MEN type 2, neurofibromatosis type 1, von Hippel–Lindau disease or SDH syndrome). Patients less than 40 years of age should undergo genetic screening for familial disease, even in the absence of a family history.

Symptoms and Signs. Hypertension, headaches, palpitations, sweating, pallor, dyspnoea, anxiety, chest pain.

Occasionally phaeochromocytoma presents with acute cardiac failure.

Investigations

- Plasma or urinary (24-h collection) metanephrines/normetanephrines
- Blood sugar may be raised.

When the biochemical diagnosis is confirmed:

- CT/MRI scans will locate approximately 90% (→Fig. 12.2)
- MIBG scanning may be used to confirm that a morphological abnormality on CT scan/MRI is indeed a phaeochromocytoma/paraganglioma.

Treatment. Treatment of phaeochromocytoma/paraganglioma is excision. It is mandatory that prior to surgery preoperative α-adrenergic blockade is maximised, e.g. phenoxybenzamine. If tachycardia is present, β-blockade may be required but only when α-blockade is complete.

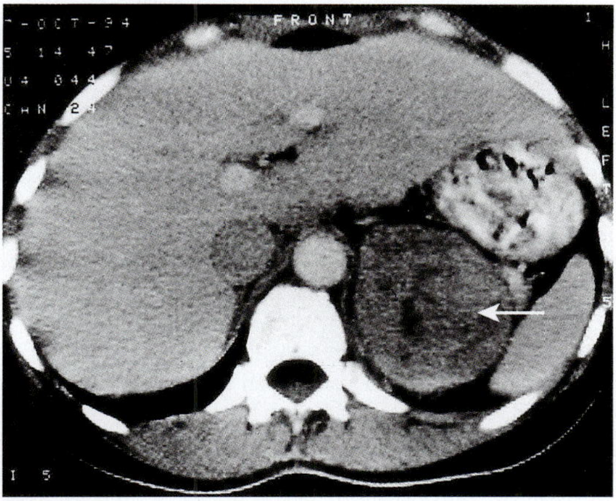

FIGURE 12.2
An abdominal CT scan showing a large phaeochromocytoma (arrow) in the left adrenal gland.

Adrenal Insufficiency

Causes

Primary

- Autoimmune
- Sarcoidosis
- Tuberculosis
- Amyloidosis
- Metastases
- Adrenal haemorrhage
- Meningococcal septicaemia (Waterhouse–Friderichsen syndrome)
- Withdrawal of long-term steroid therapy.

Secondary

- Pituitary disease.

Symptoms and Signs

Acute Adrenal Insufficiency. Shock, nausea, vomiting, hyperpyrexia, rigours, abdominal pain, coma.

Chronic Adrenal Insufficiency. Anorexia, lethargy, malaise, hypotension, weight loss, constipation, amenorrhoea, hyperpigmentation of skin.

Investigations

- If the patient is already on steroid therapy, check that the dose is adequate
- Check BP
- U&Es: $K^+\uparrow$ $Na^+\downarrow$, blood sugar$\downarrow$, serum cortisol levels reduced with inadequate response to Synacthen test

- ACTH levels high in primary disease and low in secondary causes
- Adrenal antibody screen
- CXR: may show TB
- AXR: adrenal gland calcification in TB.

Treatment. The acute case requires resuscitation with intravenous fluids and hydrocortisone. Chronic adrenal insufficiency is treated with oral steroids and fludrocortisone as mineralocorticoid replacement. Fatigue, hypotension and hyperkalaemia are signs of undertreatment. Hypertension, oedema and hypokalaemia are signs of overtreatment. Patients on replacement therapy should be warned that increased doses are required at times of stress, e.g. surgery or an acute illness.

Adrenal Incidentaloma

A mass lesion found in an adrenal gland by an imaging procedure performed for reasons other than suspected adrenal pathology. Incidentally found adrenal masses are increasingly common and are found on 0.5–5% of abdominal CTs; the frequency increases with patient's age. The majority are nonsecreting benign lesions. Once discovered, investigations are to identify:

- Is it functioning?
- Is it malignant?

Symptoms and Signs. Often none, as the name implies. History and examination may reveal signs and symptoms of an unsuspected functioning adrenal tumour, e.g. Cushing's syndrome, Conn's syndrome, phaeochromocytoma. An incidentaloma identified in a patient with a history of malignancy may be a metastasis.

Investigations

- To exclude functioning tumour, e.g. Cushing's, Conn's, phaeochromocytoma (see above)
- CT scan to assess size, morphology, and density (lipid content).

Treatment. In the absence of hormone excess, radiological signs of concern, size more than 4cm or increasing size on a follow-up scan – there is no indication for surgery.

Carcinoma of the Adrenal Gland

Adrenocortical carcinoma is rare (1–2 per million) but aggressive. It is potentially curable in the early stages, but only 30% are confined to the adrenal gland at the time of diagnosis.

Symptoms and Signs. Signs of excess hormone production, e.g. Cushing's, androgen excess. Abdominal pain. Flank pain. Signs of spread to distant organs, e.g. lungs, liver, bone.

Investigations

- U&Es
- Circulating hormone levels – tumours often produce cortisol. A tumour that produces more than one hormone (e.g. glucocorticoids and androgens) is highly likely to be malignant. In an adult, raised levels of sex hormones associated with an adrenal mass is almost always malignant.
- CT/MRI/PET.

Treatment. Surgery, chemotherapy, depending on degree of spread. Mitotane is used as adjuvant therapy after surgery.

Metastasis to the Adrenal Gland

Adrenal metastases are more common than primary adrenocortical carcinoma, primary sites include lung, breast, skin (melanoma), kidney, thyroid and colon. Metastasis from a previously unknown primary cancer is very rare. If systemic staging reveals no other evidence of disease, adrenalectomy may be appropriate.

MULTIPLE ENDOCRINE NEOPLASIA (MEN)

The MEN syndromes are inherited as autosomal dominant traits. A family history should be taken in all patients presenting with hyperparathyroidism, MTC, phaeochromocytoma and pancreatic endocrine tumours.

MEN type 1

- Hyperparathyroidism (multiglandular) (>90%)
- Duodenopancreatic tumours (>30%) with malignant potential
- Pituitary tumours.

MEN type 2A

- Medullary carcinoma of the thyroid (100%)
- Phaeochromocytoma (30–50%)
- Hyperparathyroidism (rare).

MEN type 2B

- Medullary carcinoma of the thyroid (100%)
- Phaeochromocytoma (50%)
- Multiple mucosal ganglioneuromas and marfanoid habitus.

Chapter 13

Abdominal Wall and Hernia

Bhasker Kumar • Andrew T. Raftery

CHAPTER OUTLINE

HERNIAE

Abdominal wall herniae are extremely common. Therefore, they are commonly seen in general practice, surgical outpatient clinics and unsurprisingly in OSCE examinations. This chapter will concentrate on the diagnosis and management of abdominal wall herniae.

General Description of a Hernia

Hernia (Figure 13.1A)

A hernia is an abnormal protrusion of a viscus or part of a viscus through an opening in the cavity in which it is normally contained.

Defect

The defect is in the abdominal wall, for example at the deep inguinal ring or femoral ring, or it can apply to a defect in a surgical incision (incisional hernia).

Sac

The sac is composed of peritoneum and has a neck (which may be very narrow), a body and a fundus. Not every hernia has a sac, for example paraumbilical herniae may contain extraperitoneal fat only. In some cases, the sac may be incomplete, i.e. not surrounding all of the contents as in the case of a sliding hernia.

Contents of the Sac

The contents of the sac can vary. The most common contents are bowel and omentum, in some cases it may contain ovary, appendix or a Meckel's diverticulum (Littre's hernia).

Reducible Hernia

This is a hernia in which the contents of the sac reduce spontaneously when the patient lies down or can be pushed back manually into the peritoneal cavity.

Irreducible Hernia

In the case of irreducible herniae the contents cannot be returned to the peritoneal cavity, either because there are adhesions between the sac and the contents or because

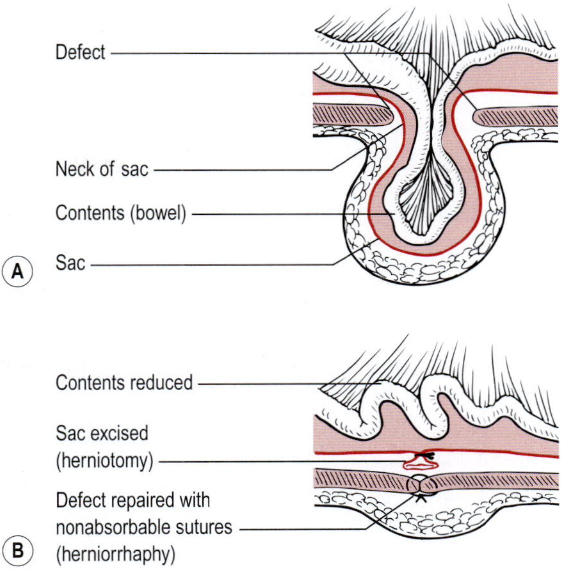

FIGURE 13.1

(**A**) General description of a hernia. (**B**) Principles of a hernia repair.

of the narrow neck of the sac. Irreducible herniae may be further subdivided as incarcerated, obstructed or strangulated.

- ***Incarcerated hernia***. In incarcerated herniae there are adhesions between the sac and the contents, but there is no obstruction and no interference with the blood supply. The hernia will simply not reduce.
- ***Obstructed hernia***. In the obstructed form a hollow viscus is trapped within the sac and obstruction occurs, the bowel contents being unable to pass the hernia site. The blood supply remains intact. This is one of the commonest causes of small bowel obstruction.
- ***Strangulated hernia***. Strangulation implies that the arterial blood supply to the contents of the sac is compromised, such that unless surgical relief is undertaken, the contents of the sac will become gangrenous.

Classification of Hernia

Herniae require a defect in the wall of the abdominal cavity for their formation. This defect may be either congenital or acquired.

Congenital

A congenital hernia develops in a peritoneal sac, which can give rise to a hernia in infancy, or it can provide a potential channel for one to occur in later life. In the latter case this could be as a patent processus vaginalis (a blind-ended tubular sac of peritoneum which accompanies the descent of the testis into the scrotum and which normally closes off after birth) in an indirect inguinal hernia, or because of the failure of the umbilical orifice to close in an umbilical hernia. These sacs represent persistent embryological channels.

Acquired

Acquired abdominal herniae occur as a result of a weakness in the abdominal wall together with predisposing factors. Weakness of the abdominal wall may occur for the following reasons:

- Due to loss of strength and elasticity, e.g. direct inguinal hernia in older patients
- Arising from surgical trauma, e.g. incisional hernia
- Due to enlargement of a foramen, e.g. an enlarged oesophageal hiatus allowing the development of a hiatus hernia
- Resulting from nerve damage with consequent weakness of the abdominal wall muscles, e.g. development of a right inguinal hernia after appendicectomy owing to damage to the right ilioinguinal nerve and consequently weakness of the muscles in the region of the inguinal canal.

If a potential weakness is present, the following factors may predispose to hernia formation by increasing intra-abdominal pressure. These include:

- heavy lifting or carrying
- coughing, e.g. asthma, COPD
- constipation
- benign prostatic hypertrophy
- pregnancy
- obesity
- ascites
- CAPD. This may unmask a persistent processus vaginalis with CAPD fluid filling a potential hernial sac and presenting as a swelling in the scrotum with scrotal oedema.

Types of Hernia (Figure 13.2)

Before learning how to examine the different types of hernia, it is important to understand the basic features of all herniae, which are:

- They occur at a weak point in the cavity.
- They reduce on lying down or with direct pressure.
- They have an expansile cough impulse.

Groin Hernia

Groin herniae are the most common type of hernia and account for approximately 75% of all herniae. They may be either inguinal or femoral; inguinal herniae may be further divided into direct and indirect herniae.

Inguinal Herniae

In an *indirect hernia* the peritoneal sac protrudes through the deep inguinal ring, passes down the inguinal canal and may extend as far as the upper pole of the testis. The defect is congenital and is due to a persistent processus vaginalis. It is more common in males. It may appear in infancy or early adult life. In infants there may be an associated hydrocele and undescended testis.

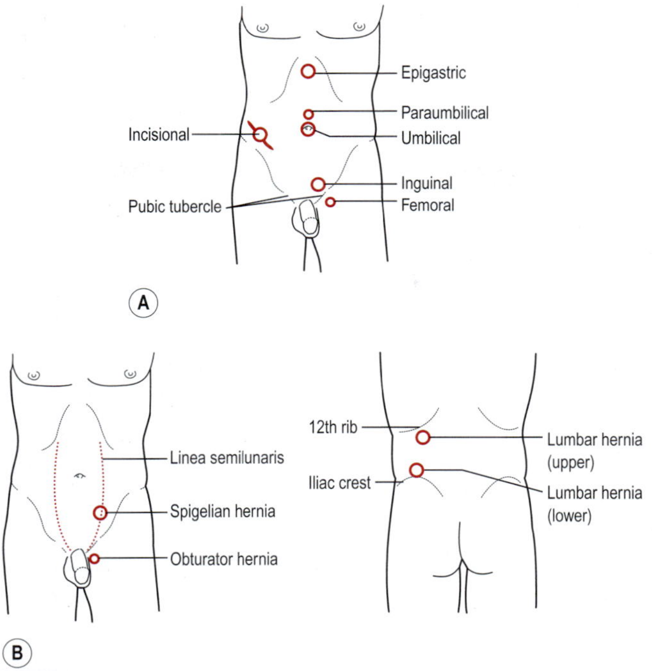

FIGURE 13.2
(**A**) Common types of herniae. (**B**) Rarer types of herniae.

A *direct hernia* is acquired. The defect occurs in the abdominal wall, in the area known as Hesselbach's triangle (bounded by the inguinal ligament inferiorly, the inferior epigastric artery laterally and the lateral border of rectus medially). The hernia results from a weakness of the transversalis fascia in the posterior wall of the inguinal canal. A direct hernia is often bilateral and occurs in older patients and may be associated with obesity, cough, constipation or prostatism.

Both direct and indirect herniae may occur together and straddle the inferior epigastric artery, the so-called 'pantaloon' hernia.

The only symptom usually is a lump in the groin. Occasionally the patient may experience an aching or dragging sensation in the groin. It is worth remembering that a pain in the groin without evidence of a lump is rarely due to a hernia – it is more likely to be due to groin strain. Some patients relate the development of the hernia to an episode of straining or lifting; others will observe that the lump disappears when they lie down, while some others will observe that they can push the hernia back into the abdominal cavity. A painful, tense, tender lump that will not reduce indicates incipient strangulation until proved otherwise and requires an urgent surgical referral.

Always start by examining while the patient is standing; it is not possible to see the true size of a hernia or to examine it properly when the patient is lying down. Look at the lump from the front. A hernia that descends into the scrotum is likely to be indirect. A diffuse bulge medially over the inguinal canal is likely to be direct. Next locate the pubic tubercle. This is essential in being able to distinguish between an inguinal and a femoral hernia. The best way to locate the pubic tubercle is to feel into the medial side of the upper thigh and follow the adductor tendons up into the groin. Once a bony ridge is located, this is the pubic tubercle. If the hernia is above and medial to this, it is an inguinal hernia; if it is below and lateral, it is a femoral hernia. You should ask the patient to cough to see if there is an expansile cough impulse.

Now ask the patient to lie down, and if the hernia does not reduce spontaneously, try and reduce it. Reduction is effected as follows: surround the swelling with the fingers of one hand to form a funnel leading to the superficial inguinal ring, while with the other hand grasp the swelling near the fundus. Gently squeeze the swelling. An indirect hernia will reduce upwards, then laterally and backwards; a direct hernia will reduce upwards and then straight backwards. Once the hernia is reduced, apply pressure over the deep inguinal ring, i.e. 1 cm above the midpoint of the inguinal ligament. Ask the patient to cough. If the hernia appears medial to the point of pressure, it is likely to be direct. If no hernia appears, release the pressure and again ask the patient to cough. If it now appears, it is likely to be indirect.

For smaller herniae it is possible to distinguish between direct and indirect by invaginating the scrotum with a little finger into the inguinal canal. Ask the patient to cough. If the hernia is indirect, the impulse hits the tip of the finger; if direct, it hits the pulp. The difference in fact is academic, since both will be carefully looked for at surgery. Complete your examination by examining the genitalia.

In males, first decide if the lump is a hernia or a true scrotal swelling by examining its upper edge. If you can 'get above it', i.e. feel its upper edge and a normal spermatic cord above it, then it must be a scrotal swelling and not a hernia.

The treatment of an inguinal hernia depends on whether it is uncomplicated or whether complications, e.g. obstruction and strangulation, have taken place. In children, an elective herniotomy (the excision of the sac) is carried out. In adults, both herniotomy and herniorrhaphy (the repair of the defect) are required (see Figure 13.1B). Inguinal herniae may be repaired in two ways. Increasingly a laparoscopic approach is preferred, but open repair is also a safe and effective operation. Either way, a tension-free mesh repair is the preferred method using polypropylene mesh. Laparoscopic repair will always need a GA. Open repair may be carried out under infiltration with local anaesthetic, spinal anaesthesia, or a general anaesthetic. The procedure is usually carried out as a day case if the patient is otherwise medically fit.

If surgery is contraindicated, e.g., patient unfit for GA, a truss may be used, but these are uncomfortable and unhygienic and are only used if the patient is unable to lie flat enough for the required period of time for the hernia to be repaired.

In the case of obstructed and strangulated hernia, emergency surgery will be required with resection of bowel if necessary, followed by excision of the sac and repair of the defect as in the case of an uncomplicated hernia.

PROCEDURE

REPAIR OF INGUINAL HERNIA

- Make an incision 2.5 cm above and parallel to the medial two-thirds of the inguinal ligament.
- Divide the superficial fascia (Camper's and Scarpa's) ligating the superficial veins (superficial epigastric vein and possibly the superficial circumflex iliac vein in the lateral end of the incision).
- Expose the aponeurotic fibres of the external oblique. Open the external oblique aponeurosis in the line of its fibres, extending the incision into the superficial inguinal ring.
- Dissect the ilioinguinal nerve off the spermatic cord and preserve it.
- Mobilise the cord. Check if there is a direct hernia (posterior to and separate from the cord). Carefully divide the layers of fascia covering the cord and check for an indirect sac. If an indirect sac is present, separate it carefully from the cord. Open the sac and reduce any contents. Twist the neck of the sac. Transfix and ligate the neck of the sac and excise redundant sac.
- Repair with Prolene mesh, attaching it to the pubic tubercle and inguinal ligament with a continuous Prolene suture and with interrupted sutures to the internal oblique and transversalis fascia, leaving an adequate opening for the cord to pass through.
- Close the external oblique with a continuous suture, making sure not to catch the ilioinguinal nerve.
- Close Scarpa's fascia and skin.
- Exert gentle traction on the testis to make sure that it is in the base of the scrotum.

As with any operation, complications can occur. Recurrence is possible, but the incidence should be less than 2%. Other complications include wound infection, ilioinguinal nerve entrapment and testicular ischaemia. Testicular ischaemia is rare after initial repair but occurs with a higher incidence after repair of a recurrent hernia due to difficulty of dissection of the spermatic cord in the scar tissue resulting from the previous operation. The patient should always be warned about the risks of testicular ischaemia because of the risk of subsequent infertility.

Femoral Hernia

In this type of hernia the defect is in the transversalis fascia overlying the femoral ring at the entry to the femoral canal. The boundaries of the femoral ring are: anteriorly, the inguinal ligament; medially, the lacunar ligament; posteriorly, the pectineal ligament; and laterally, the femoral vein. The hernia passes through the femoral canal and presents in the groin, below and lateral to the pubic tubercle. Femoral herniae are more common in females and carry a higher risk of strangulation. Femoral herniae are often of the Richter type (see below).

The patient will present with a lump below and lateral to the pubic tubercle that may be reducible. It may not be noticed, especially in obese patients, until it becomes tender and painful. This type of hernia should be carefully sought in obese patients who present with signs of intestinal obstruction without an obvious cause.

Treatment is by surgical repair because of the high risk of strangulation. An incision is made directly over the swelling. The sac is opened, the contents reduced and the sac removed. The defect is usually repaired by inserted nonabsorbable sutures between the inguinal ligament and pectineal ligament, thus closing the femoral canal, being careful not to obstruct the femoral vein. The hernia may also be repaired by inserting a mesh plug into the femoral canal. If the hernia is strangulated or obstructed, a separate abdominal incision will be required to deal with the bowel.

PROCEDURE

REPAIR OF FEMORAL HERNIA (LOW APPROACH)

- Make an incision in the line of the groin crease over the hernial sac.
- Deepen the incision to identify the hernial sac.
- Ligate superficial veins as necessary.
- Expose the sac carefully defining the neck of the sac.
- Open the sac and reduce any contents.
- Transfix and ligate the neck of the sac and excise the sac.
- Repair the femoral canal by suturing the inguinal ligament to the pectineal ligament without constricting the femoral vein.
- Place the left index finger over the femoral vein, insert a stitch into the inguinal ligament and the pectineal ligament, making sure that the most lateral stitch snugly fits around the index finger.
- Withdraw the index finger, allowing the vein to fill the space.
- Alternatively, the femoral canal may be filled with a mesh plug that is tacked in place.
- Close the wound in layers.

There is no place for a truss in the treatment of femoral hernia – it may, in fact, be dangerous by compressing the content of an incompletely emptied sac against the pubic bone. This is one reason why it is necessary to distinguish accurately between inguinal and femoral herniae on examination. The recurrence rate following surgery should be less than 3%.

HINTS AND TIPS

You may be asked to distinguish between an inguinal and femoral hernia in a clinical examination. The key to this is identification of the pubic tubercle. An inguinal hernia is above and medial to this; a femoral hernia below and lateral. You may also be asked to decide if an inguinal hernia is direct or indirect. This may be difficult especially in an obese patient. In any case, the surgical approach for both is the same, and it is always the practice to look for both during the course of the operation.

Other Types of Hernia

Umbilical Hernia

This occurs in children because of an incomplete closure of the umbilical orifice, which usually occurs spontaneously during the first year of life. It is more common in

Afro-Caribbean children and those with Down's syndrome and hypothyroidism. Surgical repair should only be carried out if the hernia has not disappeared by the age of 4 years and the fascial defect is greater than 1.5 cm in diameter.

Paraumbilical Hernia

This occurs just above or just below the umbilicus and is more common in adult females. Predisposing factors include multiple pregnancies and obesity. The neck of the sac is usually narrow and, therefore, there is a high risk of strangulation. The most common content is extraperitoneal fat followed by omentum. Treatment is by excision of the sac and a two-layer overlapping repair of the anterior rectus sheath (Mayo repair) or, if the hernia is large, by a tension-free repair with an onlay polypropylene mesh. A laparoscopic approach is also a good option.

Epigastric Hernia

This is usually a small protrusion through the linea alba in the upper part of the abdomen. Often, the hernia consists of extraperitoneal fat only, but it may contain omentum or small bowel. Treatment is by reduction of the extraperitoneal fat and simple suture of the defect with nonabsorbable sutures.

Incisional Hernia

This occurs through a defect in the scar of a previous abdominal incision. It is often broad-necked and, therefore, has a low risk of strangulation.

Aetiological factors include:

- Old age
- General debility, e.g. carcinomatosis, cirrhosis
- Obesity
- Postoperative wound infection
- Postoperative wound haematoma
- Raised intra-abdominal pressure postoperatively, e.g. coughing, straining, constipation, prostatism, ileus
- Steroid therapy
- Type of incision – midline vertical wounds have a higher incidence than transverse incisions. Incisional hernia is exceptionally rare through a Pfannenstiel incision (used for Caesarean section or hysterectomy).
- Poor suturing technique – rarely does a suture break.

Incisional herniae may occur up to 5 years postoperatively. Examination reveals a swelling protruding through the wound. They may be easily diagnosed by asking the patient to raise their head and shoulders off the couch, thus increasing intra-abdominal pressure and pushing the hernia out. Many are large and involve the whole incision, and consequently the neck of the sac is wide and the risk of strangulation rare. The smaller the defect, the greater the risk of strangulation. Small hernia may be repaired with interrupted nonabsorbable sutures. Larger hernia may be very unsightly and noticeable through the clothing. If the patient is unfit for surgery, a corset may be worn. Otherwise surgical repair should be undertaken. The old scar should be excised, the normal rectus sheath identified and the edges approximated with nonabsorbable sutures. If the edges of the defect are far apart, polypropylene mesh may be onlayed over the defect to allow closure without tension. The recurrence rate is high, being between 10% and 20%.

Richter's Hernia (Figure 13.3)

In this type of hernia, part of the circumference of the bowel becomes trapped in the defect. This is usually the antimesenteric border of the small bowel. Although a Richter's hernia is rare, it is important to know about it, as it can strangulate without obstructing and also may reduce spontaneously leaving a segment of bowel with a gangrenous area, thus resulting in perforation with resulting peritonitis. Femoral herniae are often of the Richter type.

Spigelian Hernia

This type of hernia is rare but just occasionally turns up in examinations. It occurs at the lateral border of rectus abdominis at a point a hand's breadth above the pubic symphysis at the level of the linea semicircularis (arcuate line of Douglas). This is the point at which the posterior rectus sheath becomes deficient and all aponeuroses of the abdominal muscles pass in front of the rectus muscle. Surgical repair is required.

Sliding Hernia (Hernia-en-Glissade) (Figure 13.4)

These are often seen in large/enormous inguinoscrotal herniae in older men. On the right side it may contain caecum and on the left sigmoid colon, and on both sides it may even contain bladder.

Surgical repair can be difficult, and great care should be taken to avoid damage to the bowel and structures such as bladder which may be in the sac.

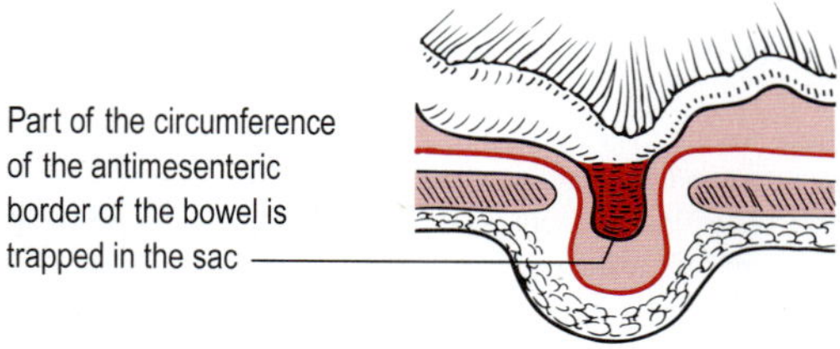

FIGURE 13.3
Richter's hernia.

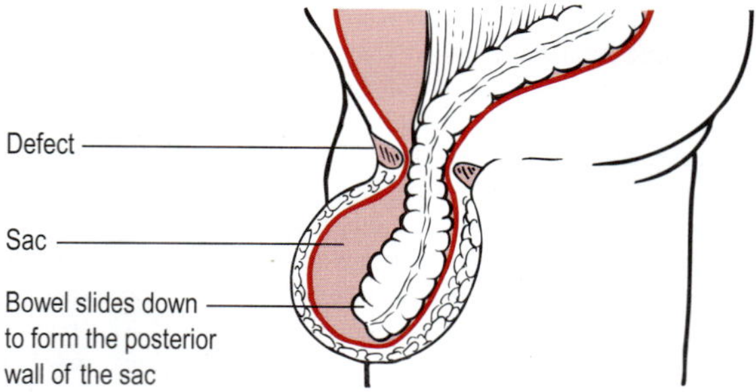

FIGURE 13.4
Sliding hernia.

Obturator Hernia

This hernia occurs through the obturator foramen and is commoner in elderly females. The diagnosis is usually made via a laparotomy for intestinal obstruction. It is difficult to feel the hernia, as it occurs in the groin deep to the pectineus muscle. The hernia may cause pressure on the obturator nerve at the obturator foramen causing referred pain down the medial side of the thigh, especially if the hernia is strangulated (Howship–Romberg sign).

Lumbar Hernia

Although lumbar herniae are very rare, it is important to know about them, as they are often mistaken for lipomas. Lumbar herniae occur through Grynfeltt's space (below the 12th rib) or Petit's triangle (just above the iliac crest). They often contain extraperitoneal fat and for that reason are often mistaken for lipomas.

Frequency of Different Types of Hernia

By far the commonest type of hernia encountered are inguinal herniae. Next in order of frequency are paraumbilical, incisional, epigastric and femoral herniae. Rarer herniae are spigelian, lumbar and obturator.

Indirect inguinal herniae are the most common herniae in both men and women. Femoral herniae, although rare, occur almost exclusively in women because of differences in pelvic anatomy. However, it should be stressed that even though femoral herniae are more common in women than in men, the commonest hernia in women remains an indirect inguinal hernia.

Are Investigations Necessary to Support the Diagnosis of a Hernia?

The diagnosis of a hernia usually depends on the history and clinical examination alone. Rarely is it necessary to carry out any investigations to diagnose an abdominal wall hernia, e.g, obese patients. However, occasionally patients present with groin pain and are referred to as having a groin hernia, but no lump is palpable. In this case it may be necessary to carry out imaging to avoid an unnecessary operation. The radiological imaging of choice would be a groin ultrasound by an expert in such scans which can be very difficult to interpret. To demonstrate the hernia, patients may be asked to do a Valsalva during the scan. Computerised tomography (CT) scan may be useful in obese patients. This is usually undertaken to confirm the presence of groin herniae (Figure 13.5) or paraumbilical herniae.

SWELLINGS IN THE GROIN AND SCROTUM

These are a common clinical problem and therefore common in examinations. A list of conditions is shown in Table 13.1. They are discussed in more detail in the relevant chapters. However, some of these lumps are more common than others and therefore more likely to enter into the differential diagnosis of a groin hernia. The student must therefore be aware of these common conditions. Before listing the conditions, it is important to reiterate factors required in making the diagnosis of a hernia.

The most important thing to remember when examining the groin for a hernia is to make sure that you examine the patient in both standing up and lying down positions. Usually, the diagnosis will be obvious. Points to remember are:

- There will be an expansile cough impulse.
- The lump will reduce.
- In some cases you may hear bowel sounds over the hernia sac.

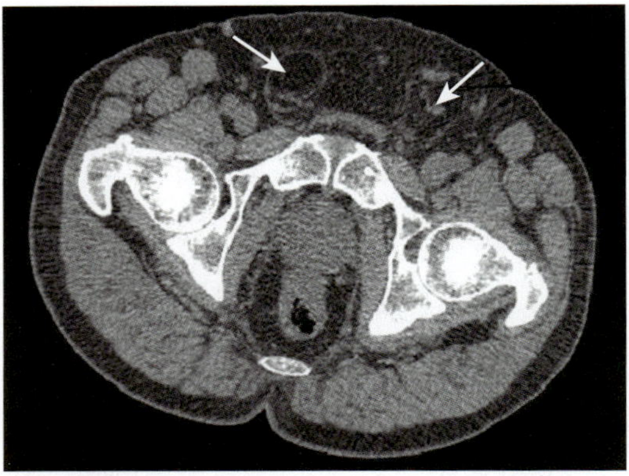

FIGURE 13.5
CT scan through the pelvis showing bilateral inguinal herniae (arrows).

These criteria will serve to distinguish a hernia from the conditions listed below which enter into a differential diagnosis of a hernia.

Saphena Varix

This is a dilated varicose vein at the saphenofemoral junction. As with a hernia, the lump disappears when the patient lies flat. There may also be a cough impulse. Diagnosis of saphena varix may be confirmed by placing the hand over the swelling and tapping the varicose veins lower down the legs. In the presence of a saphena varix there will be a palpable thrill.

Hydrocele of the Cord

This results from the processus vaginalis closing above and below, leaving a cavity between, which then fills with fluid. On examination it is possible to get above a hydrocele of the cord. Also, a hydrocele of a cord moves downwards when gentle traction is applied to the testis.

Lipoma of the Cord

There will be no cough impulse.

An Imperfectly Descended Testis

Usually, it is not possible to feel an undescended testis in the inguinal canal due to the tough overlying external oblique aponeurosis, combined with a small atrophic testis. If a testis is palpable in the inguinal canal, it may suggest that it has become malignant (imperfectly descended testes have a higher incidence of malignancy). The main clue to the diagnosis will be absence of the testis in the scrotum on that side.

Inguinal Lymph Nodes

These are usually multiple and lie below the inguinal ligament. A cause for inguinal lymphadenopathy should be sought by examining all areas drained to the inguinal lymph nodes. There will be no cough impulse.

TABLE 13.1

LUMPS IN THE GROIN AND SCROTUM

Groin	Above the inguinal ligament: • Sebaceous cyst • Lipoma • Direct inguinal hernia • Indirect inguinal hernia • Malgaigne's bulges (minor bilateral bulging of the inguinal canal – normal) • Imperfectly descended testis • Lipoma of the cord • Hydrocele of the cord (rare) • Hydrocele of the canal of Nuck (rare). Below the inguinal ligament: • Sebaceous cyst • Lipoma • Femoral hernia • Lymph nodes • Saphena varix • Femoral artery aneurysm (true or false) • Imperfectly descended testis • Neuroma of femoral nerve (rare) • Synovioma of hip joint (rare) • Obturator hernia (rare) • Psoas abscess (rare).
Scrotum	• Sebaceous cyst • Indirect inguinal hernia • Hydrocele • Epididymal cyst (spermatocele) • Epididymo-orchitis • Testicular tumour • Torsion of testes • Varicocele • Haematocele • Sperm granuloma • Torsion of testicular appendage.

Malgaigne's Bulges

These are minor bulges occurring bilaterally over the area of the inguinal canal. It is a variation of normal.

Femoral Artery Aneurysm

It is unlikely that this will be confused with a groin hernia. There will be a clear expansile pulsatile mass.

HINTS AND TIPS

It is important when examining the groin for a hernia to make sure that you examine the patient in both standing up and lying down positions. Usually, the diagnosis will be obvious. Remember that you cannot get above a hernia; the swelling will have an expansile cough impulse, and it may be reducible. These criteria will serve to distinguish herniae from the other conditions mentioned above.

OTHER CONDITIONS OF THE ABDOMINAL WALL

Umbilicus

Discharge

Patent Vitellointestinal Duct. This may result in discharge of mucus or small bowel contents. It is usually associated with a Meckel's diverticulum and usually occurs in infancy.

Patent Urachus. This may not present until early adult life or even old age and results from distension of the bladder usually because of outflow obstruction. Urine discharges through the umbilicus.

Abscess in a Urachal Cyst. This may discharge through the umbilicus.

Infection. This may occur deep in the umbilicus and cause discharge. It may be fungal. Inflammation of the umbilicus is called omphalitis.

Umbilical Calculus. This is usually black in colour and composed of inspissated desquamated epithelium and may be associated with infection and discharge. This condition is not infrequently seen in the elderly and is associated with poor hygiene.

Endometriosis. The umbilicus is usually painful and bleeds at the time of menstruation.

Mass

Umbilical Hernia. (see above)

Secondary Carcinoma. This is rare and presents as an umbilical nodule (Sister Joseph's nodule). It may be associated with carcinoma of the stomach, colon, ovary or breast.

Rectus Sheath Haematoma

This is due to tearing of the inferior epigastric vessels with haematoma in the posterior rectus sheath. It may occur in athletic, muscular young men during exercise or in thin elderly females. Occasionally it occurs during pregnancy. It is usually seen in patients on anticoagulation.

Symptoms and Signs. Sudden onset of severe lower abdominal pain in the left or right lower abdomen. Occasionally its onset is slow and progressive. Examination in the early stages reveals a tender mass in the abdominal wall. Later bruising may be detectable in the suprapubic area.

Treatment. This is usually conservative. The acute pain and discomfort should disappear within a few days. In young patients with a rectus sheath haematoma on the right side, the symptoms and signs may be mistaken for acute appendicitis.

Tumours of the Abdominal Wall

Most of these are benign lipomas. Most malignant tumours of the abdominal wall are metastatic. Musculoaponeurotic fibromatoses (desmoid tumours) may occur and are part of Gardner's syndrome (familial polyposis coli, osteomas, sebaceous cysts and desmoid tumours).

Chapter 14

Acute Abdomen

Bhasker Kumar • Andrew T. Raftery

CHAPTER OUTLINE

BASIC PRINCIPLES

Acute abdomen is the most common cause of emergency admission to a surgical unit. The term 'acute abdomen' is difficult to define, but it indicates any nontraumatic disorder of acute onset in which the symptoms are predominantly abdominal and for which, in some cases, urgent surgery may be indicated. In practice, it represents a spectrum of problems ranging from sudden onset of severe abdominal pain with a life-threatening underlying cause to minor abdominal symptoms of lengthy duration. The most important feature of the acute abdomen is to sort out the severe causes in need of urgent surgery (e.g. ruptured aortic aneurysm, perforated diverticulitis) from severe abdominal pain that does not require surgery (biliary colic, ureteric colic, pancreatitis), and also from those conditions that do not need urgent investigation and treatment (e.g. mild gastroenteritis, constipation). Prompt diagnosis is essential. A careful history and examination will indicate the cause of most acute abdomens.

History

Although it is unlikely that you will see a case of acute abdominal pain on your finals, it is important to be able to take a rapid and accurate history, as in many cases time is of the essence with a need to take a patient to theatre for urgent laparotomy. It is also important to recognise scars of previous surgery on the abdominal wall and to have an idea of what type of surgery may have been carried out through them.

Age. Certain conditions are more likely to occur in certain age groups, e.g. mesenteric adenitis in children, diverticulitis in older patients.

Pain. Abdominal pain may be one of two types: visceral pain, which is poorly localised; and parietal pain due to inflammation of the parietal peritoneum, which is well localised. Pain may also be referred into the abdomen (see below).

Visceral pain from a hollow tube gives rise to colic. When a hollow viscus with smooth muscle in its wall is obstructed, the smooth muscle contracts in peristaltic waves in an attempt to overcome the obstruction. These contractions with peristalsis give rise to intermittent spasms of pain. Visceral pain is poorly localised – pain arising from foregut structures (lower third of the oesophagus to the ampulla of Vater in the second part of the duodenum) usually gives rise to a vague pain across the epigastrium, midgut structures (second part of the duodenum to two-thirds of the way along the transverse colon) tend to give pain across the central abdomen, and a pain from hindgut structures (ending at the rectum) tends to give pain across the lower abdomen.

Parietal pain is caused by stimulation of the somatic nerves in the abdominal wall, and therefore pain from this tends to be well localised. An example of the two types of pain is readily seen in acute appendicitis. The initial vague central abdominal pain is due to distension of the lumen of the appendix (the appendix is a midgut structure). Once the appendix becomes inflamed and the inflammation spreads to the visceral peritoneum and the visceral peritoneum abuts on and inflames the parietal peritoneum in the region of McBurney's point, the result is a sharp pain well localised in the right iliac fossa. This type of pain is made worse by coughing and movement, and therefore the patient lies still. This is in contrast to the patient with colicky pain who moves about the bed in an attempt to get in a comfortable position.
Characteristics of the pain can be remembered from the mnemonic **SOCRATES**:

- **S**ite: ascertain where the pain started and if the pain moved or a new pain developed in another site. The example of acute appendicitis given above demonstrates that in acute appendicitis the pain starts across the central abdomen and a new pain develops sharply localised in the right iliac fossa when the parietal peritoneum becomes inflamed.
- **O**nset: ascertain whether the pain is of sudden or gradual onset. Colicky pains related to the gut tend to be of gradual onset. However, colic related to the biliary tract and the ureter may have a more rapid onset and be more severe. The pain associated with a perforated hollow viscus tends to be sudden and spreads rapidly. The pain associated with a ruptured aortic aneurysm tends to be sudden and extremely severe.
- **C**haracter: ascertain if it is a dull pain, whether it is vague, colicky, sharp or burning.
- **R**adiation: the pain of ureteric colic tends to radiate from loin to groin. The pain from biliary colic tends to radiate across the whole of the upper abdomen.
- **A**ssociated factors: check for vomiting, diarrhoea, fever, effect of movement, effect of micturition.
- **T**iming: is the pain constant or intermittent, and how long does the pain last? The pain may have started suddenly and be constant but getting worse. Colicky pain tends to come in bursts, causing the patient to double up for a short time, and even making them cry out with pain; the pain then wears off and gives the patient a period of relief before another attack occurs a few minutes later.
- **E**xacerbations and relieving factors: check what makes the pain better/worse. Peritonitis is made worse by moving.
- **S**everity: try to assess the severity of the pain. It is a good idea to do this on a scale of 1–10, 1 being mild and 10 the most severe. Check the severity of the pain when it initially started and also the severity of the pain when you actually are examining the patient. The pain associated with a ruptured aortic aneurysm will almost always be graded 9 or 10 even from the starting point.

Vomiting

- Did vomiting precede the pain?
- Frequency
- Character, e.g. bile, faeculent, blood, coffee grounds.

Defaecation

- Constipation: absolute constipation with colicky abdominal pain, distension and vomiting suggests intestinal obstruction.
- Diarrhoea: frequency, consistency of stools, blood, mucus, pus.

Fever. Any rigours.

Past History

- Previous surgery, e.g. adhesions may cause intestinal obstruction
- Recent trauma, e.g. delayed rupture of spleen
- Menstrual history, e.g. ectopic pregnancy.

Examination

Always try to get the patient in the most comfortable position possible. The patient should be lying flat using one pillow and should ideally be exposed from nipples to knees. Try to preserve the patient's dignity if you can with a towel.

General. It is always important to carry out a general examination looking for signs of shock or dehydration, for example sweatiness, pallor, peripheral shutdown, tachycardia and hypotension. To get the patient to relax, check the hands, mouth, eyes and neck before beginning palpation of the abdomen. You should get an idea during this time as to whether the patient looks ill. Observe if the patient is lying comfortably or is lying still but is in pain, e.g. peritonitis. If the patient is writhing in agony, it suggests that they have ureteric or biliary colic.

Pulse, Temperature, Respiration

Cervical Lymphadenopathy. (e.g. mesenteric adenitis).

Chest. (e.g. referred pain from lobar pneumonia).

Abdomen

Inspection. Moves on respiration. Scars, distended, visible peristalsis (usually chronic obstruction in patient with very thin abdominal wall). Pain on coughing. Hernial orifices. Any obvious masses, e.g. pulsatile mass to suggest aortic aneurysm.

Palpation. Patient relaxed, lying flat, with arms by side. Be gentle and start as far from the painful site as possible. Check for guarding and rigidity. Rebound tenderness is unpleasant and should not be performed in the traditional manner of palpating the abdomen deeply and then suddenly withdrawing the examining hand. The presence of rebound tenderness can be inferred from more subtle signs such as percussing the abdomen, asking the patient to cough and asking whether bumps in the road during the ambulance journey were painful (hospitals always have speed bumps and can provide much information about an acute abdomen!). Check for masses, e.g. appendix mass, pulsatile expansile mass of aortic aneurysm. Check the hernial orifices.

Percussion. For example, tympanitic note with distension due to intestinal obstruction; dullness over bladder due to acute retention.

Auscultation. Take your time (30–60s), e.g. silent abdomen of peritonitis, high-pitched tinkling bowel sounds of intestinal obstruction.

Rectal Examination. This is just as important as the abdominal examination. It should be carried out in the left lateral position. Insert a well-lubricated gloved finger posteriorly into the sacral hollow. Move the finger around in the arc of a circle until it impinges on the peritoneum of the rectovesical or rectouterine pouch. If the patient winces with pain when the finger impinges on the peritoneum, this is a sign of peritonitis in the most dependent part of the pelvis. The pain disappears when the finger comes off the peritoneum as it completes the circle and returns to the sacral hollow. The correct annotation of a positive rectal examination should be 'tender anteriorly'. 'Tender high up in the right' is inappropriate. There seems to be a misconception among medical students that you are feeling the area of the appendix. You are feeling for tenderness due to inflammation of the pelvic peritoneum caused by infected exudates draining to the most dependent part of the pelvis, i.e. the rectovesical or rectouterine pouch.

Vaginal Examination. Discharge, tenderness associated with pelvic inflammatory disease, examine the uterus and adnexa, e.g. pregnancy, fibroids, ectopic pregnancy.

HINTS AND TIPS

Carefully observe the patient while taking the history. With experience you can usually tell just by looking if the patient is unwell. Is the patient in pain, lying still, and the abdomen not moving on respiration? This is strongly suggestive of peritonitis. Is the patient constantly moving around the bed to try to get into a comfortable position with exacerbations of pain so severe as to double them up? This suggests an underlying colic. Periods of freedom from the pain with repeated exacerbations at intervals suggests intestinal colic. Unlike intestinal colic, the pain of biliary and renal colic is continuous with added more severe exacerbations.

Distinction between ureteric and biliary colic can be made by observing the patient attempting to describe the pain. With renal colic the pain radiates from loin to groin, and the patient will move their hand from loin to groin when asked to demonstrate the site of the pain. With biliary colic the pain radiates across the upper abdomen, and the patient will move their hand from side to side across the upper abdomen when asked to describe the site of the pain.

Investigations

- FBC: low haemoglobin (Hb) may indicate chronic bleeding; a raised white cell count with a neutrophil leukocytosis may indicate an inflammatory or infective process.
- U&Es: fluid loss may result in renal impairment; vomiting may cause electrolyte abnormalities.
- LFTs: may indicate gallstone pathology or hepatitis
- Amylase: a high amylase confirms the diagnosis of pancreatitis; a mildly raised amylase is also seen in ectopic pregnancy, torsion of ovarian cyst, perforated peptic ulcer and intestinal ischaemia.
- Beta-human chorionic gonadotrophin (β-HCG): pregnancy/ectopic pregnancy – must be performed in all females of childbearing age with iliac fossa pain
- CRP: inflammatory marker generally raised within 8h of an inflammatory process – can be useful in difficult cases, e.g. suspected appendicitis of 12h duration with a normal WCC and CRP is unlikely to be acute appendicitis.

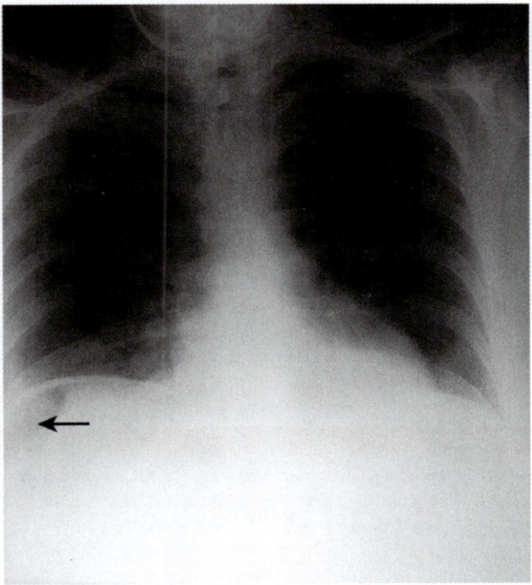

FIGURE 14.1

Gas (arrow) is seen under the right hemidiaphragm following perforation of a duodenal ulcer.

- ABG: generally only indicated in severely ill patients; it can give useful information on tissue perfusion by pH and lactate levels; PaO_2 and $PaCO_2$ can give important information for the anaesthetist prior to surgery.
- Chest X-ray (CXR): exclude referred lesion, free gas under diaphragm is known as pneumoperitoneum and may indicate hollow viscus perforation e.g. perforated duodenal ulcer (→Figure 14.1).
- AXR: distended bowel with air/fluid levels, gallstones (10% are radio-opaque); calcified aorta, e.g. aneurysm; air in biliary tree (cholecystoduodenal fistula with gallstone ileus)
- USS: e.g. ovarian cyst, ectopic pregnancy, gallstones
- Computerised tomography (CT) (Figure 14.2): useful in difficult cases – able to demonstrate free fluid, air, dilated bowel, pancreatitis
- KUB
- CT KUB for stones
- CT angiography: e.g. acute gastrointestinal (GI) haemorrhage of obscure cause, superior mesenteric embolus or thrombosis (duplex scanning may also be appropriate).

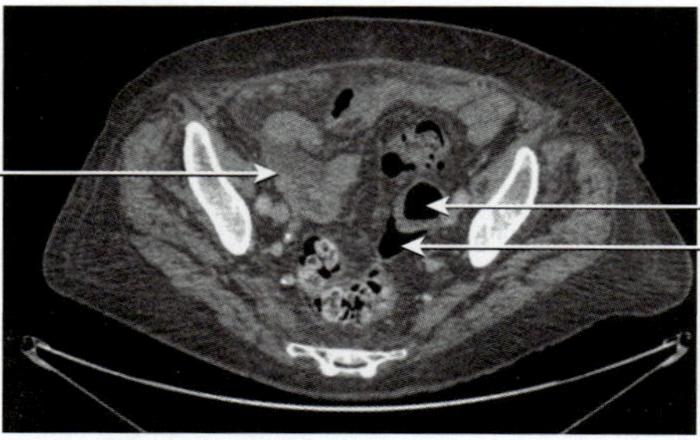

FIGURE 14.2
CT scan of the pelvis. Perforated sigmoid diverticulitis. There is free air in the pelvis at the site of perforation of a sigmoid diverticulum. There is also some free fluid.

HINTS AND TIPS

A raised serum amylase of three to four times the normal supports a clinical diagnosis of acute pancreatitis. Moderately elevated values should be interpreted with caution since abnormal levels may occur with ischaemic bowel, perforated peptic ulcer, torsion of ovarian cyst and ectopic pregnancy. Moreover, normal or even low serum amylase values may be seen with acute haemorrhagic pancreatitis. A CT scan may be obtained to confirm the diagnosis, but florid changes may not be seen for at least 5 days from onset of the attack. However, the main role for CT scanning in acute pancreatitis is to exclude any other cause for symptoms such as perforated duodenal ulcer.

Causes

Some causes of the acute abdomen are shown in Table 14.1. These conditions are covered in the relevant chapters. (For information on the site of abdominal pain in relation to suspected pathology→Table 14.2.)

Diagnosis. Diagnosing patients with an acute abdomen is the 'bread and butter' of the on-call general surgeon. The legion of causes is almost impossible to remember, but establishing a prompt diagnosis may be lifesaving. This requires a good history and examination, and avoiding over-reliance on scanning to make a diagnosis. An easy method to classify patients with an acute abdomen is given below:

- Acute abdomen + shock, e.g. ruptured abdominal aortic aneurysm, pancreatitis
- Generalised peritonitis, e.g. perforated viscus
- Localised peritonitis, e.g. acute appendicitis
- Distended abdomen, e.g. bowel obstruction
- Medical causes, e.g. lobar pneumonia.

These patients can then be divided into a number of management strategies. For example, not all patients with localised peritonitis need an operation. Indeed, not all patients with pain and shock need an operation. An unnecessary laparotomy in pancreatitis can exacerbate the condition considerably.

TABLE 14.1

CAUSES OF ACUTE ABDOMEN

Gastrointestinal	
Gut	Acute appendicitis Intestinal obstruction Perforated peptic ulcer Diverticulitis Inflammatory bowel disease Acute exacerbation of peptic ulcer Gastroenteritis Mesenteric adenitis Meckel's diverticulitis
Liver and biliary tract	Cholecystitis Cholangitis Hepatitis Biliary colic
Pancreas	Acute pancreatitis
Spleen	Splenic infarct and spontaneous rupture
Urinary Tract	
	Cystitis Acute pyelonephritis Ureteric colic Acute retention
Gynaecological	
	Ruptured ectopic pregnancy Torsion of ovarian cyst Ruptured ovarian cyst Salpingitis Severe dysmenorrhoea Mittelschmerz Endometriosis
Vascular	
	Ruptured aortic aneurysm Mesenteric embolus Mesenteric venous thrombosis Ischaemic colitis Acute aortic dissection
Peritoneum	
	Primary peritonitis Secondary peritonitis
Abdominal Wall	
	Rectus sheath haematoma
Retroperitoneal	
	Haemorrhage, e.g. anticoagulants

TABLE 14.2

SITE OF ABDOMINAL PAIN IN RELATION TO SUSPECTED PATHOLOGY

Whole abdomen	Generalised peritonitis and mesenteric infarction
Right upper quadrant	Acute cholecystitis Cholangitis Hepatitis Peptic ulceration
Left upper quadrant	Peptic ulceration Pancreatitis Splenic infarct
Right lower quadrant	Appendicitis Ovarian cyst Ectopic pregnancy Pelvic inflammatory disease Meckel's diverticulum Mesenteric adenitis Ureteric colic Rectus sheath haematoma Right-sided lobar pneumonia
Left lower quadrant	Sigmoid diverticular disease Ovarian cyst Ectopic pregnancy Pelvic inflammatory disease Ureteric colic Rectus sheath haematoma Left-sided lobar pneumonia
Radiating pain:	
• Back	Peptic ulcer Pancreatitis Aortic aneurysm Acute aortic dissection
• Groin	Ureteric colic Testicular torsion

Management. Strategies include:

- Immediate operation – these patients will die unless taken to theatre immediately, e.g. ruptured abdominal aortic aneurysm.
- Preoperative preparation and operation urgently within 6h – elderly patients may present with an acute abdomen and require urgent operation; however, preoperative dehydration and electrolyte abnormalities need to be corrected before going to theatre.
- Urgent operation (within 24h) – certain conditions, particularly in young patients, may be dealt with on a routine emergency list, e.g. acute appendicitis, small bowel obstruction with no adverse symptoms (e.g. no fever, no leukocytosis, no peritonism).

- Conservative treatment – numerous causes of an acute abdomen only require conservative treatment, i.e. nil by mouth, antibiotics (e.g. acute cholecystitis).
- Observation – many patients may have equivocal clinical signs but may be in the early stages of a condition. Time is a great diagnostic tool, and frequent re-examination may reveal evolving signs.
- Discharge.

Patients must be continually reassessed and evaluated, as they can move from one group to another; for example, a young man admitted with RIF pain and booked for urgent operation within 24h may perforate and thus display generalised peritonitis – in this instance the patient would require immediate operation.

Treatment

- Relieve pain
- Intravenous fluids and nasogastric suction
- Prompt administration of i.v. broad-spectrum antibiotics if peritonitis or sepsis
- Surgery if indicated.

Indications for Surgery in the Acute Abdomen. There are no hard and fast rules, but patients with the following symptoms will almost certainly require surgery:

- Localised peritoneal irritation with guarding or rigidity
- Progressive tenderness
- Tense or progressive distension if obstructed
- Generalised peritonitis
- Shock with bleeding or sepsis
- Free gas on radiograph (pneumoperitoneum).

MEDICAL CAUSES OF ACUTE ABDOMINAL PAIN

Occasionally, certain medical conditions may cause acute abdominal pain. The following should be considered.

Referred Pain. May be caused by degenerative disease of thoracic spine, herpes zoster, lower lobar pneumonia, pleurisy, MI.

Haematological. This may be due to sickle cell crisis.

Infective and Inflammatory. These medical conditions are possible: tabes dorsalis, Henoch–Schönlein purpura.

Endocrine and Metabolic. These conditions include uraemia, hypercalcaemia, diabetic ketoacidosis, Addison's disease, acute intermittent porphyria.

HINTS AND TIPS

Patients with medical causes of acute abdominal pain occasionally present as acute surgical emergencies. With the exception of referred pain, the other causes are extremely rare but should be borne in mind. A medical cause should be suspected if there are no abdominal signs in the presence of abdominal symptoms. A CXR and ECG will help rule out the majority of cases of referred pain.

PERITONITIS

Peritonitis is an inflammatory or suppurative response of the peritoneal lining to direct irritation. It may be localised or generalised, bacterial or chemical. Localised peritonitis is due to transmural inflammation of a viscus, e.g. appendicitis, cholecystitis, diverticulitis. It may remain localised through being contained by omental wrapping or adhesion of adjacent structures. In many cases, however, it becomes generalised, spreading to involve the whole peritoneum. Sudden perforation of a viscus usually results in generalised peritonitis. With the latter the patient is seriously ill. Hypovolaemia results from massive exudation into the peritoneal cavity, and septicaemia may result if the cause is infective, e.g. faecal peritonitis from perforated diverticulitis. Chemical peritonitis results from gastric or pancreatic juice, bile, urine or blood in the peritoneal cavity. Bile causes little reaction if sterile but causes severe peritonitis if infected or mixed with pancreatic juice. Blood and urine cause little reaction if sterile, but a severe reaction occurs if they are infective. (For a classification of peritonitis→Table 14.3.)

Symptoms and Signs. These depend on the degree of peritonitis and the precipitating cause. They also relate to the abdominal signs from the original pathology and manifestations of systemic infection. Usually there is sudden onset of abdominal pain made worse by coughing and movement. Initially it may be localised (and it may remain so in some cases) but often gradually spreads to involve the whole abdomen. Nausea, vomiting, fever, abdominal tenderness (localised or generalised), guarding, rigidity, distension, absent bowel sounds develop when ileus supervenes. Always inspect from the end of the bed and check the patient's observations chart. Patients with peritonitis are often very still in bed, as the pain is worse with movement. Manifestations of systemic infection include tachycardia, sweating, rigours, tachypnoea, oliguria, disorientation, shock and Gram-negative septicaemia. In advanced cases, and with delay in presentation, renal, respiratory, and cardiac failure may result. Don't forget to palpate the groins for an incarcerated hernia (often missed in patients presenting with vomiting).

TABLE 14.3

CAUSES OF PERITONITIS

Acute	
Bacterial	Primary (rare): • Streptococci, pneumococci • Haematogenous spread • Occurs in young girls, ascites, nephrotic syndrome and postsplenectomy Secondary (common): • Related to perforation, infection, inflammation or ischaemia of GI or GU tract
Chemical	Gastric juice (e.g. perforated gastric ulcer) Pancreatic juice (e.g. acute pancreatitis) Bile (e.g. perforation of the gall bladder) Blood (e.g. ruptured spleen) Urine (e.g. intraperitoneal rupture of the bladder)
Chronic	
	Tuberculosis Starch (immunological reaction)

Investigations

- Hb
- PCV
- WCC
- U&Es: dehydration, ARF
- LFTs
- Amylase
- CXR: gas under diaphragm, small pleural effusion
- AXR: distended bowel (ileus), local ileus ('sentinel' loop – acute pancreatitis)
- USS: free fluid, localised collections
- CT – pancreatitis, perforation/ ischaemia etc.

Complications

Systemic. Hypovolaemic shock, septic shock, ARDS, DIC, multiorgan failure, immunological failure.

Local. Intraperitoneal sepsis: residual abscesses, e.g. subphrenic or pelvic, wound infection, anastomotic breakdown, fistula formation, adhesions.

Prognosis. Overall mortality in generalised peritonitis is around 40%. Factors affecting mortality include late presentation and diagnosis, advanced age (elderly patients with faecal peritonitis have a high mortality), causation, duration of symptoms, degree of bacterial contamination, concomitant disease processes, e.g. ischaemic heart disease and end organ failure.

Treatment. Principles of treatment involve the following:

Resuscitation. This requires pain relief with narcotic analgesics, i.v. fluids, NG aspiration, correction of electrolyte imbalance, catheterisation. UO and CVP (especially in elderly) should be monitored. Oxygen and antibiotics. Liaise closely with the anaesthetist at all times.

Treatment of Causative Lesion. In generalised peritonitis this almost invariably requires surgery. Acute pancreatitis is the exception. Principles of operative treatment involve removal of all infected material from the peritoneal cavity, correction of the underlying cause, and attempts to prevent complications. Swab for C&S. Thorough examination of the peritoneal cavity, debridement of serosal surfaces, removal of affected organ, e.g. appendicectomy, colectomy. Formation of stomas rather than a primary anastomosis, which may leak in the presence of infection and unprepared bowel. Peritoneal lavage. Peritoneal drains. Occasionally, the abdomen should be left open, and the exposed bowel covered with moist swabs (laparostomy).

Postoperative Care. Attention should be paid to fluid and electrolyte balance. UO should be monitored. Antibiotic therapy, nutritional support and surveillance for sepsis. Ventilation may be necessary. CVVH or dialysis may be required for ARF.

INTRA-ABDOMINAL ABSCESSES

An abscess is a localised collection of pus. Intra-abdominal abscesses can be divided into intraperitoneal and extraperitoneal. Following peritonitis, pus may collect in either the subphrenic spaces, the pelvis or in locules between loops of bowel. Intra-abdominal abscesses tend to be less common due to the widespread use of prophylactic antibiotics. However, they may still occur in the elderly, debilitated, patients on steroid and immunosuppression. They are more commonly associated with perforations of the lower gastrointestinal tract. The mortality rate tends to be high.

Intraperitoneal Abscesses

These tend to arise in dependent areas of the abdomen where fluid may collect. They include:

- Subphrenic – occur following anastomotic leaks in gastric or hepatobiliary surgery, after splenic surgery, perforated peptic ulcer, acute cholecystitis and acute appendicitis
- Paracolic – occur with perforations secondary to inflammatory bowel disease, diverticulitis, malignancy or anastomotic leaks
- Right iliac fossa – occur with appendicitis, perforated peptic ulcer, inflammatory bowel disease
- Pelvic – as the most dependent part of the abdomen, pelvic abscesses are the most common type of intra-abdominal abscesses and can be caused by all the above plus gynaecological causes.

Extraperitoneal Abscesses

These are much less common than intraperitoneal abscesses; they most frequently follow infections of organs in the retroperitoneum or where peritoneal organs have perforated into the retroperitoneum. Extraperitoneal abscesses are most commonly associated with:

- pancreatitis
- posterior perforation of duodenal ulcer
- posterior colonic perforations
- pyelonephritis
- spinal infections, e.g. osteomyelitis.

Extraperitoneal abscesses can also present as a psoas abscess; these can occur primarily due to haematogenous spread, tuberculosis of the thoracolumbar spine or secondary to local infections, e.g. Crohn's disease.

Symptoms and Signs. General signs include malaise, swinging pyrexia, tachycardia, localised pain and tenderness, prolonged ileus. Signs specific to the position of the abscess include:

- Subphrenic – chest pain, shortness of breath (secondary to basal atelectasis), shoulder tip pain (referred from diaphragmatic irritation), hiccups
- Pelvic – diarrhoea, urinary frequency, passage of mucus PR, boggy fluctuant mass on PR or PV examination
- Psoas – pain on extension of the hip (patients tend to hold their hip in flexion); palpable psoas abscess below the inguinal ligament.

Investigations

- Hb
- WCC
- ESR
- LFTs: occasionally raised
- Blood culture may be positive.
- CXR: pleural effusion, raised hemidiaphragm, atelectasis
- AXR: ileus, air/fluid levels in abscess cavities (rare)
- USS
- CT
- Indium-labelled white cell scan.

Treatment. For well-localised, non-loculated abscesses, percutaneous drainage under US or CT control. If there are multiple abscesses or they are multiloculated, open drainage at laparotomy will be required.

PROCEDURES

LAPAROTOMY

The following description relates to laparotomy for peritonitis of unknown origin (rather than trauma).

- Incision – 'incision of indecision' approximately 10 cm centred on the umbilicus. Depending on the findings, the incision may then be extended up (bile) or down (faeces). The skin is incised with a knife and continued down to the linea alba with diathermy.
- Opening the peritoneum – the linea alba is opened along the length of the incision. Using two clips, the peritoneum is tented up and incised with scissors. The peritoneal opening is extended to allow the operator and assistant to insert a finger and lift up the abdominal wall so that the remaining peritoneum may be incised under direct vision.
- Examination of the peritoneal cavity – once inside the abdomen, a thorough and stepwise search of its contents is undertaken as follows:
  - Liver from right to left (including gallbladder)
  - Spleen
  - Oesophagus, stomach from proximal to distal and then to the duodenum
  - Kocher's manoeuvre will be required to visualise the remainder of the duodenum and head of pancreas.
  - The right kidney is palpated.
  - The lesser sac will need to be opened to visualise the body and tail of the pancreas.
  - The left kidney is palpated.
  - Small bowel is examined from the ligament of Treitz to the ileocaecal valve taking care to examine both sides and the mesentery.
  - As the small bowel is out of the abdomen, the retroperitoneum can be palpated taking particular note of an aortic aneurysm.
  - The caecum and appendix are then examined and follow onto the rest of the colon.
  - Female reproductive organs
  - Hernial orifices
- Abdomen closure – the commonest technique is to use looped monofilament suture such as 0 PDS or 0 Nylon, one from the top of the incision and the other from the bottom and meeting approximately halfway down (do not tie the knot at the umbilicus). The bites of linea alba should be 1 cm deep and 1 cm apart. The skin may be closed with clips or a subcuticular suture (clips are better after a contaminated procedure, as some clips may be removed in the postoperative period in the event of wound infection).

PERFORATED PEPTIC ULCER

If the diagnosis is known preoperatively, an upper midline incision may be used. A laparoscopic approach is increasingly popular if the surgeon has the expertise.
The following are the steps in the procedure:

- Perform a laparotomy as above. With a perforated viscus, a hiss of air may be heard as the peritoneum is incised.

PROCEDURES—Cont'd

- Send fluid for culture and sensitivity.
- Examine the duodenum (perforations are usually in D1) and stomach for perforations (if gastric ulcer, it will need to be biopsied from the ulcer edge to rule out malignancy).
- Using 3/0 Vicryl close the ulcer defect with two or three interrupted sutures, starting 1 cm from the medial edge and exiting 1 cm from the lateral edge (take care not to catch the back wall). These sutures are then tied to approximate the edges of the ulcer. Do not tie the sutures too hard, as the tissues will be friable, and the suture will cut through. Do not cut the ends of the sutures at this point.
- Fashion a pedicle of omentum and lay across the perforation. Tie the sutures over the omentum to secure it in place.
- Wash out the abdomen thoroughly with copious amounts of warm saline, particularly above and below the liver and in the pelvis.
- Close the abdomen as for laparotomy.
- A drain is not usually needed.

APPENDICECTOMY

Many appendicectomies are now performed laparoscopically. However, it is still important to understand the principles of laparoscopic appendicectomy:

- A Lanz skin crease incision is made across McBurney's point (junction of the middle and outer third of a line joining the anterior superior iliac spine and the umbilicus).
- The incision extends down to the external oblique, which is incised in the line of the incision. The muscles can then be split in the direction of their fibres.
- The peritoneum is picked up between clips (once the second clip is applied, reapply the first clip so as to drop any bowel that may have been picked up). Open the peritoneum in the line of the wound.
- Any free fluid is sent for culture and sensitivity.
- The appendix can be delivered into the wound by: (1) following the taenia coli down to the caecum where they converge on the appendix; (2) sweeping the finger from medial to lateral under the caecum, feeling for the inflamed appendix and pulling it up into the wound.
- Make a window in the mesoappendix at the point where the appendix meets the caecum. Place two clips across the mesoappendix and divide it. Suture ligate both ends.
- The base of the appendix is crushed with a haemostat. Another haemostat is placed below the crushed segment, and the crushed segment is then ligated.
- Place another haemostat above the tie and divide the appendix with a knife.
- Place a seromuscular purse string suture around the base of the appendix and bury the stump by tying it.
- If the appendix is normal, look for another cause of abdominal pain, e.g. Crohn's disease, Meckel's diverticulum or ovarian pathology.
- Wash out the abdomen (especially the pelvis) with copious amounts of saline.
- Close the peritoneum with 3/0 Vicryl, the external oblique aponeurosis with 2/0 Vicryl and then close the skin with either clips or subcuticular suture.

Chapter 15

Alimentary Tract

Vam Jagadesham • Rina George • Bhaskar Kumar

CHAPTER OUTLINE

OESOPHAGUS

Dysphagia, defined as difficulty in swallowing, is the cardinal symptom of oesophageal pathology. Progressive dysphagia is of particular significance, as it may be indicative of an underlying neoplasia. However, dysphagia may be due to numerous benign causes either of local or general origin (Table 15.1).

Investigation of Dysphagia

History

- Progressive dysphagia (solids then liquids), particularly associated with weight loss, is suggestive of malignancy.
- Malignant causes of dysphagia may be associated with odynophagia (painful swallowing) and regurgitation.
- In younger patients, a peptic stricture from oesophagitis may lead to dysphagia.
- Achalasia, a rare motility disorder of the oesophagus, is often associated with dysphagia, regurgitation, chest pain and weight loss. Patients often wait for food to "go through" after swallowing.
- There may be an obvious cause, e.g. foreign body, ingestion of caustic substance.
- Patient may complain of a sensation of a lump in the throat with no weight loss or other alarming symptoms. This is known as globus pharyngeus and is often mistaken for true dysphagia.

Examination. Often physical examination is normal in these patients. However, careful palpation for supraclavicular lymph nodes is particularly important, as it may be indicative of malignancy. An epigastric mass should always be palpated for which may be from a malignancy of the stomach or oesophagogastric junction. The liver

TABLE 15.1

CAUSES OF DYSPHAGIA

Local	
In the lumen	Foreign body
In the wall	Congenital atresia Inflammatory stricture – reflux oesophagitis Caustic stricture Achalasia Carcinoma Plummer–Vinson syndrome (oesophageal web) Scleroderma Irradiation
Outside the wall	Mediastinal lymphadenopathy Bronchial carcinoma Retrosternal goitre Pharyngeal pouch Paraoesophageal (rolling) hiatus hernia Thoracic aortic aneurysm Dysphagia lusoria (vascular ring)
General	
	Myasthenia gravis Bulbar palsy Bulbar poliomyelitis Hysteria

should be palpated for secondaries. Rare physical signs include koilonychia, which is associated with Plummer–Vinson syndrome. A lump may be palpable in the posterior triangle of the neck with pharyngeal pouch. This may gurgle when full of food.

Investigations

- FBC including Hb
- U&Es
- LFTs
- CXR: aspiration into the lung fields, bony erosions from secondaries, effusion may all be suggestive of malignancy. Rarely mediastinal mass, bronchial carcinoma, thoracic aortic aneurysm, retrocardiac air fluid level may be seen with hiatus hernia.
- Fibreoptic OGD with biopsies of suspicious lesions (should be used cautiously if pharyngeal pouch is suspected)
- Barium swallow
- Computerised tomography (CT) scan of neck/chest/abdomen – if malignancy suspected.

Treatment. Is directed at the underlying cause but may require specialist multidisciplinary team discussion.

Foreign Body

This is usually accidental and commonly occurs in young children with the ingestion of batteries and coins. Deliberate ingestion of foreign bodies may be seen in institutionalised patients such as those with mental illnesses. Foreign bodies often impact at sites of pathology such as strictures or at the narrowest parts of the oesophagus, of which there are three: (1) at its commencement at the cricopharyngeus, (2) where it is crossed by the aortic arch and the left main bronchus, and (3) where it passes through the diaphragm. Smooth objects will usually pass into the stomach. Sharp and irregular objects impact.

Symptoms and Signs. History of ingestion and acute dysphagia with clinical signs being limited. Mediastinitis with systemic signs if perforation occurs.

Investigations

- CXR/AXR may show radio-opaque foreign body.
- CXR may demonstrate pneumomediastinum if perforation has occurred.
- Water-soluble contrast swallow (especially if perforation suspected or foreign body is non-radio-opaque)
- OGD (which also forms the basis of treatment).

Treatment. The vast majority of foreign bodies will pass through the gastrointestinal tract, and therefore initial management is observation with serial radiographs in asymptomatic patients. Failure to progress (impaction) may require an OGD and removal using specialised endoscopic equipment such as a Roth net and graspers or even an over-tube. The development of signs of sepsis, chest pain and total obstruction are concerning and should prompt urgent intervention.

Oesophageal Perforation

Oesophageal perforation can be spontaneous or iatrogenic. Iatrogenic perforations are commonly related to endoscopic instrumentation but can also be caused by ingestion of foreign bodies/corrosives or following anti-reflux surgery. Spontaneous perforation, termed Boerhaave's syndrome, is rare and is related to violent retching or vomiting.

Symptoms and Signs. History of foreign body/corrosive ingestion, endoscopy or violent vomiting/retching depending on the underlying cause. Sudden or gradual onset of pain in chest, neck and upper abdomen. Other clinical features include surgical emphysema or frank signs of mediastinitis resulting in septic shock.

Investigations

- CXR: pneumomediastinum, pneumothorax, surgical emphysema, pleural effusion
- CT chest/abdomen with i.v. and oral contrast
- Upper gastrointestinal (GI) endoscopy is safe to perform and may visualise the defect and pathology.
- Water-soluble contrast swallow may confirm the diagnosis and demonstrate the site but nowadays is superseded by CT.

Complication. Mediastinitis.

Treatment

Conservative. Small perforations with minimal mediastinal contamination can be managed using broad-spectrum antibiotics and antifungals and endoscopic placed nasojejunal feeding tube.

Surgical. Large perforations with significant contamination and systemic upset require emergency thoracotomy, lavage, debridement ± repair of perforation and a laparotomy for feeding jejunostomy.

HINTS AND TIPS

Iatrogenic perforation is usually associated with less morbidity due to fasting prior to the procedure, e.g. endoscopy, therefore resulting in far less mediastinal contamination. However, mediastinal collections may develop over time and may still be associated with significant morbidity and mortality.

Oesophageal Stricture

Over 75% of oesophageal strictures are related to prolonged acid reflux and are termed 'peptic strictures'. Reflux occurs secondary to an incompetent lower oesophageal sphincter and is often associated with a sliding hiatus hernia or a lax OG junction. Oesophagitis may be seen with prolonged vomiting, prolonged nasogastric intubation and procedures that remove the lower oesophageal sphincter mechanism, e.g. oesophagectomy, total gastrectomy, Roux-en-Y bypass for weight loss.

Gastro-Oesophageal Reflux Disease (GORD)

GORD is increasingly common. Patients with GORD can present with typical symptoms including heartburn and regurgitation. Atypical symptoms (extraoesophageal) include sore throat, cough and incomplete throat clearing. Patients with suspected GORD should undergo endoscopy which may demonstrate oesophagitis and a sliding hiatus hernia or lax OG junction. Oesophageal studies, including manometry, 24-h pH monitoring and manometry studies, are indicated if anti-reflux surgery is to be considered. A DeMeester score >14.72 and a pH <4 for greater than 4.4% over a 24-h period is suggestive of abnormal reflux. Manometry is performed to exclude significant dysmotility from conditions such as achalasia.

Hiatus Hernia

There are four types of hiatal hernia. By far the commonest type of hiatal hernia is a sliding type I hernia. A less common type of hiatal hernia is a paraoesophageal (type III). A type IV hernia is a combination of a type III hernia with a viscus most commonly colon.

SLIDING HIATUS HERNIA. The gastro-oesophageal junction migrates through the hiatus, leading to an incompetent lower oesophageal sphincter which may result in GORD (→Figure 15.1).

Symptoms and Signs. Symptoms can be divided into typical and atypical. Typical symptoms include retrosternal burning pain ('heartburn') worse on bending, stooping, or lying supine, which could be associated with acid regurgitation into mouth. Chest pain may mimick angina. These typical symptoms are usually responsive to anti-reflux medications to a variable extent. Atypical symptoms include throat clearing, cough, sinusitis and hoarse voice. Complications of severe reflux oesophagitis include ulcerative ulceration, peptic stricture formation and Barrett's oesophagus.

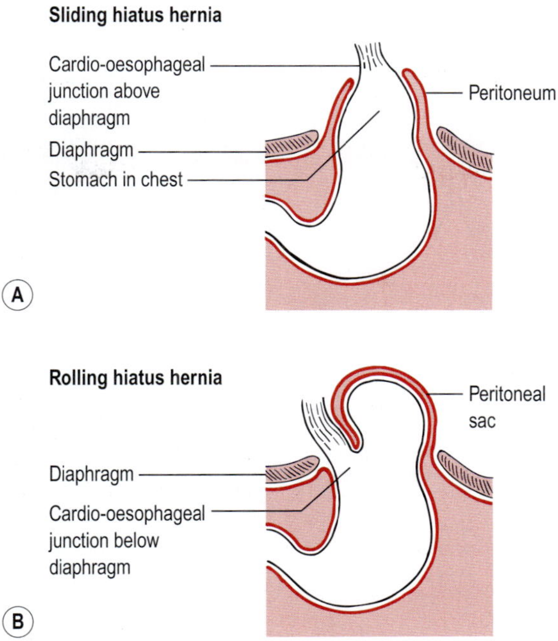

FIGURE 15.1

(**A**) Sliding hiatus hernia. The stomach slides up into the chest. Reflux occurs. (**B**) Rolling (paraoesophageal) hernia. The stomach rolls up alongside the oesophagus and dysphagia occurs. The cardio-oesophageal mechanism is intact, and therefore reflux does not occur.

Investigations.

- FBC including Hb
- U&Es
- Upper GI endoscopy is the first-line investigation of choice in patients with GORD and a suspected hiatus hernia. Biopsy can be performed if a stricture is observed or diagnosis of oesophagitis is in doubt.
- Barium swallow: confirms hiatus hernia and may demonstrate reflux, dysmotility or the presence of a stricture (→Figure 15.2)
- Oesophageal physiology (manometry and 24-h pH monitoring) should be requested only for patients who are potentially being considered for anti-reflux surgery.

Treatment

Conservative. Lifestyle modification can be adopted by encouraging weight loss, reduction in caffeinated drinks/alcohol consumption and not eating soon before going to bed. Sleeping in a more upright position may also be beneficial.

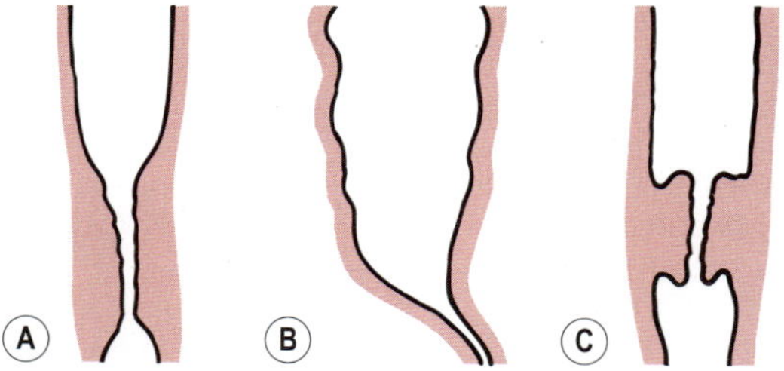

FIGURE 15.2

Types of oesophageal stricture.(**A**) Peptic stricture associated with reflux. (**B**) Tortuous dilated oesophagus with 'rat's tail' stricture of achalasia. (**C**) The irregular 'shouldered' stricture of carcinoma.

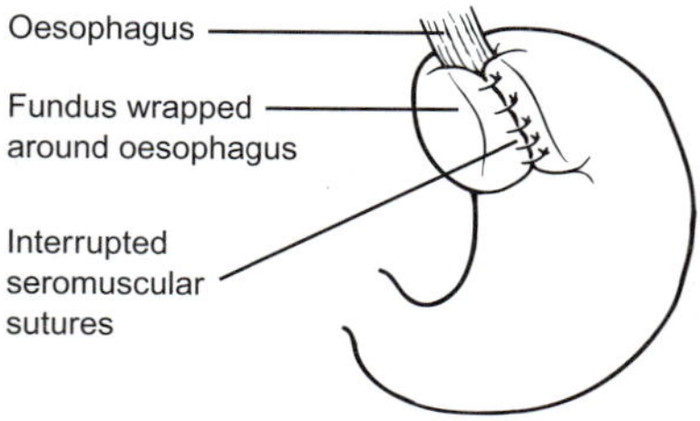

FIGURE 15.3

Nissen fundoplication.The fundus of the stomach is mobilised, wrapped around the lower oesophagus and held with seromuscular sutures.

Over-the-counter antacids can be used, but PPIs, including omeprazole or lansoprazole, are the most effective treatment. Many patients obtain symptomatic relief with this regimen.

Surgical. Anti-reflux surgery is indicated for failed medical treatment, reluctance to take medication lifelong or complications, e.g. peptic stricture. Fundoplication is the operation of choice, and these are classified into full (Nissen (360°) fundoplication (→ Figure 15.3)) or partial (Toupet (partial posterior) fundoplication and a Dor (partial anterior) fundoplication). Following oesophageal mobilisation and hiatal dissection, the crura are approximated and the fundus of the stomach is wrapped around the gastro-oesophageal junction according to the repair chosen. This is almost invariably performed laparoscopically.

HINTS AND TIPS

It is crucial to take a detailed history in patients with suspected GORD to differentiate between typical and atypical symptoms. It is important that all patients being considered for anti-reflux surgery are aware of the risk of dysphagia, gas-bloat syndrome, early satiety, weight loss, increased flatulence, failure to improve symptoms (especially with atypical symptoms) and recurrence.

Rolling or Paraoesophageal Hiatus Hernia. The gastro-oesophageal junction remains in its normal position, and the fundus herniates up into the chest alongside the oesophagus. Symptoms are usually obstructive, but some patients experience GORD in addition (→Figure 15.1).

Symptoms and Signs. Intermittent dysphagia, postprandial vomiting, chest pain due to distension, postprandial shortness of breath, epigastric pain and anaemia secondary to ulceration (Cameron ulcers). Presentation may be acute, particularly if symptoms of a gastric volvulus develop.

Investigations

- CXR: air/fluid level in mediastinum
- OGD: this can be difficult, especially in large herniae
- Barium swallow
- CT scan: can help delineate the extent of the hernia and is useful in acute presentation. Some of these herniae may even involve colon, small bowel and rarely the pancreas.

Complications. Can result in acute gastric volvulus presenting with Borchardt's triad: severe epigastric pain, unproductive retching and the inability to pass a nasogastric tube. Rarely, strangulation of the stomach may occur, which is life-threatening.

Treatment. It is generally recommended in fit patients that paraoesophageal herniae should be repaired due to the risk of gastric volvulus and subsequent mortality. Hiatal repair can be combined with either a fundoplication or a gastropexy. Large hiatal defects may require reinforcement with a biological mesh.

HINTS AND TIPS

Acute gastric volvulus is a rare entity, associated with significant morbidity and mortality, predominantly due to concomitant comorbidities. The stomach rotates >180° resulting in a closed-loop obstruction, which can lead to strangulation and necrosis. The stomach can rotate around an axis connecting the gastro-oesophageal junction and pylorus, which is known as organoaxial type. This is the most common type of gastric volvulus with mesenteroaxial type being far less common.

Achalasia

This is due to aperistalsis of the oesophagus and a lower oesophageal sphincter that fails to relax. It presents between 30 and 50 years, affects sexes equally, and the incidence is approximately 1/100,000 people per year. The cause is unknown but is due to progressive degeneration of Auerbach's myenteric plexus.

Symptoms and Signs. Typically, intermittent dysphagia that progressively worsens. Affects both liquids and solids. As a result, patients may experience weight loss.

Investigations

- OGD: may demonstrate food and fluid residue. Sometimes a tight cardia may be detected. Also to exclude pseudoachalasia secondary to benign stricture or malignant lesion.

- Barium swallow: dilated tortuous oesophagus above smooth tapering stricture ('bird's beak' appearance → Figure 15.2)
- Oesophageal manometry: 'gold standard', as both OGD and barium swallow may appear 'normal'. Manometry demonstrates a hypertensive lower oesophageal sphincter with an aperistaltic oesophagus.

Complications. Aspiration pneumonitis, recurrent chest infections and oesophageal erosions. Carcinoma, usually squamous cell, may develop even after treatment, although this is rare.

Treatment

Botulinum Toxin. Injection of botulinum toxin into the lower oesophageal sphincter is reserved for elderly patients with significant comorbidities.

Oesophageal Pneumatic Dilatation. This is achieved by stretching the cardia under fluoroscopic guidance using a plastic balloon (30–40 mm diameter). The procedure is associated with the risk of perforation, especially with repeated dilatations.

Heller's Operation (i.e. Cardiomyotomy). This procedure is commonly performed laparoscopically and involves cutting the muscle layer of the lower oesophagus longitudinally (6 cm) down to the mucosa and extending at least 2 cm on to the stomach. Due to resultant gastro-oesophageal reflux, the cardiomyotomy is combined with a fundoplication. It is a similar principle to Ramstedt's pyloromyotomy operation for pyloric stenosis in infancy.

HINTS AND TIPS

Patients with achalasia may also present with symptoms of GORD including heartburn and regurgitation, and thus can be misdiagnosed. It is, therefore, imperative that patients with suspected GORD who are being considered for anti-reflux surgery undergo oesophageal manometry. Failure to do so could result in complete dysphagia if fundoplication is performed in a patient with achalasia.

It is important to appreciate the concept of pseudoachalasia where patients can present similarly to 'true' achalasia. It is commonly due to a neoplasm at oesophagogastric junction, which may infiltrate the myenteric plexus. This underpins the importance of endoscopic examination in patients with dysphagia.

Barrett's Oesophagus

Barrett's oesophagus is an acquired condition which represents an adaptive change to chronic GORD. It is characterised by the presence of columnar mucosa within the oesophagus, which demonstrates specialised intestinal metaplasia. Endoscopy reveals areas of 'salmon' pink columnar mucosa replacing pearly white squamous epithelium. It occurs in 5–15% of patients with GORD. The risk of progression to dysplasia/malignancy (adenocarcinoma) in patients with Barrett's oesophagus is increased and, therefore, regular endoscopic surveillance with biopsy may be necessitated. Preventative measures include management of GORD with PPIs ± anti-reflux surgery. Treatment of established (high-grade) dysplasia can include endoluminal therapy (endoscopic mucosal resection, radiofrequency ablation).

HINTS AND TIPS

Despite the association, patients with Barrett's oesophagus may not have any symptoms of GORD. Similarly, patients with symptoms of GORD may not have any evidence of Barrett's oesophagus. It is, however, the chronic reflux of gastric acid that results in the metaplastic changes.

The absolute annual risk of Barrett's oesophagus becoming an adenocarcinoma is 0.12%.

Carcinoma of the Oesophagus

Carcinoma of the oesophagus is the seventh leading cause of cancer-related death and commonly occurs in men. In the West, the commonest site is the lower third of the oesophagus, with adenocarcinoma being the most frequent histological subtype in this region. Squamous cell carcinoma frequently affects the upper/middle oesophagus, with this subtype accounting for the overall majority of oesophageal cancers worldwide. Postcricoid carcinoma usually occurs in females and is associated with Plummer–Vinson syndrome. Achalasia of the cardia is also a predisposing cause for squamous cell carcinoma. Adenocarcinoma is associated with GORD and Barrett's oesophagus. Spread occurs by the following routes:

- Haematogenous to the liver and lung
- Lymphatic to paraoesophageal nodes, carinal, bronchial, supraclavicular and abdominal nodes
- Local invasion into surrounding structures; e.g. aorta, trachea, aorta.

Symptoms and Signs. Progressive dysphagia should be considered to be from a malignancy until proven otherwise. It is usually insidious in nature. Initially for solids, then fluids. Other than weight loss, patients often do not many more clinical features, but palpable supraclavicular nodes may be a sign of metastatic disease.

Investigations

- FBC including Hb
- U&Es
- LFTs
- OGD with biopsy remains the investigation of choice.
- CT scan for staging, to define local invasion, the presence of metastatic disease and indicate operability. Also to define the presence of progression following neoadjuvant therapy.
- Barium swallow: 'shouldered' stricture (→Figure 15.2). However, a bariums swallow should only be used for cases where the patient cannot undergo endoscopy, e.g. frail.
- Endoluminal ultrasound (EUS) to determine staging and local lymph node status. Also allows fine-needle aspiration of suspicious lymph nodes.
- PET-CT to demonstrate the presence of small-volume metastatic disease not seen on CT.

Treatment. Can be curative or palliative depending on operability and patient fitness. Patients undergoing curative treatment may be offered neoadjuvant chemotherapy (FLOT4) or chemoradiotherapy prior to resection. The tumour can be resected via a transhiatal, transthoracic, laparoscopic-assisted or minimally invasive approach. Principally the stomach is mobilised based on the right gastroepiploic artery, tabularised and brought up into the mediastinum and anastomosed to the remaining oesophagus in either the thorax or neck.

If the tumour is inoperable, palliation could be offered using an endoscopic stent, palliative chemotherapy or radiotherapy, all depending on the patients' symptoms.

Prognosis. Although outcomes are improving, overall prognosis is poor with a 25–30% 5-year survival following curative treatment. Most patients survive less than 6 months if the primary is inoperable.

Caustic Oesophagitis

The accidental (children) or deliberate (adults) ingestion of caustic agents causes severe chemical oesophagitis. Common substances include household agents such as caustic soda, hydrochloric acid, bleach and sulphuric acid. Extensive damage can occur to the aerodigestive tract.

Symptoms and Signs. Airway compromise with stridor is the immediate acute risk. This may require intubation. Perforation of the oesophagus or stomach is a risk depending on the substance and volume. Burning pain from mouth to stomach. Dyspnoea can occur in the presence of aspiration (chemical pneumonitis). Dysphagia and odynophagia are related to oesophageal injury. Patients may present with shock and respiratory distress.

Investigations. Early fibreoptic endoscopy (within 24h) to assess degree of damage to the oesophagus and stomach. A nasoenteral feeding tube can be placed at the same time if supplemental nutrition is anticipated.

Complications

Early. Airway compromise, oesophageal (and gastric) perforation and haematemesis.

Late. Oesophageal stricture.

Treatment

Emergency. Establishment and maintenance of the airway with prompt resuscitation is key. Following a perforation, patients may require an OGD with delayed reconstruction.

Medical. Broad-spectrum antibiotics for aspiration pneumonitis or perforation. Steroids may have a role in reducing stricture formation. Nutrition, either enteral or parenteral. Antisecretory medication. Attention must be given to any underlying mental health issues and involvement of appropriate teams for support.

Endoscopic Dilatation of Strictures. Gentle dilatation may be undertaken >6 weeks following the injury if a contrast swallow or endoscopy demonstrates a stricture. Repeated dilatation increases the risk of perforation.

Surgery. Young patients with a significant stricture(s) may require oesophageal replacement using a colonic interposition graft. Rarely stomach may be used if it has been spared from the effects of the caustic injury.

Prognosis. Appropriate early treatment of caustic burns usually gives good results. Extensive burns with strong acid or strong alkali can progress to stricture formation, which requires repeated dilatations or surgery. Following a caustic injury, patients are at increased risk of squamous cell carcinoma of the oesophagus.

HINTS AND TIPS

It is a general misconception that alkalis are more corrosive than acidic agents. It is the caustic properties, amount and duration of contact that are crucial in determining the severity of injury. Furthermore, patients should not undergo gastric lavage, induced emesis or neutralisation of the caustic agent. The key principles are airway management and resuscitation.

Plummer–Vinson Syndrome (Syn. Paterson–Brown–Kelly Syndrome)

This more commonly occurs in middle-aged females and is associated with postcricoid dysphagia, upper oesophageal webs and iron deficiency anaemia. Patients can also present with glossitis, angular cheilitis and koilonychia (spoon-shaped nails). The condition is thought to be premalignant, and patients have an increased risk of malignant transformation. Sideropenic dysphagia is associated with iron deficiency (sideropenia) but in the absence of anaemia.

Treatment. Oesophageal dilatation if dysphagic symptoms are significant from web. Follow-up to check for malignant transformation.

STOMACH AND DUODENUM

Peptic Ulceration

This occurs anywhere where pepsin and acid occur together. It is caused by an imbalance between secretion of acid and pepsin and mucosal defence mechanisms. An acidic environment and reduced mucosal defences provide ideal circumstances for pepsin to cause mucosal ulceration. Over-secretion of acid is associated with duodenal ulceration. Breakdown of the mucosal defences occurs in gastric ulceration. Exacerbating factors in peptic ulceration include stress, smoking, alcohol, NSAIDs, steroids, hyperparathyroidism, Zollinger–Ellison syndrome (ZES). Infection with *Helicobacter pylori* may impair mucosal defences and is associated with duodenal ulcer and gastritis and, to a lesser extent, gastric ulcers. Common sites for peptic ulcer are the stomach and duodenum, the anterior wall of the first part of the duodenum and the lesser curve of the stomach being the most common sites. The overall incidence, however, of peptic ulcer disease is decreasing, in particular duodenal ulcers.

Symptoms and Signs

Duodenal Ulcer (DU). Epigastric pain. May radiate through to back. Relieved by eating. Worse at night. Symptoms are periodic and last about 14 days and recur at 3–4-monthly intervals. They are often worse in spring and autumn. Vomiting is rare. If it occurs, pyloric stenosis should be suspected. Examination may reveal tenderness in epigastrium.

Gastric Ulcer (GU). Epigastric pain. Not periodic. Food may precipitate pain. Pain may be relieved by vomiting. Patient may be afraid to eat, and weight loss results. Examination reveals tenderness in epigastrium.

Investigations

- OGD and biopsy: risk of malignancy with GU and therefore require re-endoscopy after course of acid suppression therapy; antral biopsy for rapid urease test (campylobacter-like organism (CLO) test)

- Histology, faecal antigens, C14-urea breath test and serology for *H. pylori*
- Barium meal is rarely used nowadays, but if a GU is diagnosed on a barium study, OGD and biopsy should be carried out.
- Other routine investigations include Hb, FBC, U&Es, Ca, PO_4 and occasionally serum gastrin if ZES is suspected.

Treatment

Medical

- Antacids (e.g. Gaviscon) are preparations designed to neutralise gastric acid and provide mucosal protection. Relieve pain but have limited long-term efficacy.
- PPIs have revolutionised the management of peptic ulceration. They reduce gastric acid secretion by inhibiting the proton pump in parietal cells and result in greater inhibition of acid than H_2-receptor antagonists. Omeprazole and lansoprazole may be used. Patients with proven *H. pylori* infection require eradication therapy: 7-day course of amoxicillin (500mg tds), metronidazole (400mg tds) and omeprazole (20mg bd). Clarithromycin can be used in patients with a penicillin allergy. Eradication is not routinely checked for unless symptoms do not improve.

In addition to the above specific therapies, lifestyle modification advice should be provided regarding smoking cessation and avoidance of NSAIDs.

Surgical. Indications are the following:

- Failed medical treatment (rare nowadays)
- Complications – haemorrhage, perforation, pyloric obstruction. Operations in the past have included vagotomy and drainage and highly selective vagotomy. These operations are rarely performed nowadays, and the most common operation is pyloromyotomy (Figure 15.4) with oversewing of bleeding DU. Partial gastrectomy (Figure 15.5) may be required for bleeding GU.

Complications of Peptic Ulceration

Haemorrhage. Posterior duodenal ulcers erode the gastroduodenal artery. OGD is required to locate the site of the ulcer. An actively bleeding ulcer (active spurting, oozing) often can be treated endoscopically with a combination of adrenaline, clips, bipolar electrocoagulation or heater probe. If the ulcer is not actively bleeding, a course of intravenous PPI may be given. If bleeding is massive or recurrent, interventional radiology with transcatheter arterial embolisation is often successful. Surgery these days is a salvage procedure. At surgery the bleeding vessel in the base of the ulcer is oversewn to stop the bleeding. All GUs should have a biopsy taken from the edge of the ulcer to exclude malignancy. The pylorus is opened for treating a bleeding DU and is closed as a pyloroplasty (transversely). The patient is treated with long-term PPIs.

Perforation. Anterior DUs and GUs may perforate causing generalised chemical peritonitis. Surgery, which can be performed laparoscopically, involves suturing the ulcer and reinforcement with an omental patch (Graham repair). A biopsy should be taken from the edge of a GU, as there is a risk of malignancy. GU in atypical locations or with features of malignancy should undergo wedge resection rather than omentopexy. Check *H. pylori* status and eradicate appropriately. Long-term PPIs for chronic ulceration.

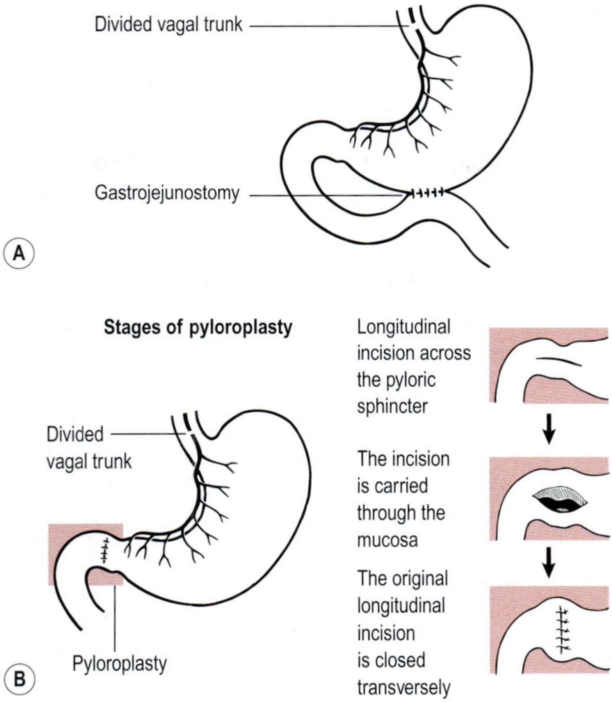

FIGURE 15.4

(**A**) Truncal vagotomy and gastrojejunostomy. (**B**) Truncal vagotomy and pyloroplasty. The pylorus is opened longitudinally and sutured transversely, thus destroying the pyloric sphincter.

Pyloric Obstruction. Late complication. Rare nowadays. Vomiting of large amounts of foul-smelling vomit often containing food eaten several days previously. Gastric succussion splash on examination. Empty stomach with wide-bore nasogastric tube. Confirm by OGD and CT scan. Management can be endoscopic using pneumatic balloon dilatation or surgical, e.g. gastrojejunostomy, antrectomy with reconstruction (Roux-en-Y reconstruction). Hypokalaemia, hypochloraemia and metabolic alkalosis may be present and require correction prior to intervention.

Zollinger–Ellison Syndrome (ZES)

ZES is a rare cause of peptic ulcer disease secondary to hypergastrinaemia. Peptic ulcers may occur in unusual sites, e.g. the third part of the duodenum. There is usually a non-beta islet cell gastrin-secreting tumour of the pancreas (gastrinoma); 60% are malignant; 30% associated with the autosomal dominant familial multiple endocrine neoplasia (MEN) type 1.

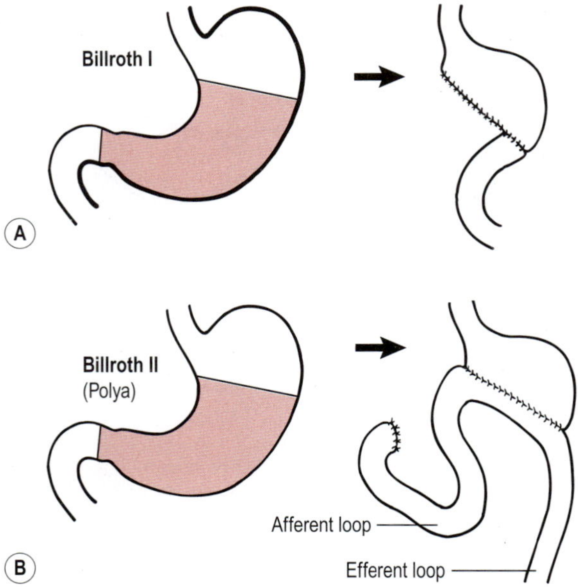

FIGURE 15.5
Types of partial gastrectomy. (**A**) Billroth I. The gastric remnant is anastomosed directly to the first part of the duodenum. (**B**) Billroth II (Polya). The duodenal stump is oversewn and continuity re-established by gastrojejunostomy.

Symptoms and Signs. Typical signs and symptoms of peptic ulcer. Diarrhoea and malabsorption may occur from overproduction of acid. Bleeding. Perforation. Recurrent ulcers after surgery for peptic ulcer. Ulcers resistant to medical treatment. May be family history of peptic ulcer although 70% of cases are sporadic. If associated with MEN type 1, can also have hyperparathyroidism with hypercalcaemia.

Investigations

- ↑Serial fasting serum gastrin
- Basal acid output elevated
- SRS: most sensitive modality
- CT scan especially for metastatic disease
- Endoscopic ultrasound.

Treatment. Excision of tumour if spread to liver has not occurred. If tumour cannot be localised or has spread, acid secretion should be controlled using a PPI, which is superior to H_2-receptor antagonists. Rarely total gastrectomy may be needed to stop bleeding.

Carcinoma of the Stomach

The incidence of gastric cancer is declining, but it still remains the second most common cause of cancer-related death worldwide. Widespread geographical variation occurs, the incidence being highest in Asia (Japan, China). *H. pylori* is a class I carcinogen associated with gastric cancer through induction of chronic atrophic gastritis. Other associations include blood group A (suggesting a genetic factor), pernicious anaemia, previous gastric surgery and GUs. Greater than 90% of gastric cancers are adenocarcinomas.

Symptoms and Signs. Onset silent and insidious. Vague dyspepsia, epigastric pain, weight loss, early satiety, dysphagia (tumours of the cardia), vomiting (pyloric area), anaemia, lassitude. Epigastric mass, hepatomegaly, ascites, left supraclavicular gland palpable (Virchow's node, Troisier's sign), gastric succussion splash, acanthosis nigricans. A smaller proportion of cases present as an emergency with haematemesis, melaena, obstruction or perforation.

Investigations

- Hb
- FBC
- ESR
- LFTs: alkaline phosphatase raised with liver secondaries
- OGD with biopsy
- CT for staging – to exclude distant metastases and assess for regional involvement. Diffuse thickening of the whole stomach may suggest linitis plastica.
- Laparoscopy and washings (for cytology) to exclude low-volume peritoneal metastases.

Treatment

Curative. Usually, a total gastrectomy with D2 lymphadenectomy. For distal tumours, a subtotal gastrectomy is appropriate as long as a proximal 5 cm resection margin can be achieved. For more proximal tumours, total gastrectomy is preferred, as it offers better functional outcomes. Patients may undergo perioperative chemotherapy (FLOT4) prior to surgery.

Palliative. Endoscopic stent for tumours causing obstruction. Surgical bypass through a gastrojejunostomy for antral tumours or resection are also options. Most units would not perform a total gastrectomy as a palliative procedure.

Prognosis. In Japan, where screening programmes are undertaken because of the high incidence, the 5-year survival for early gastric cancer is around 90%. In the Western world at least 60% of cases present too late for curative surgery. Despite improvement in outcomes, overall survival is approximately 20% at 5 years.

Gastric Surgery and Its Complications

Carcinoma and complications of peptic ulcer are the commonest indications for gastric surgery. The operations of vagotomy, vagotomy and pyloroplasty, vagotomy and gastrojejunostomy and highly selective vagotomy are described but are largely of historical interest. Patients are still seen who have had these operations and have suffered the complications of them but are increasingly rare. Vagotomy is rarely, if ever, carried out nowadays.

PYLOROPLASTY. The pylorus is cut longitudinally and sewn up transversely. The pyloroplasty is performed to allow gastric drainage.

GASTROENTEROSTOMY (FIGURE 15.4). The most dependent part of the stomach is anastomosed to a loop of jejunum. This diverts acid away from the duodenum and allows the ulcer to heal.

GASTRECTOMY (FIGURE 15.5). This may be partial or total. Partial gastrectomy usually involves removal of about seven-eighths of the stomach. The gastric remnant may be re-anastomosed directly to the first part of the duodenum (Billroth I) or the duodenal stump oversewn and the continuity re-established by a gastrojejunostomy (Billroth II or Polya gastrectomy). If partial gastrectomy is used for GU, the ulcer is removed together with the segment of stomach. For DU, removal of the bulk of the acid-secreting area of the stomach allows the ulcer to heal. The ulcer is not usually removed.

Complications

RECURRENT ULCERATION. Symptoms are similar to those experienced preoperatively. Treatment is difficult. ZES and hypercalcaemia should be excluded.

EPIGASTRIC FULLNESS. Particularly after partial gastrectomy. Treatment is to take small meals frequently. The symptom tends to improve with time.

BILIOUS VOMITING. Sudden emptying of the afferent loop with Billroth II. Associated biliary gastritis. May respond to metoclopramide. Severe cases need revisional surgery, e.g. Roux-en-Y anastomosis so that bile enters the GI tract lower down in the jejunum (→Figure 15.6).

DUMPING

Early. Fainting, sweating and dizziness shortly after eating. May be a reflex caused by osmotic effect of large volumes of food 'dumped' into the jejunum. Patient may need to lie down and rest for half an hour. Symptoms may be improved by eating small dry meals frequently and avoiding heavy carbohydrate meals. Early dumping may subside spontaneously with time.

Late. Due to hypoglycaemia and occurs 1–3h after a meal. Responds to glucose (sucking barley sugars).

DIARRHOEA. This may be disabling after vagotomy. Codeine phosphate, loperamide and small dry meals may help. The incidence is less after highly selective vagotomy.

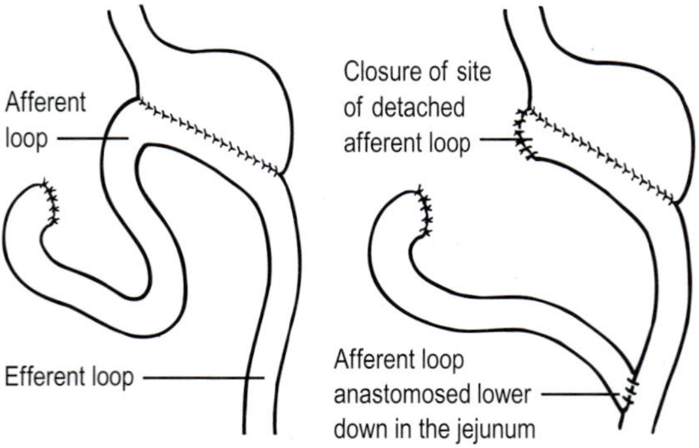

FIGURE 15.6
Roux-en-Y conversion for bilious vomiting. The afferent loop is detached and reanastomosed lower down the jejunum.

NUTRITIONAL DISTURBANCES

Weight Loss. May be due to reduced caloric intake or poor absorption.

Steatorrhoea. Due to poor mixing of food and enzymes, e.g. long afferent loop where food passes into the jejunum before it is adequately mixed with digestive enzymes coming from the afferent loop. Blind loop syndrome may be responsible, i.e. stasis in the long afferent loop with colonisation with abnormal bacteria, which restricts digestion and absorption of food. Surgical correction of the afferent loop may be necessary.

Anaemia. Iron deficiency anaemia due to reduced hydrochloric acid, which is required for oxidation of iron (Fe^{2+} to Fe^{3+}) to aid absorption in the duodenum and upper jejunum. With total gastrectomy, megaloblastic anaemia may occur, owing to loss of intrinsic factor and subsequent B_{12} deficiency. Vitamin B_{12} injections are required.

Bolus Obstruction. Destruction of the pylorus allows unmasticated food to pass into the small intestine. This may swell and lodge in the terminal ileum. This occurs particularly with orange pith and dried fruits. Patients should be warned not to eat these foods if the pylorus is not intact.

CARCINOMA. May occur in the gastric remnant. This is rare.

Obesity and Bariatric Surgery

There is increasing recognition of the role of bariatric surgery in the treatment of obesity. It has been shown to produce clinically significant weight loss and treating a range of obesity related comorbidities such as type 2 diabetes mellitus, cardiovascular disease, sleep apnoea, infertility, chronic kidney disease while also lowering the incidence of several cancers. Ninety-seven percent of all bariatric procedures worldwide are now performed laparoscopically.

Bariatric Procedures

Bariatric surgical procedures were traditionally classified according to the early understanding of their mechanism of action as either 'restrictive' or 'malabsorptive'. Although each procedure varies somewhat in their mechanism of action, studies have now established that bariatric procedures primarily act through alterations in gut hormone signalling.

LAPAROSCOPIC ADJUSTABLE GASTRIC BAND. Laparoscopic adjustable gastric banding (LAGB) was once the most common procedure performed; however, it has become significantly less popular in light of lack of weight loss and related complications. Within most healthcare settings, the management of AGB can be challenging, as it requires regular monitoring and adjustment of the band to produce clinically significant weight loss. However, it does still have a role in selected cases, as it is relatively lower risk and can be removed. The mechanism of action is not completely understood, but it produces increased satiety thereby reducing caloric intake, which is thought to be mediated primarily by the vagus nerve. Complications of AGB include dysphagia and band slippage or erosion which can require urgent surgical intervention and removal.

LAPAROSCOPIC SLEEVE GASTRECTOMY. Laparoscopic sleeve gastrectomy (LSG) is currently the most widely performed bariatric procedure worldwide, as it is a less technically demanding operation to undertake. LSG involves division of the stomach along the greater curvature to produce a smaller tubularised remnant stomach. Although this does in theory reduce the stomach volume, the primary mechanism of action resulting in weight loss is through an alteration in gut hormone signalling. The resected stomach is removed, which makes this procedure irreversible; however, it can be further modified to a Roux-en-Y gastric bypass which is primarily used in patients who develop severe gastro-oesophageal reflux following SG, which is a recognised complication. In addition to reflux, other complications include staple line leak or bleeding and stricture in the long term. Long-term regular surveillance endoscopy is recommended in light of the potential risk of developing Barrett's in the context of increased reflux (→Figure 15.9).

Laparoscopic Roux-en-Y Gastric Bypass. Laparoscopic Roux-en-Y gastric bypass (RYGB) is now the second most commonly performed bariatric procedure worldwide. RYGB involves the formation of a small gastric pouch with a loop of jejunum brought up and anastomosed to this pouch to bypass a segment of the duodenum, preventing the mixing of ingested food from biliary secretions. A second anastomosis is performed further down the jejunum with the bypassed segment to allow for the mixing of food and bile to facilitate the absorption of nutrients. As a result of duodenal bypass, there are important neurohormonal changes which increase satiety, slow gastric emptying and improve glucose homeostasis. Early complications include staple line bleed and anastomotic leak and, in the longer term, internal herniation and chronic abdominal pain It may also complicate procedures such as endoscopic retrograde cholangiopancreatography (ERCP) (→Figure 15.8).

Biliopancreatic Diversion and Duodenal Switch. Although biliopancreatic diversion and duodenal switch (BPD/DS) is the bariatric procedure which leads to the greatest weight loss and improvement in glycaemic control resulting in remission of T2DM, this procedure is rarely undertaken in the UK. BPD/DS requires the formation of a gastric sleeve combined with the bypass of a long segment of small intestine, leaving only a short channel for the absorption of nutrients. As a result, the procedure is associated with a high risk of nutritional complications which require close, lifelong supplementation and monitoring to avoid the development of severe and potentially irreversible complications.

One Anastomosis Gastric Bypass. This procedure is increasing in popularity in recent years given the mounting evidence that it produces weight loss and resolution of obesity-related comorbidities on par with that RYGB. One anastomosis gastric bypass (OAGB) which is also called a 'mini bypass' involves the formation of a small gastric pouch which is then anastomosed to a loop of jejunum to bypass the duodenum and proximal jejunum. Complications include higher rates of biliary reflux and nutritional deficiencies as compared to RYGB (→Figure 15.7).

Upper Gastrointestinal Tract Bleeding

Is defined as any bleeding derived from a source proximal to the ligament of Treitz. This causes either haematemesis (vomiting of blood) or melaena (passage of altered

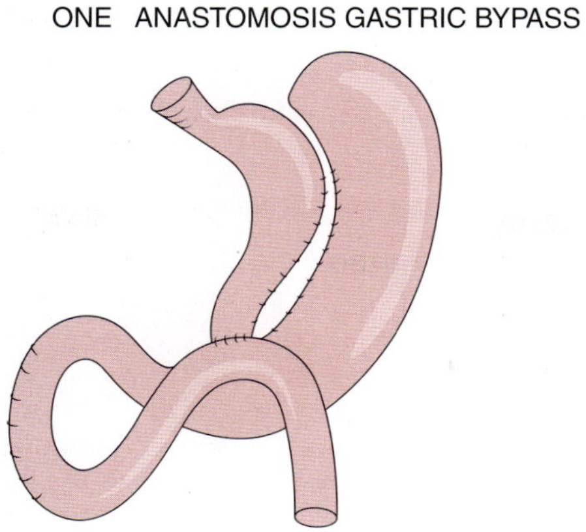

FIGURE 15.7
One Anastomosis Gastric Bypass.

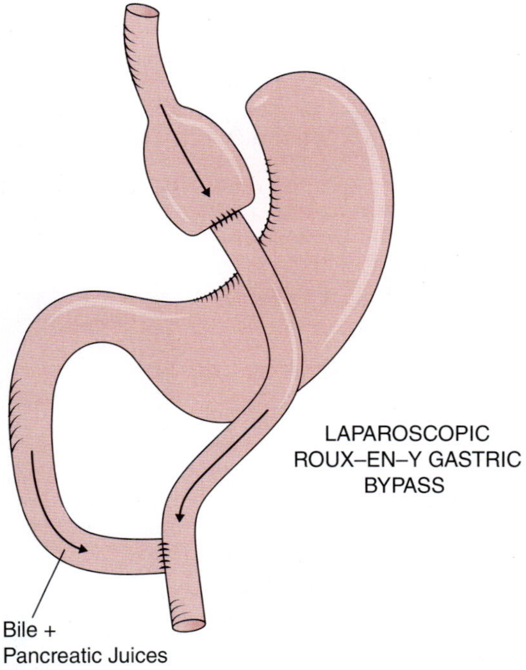

FIGURE 15.8
Laparoscopic Roux–En–Y Gastric Bypass.

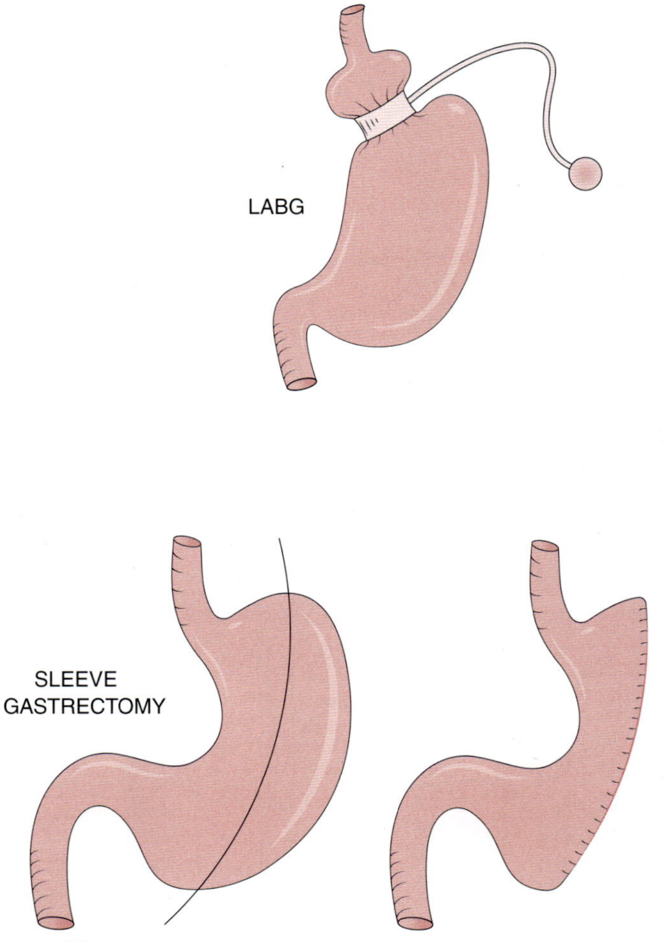

FIGURE 15.9
Sleeve Gastrectomy.

blood PR – usually black and tarry with a characteristic smell), or both. Causes include peptic ulceration, acute gastric erosions, neoplasia (usually gastric adenocarcinoma) or oesophageal varices, oesophagitis, Mallory–Weiss syndrome. Rarer causes include gastrointestinal stromal tumour (GIST), angiomatous malformations, haemobilia and bleeding disorders. Drugs that may precipitate bleeding include steroids, NSAIDs and anticoagulants. Principles of treatment include resuscitation, replacement of circulating blood volume, diagnosis and treatment of the cause.

Symptoms and Signs. Clinically anaemic. With severe bleed, haemorrhagic shock will occur. History of aspirin, NSAIDs, steroid or anticoagulant. Stigmata of liver failure. Abdominal mass.

Investigations

- Hb
- FBC
- U&Es
- LFTs
- Clotting screen
- Crossmatch blood
- OGD
- CT angiography if source of bleeding is not demonstrated at OGD.

Treatment

- Adhere to principles of A, B and C.
- Focused assessment with concomitant resuscitation
- Gain intravenous access (large bore cannulae) and treat shock – crystalloids, colloids and blood.
- Catheterise.
- Establish diagnosis with urgent endoscopy – treat accordingly with combination therapy.
- Give intravenous PPI only after endoscopy in patients with bleeding secondary to an ulcer.
- Eradication of *H. pylori* if appropriate
- Re-endoscopy is not routinely performed. Patients who rebleed should be re-endoscoped or undergo angiography. If unstable, then operative intervention may be required.

Indications for Surgical Intervention

- Massive uncontrolled bleeding in an unstable patient
- Rebleeding that is not manageable at re-endoscopy or controlled with angiography, especially if bleeding vessel or clot on ulcer has been seen at index endoscopy.

Interventional Options Are Nonoperative or Operative

Nonoperative

- Dual endoscopic therapy is recommended with clips, adrenaline, heater probe, bipolar electrocoagulation, argon beam or haemospray.
- Control varices with endoscopy and banding as first-line therapy. Recurrent variceal bleeding may require a re-scope, a Sengstaken tube or a shunt procedure. Bleeding may also be managed with transcatheter arterial embolisation.

Operative

- Peptic ulcer: underrunning of the bleeding vessel or resection + PPIs + eradication therapy for *H. pylori* if appropriate. Partial gastrectomy may be necessary.

- Oesophageal varices: oesophageal transection (very rare). Portacaval or distal splenorenal shunting. Usually managed effectively with endoscopic banding.
- Carcinoma: partial or total gastrectomy.

Prognosis. The overall mortality for an upper GI bleed is 10%. Adverse prognostic factors include age >60 years, shock at presentation, significant comorbidities, in-patient at the time of the event, rebleeding and oesophageal varices.

HINTS AND TIPS

Be wary of the patient who has undergone previous open aortic surgery who presents with symptoms and signs of an upper GI tract bleeding. An aortoenteric fistula must be considered in your differential and can be diagnosed by CT angiography. Massive upper gastrointestinal (UGI) bleeding can present with bright red rectal bleeding due to rapid transit through the GI tract. Therefore, always consider OGD in patients with bright red rectal bleeding who are in hypovolaemic shock. Passing a nasogastric tube in such cases may reveal the presence of blood in the upper tract prompting an urgent OGD.

Other Conditions of the Stomach and Duodenum

Stomach

GASTROINTESTINAL STROMAL TUMOUR (GIST). These are rare mesenchymal tumours and account for approximately 1% of all tumours in the GI tract. They commonly occur in the stomach (and small bowel). Submucosal tumours are characterised by the markers CD117 (*c-KIT*) and CD34. Can present with epigastric discomfort, indigestion, haematemesis or melaena due to ulceration of mucosa overlying tumour. Investigations include OGD, EUS and CT scan. Metastases rarely occur, and surgical excision is required with a small resection margin. Grading is based on tumour size, CD117 positivity and mitotic rate. Imatinib/sunitinib (tyrosine kinase inhibitor) is recommended for adjuvant therapy, incomplete removal, recurrence or metastatic disease.

LYMPHOMA (MUCOSAL ASSOCIATED LYMPHOID TUMOUR, MALT). Symptoms are non-specific but can mimic those of peptic ulcer or gastric carcinoma. Intimate association between gastric MALT and *H. pylori*. OGD and biopsy to confirm diagnosis. Treatment involves eradication of *H. pylori*, and this can lead to regression of low-grade lymphoma. Chemotherapy, radiotherapy and/or monoclonal antibody therapy can also be used. Surgical resection has a limited role and is rarely required. Prognosis is good, especially in patients with low-grade tumours that respond to *H. pylori* eradication.

Duodenum

Other than ulceration, conditions of the duodenum are rare. A duodenal diverticulum may occur on the medial wall near the ampulla of Vater. Most are asymptomatic. Rarely bleeding and perforation may occur. Symptomatic diverticulae should be excised. Tumours of the duodenum are rare and can include adenocarcinomas, carcinoids and GISTs. Adenocarcinoma does *not* occur in duodenal ulcers. A tumour that arises near the ampulla (second part of the duodenum) may cause obstructive jaundice.

CONDITIONS OF THE SMALL BOWEL

Meckel's Diverticulum

A remnant of the vitellointestinal duct of the embryo. Classically it occurs in 2% of patients, is 2 inches long, and 2 feet from the ileocaecal junction ('rule of 2s'). It occurs on the antimesenteric border of the terminal ileum.

Symptoms and Signs. Symptomless. Incidental finding at laparotomy. Symptoms typical of acute appendicitis may occur. Rectal bleeding (ectopic gastric mucosa). Rarely umbilical discharge (fistula), intestinal obstruction (due to entrapment around the band from the apex of the diverticulum to the back of the umbilicus), small bowel volvulus or intussusception (ileoileal).

Investigations

- Technetium scan for GI bleeding may show gastric mucosa in a Meckel's.
- Laparotomy is required for complications of Meckel's – the cause is not usually apparent until laparotomy is undertaken.

Treatment. Excision of the diverticulum.

Crohn's Disease

This is dealt with in the section on inflammatory bowel disease (p. 288).

Typhoid

Caused by *Salmonella typhi*. About 200 cases occur in the UK annually. It may occur in the immigrant population and in those who have travelled to countries where the disease is endemic. The organism enters Peyer's patches and may result in perforation or bleeding usually involving the ileum. This usually occurs during the third week of the disease. The patient shows signs of perforation with peritonitis. Surgical closure of the perforation is required. The bowel is very friable. Chloramphenicol i.v. is given for 2 weeks postoperatively.

Tuberculosis

This may present as an acute abdomen in recent immigrants. It chiefly affects the terminal ileum and the ileocaecal region. Differentiation from Crohn's disease is essential.

Symptoms and Signs. Ill patient: fever, diarrhoea, colicky abdominal pain. Weight loss. May be history of pulmonary TB. Mass in right iliac fossa (RIF). Chest signs.

Investigations

- CXR
- Mantoux
- Sputum culture
- AXR: small bowel obstruction
- Barium studies show thickening, ulceration and narrowing of terminal ileum.
- USS: may show mass
- CT: may show abscess
- Diagnosis may be made only at laparotomy.

Treatment. Antituberculous therapy for 6 months to 2 years. Surgery is required if diagnosis is unclear, for perforation, abscess, bleeding or obstruction.

TUMOURS OF THE SMALL INTESTINE

These form less than 5% of all tumours of the GI tract. Obstruction and bleeding are the usual symptoms.

Benign

These include adenomas, leiomyomas and lipomas. Obstruction, intussusception or bleeding may occur. Polyposis of the small bowel (mainly jejunum) may occur in association with pigmentation of the lips and mouth (Peutz–Jeghers syndrome). Bleeding or intussusception may occur.

Malignant

Adenocarcinoma is rare and usually affects the jejunum. Bleeding and obstruction may occur. Lymphoma may present as intestinal obstruction or a palpable mass. Consider lymphoma in patients with coeliac disease. Palliation of these tumours is by radiotherapy or chemotherapy.

Carcinoid Tumour

These occur most commonly in the appendix but can occur anywhere in the GI tract and occasionally in the lung. Those in the small bowel grow slowly, but most of those greater than 2cm have metastasised at the time of surgery. The tumours arise from argentaffin cells.

Symptoms and Signs. May be none before metastases occur. Carcinoid syndrome is associated with liver metastases. Flushing (caused by alcohol, coffee), diarrhoea, bronchospasm, pulmonary stenosis. Loud borborygmi may be heard on auscultation. Hepatomegaly, palpable abdominal mass.

Investigations

- Raised 24-h excretion of 5-HIAA
- USS
- CT.

Treatment. Resection of primary tumour. Partial hepatectomy if metastases confined to one lobe. Methysergide blocks 5-HT and may be beneficial in patients with metastases. Phenoxybenzamine may be helpful in reducing flushing. Other procedures include hepatic embolisation, systemic chemotherapy and hepatic infusion chemotherapy.

Prognosis. Malignant carcinoid of the small bowel has a 25% 5-year survival.

SMALL BOWEL OBSTRUCTION

Mechanical obstruction of the small bowel may be simple (one point of obstruction) or closed loop (obstruction at two points enclosing a segment of bowel). If the bowel is viable, the obstruction is termed non-strangulating. If the blood supply is compromised, strangulating obstruction occurs with subsequent infarction of the bowel. Strangulation occurs when the obstructing mechanism cuts off the mesenteric arterial blood flow, e.g. the neck of the sac with a loop of bowel trapped in a hernial sac, or the twist of a volvulus. Mechanical obstruction is more common in the small bowel than in the large bowel.

Causes. Causes may be found:

- In the lumen: gallstone ileus, food bolus (following pylorus-destroying operations, i.e. gastrojejunostomy or pyloroplasty)

- In the wall: congenital atresia, Crohn's disease, tumours, e.g. lymphoma or carcinoma
- Outside the wall: herniae, adhesions, volvulus, intussusception.

Symptoms and Signs. Colicky abdominal pain. The patient cannot get into a comfortable position. Vomiting. Constipation. Symptoms depend on whether the obstruction is high or low. High obstruction is characterised by early vomiting (bilious) and late constipation. Low obstruction is characterised by early constipation and late vomiting (faeculent). Distension, marked with low obstruction, tympanitic abdomen, high-pitched tinkling bowel sounds. Hernial orifices should be carefully examined. Pyrexia, tachycardia, continuous pain and localised tenderness suggest actual or impending strangulation.

Investigations

- Hb
- FBC
- WCC with neutrophilia may indicate strangulation
- U&Es
- AXR: distended loops of small bowel in central abdomen (→Figure 15.10). Erect films show air/fluid levels. Absent or diminished colonic gas. Dilated proximal small bowel shows lines close together (valvulae conniventes) crossing completely the lumen of the bowel. These get progressively fewer the more distal the distended loop and are absent in the terminal ileum. Look for gas in the biliary tree (gallstone ileus with cholecystoduodenal fistula).

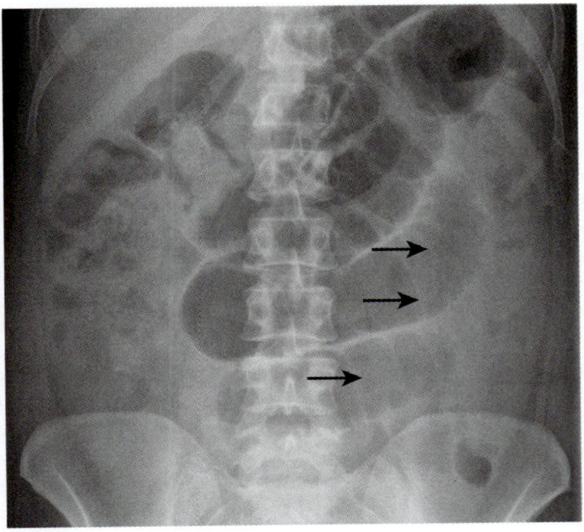

FIGURE 15.10
Small bowel obstruction. Distended loops of small bowel are visible in the central abdomen. These are identifiable as small bowel as the valvulae conniventes (arrows) cross the entire lumen.

Treatment

Conservative

- Intravenous fluids and nasogastric aspiration
- Nil orally
- 2-hourly temperature and pulse
- Abdominal examination 8-hourly
- Some cases of simple mechanical obstruction, e.g. due to adhesions, will settle on this regimen.

Indications for Surgery. Strangulating obstruction, e.g. a tender irreducible hernia requires urgent surgery. If a conservative 'drip and suck' regimen has been undertaken for obstruction, surgery is indicated for signs of incipient strangulation (pyrexia, tachycardia, localised tenderness). Surgery is also required for simple obstruction that fails to settle, e.g. adhesions, gallstone ileus. At surgery, the affected bowel is inspected for viability. Indications of nonviability include:

- Absence of peristalsis
- Loss of normal sheen
- Loss of pulsation in bowel mesentery
- Colour: green or black bowel is nonviable and resection is required. Plum-coloured bowel may respond to wrapping for a few minutes in warm saline-soaked packs. If colour returns and it will transmit a peristaltic wave, it is viable.

Prognosis. Small bowel obstruction has a very low mortality rate if it is simple. Strangulating obstruction increases the mortality and if small bowel resection is required, especially in the elderly, the mortality rate may reach 25%.

APPENDICITIS

This is the commonest cause of the acute abdomen in the UK. It usually occurs when there is an obstruction in the lumen of the appendix either by a faecolith or foreign body or by enlargement of lymphoid follicles in its wall. It most often affects children, teenagers and young adults. It is rare at the extremes of life. In the infant, the lumen of the appendix is wide in relation to the remainder of the bowel and the diet is soft; hence, obstruction within the lumen is less likely. In the elderly, the lumen tends to be obliterated. Rarer causes of appendicitis include carcinoma of the caecum obstructing the appendiceal lumen, carcinoid tumour and obstructing fibrous bands. Occasionally a carcinoma obstructing the lumen of the appendix will cause it to distend and fill with mucus, i.e. a mucocele of the appendix.

Symptoms and Signs. Central abdominal cramping or colicky pain. Nausea. Vomiting is uncommon. Occasionally the patient may pass a loose stool. Frank diarrhoea is uncommon. Central abdominal pain lasts approximately 8 h. It is followed by the development of a sharp, stabbing somatic type of pain in the RIF made worse by coughing or moving. Low-grade pyrexia (37.2–37.8°C). Flushed. Characteristic fetor (sweet faecal smell to breath). White furred tongue. Tachycardia (100 bpm in first 24 h). Tender with guarding in RIF over McBurney's point. Examination PR: tender anteriorly in the rectovesical or rectouterine pouch.

HINTS AND TIPS

In infants, diarrhoea and vomiting may be the only symptoms. This may lead to difficulty in diagnosis and confusion with gastroenteritis. In elderly patients there may be confusion and, later, shock may develop.

Investigations

- WCC: usually $>10\times10^9$/L with neutrophil leukocytosis
- USS: may show a mass or abscess; usefulness in early appendicitis depends on the experience of the ultrasonographer
- CT: may confirm diagnosis of appendicitis; useful in excluding other causes of abdominal pain
- Diagnostic laparoscopy.

Differential Diagnosis. In the classical case of acute appendicitis there are few conditions that enter into the differential diagnosis. These include mesenteric adenitis, Meckel's diverticulitis, Crohn's disease (regional ileitis), mesenteric embolus and right-sided colonic diverticulitis. All these conditions will initially cause central abdominal cramping pain with subsequent tenderness in the RIF.

In the atypical case, other causes of intra-abdominal pathology, urinary tract disease, gynaecological problems (see Ch. 23) and extra-abdominal conditions must be considered.

Abdominal Disease. Cholecystitis, gastroenteritis, pancreatitis, perforated DU, intestinal obstruction, diverticulitis, nonspecific abdominal pain.

Urinary Tract. Acute pyelonephritis, renal colic, cystitis. An inflamed appendix adherent to the bladder may cause frequency and pyuria. Organisms will be absent on urinary microscopy.

Gynaecological Causes. (See Ch. 23). Salpingitis. Ectopic pregnancy. Degeneration of a fibroid. Mittelschmerz. Pelvic inflammatory disease.

Extra-Abdominal Causes. Referred pain from nerve roots, e.g. herpes zoster, degenerative and malignant disease affecting roots T11, T12. Referred pain from right lower lobar pneumonia. Referred pain from a right-sided testicular torsion.

Treatment. The treatment of acute appendicitis is appendicectomy. Prophylactic antibiotics should be given on induction of anaesthesia according to local protocols.

Complications. Appendicitis may resolve spontaneously. The appendix may become surrounded by adjacent small bowel and omentum and give rise to an appendix mass. It may perforate, giving rise to generalised peritonitis or it may perforate amidst local adhesions giving rise to an appendix abscess. Often it is difficult to diagnose appendicitis. If the symptoms have been present for 48h ('48h rule') and the diagnosis is truly appendicitis, then the patient should either have developed an appendix mass or generalised peritonitis. If neither of these two is present, then the diagnosis of appendicitis should be reviewed.

Appendix Mass

Omentum and small bowel adhere to the inflamed appendix. This usually happens 2–5 days after onset of initial symptoms. This should be initially treated conservatively. Mark out the size of the mass on the abdominal wall; i.v. fluids, analgesia and antibiotics (cefuroxime and metronidazole) should be administered. If the mass resolves, it is usual to carry out an interval appendicectomy after 3 months. If the mass gets bigger, it is likely that an abscess is forming, i.e. the appendix has perforated within the appendix mass.

Appendix Abscess

If an appendix mass enlarges and the temperature fails to settle, an appendix abscess is developing. The patient may appear toxic with a tachycardia. An appendix abscess requires either surgical drainage and appendicectomy, or percutaneous insertion of a drain under ultrasound control. Interval appendicectomy is required subsequently.

Other complications include subphrenic abscess, pelvic abscess, paralytic ileus, septicaemia, portal pyaemia (rare). Long-term complications may be due to adhesions resulting in intestinal obstruction in a small proportion of patients. Tubal adhesions with infertility may occur in females.

Appendicitis in Pregnancy

This is no commoner than at other times. Pain and tenderness are higher because of displacement of the appendix by the enlarging uterus. Prompt assessment and intervention are essential. There is a risk of spontaneous abortion in the first trimester, but if treatment is delayed until perforation occurs, the risk is considerably higher (approximately 25%).

CONDITIONS OF THE COLON, RECTUM AND ANUS

Colonic Polyps

A polyp is a sessile (broad-based) or pedunculated (on a stalk) protrusion from a body surface. In the colon, it is a lesion that projects into the lumen.

Hamartomas

Juvenile Polyps. May occur in large or small bowel. Cause bleeding or obstruction. May autoamputate in adolescence.

Peutz–Jeghers Syndrome. Diffuse GI polyposis with mucocutaneous pigmentation of lips and gums. The polyps have no malignant potential. Surgery is indicated only for symptoms, i.e. obstruction or bleeding.

Hyperplastic polyps: common finding on colonoscopy. Normally have no malignant potential. There is some evidence that large hyperplastic polyps can undergo malignant change.

Neoplastic Polyps

Adenomatous Polyps and Villous Adenomas. These have malignant potential, especially the villous adenoma. The risk of malignancy developing within a polyp increases with the size of the polyp. Once detected, patients are offered colonoscopic screening to detect further polyp formation.

Familial Polyposis Coli. This is an autosomal dominant condition with multiple polyps involving colon and rectum. Duodenal adenomas may also occur and progress to malignancy. It first appears in adolescence. If untreated, malignancy will develop before the age of 40 years. The aim of treatment is to offer prophylactic surgery before a cancer develops. The options are:

- *Ileorectal anastomosis*: preserves sexual and reproductive function. The remaining rectum is easy to survey and continence is maintained.
- *Restorative proctocolectomy (ileoanal pouch formation):* normally a two-stage procedure that is technically demanding. Although rare, adenoma and/or cancer formation can still occur in the 'cuff' of the rectum that remains at the anastomosis. A mucosectomy can be performed at the time of the operation, which removes this risk, but it often results in a poorer outcome. There is also a 10% pouch failure rate which would result in a permanent end ileostomy.
- *Panproctocolectomy and end ileostomy*: often reserved for patients with a low rectal cancer at presentation.
- There is a need for upper GI surveillance as most of the mortality is from development of ampullary/duodenal carcinomas developing from duodenal adenomas.

GARDNER'S SYNDROME. A variant of familial polyposis, it is associated with desmoid tumours, osteomas of the mandible and multiple sebaceous cysts.

INFLAMMATORY PSEUDOPOLYPS. These may arise in ulcerative colitis. Lymphoid hyperplasia may also be apparent as a polyp.

Symptoms and Signs of Polyps. Passage of blood and mucous PR. Rarely obstruction or intussusception.

Investigations

- Sigmoidoscopy and biopsy
- Colonoscopy
- CT colonography (virtual colonoscopy) (→Figure 15.11): is less invasive than colonoscopy and barium enema. Still requires bowel preparation and a small rectal tube insufflates air into the rectum. The image generated is a 3D model of the lumen of the large bowel, as well as the abdomen and pelvis. It is about 80% accurate at detecting polyps greater than 6mm. It is most useful for investigating the bowel in frail patients or when colonoscopy could not be completed
- Barium enema (→Figure 15.12). Almost obsolete for polyp detection.

Treatment. Pedunculated polyps or small sessile polyps may be removed at sigmoidoscopy or colonoscopy. If invasive carcinoma is found, it is staged according to the Haggitt classification for pedunculated polyps or the Kikuchi classification for sessile polyps. The level of invasion into the polyp has been shown to correlate well with prognosis and forms an important guide to treatment of colorectal neoplasms. If the lesion has been completely removed, with a margin, the options are close endoscopic surveillance or colectomy.

Colorectal Cancer

Commonest GI cancer. Usually presents after middle life but can occur earlier. The highest incidence of colorectal cancer is seen in Western Europe and North America; the lowest incidence occurs in Asia and South Africa. The precise cause is unknown but is probably due to a complex interplay between environmental and genetic factors. Being overweight and being underactive (with the lifestyle choices that accompany these conditions) are clear risk factors. Other predisposing factors include inflammatory bowel disease, familial polyposis coli, colorectal polyps, previous irradiation and family history.

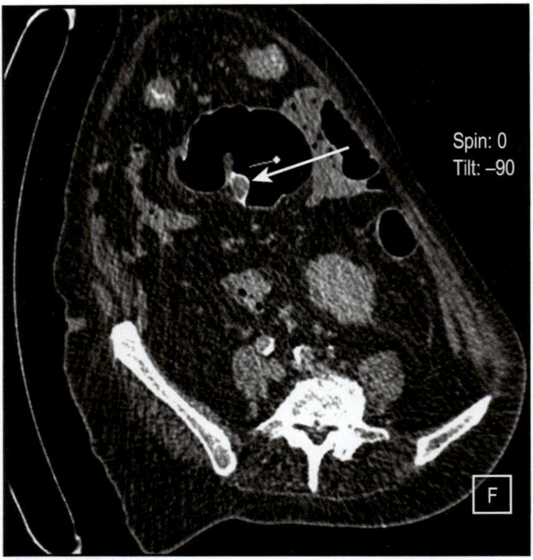

FIGURE 15.11
Image from a CT colonography study showing a soft tissue polyp arising from the medial wall of the caecum adjacent to the ileocaecal valve (arrow).

Apart from familial adenomatous polyposis, there are other groups of patients who have hereditary predisposition to develop large bowel cancer.

Lynch syndrome is the commonest inherited bowel cancer syndrome and accounts for about 2% of all colorectal cancer cases. It is inherited in an autosomal dominant fashion and is characterised by an increased risk of developing colon cancer than the normal population and the onset of the disease is at an earlier age (about 45 years). The syndrome also confers a risk of cancers to the endometrium, ovary, stomach, small bowel, hepatobiliary tract, urinary tract, brain and skin.

The diagnosis is made by a combination of factors:

- ***Family history***: Amsterdam II criteria. At least three family members, over two generations, affected with Lynch syndrome-associated cancers.
- ***Tumour analysis:*** evidence of MSI (short sequences of DNA that are repeated in an abnormally high number).
- ***Genetic mutation***: if the patient tests positive for an *MMR* gene mutation.
- There is a subgroup of patients who only fulfil part of the above criteria i.e. family history, but absence of MSI/MMR. In this situation, the patient and at-risk family members should be offered screening.
- The relative sites of distribution of carcinoma in the colon are rectum, 40%; sigmoid colon, 25%; descending colon, 5%; transverse colon, 10%; caecum and ascending colon, 20%.

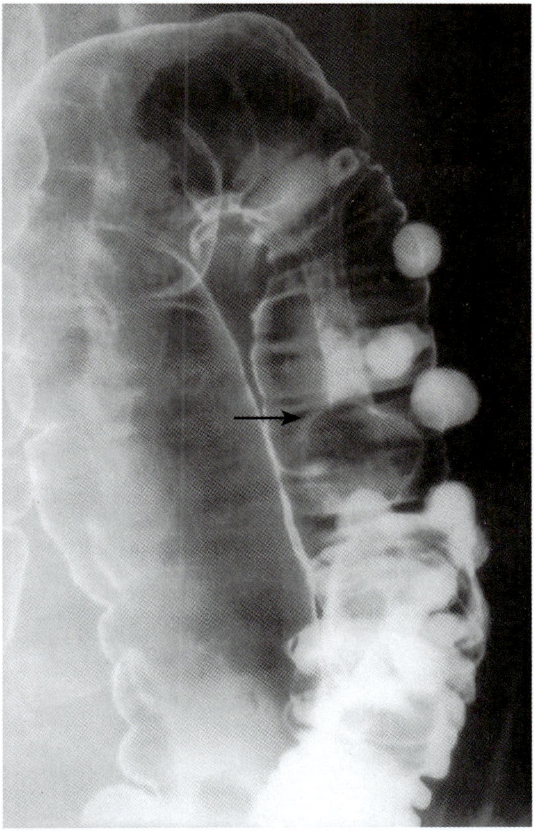

FIGURE 15.12
A barium enema showing part of the sigmoid colon. A large pedunculated polyp is seen (arrow). There is also marked diverticular disease.

Symptoms and Signs. Clinical features depend upon the site. Right colon: anaemia, palpable mass, change in bowel habit. Left colon: change in bowel habit, lower abdominal colicky pain. Blood or mucus on or mixed with stool. With sigmoid cancers, spurious diarrhoea may occur. Rectal cancers present with frequency of defaecation because of tenesmus (a sense of incomplete evacuation). Blood and mucous PR. Patients may present with symptoms due to direct spread, and sacral pain or sciatica due to direct invasion of the nerve. Jaundice due to liver or porta hepatis node metastases. Examination may reveal an abdominal mass or hepatomegaly. Examination PR may show blood on examining glove or mass may be palpable.

Some 25% of large bowel cancers present as emergencies. Obstruction may occur, e.g. small bowel obstruction with caecal cancers growing over the ileocaecal valve or obstruction occurring on the left side where the bowel lumen is narrow and the faeces are more formed. Perforation may occur because of either direct perforation of the cancer or perforation of the caecum with a closed-loop obstruction where the ileocaecal valve is competent. Massive haemorrhage is rare.

Investigations

- Hb
- FBC
- U&Es (ureteric involvement)
- LFTs (liver secondaries, alkaline phosphatase raised)
- Carcinoembryonic antigen (CEA) tumour marker, which is useful for monitoring known colorectal cancer but NOT used to detect the disease
- Colonoscopy and biopsy (to make diagnosis and rule out a synchronous lesion)
- CT colonography (→Figure 15.13): to exonerate the rest of the large bowel if colonoscopy not complete or unable to be performed
- USS: liver secondaries, ureteric obstruction
- CT/PET: secondaries

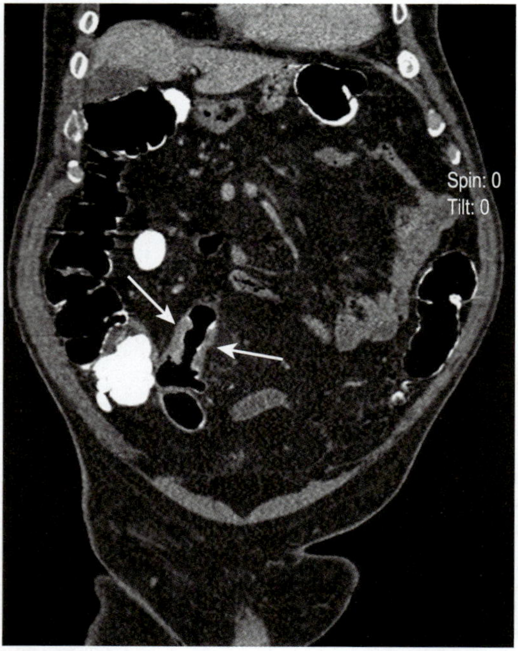

FIGURE 15.13

Coronal image from a CT colonography study in a patient with sigmoid adenocarcinoma. The CT shows an area of circumferential thickening (arrow) with an irregular mucosal surface, in keeping with the known tumour.

- Magnetic resonance imaging (MRI) pelvis: to accurately stage rectal cancer (→Figure 15.14)
- Endoanal USS: to accurately stage early rectal cancer if a transanal resection is possible
- MRI liver: to accurately assess the presence and respectability of liver metastases
- Barium enema (5% of tumours are metachronous); 'apple core' lesion may be visible (→Figure 15.15). Almost obsolete with the advent of CT colonography.

Treatment (→ Figure 15.16).
Elective

- Caecum and right colon: right hemicolectomy (see Procedures box, below)
- Transverse colon: extended right hemicolectomy
- Descending colon: left hemicolectomy
- Sigmoid colon: sigmoid colectomy
- Rectum and rectosigmoid: anterior resection with primary anastomosis. If low rectal tumour, abdominoperineal excision of the rectum should be carried out with a permanent colostomy
- Transanal endoscopic microsurgery (TEMS): this is a minimally invasive technique to remove rectal lesions transanally. It is indicated for curative resections of rectal polyps or early rectal cancers, as well as palliative treatment for patients who are unfit for formal surgical resection.

For any operation on the colon or rectum, the patient should be warned about a temporary or permanent stoma.

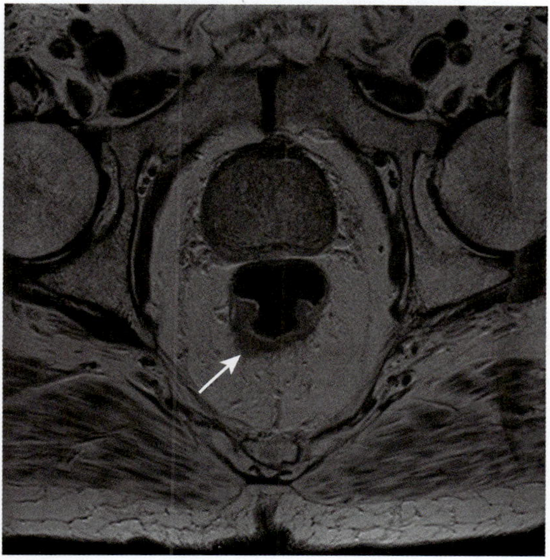

FIGURE 15.14
Sagittal image from a rectal MRI scan showing a flat ulcerated lesion (arrow) arising from the posterior wall of the low rectum in a male patient.

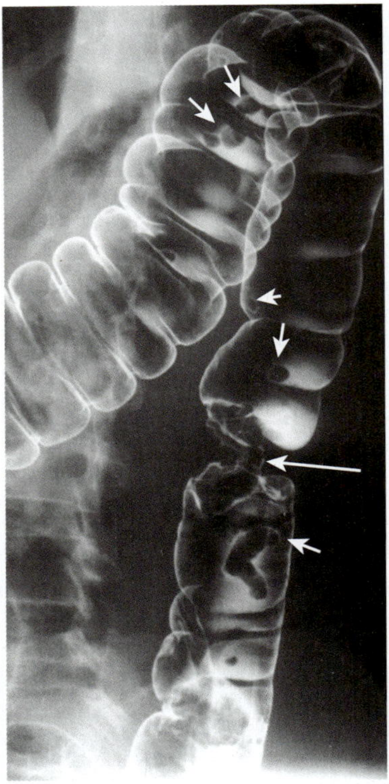

FIGURE 15.15

Image from a double contrast barium enema study showing an 'apple core' lesion within the descending colon, later proven to be an adenocarcinoma (long arrow). Multiple filling defects within the adjacent colon (short arrows) are in keeping with polyps.

HINTS AND TIPS

PREPARATION FOR BOWEL SURGERY

It has been shown that clearing the bowel of faeces before surgery (bowel preparation) does not reduce the rate of anastomotic dehiscence. There is also significant evidence to show that giving bowel preparation causes fluid and electrolyte imbalance, which would adversely affect anastomotic healing. Current practice is to omit oral bowel prep for all colonic resections, unless you plan to form a defunctioning ileostomy to protect a low anastomosis. However, a phosphate enema is given preoperatively for left-sided resections to enable a rectal anastomosis without faecal loading.

Emergency. Correct fluid and electrolytes imbalance. In closed-loop obstruction a caecum of greater than 10 cm in diameter on AXR is an indication for urgent surgery, especially if it is tender. Right-sided tumours may be treated with right hemicolectomy with primary anastomosis. Lower left-sided tumours should be treated by resection of the tumour and Hartmann's procedure, i.e. closure of the rectal stump and fashioning of an left iliac fossa (LIF) end colostomy. Continuity of the bowel is re-established some months later. Some surgeons carry out an on-table colonic lavage with primary anastomosis covered by a loop ileostomy.

HINTS AND TIPS

DIAGNOSING ANASTOMOTIC DEHISCENCE

A leak from an anastomosis is a significant and life-threatening complication of colorectal surgery. Despite adhering to good surgical technique, most specialist colorectal surgeons would quote a leak rate of about 5%. A leak can present in a number of ways, but the earlier the leak can be diagnosed and treated, the less the morbidity and mortality for the patient. Typically, a leak occurs between 5 and 10 days postsurgery, and that is when the surgeon has to be most vigilant. Common presentations are prolonged ileus, pyrexia, tachycardia or the new onset of atrial fibrillation. However, any patient who is not progressing appropriately after surgery should be investigated with a CT or water-soluble enema.

Prognosis. This is based on Dukes' classification, originally described for rectal cancer but now applied to all colorectal adenocarcinomas. Although TNM staging is used as the standard in reporting pathological specimens, Dukes' staging is still regarded as a reproducible way of discussing 5-year survival rates (Table 15.2):

- Dukes' A – 87%
- Dukes' B – 67%
- Dukes' C – 37% (cancer registry data).

Surveillance After Curative Resection. Most units follow up their patients for 5 years post cancer resection, if they are fit enough, with a programme that involves:

- 6 monthly CEA level
- CT chest/abdomen/pelvis at 1 and 3 years
- Colonoscopy at 1 and 5 years (NICE guidelines).

Bowel Screening. The purpose of bowel screening is to pick up early cancers and polyps in asymptomatic individuals. About 1 in 20 people in the UK will develop colorectal cancer in their lifetime. Regular bowel screening has been shown to reduce the risk of dying from bowel cancer by 16%.

In the majority of the UK, faecal occult blood testing is offered to men and women aged 60–75 every 2 years. If this screen is positive, the participant is offered a colonoscopy.

Other methods of screening are currently being evaluated, such as flexible sigmoidoscopy, CT colonography and faecal immunological testing (FIT).

Surveillance colonoscopy is also offered to at-risk asymptomatic patients with strong family history, previous polyps, bowel cancer syndromes and inflammatory bowel disease.

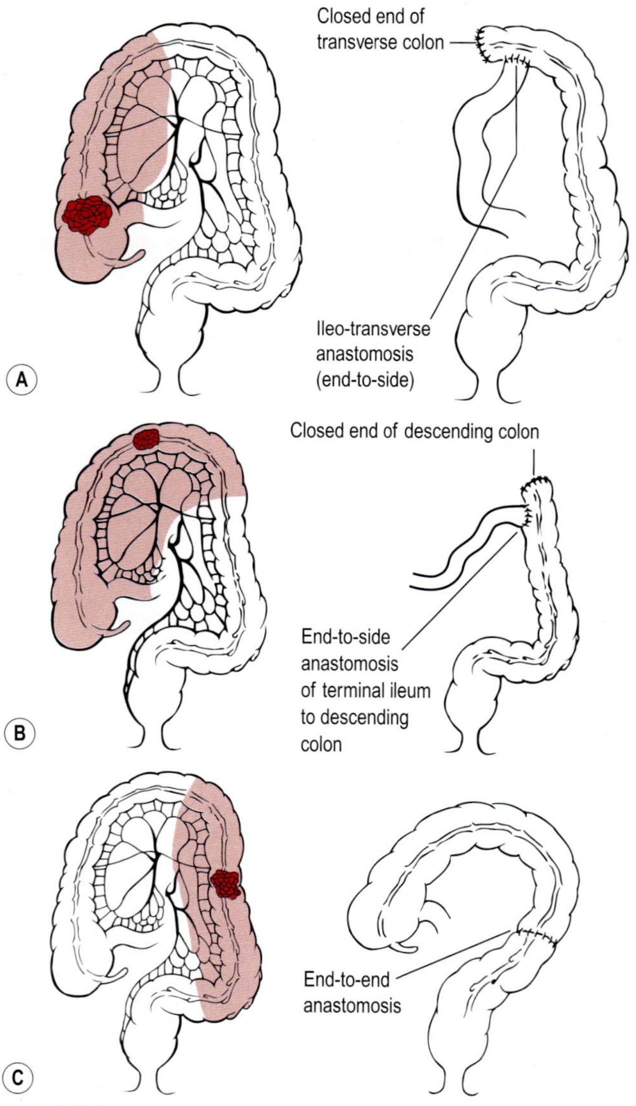

FIGURE 15.16

Operations for colorectal cancer. The diagrams indicate the extent of resection and the method of re-establishing continuity. (**A**) Right hemicolectomy. (**B**) Extended right hemicolectomy. (**C**) Left hemicolectomy.

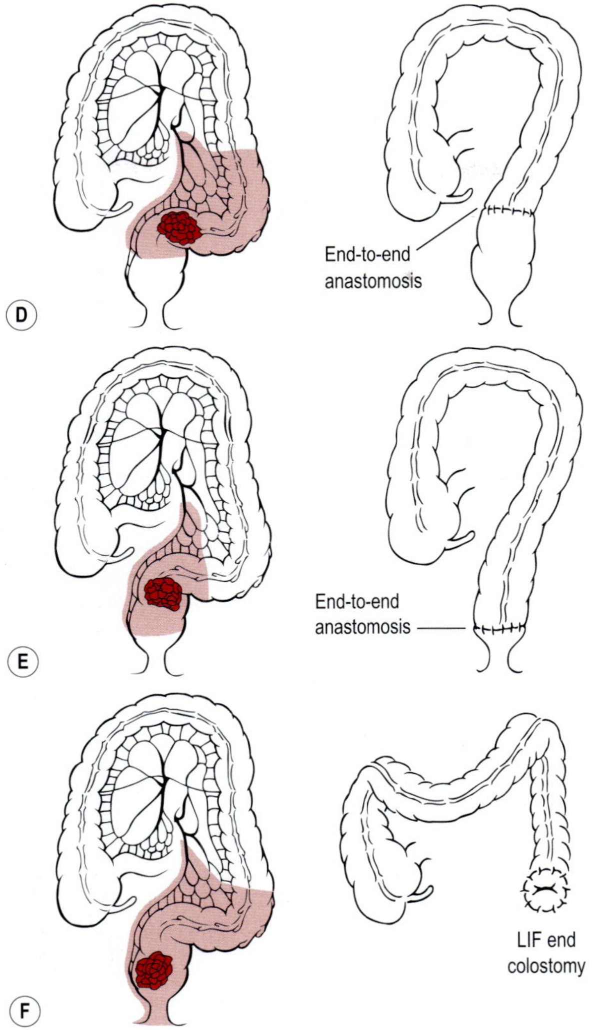

FIGURE 15.16, Cont'd

(**D**) Sigmoid colectomy. (**E**) Anterior resection. (**F**) Abdominoperineal resection of the rectum with permanent colostomy. The shaded area is the area resected. Diverticular disease. A barium enema showing numerous diverticulae in the sigmoid colon.

TABLE 15.2

DUKES' CLASSIFICATION*

A	Confined to bowel wall; 87% 5-year survival
B	Through wall into surrounding tissue; 67% 5-year survival
C	Lymph node involvement; 37% 5-year survival

*If distant metastases are present, the 5-year survival is only 5%.

Inflammatory Bowel Disease

The two main disorders are Crohn's disease and ulcerative colitis.

Crohn's Disease

This is a chronic inflammatory disorder that may occur anywhere in the alimentary tract from the mouth to the anus. Common sites include the terminal ileum (regional ileitis), colon and rectum. Unlike ulcerative colitis, the whole thickness of the bowel wall is involved. The aetiology is unknown, although smoking has been proven to exacerbate the disease. The disease occurs most commonly in the 15–35 years age group. Familial clustering occurs. Malignancy may rarely occur in both the small and large bowel.

Symptoms and Signs. Malaise, anorexia, fever, nausea, abdominal pain, weight loss, diarrhoea, rectal bleeding. Perianal inflammation with abscess, fissure, and fistulae formation may occur. Pallor, malnutrition, abdominal mass, perianal sepsis, fissures, fistulae, clubbing, erythema nodosum, pyoderma gangrenosum and uveitis.

Investigations

- Hb
- FBC
- ESR
- Folate
- B_{12}
- U&Es: electrolyte imbalances
- LFTs: albumin reduced
- CRP: elevated levels
- Faecal calprotectin: a protein that is excreted in excess into the lumen of the intestine during the inflammatory process
- Radiographs – AXR: obstruction, perforation, toxic dilatation
- MRI small bowel (enteroclysis) (→Figure 15.17): useful for defining extent of active Crohn's from 'burnt out' stricture
- Small bowel enema and barium enema: skip lesions in small bowel, strictures, 'rose thorn' ulcers, 'cobblestone' mucosa (→Figure 15.18)
- Sigmoidoscopy and biopsy
- Colonoscopy and biopsy
- CT: abscesses
- Capsule endoscopy.

Complications. Extra-alimentary manifestations (see above). Toxic dilatation. Stricture. Internal fistulae. Haemorrhage. Abscess formation. Perianal complications. Gallstones. Renal calculi. Psychological problems. Risk of carcinoma.

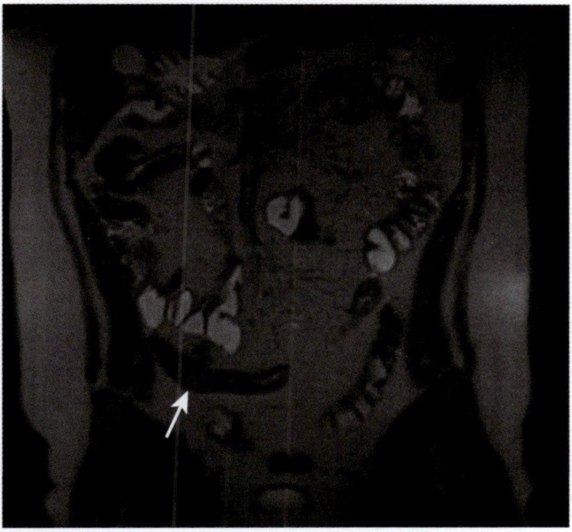

FIGURE 15.17

Coronal image from an MR enterography study in a patient with Crohn's disease showing abnormally thickened terminal ileum (arrow). Immediately above this loop is a band of low-signal fibrosis extending to an adjacent ileal loop at a site of previous fistulation.

Treatment

Medical. Correction of fluid and electrolyte imbalance. Nutritional support. Steroids: 40 mg daily of prednisolone in acute exacerbations. Budesonide is used for ileal or right colonic disease. Rectal disease may respond to Predsol enemas. Mesalazine may help colonic disease and may reduce the frequency of relapses. Other drug therapies include azathioprine (useful as steroid-sparing drug in some cases), ciclosporin, metronidazole (especially for colonic disease with perianal sepsis). Biological agents (infliximab/adalimumab) are monoclonal antibodies to TNFα (tumour necrosis factor α) and are used to treat a variety of immune diseases. Antidiarrhoeal agents may be used for symptomatic control but should be stopped if obstructed symptoms occur.

Surgical. Indicated for toxic dilatation, acute haemorrhage, perforation, obstruction, abscess formation, fistula formation, failure of medical treatment, uncertainty of diagnosis, development and prevention of carcinoma. Surgery involves segmental resection of bowel, sparing as much bowel as possible. For short strictures stricturoplasty may be carried out. Proctocolectomy with ileostomy may be required. Unlike ulcerative colitis, surgery in Crohn's disease cannot be guaranteed to be curative.

Prognosis. Acute regional ileitis may be cured by right hemicolectomy. Colonic Crohn's often responds well to medical treatment but at least 50% of patients will require surgery at some time. The mortality rate is about 14% over 30 years. The disease

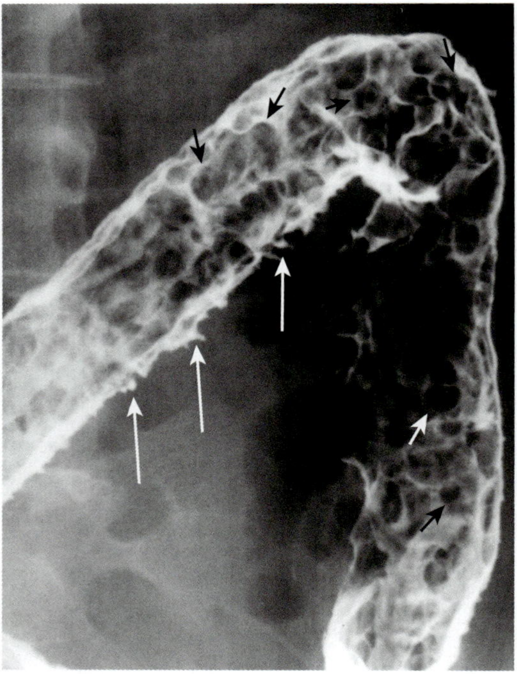

FIGURE 15.18

Selected image of the splenic flexure from a double contrast barium enema study in a patient with Crohn's disease showing 'cobblestoning' of the mucosa (short arrows) and deep ulceration (long arrows).

pursues a course of remissions and exacerbations. The only proven interventions that prevent recurrence after a Crohn's resection are smoking abstinence and maintenance 5-ASA (mesalazine).

Ulcerative Colitis

This is a chronic inflammatory disease that involves the whole or part of the colon. The inflammation is confined to the mucosa and nearly always involves the rectum, extending to involve the distal or total colon. The aetiology is unknown but immunological, dietary and genetic factors may be involved. The majority of cases present between 25 and 30 years of age. Familial clustering occurs. Malignant change occurs in the colon with time.

Symptoms and Signs. Diarrhoea, rectal bleeding, abdominal pain, fever, weight loss. The disease may be acute and fulminant, intermittent or chronic. Pallor, malnutrition, abdominal tenderness, abdominal distension, erythema nodosum, pyoderma gangrenosum, arthritis, uveitis, jaundice (sclerosing cholangitis).

Investigations

- Hb
- FBC
- U&Es: dehydration and electrolyte imbalance in severe cases
- LFTs: hypoalbuminaemia or abnormal because of complications of sclerosing cholangitis
- CRP
- AXR: acute toxic dilatation, perforation
- Sigmoidoscopy: red, inflamed mucosa, contact bleeding, pseudopolyps
- Biopsy
- Colonoscopy: assess extent of disease, exclude carcinoma
- CT to assess disease extent or complications
- Barium enema – double contrast (→Figure 15.19): loss of haustrations, mucosal distortion, colonic shortening, stricture due to carcinoma. Barium enema should not be performed on ill patients with toxic dilatation in case of perforation.

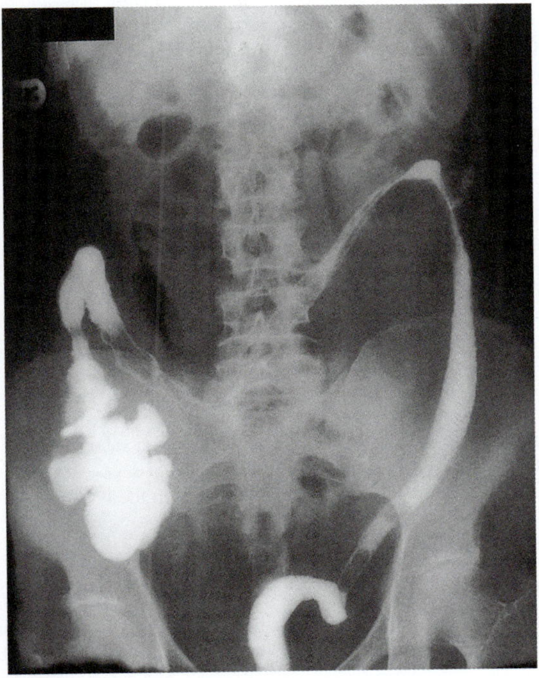

FIGURE 15.19
Ulcerative colitis. There is shortening of the colon with loss of haustrations ('lead pipe' appearance).

Complications. Local complications include toxic dilatation, haemorrhage, stricture, perforation and carcinoma. Extracolonic complications include seronegative arthritis (sacroileitis, ankylosing spondylitis), sclerosing cholangitis, chronic active hepatitis, uveitis and amyloid.

Treatment

Medical. Acute severe ulcerative colitis is treated with i.v. fluids, blood transfusion, parenteral nutrition and parenteral steroids. This regimen is instituted usually for 5 days. Regular examination of the patient is undertaken. If the patient deteriorates or toxic dilatation or perforation supervene, urgent surgery is required.

In the less ill patient, oral steroids may be given until the disease is controlled. Those who respond to the above regimens may be treated with sulfasalazine or mesalazine orally to maintain the remission. Distal colitis and proctitis may be controlled by Predsol retention enemas for relapses and sulfasalazine for maintenance. Biological agents can also be used.

Surgical. Indications for surgery include acute toxic dilatation, perforation, failure to respond to medical treatment, chronic disease, severe arthritic symptoms, carcinoma. In the acute setting, the majority of surgeons would perform a subtotal colectomy with an end ileostomy. This has the advantage of avoiding pelvic surgery in the emergency setting, with all its inherent risks, and being able to get a definitive diagnosis of ulcerative colitis before considering restorative surgery. Once UC has been proven, a completion proctectomy (± ileoanal pouch) can be undertaken.

HINTS AND TIPS

SEVERITY OF COLITIS

Ideally, patients admitted with acute severe colitis, from Crohn's or ulcerative colitis, should be reviewed by a gastroenterologist or surgeon on a daily basis. Evidence that the patient is not responding to high-dose steroids include stool frequency over six times per day, rising CRP and failing albumin or haemoglobin (Truelove and Witts classification). If the patient has not improved by day 3 of intravenous hydrocortisone, or day 4 after instigation of biological therapy, a colectomy is indicated.

Prognosis. The mortality rate with toxic dilatation or perforation is around 5%. The risk of colorectal cancer increases after 10 years duration of disease, being about 2% at 10 years and up to 30% at 30 years. The risk is greater in those with total colitis and severe disease. Dysplasia often precedes carcinoma. Colonoscopic surveillance should be carried out at least every other year after the patient has had the disease for 10 years.

Diverticular Disease

Diverticulae are outpouchings of mucosa through the bowel wall associated with increased intraluminal pressure (pulsion diverticulae). They occur between the taenia coli where vessels penetrate the bowel wall. They occur most commonly in the sigmoid colon and descending colon but may occur anywhere in the colon. They are rare before the age of 40 but thereafter there is an increase in incidence with age such that about 40% of patients over 70 have them. Diverticular disease is rare in countries where there is considerable roughage in the diet and is largely a condition occurring in Western civilised societies where the diet is refined.

Symptoms and Signs. Diverticular disease may be asymptomatic (diverticulosis).

Acute Diverticulitis. Gives rise to lower abdominal colicky pain with localising somatic pain usually in the LIF. Diarrhoea, constipation and abdominal distension may occur. Fever. Tender in LIF.

Chronic Diverticular Disease. May cause lower abdominal colicky pain, alternating constipation and diarrhoea, and excessive flatus together with abdominal distension. There may be little to find on abdominal examination.

Investigations

- FBC (WCC raised in acute but normal in chronic)
- CRP
- CT to make diagnosis and detect complications
- Sigmoidoscopy to exclude carcinoma (usually deferred for 6–8 weeks for acute inflammation to settle)
- Colonoscopy or CT colonography
- Barium enema (→Figure 15.12) – largely superseded by CT colonography.

Differential Diagnosis. Carcinoma of the colon. Crohn's disease. Ischaemic colitis.

Complications. Acute diverticulitis. Stricture formation. Perforation with either generalised peritonitis, paracolic abscess or fistula formation (vesicocolic, vaginocolic, ileocolic). Haemorrhage. Large bowel obstruction.

Treatment.

Uncomplicated, Symptomatic Diverticular Disease. Antispasmodic, e.g. Colofac. Bulking agent, e.g. Fybogel.

Acute Diverticulitis. Bed rest. Fluids only or nil orally. Analgesic. Antibiotics: cefuroxime and metronidazole i.v. When symptoms settle, treatment is as for uncomplicated symptomatic diverticular disease.

Perforation With Paracolic Abscess. Percutaneous drainage and i.v. antibiotics.

If the first presentation of diverticular disease is with inflammation or localised collection, and this has been successfully treated conservatively, the evidence is that these patients are unlikely to present again with a significant episode of sepsis related to diverticulitis. Therefore, most surgeons would not offer an elective resection after these episodes.

Perforation With Purulent Peritonitis. Options are Hartmann's or laparoscopy and copious washout with adequate drainage established and close postoperative monitoring.

Perforation With Generalised Faecal Peritonitis. Laparotomy. Peritoneal lavage. Resect perforated area. In case of sigmoid diverticulae treatment is by Hartmann's procedure (see Procedures box at end of chapter). Drain peritoneal cavity. Antibiotics as for acute diverticulitis. In the elderly, perforated diverticulitis with faecal peritonitis carries a high mortality.

Fistula Formation. This involves bladder, vagina or small bowel. A vesicocolic fistula presents with dysuria and pneumaturia (passing wind in urine), a vaginocolic fistula presents with the passage of faeces PV and ileocolic fistula with diarrhoea. Vesicocolic fistulae show gas in the bladder on a plain radiograph. Barium enema may show the communication. Primary resection and anastomosis is the treatment of choice for ileocolic and vaginocolic fistulae and vesicocolic fistulae.

Haemorrhage. Usually self-limiting. May be profuse and require transfusion. Exact site may be difficult to establish. Angiography and embolisation may be required. If haemorrhage is life threatening, total colectomy with ileostomy and preservation of rectal stump may be required. Continuity of the bowel is re-established subsequently.

Intestinal Obstruction. Progressive diverticular disease can cause stricture. Treatment is by resection with either a Hartmann's procedure followed by subsequent restorative surgery, or a primary anastomosis protected by a temporary defunctioning loop ileostomy.

HINTS AND TIPS

BOWEL OBSTRUCTION

Commonly, a patient with large bowel obstruction from any cause (malignant/benign) will present with a history of alternating constipation and diarrhoea. As the obstruction progresses they describe absolute constipation – the inability to pass flatus or stool. This is a surgical emergency, particularly if the patient has a competent ileocaecal valve. Clinically, if the patient has right-sided abdominal pain, this is an ominous sign, as the caecum is the most easily distensible part of the colon. Therefore, even if the level of obstruction is on the left side of the colon, often the caecum is the first part of the large bowel to perforate, necessitating a subtotal colectomy.

Volvulus

This is a twisting of a loop of bowel around its mesenteric axis. Partial or complete obstruction may result. Occlusion of the arteries at the base of the involved mesentery leads to gangrene and perforation. The sigmoid colon or caecum may be involved, the sigmoid being the more common.

Sigmoid Volvulus

Middle-aged and elderly males are more often affected. The twist is usually anticlockwise. A large redundant sigmoid colon and constipation are predisposing factors.

Symptoms and Signs. Sudden onset of lower abdominal colicky pain associated with gross abdominal distension. May be history of recurrent mild attacks associated with partial volvulus relieved by passage of large amounts of faeces and flatus. Distended tympanic abdomen.

Investigations

- AXR: distended loop of bowel the shape of a 'coffee bean' arising out of the pelvis on the left side
- CT to distinguish between sigmoid volvulus and pseudo-obstruction
- Barium enema may be helpful in doubtful cases – the barium column resembles a 'bird's beak' because of the way the lumen tapers towards the volvulus (→Figure 15.20).

Treatment. Decompression by sigmoidoscopy. A rectal flatus tube should be left in situ for as long as is tolerated. If the patient is fit, elective resection of the sigmoid is carried out at a later date. If decompression is unsuccessful or there are signs of

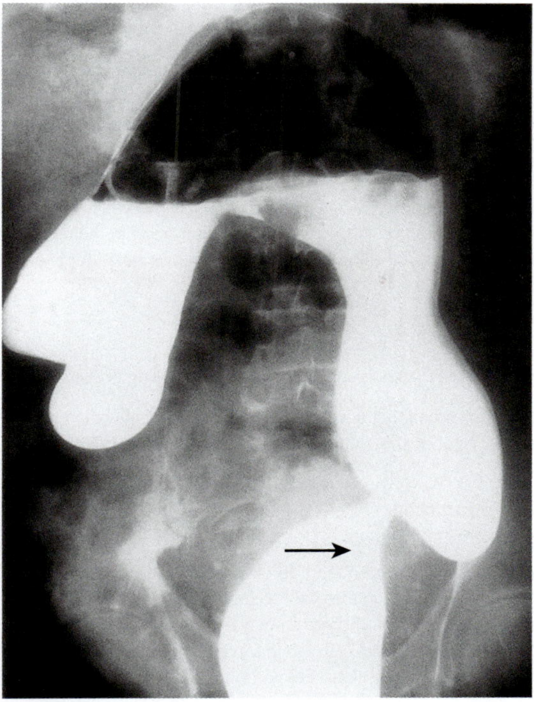

FIGURE 15.20

Barium enema showing a sigmoid volvulus. A 'bird's beak' deformity is seen (arrow). In this case, barium has passed into the volvulus – often it does not.

gangrene or perforation, a Hartmann's procedure is undertaken, or a resection with the two ends of the colon being brought out as a double-barrelled colostomy (Paul–Mikulicz procedure), which is later closed.

Caecal Volvulus

This occurs when the caecum and ascending colon are excessively mobile, or if there has been a defect in rotation, the caecum retaining its mesentery.

Symptoms and Signs. Sudden onset of abdominal pain, vomiting and constipation. Tympanitic mass in LUQ. Tender mass if impending infarction.

Investigations. AXR: dilated caecum in left upper quadrant.

Treatment. Laparotomy and right hemicolectomy with or without a primary anastomosis. This is performed whether the bowel is still viable or not as the risk of recurrent volvulus is high.

Prognosis. The mortality rate is high, usually owing to delayed diagnosis.

Irradiation Proctitis

This may complicate irradiation of pelvic lesions, e.g. cervix, uterus, bladder, prostate. Bleeding, diarrhoea and tenesmus may result. Later ulceration and stricture formation may also occur. Early symptoms appearing soon after irradiation may respond to steroid enemas. Other useful treatments are formalin application, endoscopic application of APC and hyperbaric oxygen treatment.

Angiodysplasia

Vascular anomalies that may be degenerative and may cause bleeding from the large bowel. This is most common in the elderly. It is commonest in the right colon.

Symptoms and Signs. Bleeding PR, which may be torrential but is often repeated small bleeds.

Investigations

- Colonoscopy
- Selective mesenteric angiography in the actively bleeding phase.

Treatment. Resuscitation if needed. Tranexamic acid. Coagulation with APC under direct vision at colonoscopy. Embolisation at angiography. Extensive areas require colectomy.

Large Bowel Obstruction

The major causes are carcinoma, diverticular disease and volvulus. In 20% of patients the ileocaecal valve is competent and decompression into the small bowel does not occur. Closed-loop obstruction therefore occurs, the caecum progressively distending. Ischaemia and perforation of the caecum may occur.

Symptoms and Signs. Colicky abdominal pain, constipation and vomiting (late). Constant severe pain suggests ischaemic bowel. Distended tympanitic abdomen. Obstructed bowel sounds. Collapsed, empty rectum on PR examination.

Investigations

- AXR: distended large bowel with air/fluid levels surrounding the abdomen like a picture frame (→Figure 15.21)
- CT chest/abdomen/pelvis will usually give definitive diagnosis and staging, should it be appropriate
- Sigmoidoscopy: rectosigmoid lesions may be seen (not done if acutely obstructed)
- Instant enema to exclude pseudo-obstruction
- Limited barium enema may show 'apple core' lesion.

Treatment. Drip and suck. Correct electrolyte imbalance. A caecum 10 cm or greater in diameter on radiograph is an urgent indication for surgery, especially if tender to palpation. Laparotomy with decompression of the obstruction. Right-sided lesions are treated by right hemicolectomy. Left-sided lesions may be treated by left hemicolectomy with covering loop ileostomy. Low left-sided lesions are treated by resection of the tumour with Hartmann's procedure. However, on-table lavage of the colon and primary anastomosis may be carried out in experienced hands with or without a defunctioning loop ileostomy. A carcinoma on the apex of the sigmoid loop may be treated by resection and a Paul–Mikulicz double-barrel colostomy. In a poorly patient a defunctioning colostomy or caecostomy may be carried out and elective resection delayed until a later date when the patient is fitter. Sigmoid volvulus may be treated

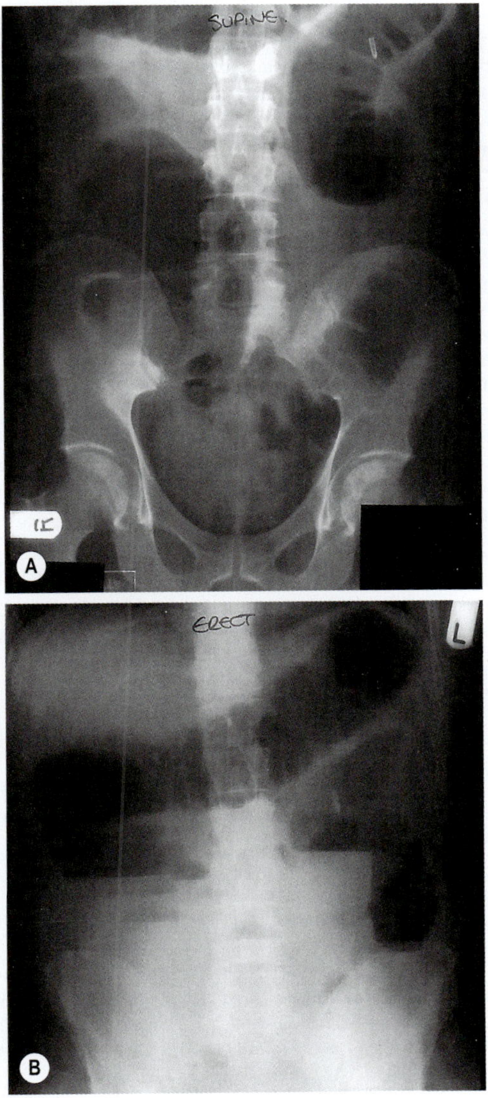

FIGURE 15.21

A plain AXR showing large bowel obstruction. (**A**) Supine film. The left colon is distended down to the pelvis where there is sharp 'cut-off' of the gas shadow. (**B**) Erect film. This shows air/fluid levels in the large bowel. Again the sharp 'cut-off' is seen in the pelvis. This represents the point of the obstructing lesion, which in this case was in the lower sigmoid colon.

by resection and a Paul–Mikulicz procedure. Colonic stenting may be carried out in those unfit for surgery or as a bridge to alleviate obstruction before definitive 'elective' surgery (with the aim of avoiding stoma formation).

Prognosis. The overall mortality rate approaches 15%. Perforation is the main cause of mortality.

ANAL CONDITIONS

Haemorrhoids

These are enlarged vascular cushions in the lower rectum and anal canal. They are not simply varicosities. At least 10% of the population will have symptomatic haemorrhoids at some time in their life. The classical position of haemorrhoids corresponds to branches of the superior haemorrhoidal artery occurring at the 3 o'clock, 7 o'clock and 11 o'clock positions with the patient in the lithotomy position.

Symptoms and Signs. Asymptomatic. Rectal bleeding (on toilet paper or drips into toilet on defaecation). Prolapse. Itching. Piles are not painful unless they thrombose. First-degree piles remain in the rectum and manifest only by bleeding. Second-degree piles prolapse on defaecation but reduce spontaneously. Third-degree piles prolapse and require manual reduction. Check Hb if bleeding is prolonged or heavy. Examine abdomen to exclude other lesions. Digital rectal examination.

Investigations

- Sigmoidoscopy to exclude other lesions
- Proctoscopy to confirm presence of piles. Remember at least 10% of population will have piles. Abdominal pain is not associated with piles
- If there is any doubt as to the cause of bleeding, carry out colonoscopy.

Treatment

Conservative

- Simple first-degree piles often respond to high-fibre diet/regular laxatives, as well as advice on avoiding straining
- Injection treatment: inject 2–3 mL of phenol in almond oil into the submucosa above the pile. This is suitable for first-degree and small second-degree piles
- Rubber band ligation.

Surgical

- HALO (haemorrhoidal artery ligation operation)
- Large second-degree piles and third-degree piles require haemorrhoidectomy (open/stapled)
- Thrombosed piles may be treated by bed rest, analgesia and ice packs. The piles may thrombose with cure or remain as skin tags, which require subsequent excision. Some surgeons advocate emergency haemorrhoidectomy. Whatever treatment is used, subsequent regulation of bowel habit with high-fibre diet and bulk laxatives is required.

Complications of Haemorrhoidectomy. Acute retention of urine. Haemorrhage (slipped ligature in the early postoperative period or secondary haemorrhage 8–10 days postoperatively). Stricture may occur with anal stenosis if too much skin has been excised.

Differential Diagnosis. Perianal haematoma, rectal prolapse, fissure-in-ano, inflammatory bowel disease, anal polyp, carcinoma, proctalgia fugax.

Rectal Prolapse

This may be partial or complete. Partial prolapse involves the mucosa alone and prolapse is usually no more than a few centimetres. Complete prolapse involves all layers of the rectal wall and is most common in elderly females.

Symptoms and Signs. Protruding mass from the anus, especially during defaecation. May reduce spontaneously. May need manual reduction and eventually becomes difficult to reduce. Blood and mucous PR from ulceration of exposed mucosa. Palpate prolapse between fingers. Mucosal prolapse reveals two layers of mucosa about 2–4 cm long with radial folds. Lax sphincter on examination PR. Complete prolapse is thick, up to 12 cm long and patient may be unable to contract sphincter muscles after prolapse reduced.

Differential Diagnosis. Prolapsing haemorrhoids, polyps, intussusception.

Treatment. Mucosal prolapse usually responds to sclerosants injected submucosally as for piles. Excision of prolapsed mucosa may be necessary. Complete prolapse can be treated by an abdominal or perineal procedure depending on the fitness of the patient. Abdominally, the majority of specialists would perform a laparoscopic ventral rectopexy, where the front of the rectum is mobilised and then hitched up and fixed to the sacrum by a prosthetic mesh. Perineal procedures include excision of mucosa and longitudinal plication of the rectal muscle (Delorme procedure), full-thickness excision of the rectal prolapse (Altmeier's procedure) and circumferential narrowing of the anus by inserting a suture subcutaneously around the anal orifice (Thiersch wire – although nylon rather than wire is used nowadays).

Complications. Abdominal rectopexy usually gives good results but residual incontinence due to chronic stretching of the sphincter may result. Thiersch wire procedure may result in infection and faecal impaction.

Rectal Prolapse in Children

Usually self-correcting. Parents require reassurance. Keep act of defaecation as short as possible and avoid straining. Repeat simple reduction is all that is required. A mild laxative may be necessary. In a few cases, subcutaneous injection of sclerosant may be required.

Perianal Haematoma

Symptoms and Signs. Acute perianal pain. Worse on sitting, walking and defaecation. Tense, smooth, tender blue lump at anal verge.

Treatment. Symptoms may subside spontaneously after 2–3 days, during which time analgesia is given. If patient presents in acute phase, incision under LA should be carried out.

Anal Fissures

This is a tear at the anal margin due to passage of a constipated stool. The fissure is usually in the midline posteriorly but may occasionally be anterior. Multiple fissures may be due to Crohn's disease.

Symptoms and Signs. Acute anal pain, severe on defaecation. Blood on toilet paper. Part the buttocks and the fissure may be apparent. Acute sphincter spasm. Examination PR impossible. Occasionally 'sentinel' pile. This is a skin tag at the anal verge external to the fissure.

Differential Diagnosis. Crohn's disease, trauma (beware abuse in children), carcinoma, herpes, TB, syphilis and psoriasis.

Treatment

Conservative. First-line treatment of anal fissures is usually topical application of 2% Diltiazem cream twice a day for 6–8 weeks. This reduces anal spasm and allows the fissure to heal. Glyceryl trinitrate 0.2% ointment is an alternative, which is applied in the same fashion for a similar time period. Attention should also be given to correcting constipation with a stool-softening laxative and high-fibre diet.

Surgical. The majority of acute anal fissures settle with conservative management. In those that do not, the first-line surgical option is botox injection into the intersphincteric plane at 3 and 9 o'clock. This temporarily reduces sphincter spasm for a period of 8–12 weeks, which is usually enough time to get the fissure to heal. This treatment can be repeated. A lateral subcutaneous internal sphincterotomy should be carried out if other methods fail. It should be undertaken with extreme caution in women. A laxative and high-fibre diet should be taken in the postoperative period. Recurrent fissures or fissures in abnormal positions should be treated by excision of the fissure, which is sent for histological examination to exclude underlying causes, e.g. Crohn's, anal carcinoma.

Anorectal Abscesses (→ Figure 15.22)

These develop in tissue spaces adjacent to the anorectal area. They may be perianal (in a hair follicle, sebaceous gland or perianal haematoma), ischiorectal (in the ischiorectal fossa), intermuscular (between internal and external sphincters), or pelvirectal (spreading from a pelvic abscess – rare). In many cases, the infection may start in the anal crypt and spread along tissue planes.

Symptoms and Signs. Constant, throbbing, perianal pain – worse on sitting. With pelvirectal abscesses, the pain may also be in the lower abdomen. Indurated tender mass perianally. Fever.

Treatment. Prompt surgical drainage to prevent fistula formation. There is no role for antibiotics except in diabetics and the immunocompromised – and then only as an adjunct to surgery. Incision, curettage and packing are required.

Complications. Fistula-in-ano occurs in up to 30% of patients.

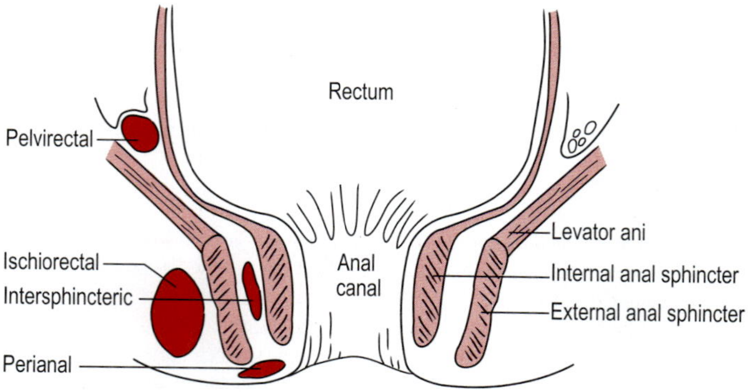

FIGURE 15.22

The anatomy of anorectal abscesses.

Fistula-in-Ano

A fistula is an abnormal communication between two epithelial surfaces. In this instance, there is an internal opening in the anal canal and one or more external openings on the perianal skin. Most arise from delay in treatment, or inadequate treatment, of anorectal abscesses. Rarer causes include Crohn's disease, tuberculosis and carcinoma. It may be difficult to locate the internal opening. Application of Goodsall's rule ('if the external opening lies anterior to a line drawn transversely through the centre of the anus, the track passes radially through a straight line towards the internal opening. If the external opening is behind this line the track curves in a horseshoe manner to open into the midline posteriorly') (→Figure 15.23). Fistulae may be classified into intersphincteric, transphincteric, suprasphincteric, extrasphincteric (Parks' classification→Figure 15.24).

Symptoms and Signs. History of abscess, which drains spontaneously or was surgically drained. Persistent drainage of pus, mucus, blood or faecal matter associated with perianal irritation and discomfort. Drainage may be intermittent if the fistula heals and opens recurrently. Single opening near anus. Examination PR reveals indurated track, pressure on which may cause discharge. Proctoscopy or sigmoidoscopy to define internal opening.

Investigations

- Examination under anaesthetic is the first-line investigation
- MRI. To delineate anatomy in complex/high fistulae
- Endoanal ultrasound.

Differential Diagnosis. Pilonidal sinus, hidradenitis suppurativa, incontinence, Crohn's disease, trauma.

Treatment. The track is identified by probing and, if low, laid open under GA, so that it heals by granulation tissue from the base. With high fistulae or pelvirectal fistulae there is a danger to puborectalis when opening the track. Incontinence may result. Therefore, first-line treatment of a high/complex fistula is the placement of a seton in the track. This prevents the track closing and further perianal sepsis recurring. An MRI would be requested to confirm anatomy and relationship to the anal sphincters. There are many ways to deal with high fistulae including plugs, glue and anal advancement flaps.

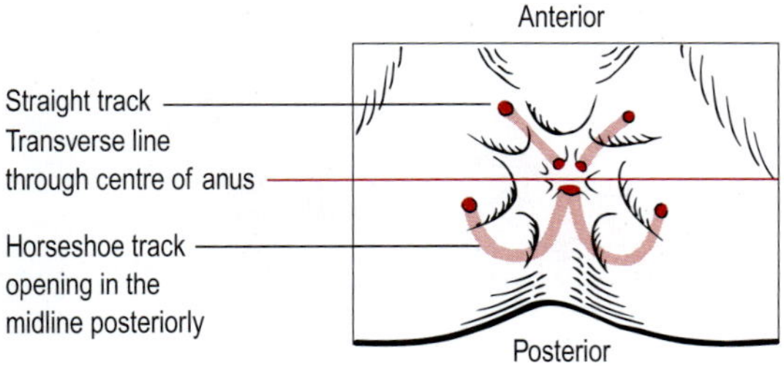

FIGURE 15.23
Goodsall's rule.

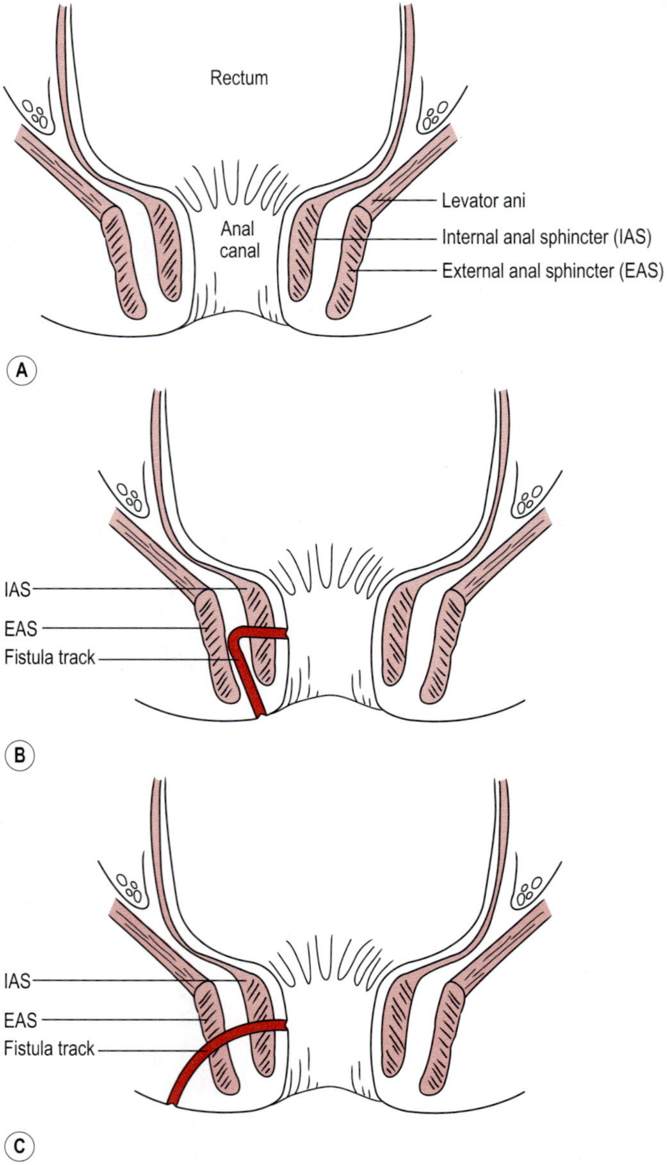

FIGURE 15.24

The anatomy of fistula-in-ano. (**A**) Normal anatomy. (**B**) Intersphincteric fistula. (**C**) Trans-sphincteric fistula.

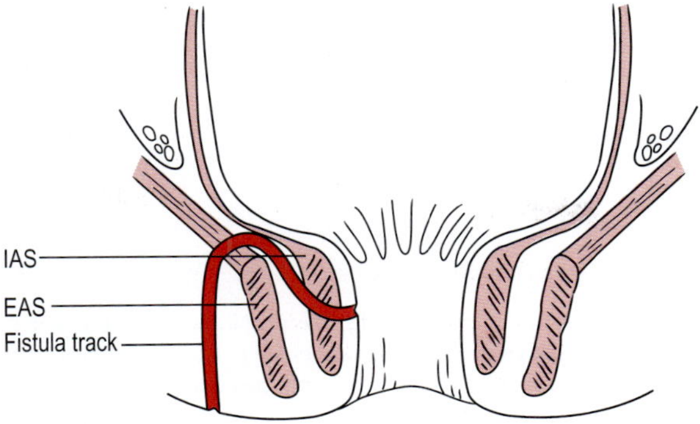

D

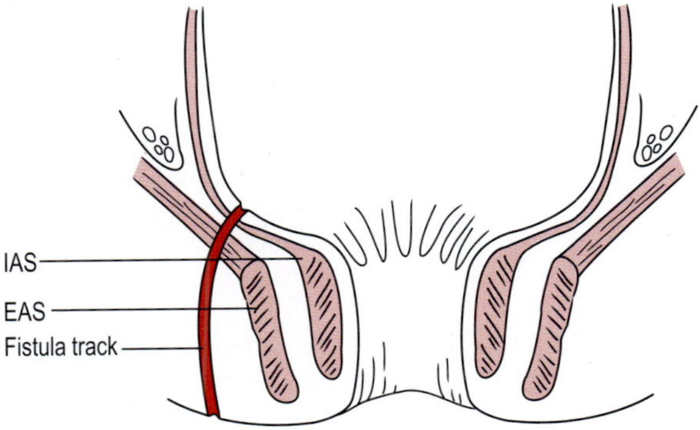

E

FIGURE 15.24, Cont'd
(**D**) Suprasphincteric fistula. (**E**) Extrasphincteric fistula.

Pruritus Ani

This is itching in the perianal area. It is a symptom of various conditions, but the most common cause is faecal residue on the perianal skin. This can be caused by faecal leakage/incontinence, the presence of skin tags making cleaning difficult, or just poor hygiene. Other local causes are sweating, fistula, haemorrhoids, neoplasia, warts, fungal infections, contact dermatitis (deodorants), worms, antibiotics (possibly via the complication of diarrhoea or fungal infection). General causes include diabetes mellitus, obstructive jaundice, Hodgkin's disease. Dermatological diseases include scabies, pediculosis, psoriasis and atopic eczema. Often an 'itch/scratch' vicious circle is created, and symptoms persist even after the initial cause has been eradicated.

Symptoms and Signs. Worse at night whatever the cause. History of precipitating cause, e.g. antibiotics, diabetes, pruritus elsewhere. Perianal skin may be normal, or inflamed, moist or macerated. Examination PR and proctoscopy to exclude anal conditions, e.g. fistulae.

Investigations

- Hb
- WCC
- Blood sugar
- Perianal scrapings and microscopy for fungus.

Treatment. Specific for the underlying disease. Nonspecific treatment includes advice on hygiene, diet, wearing loose underclothes, cleansing after defaecation with water or unscented wet wipes and using a barrier cream to protect the perianal skin. Application of hydrocortisone and local anaesthetic cream may help, but should only be used short term. Surgical measures include treating piles, excising skin tags and injecting methylene blue into the perianal skin. This numbs the perianal skin, breaking the itch–scratch cycle. Often the condition is notoriously difficult to treat.

Sexually Transmitted Diseases

Condylomata Acuminata (Anal Warts)

Caused by HPV. Usually sexually transmitted. Over 50% of patients admit to anal intercourse. May be few or a continuous carpet of warts extending into the anal canal. Symptoms include bleeding and pruritus. Small groups may be treated with topical podophyllin. Widespread lesions require surgical excision or diathermy. Recurrence is common.

Gonorrhoea

Gonococcal proctitis presents with pain, bleeding and purulent rectal discharge. Proctoscopy reveals ulcerated friable mucosa and pus in the rectal lumen. Culture confirms diagnosis. Treatment is usually by i.m. procaine penicillin and probenecid.

Herpes

Severe perianal pain, constipation, discharge and ulceration. Examination reveals vesicles and ulcers. Treatment is by topical or oral aciclovir.

Syphilis

Perianal or anal ulcers. May resemble anal fissure. Often painless. Diagnosis is confirmed by dark field examination of discharge and serology. Penicillin is treatment of choice. Contact follow-up is important.

Acquired Immunodeficiency Syndrome (AIDS)

Anorectal manifestations include fissure, perianal sepsis, ulceration, fungal or viral infections, rectal lymphoma and Kaposi's sarcoma.

Premalignant Anal Conditions

Over 80% of anal cancers are squamous cell cancers that are an end result of changes secondary to sexually acquired HPV infection. The premalignant dysplastic changes are called intraepithelial neoplasia and are graded I–III according to the depth of epithelium that has been affected. AIN I and II run a relatively benign course and can be observed. Although we are unsure about the natural history of AIN III, common practice is to excise small areas and carefully observe/biopsy larger areas regularly.

Anal Malignancies

Overall, anal tumours are rare, accounting for only 4% of lower GI malignancies, and include epidermoid tumours, malignant melanoma, lymphoma (often in association with AIDS) and Kaposi's sarcoma (associated with AIDS). Adenocarcinoma occurs in the upper part of the anal canal but may spread across the dentate line and appear at the anal margin. The most common of the tumours is the epidermoid carcinoma (squamous cell carcinoma). Patients should be checked for a history of homosexuality with penetrative anal sex.

Symptoms and Signs. Bleeding, pruritus, pain, discharge, palpable mass in anal canal. Patients may think they have haemorrhoids. Rectal examination may reveal visible tumour growing out of the anus. Hard, irregular, ulcerated mass. Palpable inguinal nodes. Hepatomegaly if secondaries.

Investigations

- Biopsy
- USS liver.

Treatment. Only very small, noninvasive lesions may be locally excised. For the vast majority of cases, first-line treatment is long course of chemoradiotherapy. A salvage abdominoperineal resection is performed if the cancer fails to respond or the cancer recurs.

Prognosis. Between 60% and 75% of patients survive 5 years.

RECTAL BLEEDING

Bleeding PR is a common clinical problem. The commonest causes are haemorrhoids, fissure-in-ano and colorectal cancer. Massive rectal bleeding may be due to diverticular disease, angiodysplasia, or a cause in the upper GI tract, e.g. peptic ulcer or an aorto-enteric fistula. If bright red rectal haemorrhage is coming from the upper GI tract, the bleeding is massive with rapid gut transit time and the patient will always be shocked. (For causes of rectal bleeding→Table 15.3.)

Symptoms and Signs. Check colour and amount of blood. Bright red bleeding in small amounts usually indicates that the source is in the anal canal or rectum. Large amounts suggest diverticular disease or angiodysplasia. Bleeding from haemorrhoids may occasionally be considerable. Blood on toilet paper suggests haemorrhoids or fissure-in-ano. Dripping into the toilet at defaecation suggests haemorrhoids. Blood streaked on stools suggests rectosigmoid or rectal carcinoma. Blood and mucus on defaecation suggest rectal carcinoma. Blood, mucus and pus associated with abdominal pain, diarrhoea and fever, suggest colitis. Bleeding associated with change in bowel habit and abdominal pain suggests colonic cancer. Bleeding associated with pain on defaecation suggests fissure-in-ano or carcinoma of the anal canal. Check for abdominal pain, anal pain, change in bowel habit, abdominal distension. Symptoms of anaemia, weight loss, jaundice. Abdominal mass, e.g. colonic tumour, hepatomegaly (metastases). Abdominal tenderness, distended abdomen – shifting dullness (ascites) – obstructed bowel sounds. Inspection PR for piles, warts, fissure, tumour. Rectal mass (90% of rectal cancers can be felt on examination PR).

TABLE 15.3

CAUSES OF RECTAL BLEEDING

Haemorrhoids
Fissure-in-ano
Carcinoma of anus
Colorectal carcinoma
Colorectal polyps
Diverticular disease
Inflammatory bowel disease:
• Crohn's disease
• Ulcerative colitis
Ischaemic colitis
Angiodysplasia
Irradiation colitis or proctitis
Rectal prolapse
Meckel's diverticulum
Intussusception
Mesenteric infarction
Aortoenteric fistula
Massive upper GI haemorrhage
Trauma
Bleeding diathesis

Investigations

- Hb
- FBC
- U&Es (ureteric involvement with colorectal tumours)
- LFTs (liver metastases)
- Clotting screen
- Proctoscopy: haemorrhoids
- Sigmoidoscopy and biopsy
- Barium enema (rarely used nowadays)
- Colonoscopy
- Selective mesenteric angiography and embolisation, preferably in bleeding phase
- Radiolabelled autologous red cells
- Technetium scanning (taken up by ectopic gastric mucosa in Meckel's)
- Gastroscopy if upper GI haemorrhage suspected.

Treatment. Principles of treatment include:

- Resuscitation if massive bleeding
- Diagnosis of the cause
- Definitive treatment of the cause.

The treatment of the various conditions is covered elsewhere in this book.

TABLE 15.4
CAUSES OF HEPATOMEGALY

Regular generalised enlargement without jaundice	Cirrhosis
	Congestive cardiac failure
	Reticuloses
	Budd–Chiari syndrome (hepatic vein obstruction)
	Amyloid
Regular generalised enlargement with jaundice	Viral hepatitis
	Biliary tract obstruction
	Cholangitis
Irregular generalised enlargement without jaundice	Secondary tumours
	Macronodular cirrhosis
	Polycystic disease
	Primary tumours
Irregular generalised enlargement with jaundice	Cirrhosis
	Widespread liver secondaries
Localised swellings	Riedel's lobe
	Hydatid cyst
	Amoebic abscess
	Primary carcinoma

LIVER

Diseases of the liver usually present to the surgeon as jaundice, hepatomegaly, or ascites. This section will deal only with liver disease as far as it concerns the surgeon. (For causes of hepatomegaly→Table 15.4.)

Infections in the Liver

Abscess

This is rare and usually caused by pyogenic bacteria (80% of cases). Causes are due to the following:

- Portal pyelophlebitis secondary to acute abdominal infection, e.g. appendicitis, diverticulitis, peritonitis
- Biliary disease, e.g. cholecystitis, ascending cholangitis
- Trauma
- Direct extension from subphrenic abscess, empyema of gallbladder
- Septicaemia

- Infection of a liver cyst
- Rarely there is no cause, i.e. cryptogenic.

Symptoms and Signs. Those of underlying disease. Fever, toxic, rigours, jaundice, upper abdominal pain, may be of acute onset with no apparent underlying cause. Tender hepatomegaly.

Investigations

- WCC
- LFTs: abnormal
- Blood cultures positive
- USS
- CT (95–100% sensitivity)
- Gallium and technetium radionuclide scan.

Differential Diagnosis. Tumour (HCC), amoebic abscess, hydatid cyst.

Treatment. Multiple small abscesses require a prolonged course of intravenous antibiotics, e.g. gentamicin and metronidazole. Prognosis is poor. These often complicate septicaemia in an immunocompromised patient. Solitary or multiple large abscesses may be treated by percutaneous drainage under radiological guidance. Surgery is rarely required, unless it is for the underlying cause (appendicitis, diverticular abscess) or failed radiological management.

Amoebic Abscess

Accounts for 10% of all liver abscesses and is due to infection with the protozoan parasite *Entamoeba histolytica*. *Entamoeba* cysts are transmitted by food and water contamination (faeco-oral spread). Liver abscesses are the most frequent sequelae of intestinal infection but >50% occur in the absence of amoebic dysentery. Abscesses may be single (common) or multiple. They may be small or very large containing up to 3L of pus. They are more common in the right lobe of the liver. Cases in Europe occur in immigrants or those who have returned from areas where the disease is endemic (Mexico, India, Asia and Africa).

Symptoms and Signs. Insidious onset. Right hypochondrial pain. Malaise. Pyrexia. Weight loss. Occasionally rigours and diarrhoea. Jaundice uncommon.

Investigations

- USS
- CT – characteristic contrast-enhancing peripheral rim.

Treatment. Metronidazole. Large abscesses (>5cm) and those failing to respond to metronidazole require percutaneous drainage under radiological guidance. Surgery is rarely required and should be avoided.

Hydatid Disease

Due to infection with an *Echinococcus granulosus* (tapeworm). The tapeworm develops in the dog intestine and ova are shed in the faeces. These contaminate grass or vegetables and are ingested by sheep, cattle or humans. The ova then pass to the liver via the portal circulation where they develop into hydatid cysts. These may also enter the kidneys and lungs. The disease occurs in sheep- and cattle-rearing countries of the world, e.g. Australia, Africa and Wales.

Symptoms and Signs. Mass without associated symptoms, or associated with abdominal pain. Hepatomegaly. Jaundice (due to pressure on ducts). Rupture into the peritoneal cavity results in peritonitis and anaphylactic shock.

Investigations

- AXR: calcified outline of cyst
- Hydatid serology
- USS
- CT – to demonstrate daughter cysts and hydatid sand.

Treatment. Medical treatment is with albendazole or mebendazole and these can be used on a perioperative basis. This may result in shrinkage in some cases but usually surgery is indicated. Care must be taken to avoid spilling cyst contents into the peritoneal cavity, which can result in seeding, secondary infestation and anaphylactic shock. The cyst is usually aspirated under direct vision and a scolicidal agent (hypertonic saline, hydrogen peroxide, chlorhexidine, cetrimide) injected into the cyst. The cyst is then carefully excised and the cavity closed.

Liver Tumours

Secondary tumours of the liver are common arising from the GI tract, lung and breast. More than 25% of patients who die of malignant disease have liver secondaries. Primary tumours are rare. The commonest malignant primary tumours are HCC and cholangiocarcinoma. Benign tumours are also rare and include adenoma and cavernous haemangioma.

Primary Malignant Tumours

HEPATOCELLULAR CARCINOMA (HCC). The vast majority of HCC occur on a background of chronic liver disease and cirrhosis. Hence, it is common in Africa and Asia where hepatitis B and hepatitis C are endemic. It is also associated with alcohol (related cirrhosis), the contraceptive pill (through its association with hepatic adenomas), aflatoxin, haemochromatosis and obesity (nonalcoholic steatohepatitis).

Symptoms and Signs. Pre-existing cirrhosis. Abdominal pain. Weight loss. Fever. Ascites. Jaundice. Hepatomegaly.

Investigations

- Hb
- Clotting screen: prothrombin time, INR
- LFTs abnormal, especially liver enzymes (ALT/AST)
- α-Fetoprotein raised (>400 ng/mL considered diagnostic). A normal value does not, however, exclude HCC
- CXR: raised diaphragm, lung secondary
- USS – allows biopsy
- CT – early enhancement during arterial phase with rapid washout during portal venous phase. Also allows volumetric analysis
- MRI.

Treatment. In the absence of cirrhosis, which makes up a small proportion, patients with unifocal HCC may undergo a major hepatectomy (>50% of total liver volume) due to the regenerative capacity of the liver. In patients with cirrhosis, multifocal tumours and the ongoing risk of recurrence in the cirrhotic liver limit surgical options.

Liver transplantation is the only surgical option, which treats the underlying liver disease and removes the HCC.

In patients not suitable for surgical intervention, radiofrequency ablation or transarterial chemoembolisation are feasible options.

Prognosis. Unifocal, small tumours (2 cm) have a good prognosis following hepatectomy, especially in patients without cirrhosis. The risk of recurrence, however, is high at 75% within 5 years.

CHOLANGIOCARCINOMA. Cholangiocarcinoma arises from the cells within the intrahepatic and extrahepatic biliary tree and histologically are adenocarcinomas (>95%). It is less common than HCC with an incidence of 1–2/100,000 per year. There is an association with primary sclerosing cholangitis, parasitic biliary infestation, Caroli's disease and choledochal cysts.

Symptoms and Signs. Usually present with symptoms and signs of obstructive jaundice. Also abdominal pain and weight loss.

Investigations

- Hb
- LFTs: bilirubin ↑, alkaline phosphatase ↑
- Clotting screen: PT
- USS-allows biopsy
- CT
- Magnetic resonance cholangiopancreatography (MRCP) ± angiography
- ERCP or percutaneous transhepatic cholangiography (PTC) – although these are more routinely used to stent the biliary tree to relieve obstruction.

Treatment. Surgical resection is rarely feasible due to advanced stage at presentation. Palliative options include stenting (plastic or metal), surgical bypass or chemotherapy. Rarely liver transplantation may be feasible.

Prognosis. Poor. Most patients are dead within 6 months of diagnosis.

Hepatic Metastases

Common as it is usually the first site of metastatic disease. Colorectal cancer is the most common primary for hepatic metastases.

Symptoms and Signs. Those of the primary tumour. Previous surgery for primary. Anorexia, vomiting, weight loss, cachexia. Upper abdominal pain or discomfort. Jaundice. Ascites. Hard, irregular, palpable liver.

Investigations

- Hb
- LFTs: alkaline phosphatase ↑, bilirubin ↑, albumin ↓
- CEA for colorectal cancer
- USS – allows biopsy
- CT (→ Figure 15.25)
- MRI
- PET.

Treatment. Hepatectomy is the only option that offers the prospect of cure and this may be preceded by portal vein embolisation (induces atrophy of the liver to be resected and hypertrophy of the liver that will remain). Chemotherapy (neoadjuvant or palliative) can be given in selected patients systemically or via the hepatic artery.

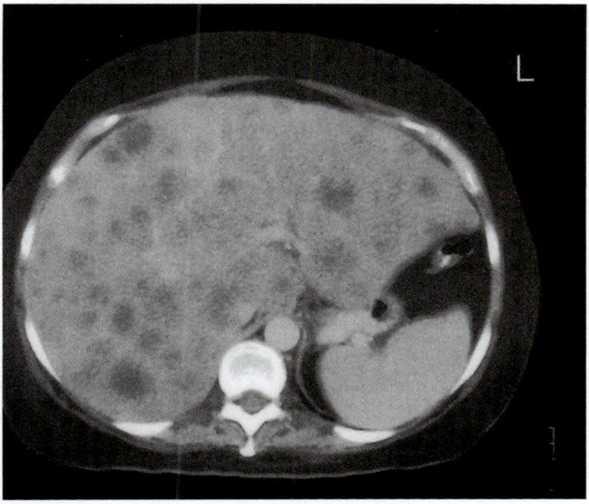

FIGURE 15.25

CT scan of abdomen. Numerous liver metastases are seen in both the right and left lobes of the liver.

Prognosis. Depends upon the primary tumour. Few patients survive 5 years but there is a 35–40% 5-year survival rate for patients with colorectal secondaries that are completely resected.

Portal Hypertension

Portal hypertension occurs when portal venous pressure >12 mmHg. Collateral channels open to divert portal blood flow and 90% is via portosystemic collaterals. The clinically most important portosystemic anastomosis is at the gastro-oesophageal junction, which results in the formation of oesophageal varices. Other consequences of portal hypertension include splenomegaly, ascites (in hepatic and posthepatic forms) and the manifestations of hepatic failure (encephalopathy).

Causes

Prehepatic. Portal vein thrombosis, congenital malformations, extrinsic compression of portal vein (tumour) neonatal umbilical sepsis. Exchange transfusion via umbilical catheter.

Hepatic. Cirrhosis, schistosomiasis, primary biliary cirrhosis

Posthepatic. Budd–Chiari syndrome (obstruction of the hepatic veins, which may be due to idiopathic hepatic vein thrombosis, congenital obliteration, or blockage of the hepatic vein by tumour), constrictive pericarditis.

Symptoms and Signs. Jaundice. Alterations in mental state. Flapping tremor. Coma. Haematemesis and melaena. Ascites. Spider naevi, palmar erythema, clubbing, gynaecomastia, testicular atrophy, caput medusae. Peripheral oedema. Leukonychia. Dupuytren's contracture. Xanthoma. Kayser–Fleischer rings. Bruising.

Investigations

- Hb
- FBC
- LFTs
- Clotting screen: PT, INR
- OGD.

Treatment of Bleeding Oesophageal Varices

Acute Bleed. Resuscitate and use appropriate monitoring. Blood volume replacement. Administer ciprofloxacin or norfloxacin early to increase the risk of survival. Vasoactive drugs (terlipressin, octreotide) reduce portal venous pressure.

Urgent endoscopy to confirm diagnosis. Variceal band ligation is considered first-line therapy although injection of sclerosant can also be used. If a patient rebleeds or continues to bleed, balloon tamponade (Sengstaken–Blakemore tube) can be used as temporary measure until definitive treatment can be offered. Patients who fail to respond should be considered for transjugular intrahepatic portosystemic shunt. Oesophageal transection is very rarely performed.

Definitive Treatment After Bleeding

- Variceal band ligation, β-blocker therapy or a combination of the two
- Portosystemic shunting. Splenoportogram and CT are carried out to assess the patency of the portal vein. Shunts may be portocaval, mesocaval, or splenorenal. They are rarely performed in emergency cases due to the success of endoscopic variceal band ligation. Shunting is usually carried out in the elective stage when there have been previous bleeding episodes. For a successful shunt operation, hepatic function needs to be reasonably good. Jaundice, hypoalbuminaemia, ascites and encephalopathy indicate a poor prognosis with shunt operations. Liver transplantation is preferable except when the obstruction is prehepatic with good liver function.

Prophylaxis. Many patients with varices never bleed unless the hepatic venous pressure gradient exceeds 12 mmHg. If varices are known to be present, oral (nonselective) β-blockade with propranolol significantly decreases the bleeding risk. Those intolerant to β-blockade or have a contraindication can undergo variceal band ligation.

Prognosis. The mortality rate for the first variceal bleed is as high as 30–50%. Long-term survival after portocaval shunt operations is poor. The 5-year survival after portocaval shunting for alcoholic liver disease is about 45%. Some degree of encephalopathy develops in 14–30% of patients.

HINTS AND TIPS

Always suspect variceal bleeding in patients who present with haematemesis on a background of chronic liver disease/cirrhosis. Early intervention using a multidisciplinary approach can reduce morbidity and mortality. As with all acute conditions, adherence to the principles of ABC are integral to successful management.

EXTRAHEPATIC BILIARY SYSTEM

Cholelithiasis (Gallstones)

This is common and present in 10% of the population over 50 years. It is more common in females, especially in multiparous women. Obesity, drugs, contraceptive pill, clofibrate, haemolytic disorders, ileal disease (resection, Crohn's disease) are aetiological factors. Factors that may produce lithogenic bile include increased cholesterol content, reduced bile acids, biliary stasis. Classically three types of stone are described:

- Cholesterol stones: (may be solitary), cholesterol 'solitaire' – radiolucent
- Pigment: occur with haemolysis – small, black, irregular and friable – radiolucent
- Mixed: often faceted – contain calcium, pigment and cholesterol – 10% are radio-opaque (→Figure 15.26).

About 80% of stones are asymptomatic. Symptoms are related to the complications they cause.

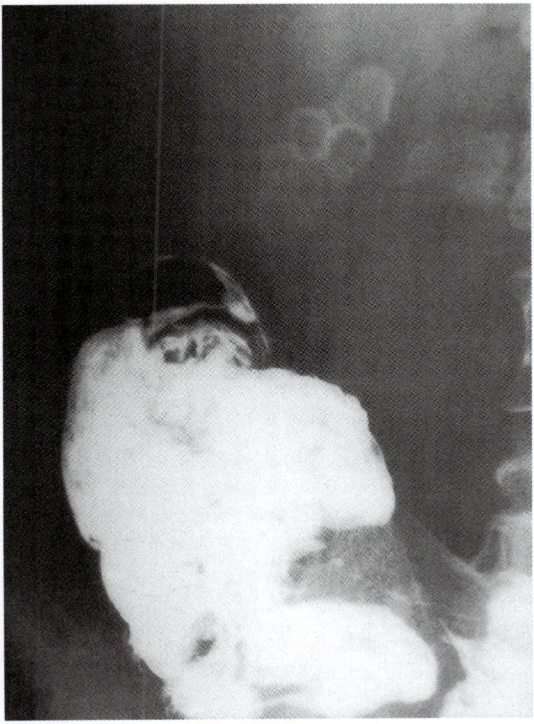

FIGURE 15.26

Gallstones. An incidental finding on barium enema. There are several radio-opaque gallstones in the right hypochondrium.

Complications

Gallbladder. Acute cholecystitis, chronic cholecystitis, acute-on-chronic cholecystitis. Empyema (pus in the gallbladder). Mucocele (mucus in the gallbladder). Carcinoma. Perforation of gallbladder.

In the Ducts. Obstructive jaundice, cholangitis, pancreatitis.

In the Gut. Gallstone ileus (associated with cholecystoduodenal fistula).

Acute Cholecystitis

Gallstones are the most common cause. Rarely, acalculous cholecystitis may occur. Sometimes it is associated with typhoid fever. Most cases are in fact acute-on-chronic, many patients having demonstrated symptoms of chronic cholecystitis in the past.

Symptoms and Signs. Nausea, fever, vomiting. RUQ pain radiating under ribs to right scapula. Tender with guarding in the right hypochondrium. Positive Murphy's sign.

Investigations

- Hb
- WCC
- LFTs
- USS.

Treatment. Acute cholecystitis can be managed with i.v. antibiotics (covering Gram-negative bacteria and anaerobes) and analgesia. Acute cholecystectomy can be performed safely (within 48–72h of symptom commencement) in these patients and is not associated with an increased risk of complications. Alternatively, patients can undergo an elective cholecystectomy after 6 weeks. Patients failing to respond to medical management may undergo a percutaneous cholecystostomy or an emergency cholecystectomy.

Chronic Cholecystitis

Virtually always associated with gallstones. Repeated episodes of infection cause chronic thickening and fibrosis.

Symptoms and Signs. Flatulent dyspepsia. The classical case is the middle-aged obese female patient who gets upper abdominal discomfort and distension relieved by belching. Intolerance of fatty food. Often little to find on clinical examination.

Investigations. USS.

Treatment. Cholecystectomy, which is frequently performed laparoscopically. Unfit patients may be placed on a low-fat diet to control symptoms or treated by extracorporeal shock wave lithotripsy if suitable. Dissolution of stones that are small and non-radio-opaque in a functioning gallbladder may be attempted with chenodeoxycholic acid given orally.

Biliary Colic

This is a symptom rather than a complication of gallstones. It is produced by impaction of a stone in the neck of the gallbladder or in the cystic duct. The stone may either fall back into the gallbladder or pass through the cystic duct into the CBD, whence the pain abates.

Symptoms and Signs. Sudden onset of severe pain across the epigastrium (it is not confined to the RUQ). Severe spasms of colic against the background of continuous severe pain. The patient rolls around in agony and cannot get into a comfortable position. Tachycardia, sweating and vomiting. Examination may reveal rigidity in the upper abdomen (beware of making a diagnosis of peritonitis – in peritonitis the patient does not roll around but remains still). An attack may last 2–4 h. Following an attack, jaundice may occur owing to the passed stone impacting in the CBD (known as choledocholithiasis).

Treatment. Morphine i.v. Subsequent investigations for gallbladder disease and cholecystectomy if appropriate.

Mucocele

This may follow an attack of biliary colic. Stone impacts in neck of gallbladder. Bile absorbed. Mucus secretion continues.

Symptoms and Signs. Previous history of biliary colic. RUQ discomfort. Occasionally patient feels lump. Large, tense globular mass in RUQ.

Investigations. USS.

Treatment. Cholecystectomy.

Empyema

This follows an attack of cholecystitis. Infection develops after impaction of a stone in the neck of the gallbladder. Obstruction leads to stasis, overgrowth of bacteria and the gallbladder fills with pus.

Symptoms and Signs. Attack of acute cholecystitis or biliary colic. Fever, toxicity. RUQ pain. Tender mass in RUQ.

Investigations

- WCC
- USS
- CT – may demonstrate gas within the wall (emphysematous gallbladder).

Treatment. Give i.v. fluids and i.v. antibiotics (covering Gram-negative bacteria and anaerobes). Patients with confirmed empyema may be managed conservatively with percutaneous drainage (cholecystostomy), which is under radiological guidance. Surgery is rarely indicated as patients are usually too unwell. Cholecystectomy, if indicated, may be undertaken at a later date.

Perforation of the Gallbladder

This is rare and usually presents either as generalised biliary peritonitis or leakage of pus from a perforated empyema. Infected biliary peritonitis has a high mortality especially as this condition is most common in the elderly. Treatment can involve i.v. antibiotics, percutaneous drainage or laparotomy with peritoneal lavage and cholecystectomy.

Carcinoma

Is a rare disease and is associated with long-standing gallstone disease, adenomatous polyps and is three times commoner in females. Local invasion of the liver and bile ducts occurs. Jaundice occurs owing to direct extension into the bile duct together with secondaries in the nodes at the porta hepatis. Small tumours may be an incidental finding at cholecystectomy for gallstones. In the latter case, long-term survival may be expected. Many cases present late when local spread and lymph node metastases have occurred. In this case, prognosis is poor – 90% of patients surviving less than 1 year.

Cholangitis

This is a serious condition caused by complete or partial biliary obstruction (gallstones, tumour) in association with ascending infection of the biliary tree. It may be complicated by septicaemia and liver abscesses.

Symptoms and Signs. RUQ pain, fever (with rigours), jaundice – known as Charcot's biliary triad. When in combination with hypotension and mental state changes, it is known as Reynold's pentad.

Investigations

- WCC
- LFTs
- Blood cultures
- USS
- MRCP.

Treatment. Antibiotics – cefuroxime/metronidazole/gentamicin. Acute suppurative cholangitis may occur with pus under tension in the biliary tree. Urgent decompression of the biliary tree is required and can be performed endoscopically (ERCP) or radiologically (PTC) depending on the underlying pathology.

Gallstone Ileus

This results from a fistula occurring between the fundus of the gallbladder and the adjacent duodenum. A stone passes through the fistula and may impact in the terminal ileum causing obstruction to the small bowel.

Symptoms and Signs. Colicky abdominal pain, vomiting and distension. History of flatulent dyspepsia. The diagnosis should be suspected in middle-aged to elderly females with symptoms of small bowel obstruction in the absence of a hernia or previous abdominal surgery to suggest adhesion formation.

Investigations. AXR: dilated loops of small bowel, air in the biliary tree (→ Figure 15.27A). CT, dilated small bowel, gallstone in lumen, air in biliary tree (Figure 15.27B).

Treatment. Laparotomy. Removal of stone from small bowel lumen by 'milking' through ileocaecal valve or removal by enterotomy proximal to where gallstone has impacted. Enterotomy closed transversely to avoid stricturing the small bowel. Cholecystectomy at a later date if symptoms referable to gallbladder continue.

Acalculous Cholecystitis

Acute cholecystitis without gallstones may occur in a variety of conditions but invariably occurs in sick patients on critical care. It may be due to infection, e.g. typhoid, or may occur following sepsis, burns, TPN, multiple injuries, in the puerperium and after unrelated surgery. Treatment is the same as for calculous acute cholecystitis, using i.v. antibiotics ± percutaneous drainage.

Treatment of Gallstones

Nonsurgical Treatment

Oral Dissolution Therapy. Suitable for small (<1 cm) radiolucent cholesterol stones in a functioning gallbladder. Ursodeoxycholic acid can be given orally. Side effects include diarrhoea, pruritus and transient rise in serum transaminases. Treatment must be continued for >6 months. Recurrence rates are high.

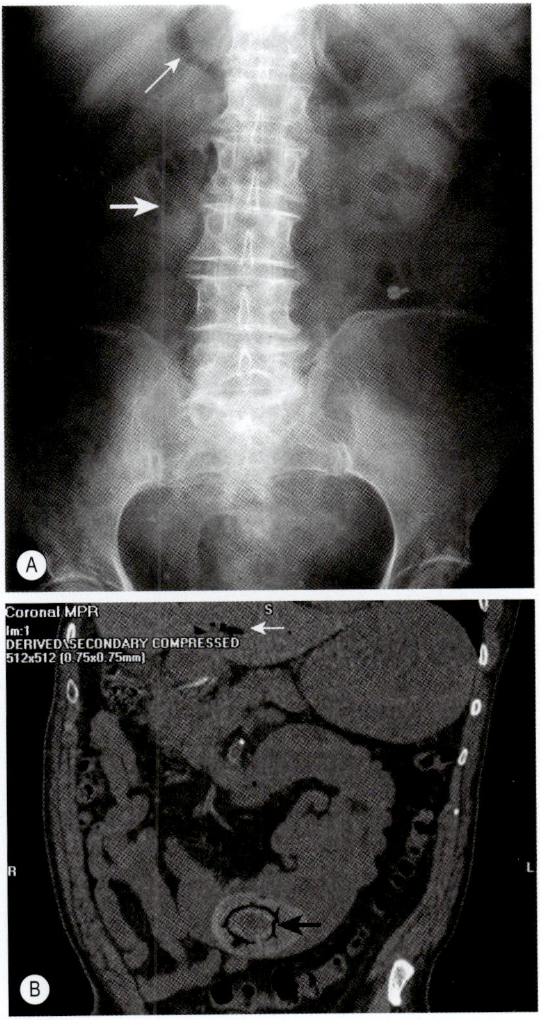

FIGURE 15.27

(**A**) Plain AXR showing gallstone ileus. In this case, a large non-radio-opaque stone was obstructing the upper jejunum. Only one small loop of distended bowel is seen in the abdomen (large arrow). Gas is clearly seen in the biliary tree (small arrow) indicating the presence of a cholecystoduodenal fistula. (**B**) CT abdomen showing gallstone ileus. A large gallstone (large arrow) is seen in a dilated loop of small bowel. Gas is seen in the intrahepatic biliary tree (small arrow).

Extracorporeal Shock Wave Lithotripsy. Suitable for medium-sized, radiolucent stones in a functioning gallbladder. Concurrent treatment with ursodeoxycholic acid is required. Treatment by this method requires further evaluation. Biliary colic may occur as fragments are passed through the cystic duct.

Endoscopy. Stones in the CBD (choledocholithiasis) may be managed with ERCP, which involves a sphincterotomy and stone extraction. This treatment is suitable for patients with CBD stones and preventing recurrence of gallstone pancreatitis in patients who are unfit for a cholecystectomy. It allows jaundice to settle even if there are residual stones in the gallbladder; further treatment is required if the patient is fit for a cholecystectomy. It is useful also for removing retained stones postcholecystectomy or stones forming in the CBD (secondary stones).

Treatment of Asymptomatic Gallstones. These may be seen on AXR or USS carried out for other conditions, or they may be discovered at laparotomy for another condition. Generally intervention is not recommended in patients who are asymptomatic as <25% will develop symptoms within 10 years.

Obstructive Jaundice

Jaundice occurs when the serum bilirubin exceeds 35 mmol/L. Obstructive jaundice, known as posthepatic jaundice, occurs because of obstruction of the extrahepatic biliary tree.

Causes

In the Lumen. Gallstones (common), roundworms (rare), blood clots in haemobilia.

In the Wall. Congenital biliary atresia, traumatic stricture, sclerosing cholangitis, cholangiocarcinoma, choledochal cysts.

Outside the Wall. Carcinoma of the head of the pancreas, carcinoma of the ampulla of Vater, malignant nodes in the porta hepatis, Mirrizi's syndrome (a rare complication in which a gallstone becomes impacted in the neck of the gallbladder causing compression of the adjacent common hepatic duct).

Symptoms and Signs. Previous history of cholecystectomy. Previous history of malignancy. Painless jaundice suggests malignancy. Jaundice preceded by severe upper abdominal pain suggests gallstones. Gradual onset of jaundice associated with dark urine and pale stools. Pruritus. Smooth palpable liver. Palpable gallbladder (carcinoma of pancreas or ampulla of Vater); Courvoisier's law states that 'if in the presence of jaundice the gallbladder is palpable, the cause of the jaundice is unlikely to be due to stones'. The reason for this is that with gallstone disease the gallbladder is usually fibrotic and unable to distend and thus become palpable.

Investigations

- Hb
- FBC
- U&Es
- LFTs: conjugated bilirubin and alkaline phosphatase markedly raised
- PT: may be clotting defect due to poor absorption of vitamin K (fat-soluble vitamin)
- USS: may show dilated ducts and site of obstruction, gallstones in gallbladder; the technique is poor for the lower end of the bile duct and head of pancreas as gas may obscure view

- CT: shows intrahepatic lesions, pancreatic lesions, demonstrates invasion of adjacent structures
- MRCP
- ERCP (→Figure 15.28): allows biopsy and brush cytology, defines level of lesion, allows stenting and relief of jaundice
- PTC (→Figure 15.29) if ERCP impossible
- Liver biopsy.

Treatment. Check PT. Correct any clotting derangement with parenteral vitamin K ± fresh frozen plasma. Provide i.v. crystalloids to reduce risk of hepatorenal syndrome. Mannitol (i.v.) may be used as a renal protective agent. Antibiotics should be given if there is evidence of cholangitis. Subsequent treatment depends on the cause of jaundice:

Gallstone in CBD. Explore duct at time of cholecystectomy or remove pre- or postoperatively with ERCP.

Congenital Biliary Atresia. (→Ch. 21).

Traumatic Stricture. Needs bypass via Roux loop of intestine anastomosed to the proximal dilated duct.

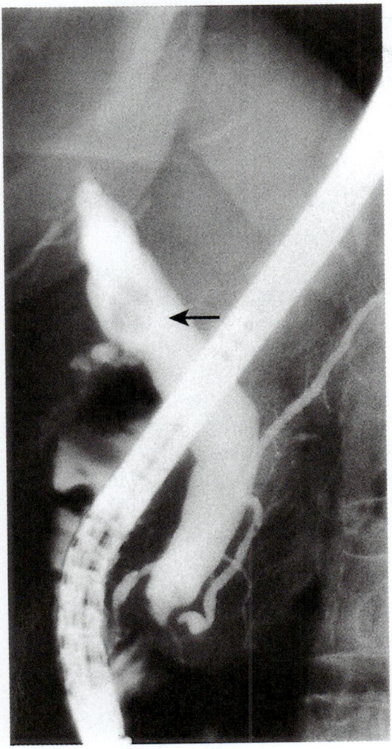

FIGURE 15.28
ERCP. A gallstone (arrow) is seen in the dilated bile duct.

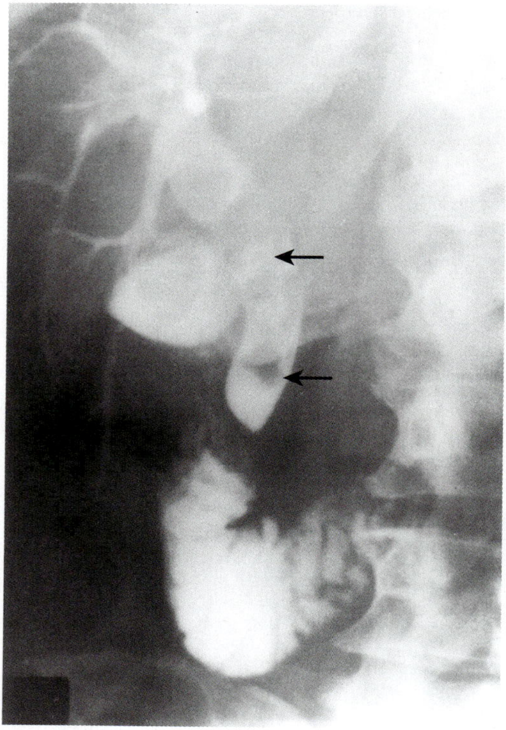

FIGURE 15.29

A percutaneous transhepatic cholangiogram. At least two stones (arrows) are seen within a grossly dilated bile duct. There is free flow of contrast into the duodenum.

Sclerosing Cholangitis. Hepaticojejunostomy, i.e. anastomose a loop of jejunum to a dilated duct at the hilum of the liver. Stenting by endoscopic retrograde route or percutaneous transhepatic route may be of benefit. The prognosis is poor.

Cholangiocarcinoma. Primary resection is rarely possible and has a high mortality. Stenting combined with palliative chemotherapy can prolong life to a degree, but overall survival is poor.

Choledochal Cyst. Excision of cyst with Roux-en-Y choledochojejunostomy.

Carcinoma of the Head of the Pancreas or Ampulla of Vater. Attempted curative resection may be carried out via a pancreaticoduodenectomy (Kausch–Whipple procedure). Relatively few tumours are curable due to late presentation. Recurrence rates are high. If the tumour is inoperable due to local invasion of adjacent structures or the presence of liver metastases, stenting may be carried out (either by ERCP or PTC). If the tumour is found to be inoperable at laparotomy, a 'triple bypass' is carried out (→ section on pancreas).

Nodes at the Porta Hepatis. Stenting is the treatment of choice. Palliative chemotherapy may help depending upon the type of tumour invading the nodes.

Complications of Surgery on the Jaundiced Patient. Coagulation disorders. Hepatorenal failure. GI tract haemorrhage (stress ulcers). Delayed wound healing.

HINTS AND TIPS

Obstructive jaundice invariably results in a coagulopathy. The poor absorption of vitamin K secondary to the absence of bile salts in GI tract results in reduced synthesis of factors II, VII, IX and X. Vitamin K is an essential cofactor in the synthesis of these factors. This results in a prolonged PT and can be reversed with the administration of parenteral vitamin K. In patients with a haemorrhagic diathesis the provision of fresh frozen plasma or prothrombin concentrates may be necessitated.

PANCREAS

Pancreatitis

Pancreatitis may be divided into acute and chronic. Acute pancreatitis is a condition presenting with acute onset of abdominal pain associated with raised levels of pancreatic enzymes in the blood and urine. The gland normally returns to functional and anatomical normality. Recurrent attacks may occur (relapsing acute pancreatitis). Chronic pancreatitis is a continuing inflammatory disease characterised by irreversible functional and anatomical abnormalities in the gland, resulting in fibrosis of the gland and pancreatic insufficiency.

Acute Pancreatitis

Aetiological factors include gallstones (40%), alcohol (35%). Other causes include hyperlipidaemia, hyperparathyroidism (hypercalcaemia), viral infections (mumps, Coxsackie virus), hypothermia, trauma, pancreatic divisum, drugs (steroids, oestrogen-containing contraceptives, azathioprine, thiazide diuretics), hereditary, scorpion bites, idiopathic (10%), autoimmune (IgG4-related), post-ERCP, pancreatic carcinoma.

Symptoms and Signs. Severe epigastric pain radiating through to back. Nausea, vomiting, shock. Tender in epigastrium initially spreading to whole abdomen. Abdominal distension. Absent bowel sounds. Bluish discoloration in flank (Grey Turner's sign) or periumbilical area (Cullen's sign) – due to severe haemorrhagic pancreatitis with spread of blood retroperitoneally to these areas.

Investigations

- Hb
- Hct – >0.47 on admission is measure of severe disease
- WCC↑
- U&Es
- LFTs: bilirubin↑, mild derangement of others
- Amylase raised >1000 μ/L (three times the reference range is diagnostic)
- Urinary amylase if delayed presentation
- Lipase (more specific than amylase)

- Ca^{2+}↓
- Blood sugar↑
- ABG – PO_2↓
- ECG changes may occur, diminished T waves. Beware the patient with haemorrhagic pancreatitis who presents late and in whom the amylase is normal because of extensive destruction of the pancreas
- AXR: absent psoas shadows, 'sentinel loop' adjacent to pancreas because of local ileus
- CXR: small pleural effusions
- USS: should be performed in all patients with acute pancreatitis to look for gallstones
- CT: only indicated if no clear diagnosis or absence of clinical improvement – may demonstrate necrosis, peripancreatic collections, abscess. Severity can be determined using Balthazar grading.

Complications. ARF. ARDS. Gastric erosions (haematemesis and melaena). Disseminated intravascular coagulation. Psychosis. Diabetes. Local complications include pancreatic necrosis, abscess formation, pseudocyst formation. Relapsing acute pancreatitis. Chronic pancreatitis.

Differential Diagnosis. Perforated peptic ulcer. Acute exacerbation of peptic ulcer. Cholecystitis. Mesenteric infarction. MI.

Treatment

Mild Case. Supportive care with provision of i.v. fluids and appropriate analgesia. Antibiotics are not indicated. Nutrition is key and patients can take oral diet with supplements. Enteral feeding can also be used. Regular blood tests provide evidence of recovery (WCC, CRP).

Severe Case. Severity is indicated by Ranson's criteria:

- At presentation, age >55 years, WCC >16×10^9/L, glucose >11 mmol/L, LDH >350 IU/L, AST >200 IU/L
- During first 48 h: PCV: fall >10%, urea >16 mmol/L, Ca^{2+} <2 mmol/L, PaO_2 <8 kPa, base deficit <4. The more criteria present the greater the mortality
- Patients with organ dysfunction >48 h are defined as severe pancreatitis (American College of Gastroenterologists).

Patients with severe pancreatitis need supportive care in a critical care unit. Treatment involves provision of i.v. fluids, catheterisation to measure hourly urine output, analgesia and early enteral feeding (NG or nasojejunal (NJ)). Stress-ulcer prophylaxis should be used and include PPIs or H_2-receptor antagonists. Unwell patients may need organ support in the form of inotropes/vasopressors, calcium gluconate for hypocalcaemia, intubation and ventilation for ARDS, dialysis for ARF. Antibiotics are not recommended unless there are signs of sepsis related to the pancreatitis (e.g. infected pancreatic necrosis/peripancreatic collections).

Indications for Surgery

- Patients who continue to deteriorate with CT evidence of necrosis may require a necrosectomy, which is associated with a high mortality rate. Percutaneous and minimally invasive necrosectomies are favoured.
- Drainage of pseudocyst – wait >6 weeks to mature. Cystogastrostomy can be performed if pseudocyst is symptomatic.
- Early cholecystectomy is recommended if gallstones are the cause.

Prognosis. Mortality rate overall is about 10%, especially those with biliary pancreatitis. Patients with severe pancreatitis have a mortality of 30%.

HINTS AND TIPS

Acute pancreatitis can be diagnosed based on the presence of two out of three of the following: (1) serum amylase/lipase greater than three times upper limit of normal, (2) abdominal pain consistent with pancreatitis, (3) characteristic findings from abdominal imaging (American College of Gastroenterology).

Chronic Pancreatitis

Defined as chronic inflammation of the pancreas with irreversible morphological changes.

Alcohol abuse is responsible for most cases (~60–70%). Less common causes include autoimmune, hereditary, cystic fibrosis, hyperlipidaemia and idiopathic pancreatitis (20–30%). Direct trauma with subsequent duct stricture may also result in chronic pancreatitis.

Damage to acini occurs with destruction of the parenchyma leading to atrophy, fibrosis, calcification and ductal stenoses with dilatation distally.

Symptoms and Signs. Intermittent upper abdominal/epigastric pain with radiation through to the back. Weight loss. Nausea, vomiting, steatorrhoea. A range of 30–40% develop diabetes. A few patients may become addicted to narcotic analgesics because of the severity of the pain. Upper abdominal tenderness. Occasionally jaundice if CBD obstructed.

Investigations

- AXR: speckled pancreatic calcification (only observed in 25–30%)
- Blood glucose may be raised
- Ca may be raised
- Lipid profile (hyperlipidaemia)
- Amylase elevated during acute exacerbations. In the late stages, atrophy of the pancreas can result in 'normal' serum amylase levels
- Faecal elastase-1: <200 μg/g
- USS: cystic change and duct dilatation
- CT: atrophic pancreas, calcification, dilated pancreatic duct, pseudocysts
- MRCP/ERCP: assess duct dilatation and stenoses.

Treatment

Medical. Stop alcohol and smoking. Low-fat diet. Pancreatic extracts given orally (Pancrex or Creon). Treat diabetes mellitus. Fat-soluble vitamins. Adequate analgesia (opiates may be required). Coeliac plexus blockade may be necessary.

Surgical. Largely carried out for pain to improve duct drainage. Decompression of the duct by endoscopic sphincterotomy and insertion of pancreatic duct stent at ERCP. Longitudinal, lateral pancreaticojejunostomy (Frey procedure) may be carried out. Other operations include resection of the head, body and tail or whole gland. If total pancreatectomy is required, brittle diabetes results – consider isolating the islets cells from the pancreas and carrying out islet autotransplantation.

Prognosis. Depends upon ability to abstain from alcohol and smoking. Thirty percent of patients die within 10 years. There is a small risk of developing pancreatic cancer. Some patients have a miserable life with narcotic addiction, diabetes mellitus and malnutrition.

Pancreatic Cysts

True cysts are rare and may be associated with congenital polycystic disease, retention cysts, hydatid disease and tumour (cystadenoma and cystadenocarcinoma). Pseudocysts are more common and are a consequence of acute pancreatitis, pancreatic trauma or, rarely, posterior perforation of a gastric ulcer.

Pancreatic Pseudocyst

This is a localised collection of fluid (typically the lesser sac) rich in pancreatic enzymes (e.g. amylase) with a nonepithelialised wall that is related to a recent attack of acute pancreatitis (>6 weeks).

Symptoms and Signs. Pancreatic trauma. Acute pancreatitis. Perforated posterior GU. Rarely no history. Development of a tender epigastric mass. Fever, weight loss, nausea and vomiting (gastric outlet obstruction).

Investigation

- WCC
- Amylase – elevated
- Bilirubin occasionally elevated (with compression of extrahepatic biliary tree)
- USS
- CT: collection of fluid in lesser sac. Also allows assessment of wall thickness, which is relevant in planning treatment.

Complications. If left, most pseudocysts will resolve spontaneously. Rarely infection (10%), rupture, or haemorrhage into the cyst may occur.

Treatment. Indications for intervention include symptomatic pseudocysts or those causing complications.

Percutaneous drainage (USS or CT guidance) especially for infected pseudocysts. Endoscopic drainage, which can be transmural (through posterior wall of stomach) or transpapillary (stenting pancreatic duct). Surgical drainage can be performed laparoscopically and involves formation of a cystogastrostomy (posterior gastric wall).

Tumours of the Pancreas

Carcinoma of the Pancreas

Adenocarcinoma of the pancreas is increasing in frequency in the age range 40–60 years and is the eighth leading cause of cancer-related death worldwide. It is rarely curable because of local invasion or lymph node metastases before it has been detected. Early diagnosis is difficult due to nonspecific symptoms. Some 75% occur in the head of the pancreas, 15–20% in the body and the remainder in the tail. Risk factors include diabetes mellitus, alcoholism (related to chronic pancreatitis), cigarette smoking.

Symptoms and Signs. Epigastric pain. Deep, boring back pain. Obstructive jaundice (head of pancreas, secondaries in porta hepatis). Weight loss, fatigue, malaise, indigestion, pruritus. Palpable epigastric mass. Palpable gallbladder (Courvoisier's law – 'if in the presence of jaundice the gallbladder is palpable, the cause of the jaundice is unlikely to be stones'). Hepatomegaly. Thrombophlebitis migrans. Rarely splenomegaly due to splenic vein thrombosis from direct invasion of latter. Virchow's node.

Investigations

- Hb
- FBC
- ESR
- LFTs
- Blood sugar
- CA 19–9: elevated in ~75%
- USS: often small mass obscured by bowel gas
- CT scan (→Figure 15.30) degree of invasion, metastases, guided biopsy, assess tumour resectability
- EUS – complements CT. Allows FNA and assesses resectability
- PET scan: metastases
- MRCP
- ERCP: although can be diagnostic (brush cytology, biopsy), frequently reserved for biliary decompression.

Treatment

- Pancreaticoduodenectomy (Kausch–Whipple procedure) for carcinoma of the head of the pancreas (→Figure 15.31). This involves a partial gastrectomy, partial pancreatectomy (head of pancreas), distal choledochectomy and cholecystectomy. All above share the same common blood supply, hence the extensive resection. A pylorus-preserving pancreaticoduodenectomy can also be performed.

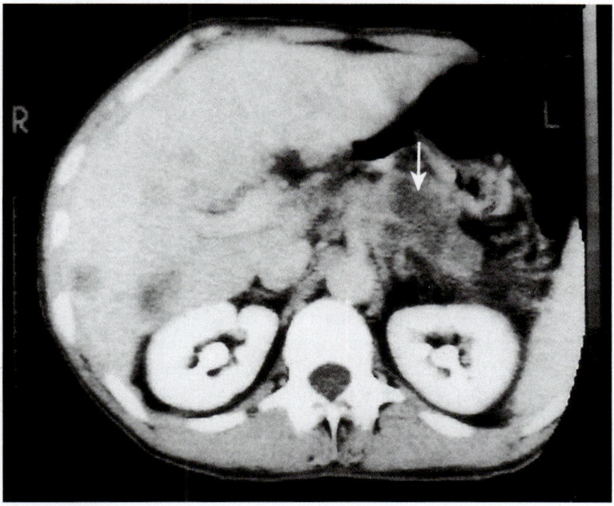

FIGURE 15.30
CT scan of the upper abdomen. There is a carcinoma in the pancreas (arrow).

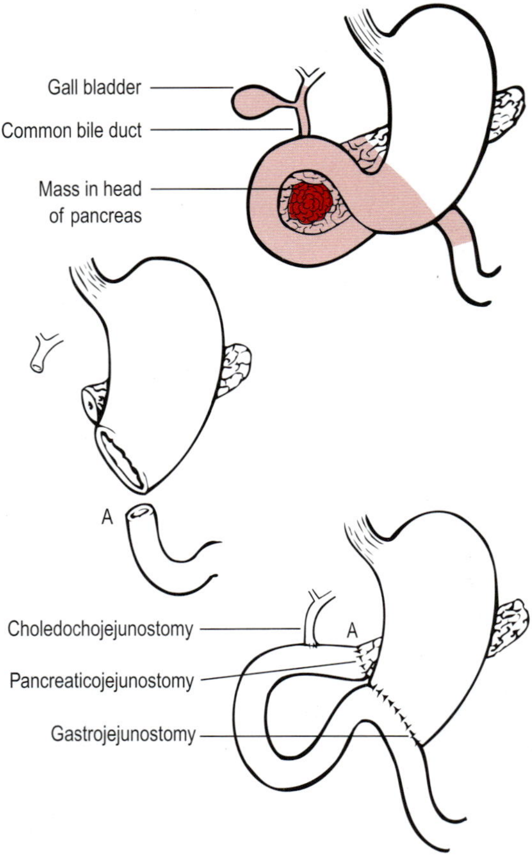

FIGURE 15.31

Pancreaticoduodenectomy (Whipple's operation). The shaded area is excised.

Continuity is re-established via a Roux-en-Y choledochojejunostomy, pancreaticojejunostomy and gastroenterostomy. Operative mortality is high (~5%). Relatively few cases are suitable for this operation due to local invasion (portal vein, superior mesenteric vessels).

- Total pancreatectomy for extensive tumour.
- Tumours in the tail may be treated by distal pancreatectomy.
- Palliative decompression and relief of jaundice can be treated by 'triple bypass', i.e. cholecystojejunostomy (to drain bile past the obstruction from gallbladder to jejunum), jejunojejunostomy (to prevent food passing up into the gallbladder),

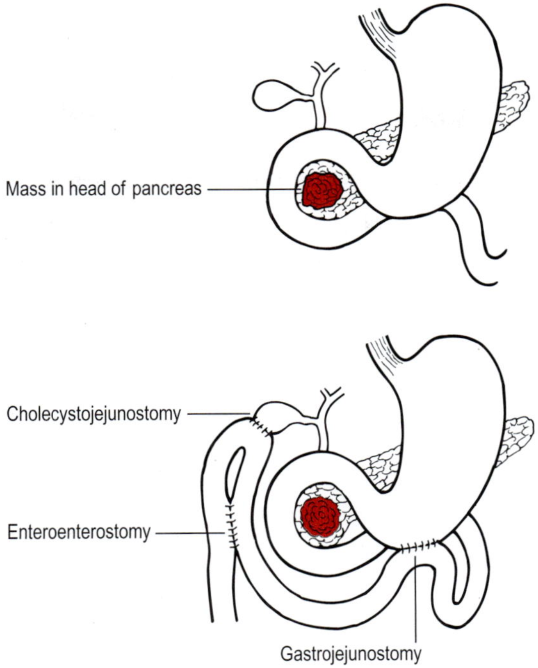

FIGURE 15.32
Triple bypass for carcinoma of the head of the pancreas.

and gastrojejunostomy (to ensure adequate drainage of food from the stomach should the tumour invade the duodenum) (→Figure 15.32).

- As the prognosis is poor and many cases are inoperable at presentation, biliary stenting (ERCP/PTC) to relieve the jaundice is becoming the treatment of choice.

Prognosis. The 5-year survival rate following curative surgery is 15–20%. The overall 5-year survival, however, is poor at 5%.

HINTS AND TIPS

The retroperitoneal location of the pancreas accounts for the back pain or radiation through to the back associated with pancreatic pathology. However, due its retroperitoneal position, pancreatic cancer can be associated with insidious symptoms of malaise or back pain alone. Back pain with pancreatic cancer is an ominous sign suggesting local infiltration. As a consequence, pancreatic cancer presents late with weight loss or obstructive jaundice usually when it is inoperable.

Endocrine Tumours of the Pancreas

Rare. Include gastrinomas (see ZES, above), insulinomas and, more rarely, glucagonomas and VIPomas (vasoactive intestinal peptide).

Insulinoma

Some 80% are solitary benign tumours of the β cells; 10% are malignant and 10% are multiple. Insulinomas are associated with MEN type 1. They result in hyperinsulinaemia and the symptoms are related to the subsequent hypoglycaemia.

Symptoms and Signs

Related to Cerebral Glucose Deprivation. These include weakness, diplopia, sweating, palpitations, memory lapse, bizarre behaviour, seizures and coma.

Related to GI Tract. These are hunger, abdominal pain and diarrhoea. Symptoms relieved by eating. Often excessive appetite with weight gain. The classical diagnostic criteria are known as 'Whipple's triad':

- Symptoms of hypoglycaemia
- Low blood sugar at the time of symptoms
- Symptoms are relieved by the administration of glucose.

Investigations

- Prolonged (72h) fasting blood sugar (inappropriate levels of insulin with hypoglycaemia is hallmark)
- Plasma insulin and proinsulin
- C-peptide levels
- EUS
- CT scan to localise tumour
- SRS (Octreoscan)
- Rarely, selective angiography may be required
- Intraoperative ultrasound.

Treatment. Diazoxide to reduce insulin secretion. Octreotide may have benefit. Because of malignant potential, treatment should be surgical exploration and excision.

SPLEEN

Splenomegaly

The spleen must be enlarged to about three times its normal size before it becomes clinically palpable. The lower margin may feel notched to palpation. It may become so large that it is palpable in the RIF. Massive splenomegaly in the UK is likely to be due to CML, myelofibrosis or lymphoma. Splenomegaly may lead to hypersplenism, i.e. pancytopenia as cells become trapped in an overactive spleen and are destroyed. Anaemia, infection, or haemorrhage may result. (For causes of splenomegaly→ Table 15.5.)

INDICATIONS FOR SPLENECTOMY. These are: trauma; as part of other operative procedures, e.g. radical gastrectomy, splenorenal shunting; haematological disease, e.g. haemolytic anaemia, ITP; tumours; cysts; occasionally for diagnosis.

TABLE 15.5
CAUSES OF SPLENOMEGALY

Infective:	
• Bacterial	Typhoid Typhus Tuberculosis Septicaemia Abscess
• Viral	Glandular fever
• Spirochaetal	Syphilis Leptospirosis
• Protozoal	Malaria
• Parasitic	Hydatid cyst
Inflammatory	Rheumatoid arthritis Sarcoid Lupus Amyloid
Neoplastic	Leukaemia Lymphoma Polycythaemia vera Myelofibrosis Primary tumours Metastases
Haemolytic disease	Spherocytosis Acquired haemolytic anaemia Thrombocytopenic purpura
Storage diseases	Gaucher's disease
Deficiency diseases	Pernicious anaemia Severe iron deficiency anaemia
Splenic vein hypertension	Cirrhosis Splenic vein thrombosis Portal vein thrombosis
Nonparasitic cysts	

Effects of Splenectomy

Haematological

- Leukocytosis
- Thrombocytosis – platelet counts rise after splenectomy and may reach 1000×10^9/L. Peak rises usually at 7–10 days. There is little evidence to support an

increased risk of thromboembolic disease. Full anticoagulation is not indicated, although prophylactic aspirin may be given if the platelet count is very high
- Abnormal blood film:
  - nuclear remnants (Howell–Jolly bodies)
  - denatured haemoglobin (Heinz bodies)
  - iron granules (Pappenheimer bodies).

Immunological. Splenectomy removes secondary lymphoid tissue. The spleen is a major site of phagocytosis, antibody production (↓IgM), opsonisation of bacteria. It is also a major reservoir for lymphocytes.

Postsplenectomy Management. Patients who have undergone splenectomy are more susceptible to infection from capsulated organisms, e.g. *Streptococcus pneumoniae, Haemophilus influenzae* and *Neisseria* species. Infections with these organisms can lead to overwhelming postsplenectomy infection. This has an insidious presentation with a prodromal illness, confusion, nausea and collapse; >50% are due to *S. pneumoniae*. The risk is greatest in young children. In patients in whom splenectomy is a planned procedure, vaccination against pneumococcal, meningococcal (groups A, C, W and Y) *H. influenzae* type b infections should be given at least 2 weeks prior to splenectomy. Lifelong prophylactic antibiotics (penicillin or erythromycin) should be offered to those at high risk of pneumococcal infection, which includes children under 16 years of age and those over 50 years. In patients having emergency splenectomy, vaccines should be administered 2 weeks postoperatively. Protection from the polyvalent pneumococcal vaccine (Pneumovax) lasts 4–5 years, after which revaccination is advisable. Patients should also be informed of the increased risk of infection in areas where malaria is endemic.

Rupture of the Spleen (→ Ch. 4)

Spontaneous Rupture. May occur when the spleen is the site of disease, e.g. infectious mononucleosis, malaria, lymphoma, leukaemia, typhoid. In any disease where there is splenomegaly trivial trauma may cause splenic disruption.

PROCEDURES

RIGHT HEMICOLECTOMY

- Make a midline incision centred on umbilicus.
- Carry out a laparotomy. Check for liver metastases.
- Incise the lateral peritoneal attachment of the right colon and mobilise it from the posterior abdominal wall.
- Identify and preserve gonadal vessels, the ureter and second part of the duodenum.
- Mobilise the hepatic flexure by dividing the greater omentum from the right extremity of the transverse colon.
- Once the right colon is mobilised, identify the ileocolic and right colic vessels. Ligate and divide them close to their origins so as to remove any affected lymph nodes.
- Mobilise the terminal ileum up to 15cm from the ileocaecal valve.
- Divide the transverse colon and terminal ileum between clamps.
- Close the end of the transverse colon with either staples or two layers of PDS sutures.
- Close the end of the terminal ileum in similar fashion.
- Re-establish continuity by side-to-side ileotransverse anastomosis using a staple gun or PDS sutures.
- Bring out a drain through a separate stab incision in the abdominal wall.
- Close the abdomen in layers.

HARTMANN'S PROCEDURE

- Long midline incision.
- Carry out a full laparotomy to determine the nature of the lesion, e.g. malignancy or diverticular disease.
- Depending on the degree of contamination, consider resection and primary anastomosis with covering loop ileostomy. If not feasible, proceed to Hartmann's procedure.
- Mobilise left colon to sacral brim.
- Identify ureter and gonadal vessels.
- Ligate inferior mesenteric artery, preserving left colic artery.
- Ligate inferior mesenteric vein.
- Carry out radical excision if carcinoma, i.e. ligating inferior mesenteric artery close to aorta.
- Resect specimen.
- Oversew or staple rectal stump.
- Create a site for colostomy.
- Construct colostomy in left iliac fossa.
- If contamination, carry out copious lavage with normal saline.
- Insert drain through a separate stab incision to pelvis.
- Close incision.

Chapter 16

Vascular Surgery

Katherine I. Bridge • Michael S. Delbridge • Eleanor Atkins

CHAPTER OUTLINE

Vascular disease, encompassing both arterial and venous disease, is a common problem spanning a wide patient population. Vascular disorders may be referred from GPs or present more acutely via the Accident and Emergency department; in addition, other hospital specialties such as acute medicine, diabetology and cardiology may refer patients. While reconfiguration of vascular services has led to procedures mainly being carried out in tertiary referral centres, the ability to properly examine and correctly diagnose these problems remains a vital skill for medical students and junior doctors in all specialties and GPs alike.

ARTERIAL

History

Peripheral arterial disease usually affects the lower limbs but may affect any arterial tree, including the upper limb, gastrointestinal (GI) tract, cerebral vessels and renal vessels. The usual cardiovascular risk factors apply and include smoking, hypercholesterolaemia, hypertension, family history, diabetes and thrombophilia.

The classic initial symptom of a patient with peripheral arterial disease affecting the lower limbs is intermittent claudication. This is pain in the muscle due to ischaemia, brought on by exercise and relieved by rest. It is consistently brought on by the same degree of exercise (the 'claudication distance'), a surrogate measure of disease status that can be monitored over time. Patients typically describe a pain that is cramping in nature, most commonly in the calf (because of superficial femoral artery disease) or buttock and thigh (aortoiliac disease), which is worse in the cold or when walking uphill. Males with aortoiliac disease may complain of impotence in addition to buttock claudication (Leriche's syndrome).

The main differential diagnoses are spinal claudication (the pain is still present at rest and relieved by leaning forward, i.e. often improves when walking uphill) and venous claudication (the pain is 'bursting' and takes longer to resolve). Any sudden deterioration in the claudication distance requires urgent assessment.

Rest pain should be a red flag symptom and indicates the presence of more severe disease. This is a constant pain, typically in the feet and occurring at night whilst in bed ('night pain'). It occurs as a result of decreased cardiac output, with decreased blood pressure and peripheral vasodilatation, all of which leads to decreased blood supply to the peripheries. The pain is relieved by hanging the leg out of bed or walking. This is due to the effect of gravity increasing blood flow, coupled with cooling of the limb outside of the covers, reducing metabolic demand such that less blood flow is required. Rest pain and night pain, coupled with gangrene (i.e. tissue necrosis), or a wound that does not show signs of healing over a 2-week duration, signify the progression to chronic limb-threatening ischaemia.

Other Systems

In addition to the presenting lower limb symptoms, a history should be sought for symptoms involving other areas of the vascular system, e.g. cardiac (myocardial infarction (MI), angina); GI system (upper to central abdominal cramping pain coming on about 20min after a large meal – 'mesenteric angina'); cerebrovascular: (1) carotid (anterior circulation): stroke, TIAs, transient blindness, i.e. amaurosis fugax; (2) vertebral (posterior circulation): dizziness, drop attacks, bilateral blindness, diplopia, vertigo, problems with stance/gait; and (3) renal (hypertension).

Examination

The patient's limbs should be examined in a warm room, using the conventional system of inspection palpation and auscultation.

Upon inspection, check for the colour of the limb. Arterial disease may be present as a whole range of colours, from marble white (acute ischaemia) to purple/blue/cyanotic, or have a red shiny appearance known as a 'sunset foot' (chronic ischaemia). Take note of any scars from previous vascular procedures. In males, the ischaemic leg is typically hairless. Inspect the veins; in a normal limb, the veins should look full even if the limb is horizontal. In an ischaemic foot, veins will be collapsed and look like pale blue gutters in the subcutaneous tissue ('guttering of the veins'). Inspect the pressure areas (heels, tips of toes, ball of foot, head of fifth metatarsal) for any signs of ulceration or gangrene. Do not forget to look between the toes for any small ulcers or evidence of infection.

Lift the straightened limb off the couch. The vascular angle (Buerger's angle) is the angle to which the leg must be raised before it becomes white. A normal leg can be lifted to 90°, and the toes will stay pink. In a severely ischaemic leg, elevation to 15° may cause pallor. Following elevation, the limb is placed in the dependent position, and in the presence of severe ischaemia a purple/red colour occurs as the foot is reperfused. This occurs due to vasodilatation caused by ischaemic metabolites (reactive hyperaemia).

Next, check the temperature of the skin, comparing both legs. Check the capillary refill time by pressing the tip of the nail or pulp of the digit for 2s and observe the time taken for the blanched area to turn pink. In a normal limb, this should happen immediately. Delay (>2s) will occur in the ischaemic digit. Palpate and record all pulses bilaterally. They should be assessed for strength (normal, weak or absent) and recorded as shown in Table 16.1. Be sure to palpate the abdomen for the abdominal aorta. The presence of aneurysmal dilatation of any artery should be noted.

Listen over the groins, iliac fossa, abdomen and neck for the presence of a bruit. Measure the blood pressure in both arms to exclude subclavian disease. The ankle–brachial pressure index (ABPI) should be measured in the lower limbs.

TABLE 16.1

TABULATION OF PULSES

Pulses	R	L
Radial	++	++
Brachial	++	++
Subclavian	++	++
Carotid	++ (bruit)	++
Femoral	++	++ (bruit)
Popliteal	+	–
Posterior tibial	–	–
Dorsalis pedis	–	–

++Normal volume; +diminished volume; –absent.

HINTS AND TIPS

Always examine the vascular patient in a warm room. Examine the patient standing upright to assess for evidence of venous disease (such as varicose veins) before asking the patient to lie supine on the couch. Palpate peripheral pulses gently using only the tips of your fingers; in patients with ischaemia, distal pulses may be weak and are often difficult to feel. Pressing harder in this instance may occlude the artery as it is pressed against the underlying bone and will only make it harder to feel the patient's pulse. The same applies when using a hand-held Doppler; don't be tempted to press harder to elicit a weak pulse. Don't be afraid to record a pulse as absent!

PROCEDURE

HOW TO PERFORM ABPIS

The ABPI provides a measure of the severity of peripheral vascular disease. A ratio of 0.9–>1.2 is considered normal; 0.4–0.8 equates to the presence of intermittent claudication and <0.4 is defined as severe ischaemia. Ratios greater than 1.2 indicate incompressibility of vessels and do not exclude significant arterial disease. ABPIs are measured by placing a cuff around the patient's ankle and using a hand-held Doppler probe, the DP and/or PT pulses are detected. The locations of these pulse points are illustrated in Figure 16.1. The cuff is then inflated above the systolic pressure and deflated until the signal returns. This is repeated for both DP and PT pulses. Brachial artery pressure is then measured and the ratio calculated by dividing the highest pressure measured at the ankle by the highest pressure measured in the arm. In diabetic patients, the arteries may be incompressible and lead to falsely elevated levels.

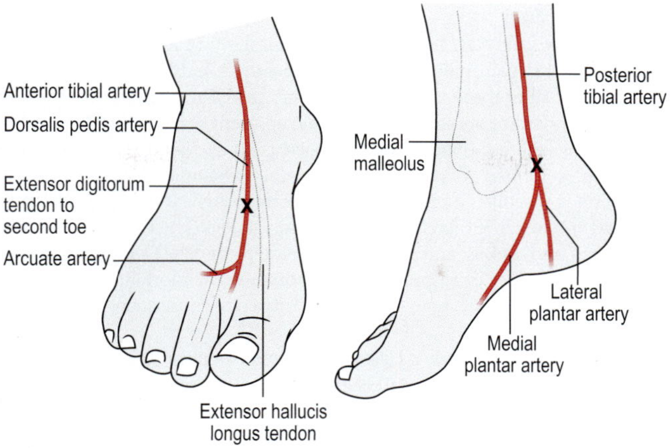

FIGURE 16.1
The location of the pulses of the foot. The pulse of dorsalis pedis can be felt between the extensor tendons of the first and second toes (this pulse is absent in approximately 10% of normal individuals). The posterior tibial pulse is felt on the medial side of the ankle, inferior and posterior to the medial malleolus.

Arterial Occlusive Disease

Acute Arterial Occlusion

Definition – a deterioration in the blood supply of the leg that leads to rest pain or signs of severe ischaemia of less than 2 weeks' duration.

This may range from a patient without PVD who has an embolic occlusion and presents with a dramatically ischaemic limb (the 'acutely ischaemic limb') to a patient with PVD who develops severe new onset rest pain ('acute-on-chronic ischaemia').

Causes

Embolus. This may come from the heart (left ventricular thrombus in AF, mural thrombus following MI, vegetation secondary to valvular lesions, atrial myxoma) or it may come from proximal atherosclerotic plaques or thrombus within aneurysms.

Thrombosis. This usually occurs in an area of arteriosclerotic narrowing due to plaque rupture. There is usually a history of claudication or rest pain prior to the acute event. It may also occur with popliteal aneurysm, a blocked bypass graft and thrombotic conditions, e.g. antiphospholipid syndrome.

Trauma. This may be: (1) penetrating: as a result of arterial catheterisation or angioplasty; following a limb fracture, e.g. popliteal artery damage following supracondylar fracture of the femur; brachial artery damage following a supracondylar fracture of the humerus in a child; (2) blunt: as a result of a joint dislocation (especially posterior dislocation of the knee); and (3) iatrogenic: accidental intra-arterial injection.

Symptoms and Signs

Acute Embolus in a Normal Limb. While the classical symptoms are easily remembered as the six'Ps' (pain, pallor, paraesthesia, paralysis, pulselessness and perishingly cold), not all of these are present in every case. Paralysis and paraesthesia are the most important of these signs, as they represent how salvageable the limb is. In a patient with an embolic source of occlusion and with no previous PVD and thus no preformed collateral circulation, the ischaemia is sudden and profound. This is a vascular emergency, as muscle may only survive for 6 h from the onset of symptoms. It is therefore necessary to establish the exact time of onset of symptoms and assess and treat the patient promptly. Delay in treatment increases the incidence of amputation and mortality. The mortality from embolic episodes is 20–30% irrespective of treatment, often as a consequence of comorbid conditions.

Acute-on-Chronic Ischaemia in a Limb With Peripheral Vascular Disease. In contrast, a patient with pre-existing arterial disease may not present as acutely, and the limb will survive longer periods of ischaemia. Presentation is more often with a sudden deterioration in claudication distance or onset of rest pain.

In either group, the presence of sensory or motor changes in the foot, or calf tenderness on squeezing or passive dorsiflexion of the foot and toes indicates impending muscle infarction and requires immediate revascularisation. After 6 h without treatment there is vasodilatation and release of deoxygenated blood as a result of tissue hypoxia. This leads to a more mottled appearance that still blanches on pressure. At this stage, the leg may be saved by prompt surgery. After 12 h, the arteries and veins thrombose, capillaries rupture, and there is fixed staining that does not blanch. At this stage, the limb is unsalvageable and revascularising the limb is inappropriate and may lead to mortality due to release of potassium, lactic acid and other toxic metabolites.

Investigations

- FBC
- U&Es
- VBG including glucose and lactate
- Clotting screen
- Crossmatch
- ECG
- Duplex ultrasound or CT/MR angiogram depending on local availability
- Include aortic arch if performing a CT/MR angiogram to identify proximal aortic disease as a source of embolus
- Echocardiogram – usually performed at a later date to identify cardiac sources of emboli
- 24 h ECG – to identify cardiac arrhythmias.

Treatment. As with any unwell patient, the initial management involves A, B and C – in particular, patients may be compromised secondary to arrhythmias or other cardiac events and often have significant comorbidities. Anticoagulate with intravenous heparin. Administer analgesia. Administer oxygen via facemask. Keep nil by mouth and call the vascular surgeons as soon as acute limb ischaemia is identified to discuss further investigation and management.

The further management depends on the clinical condition of the limb. Options include:

Embolus in a Normal Limb. The diagnosis is clinical (CT/MR angiogram can be unnecessary) and the patient should be taken to theatre immediately for embolectomy. If known peripheral vascular disease or previous vascular surgery/ intervention, imaging can be much more useful to diagnose the problem.

Thrombosis in a Limb With Peripheral Vascular Disease. In these patients the presentation may not be as dramatic. CT/MR angiography can provide much information about the cause of ischaemia. Treatment options include: surgical thrombectomy; bypass grafting; thrombolysis – provided that the limb will survive for at least 12 h to give time for clot dissolution.

In all patients, fasciotomy should be considered to prevent compartment syndrome after revascularisation. In some patients where ischaemia is considered irreversible, a primary amputation may be performed. However, in cases with major comorbidities, palliative care may be more appropriate.

Prognosis. Surgery should be undertaken within 6–8 h of onset of symptoms. Delay in treatment increases the incidence of amputation and mortality. Mortality is more a consequence of the comorbid conditions than the result of the emboli.

HINTS AND TIPS

Acute arterial embolus in a normal limb is an emergency. To save the limb, urgent embolectomy is required. As a junior doctor on call, if you suspect an acutely ischaemic limb, request senior review immediately. Remember A, B, C. Administer oxygen, gain i.v. access, request routine blood tests including clotting and G&S. Treatment is on the basis of clinical diagnosis; time should not be wasted on unnecessary investigations.

Chronic Arterial Occlusion

Lower Limb (Aorto-Ilio-Femoral Disease)

Causes. This is invariably due to arteriosclerosis and is most commonly a consequence of smoking. Arteriosclerosis may affect a single artery or several in combination; typical patterns include aortoiliac disease, isolated iliac stenoses and superficial femoral occlusion.

Other causes include multiple recurrent small emboli, vasculitis, fibromuscular dysplasia, Buerger's disease, cystic adventitial disease (especially in the young), popliteal entrapment (especially in the young), polycythaemia and Takayasu's disease (rare).

Symptoms and Signs. Patients present with a history of intermittent claudication progressing to rest pain, and then ischaemic ulcers and gangrene may supervene. Ischaemic ulcers tend to develop at pressure areas, e.g. bunion area, tips of toes, lateral aspect of head of fifth metatarsal and around the heel. The foot may be cold, pale and show venous guttering and dependent rubor. Pulses will be absent or reduced. Palpable thrills or bruits may be present.

Investigations

- FBC
- ESR
- U&Es

- HBA1c
- Lipids
- ECG
- Duplex ultrasound – noninvasive; gives information about the degree of stenosis by visual estimation and velocity measurement
- ABPIs. Normally, this is between 0.9 and 1.2. Pressures around 0.8 are compatible with claudication and pressures around 0.4 with rest pain. Pressures below 0.4 indicate severe ischaemia and are usually associated with ulceration and gangrene. Pressures >1.2 indicate vessel incompressibility and do not exclude significant arterial disease.
- Toe pressures (TPs). These can be helpful especially in patients with diabetes who are more likely to have incompressible vessels, or in oedema, large legs or other reasons wherein ABPI may be challenging to obtain.
- CT/MR angiogram (Figures 16.2, 16.3) – noninvasive but does not allow intervention
- Angiography (by direct arterial puncture) – invasive and thus has complications (haem atoma, dissection, emboli, false aneurysm, contrast reaction and contrast nephrotoxicity) but allows therapeutic interventions to be performed (see below).

Treatment

Medical. Mild to moderate claudication that is not disabling does not require surgical treatment and can be managed in primary care. Patients are advised to stop smoking and exercise regularly within their claudication distance to aid in the development of a collateral circulation. Supervised exercise programmes are helpful if available. Advice is also given on foot care, particularly podiatry. All patients should be prescribed an antiplatelet agent (aspirin or clopidogrel) and

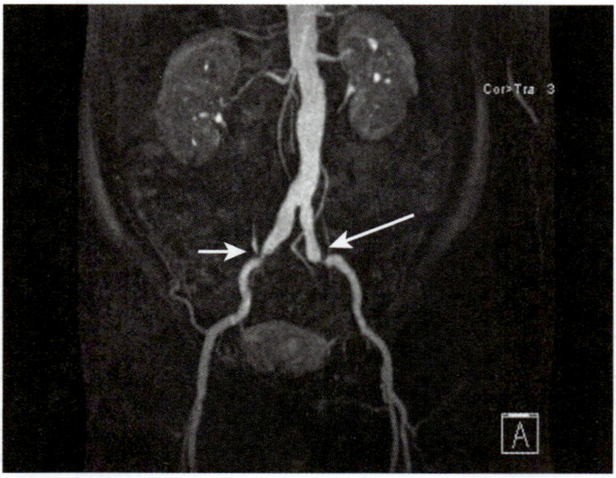

FIGURE 16.2

MRA aorta and iliac vessels. There is a tight stenosis at the origin of the left external iliac artery (large arrow) involving the origin of the internal iliac artery which is occluded. There is also a stenosis at the origin of the right external iliac artery (small arrow).

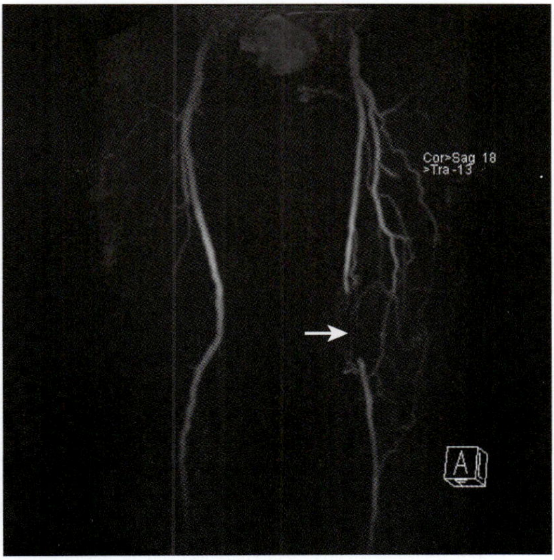

FIGURE 16.3
MRA femoral vessels. There is a block in the left (superficial) femoral artery in the adductor canal (arrow). The distal artery fills via numerous collaterals.

a statin for secondary prevention of cerebrovascular and cardiac disease; there is evidence that cardiac events can be reduced by up to one-third by reducing low-density lipoproteins/cholesterol by one-third, regardless of the baseline cholesterol, down to a total cholesterol of 3.5 mmol/L. Control hypertension. Ensure diabetic control is optimal. Nicotine replacement to help stop smoking. Drugs such as naftidrofuryl may increase pain-free walking distance. Infusions of iloprost (a prostacyclin analogue) are occasionally used in chronic limb-threatening ischaemia with no hope of reconstruction but are rarely helpful. Patients should be encouraged to seek medical advice if claudication suddenly deteriorates or rest pain develops.

In patients with severe disease that is unreconstructable (not amenable to surgery or endovascular intervention), chemical lumbar sympathectomy with injection of phenol under radiological guidance can be used in an attempt to control pain.

Medical. NICE guidelines suggest that naftifofuryl oxalate can be used for 3–6 months if supervised exercise programme has not led to an improvement or the patient does not want to undergo intervention or bypass.

Endovascular. Intervention consists of angioplasty ± stenting. Potential success can be estimated in relation to anatomical location i.e iliac lesions do better than SFA. Current NICE guidelines state that angioplasty/stenting should be offered when advice on risk modification has been given, a supervised exercise programme has been completed and not shown improvement and the lesion is suitable. Primary stenting is only indicated in occlusive lesions of the SFA and iliacs. Generally most radiologists will stent iliac lesions with uncovered self-expanding metal stents (i.e. Luminexx stent) only using covered stents for complications such as rupture. In the SFA there has been a move to angioplasty alone with stenting only used for residual wasting or flow limiting dissection.

In critical ischaemia subintimal angioplasty is a technique where the lesion is crossed between the layers of the wall rather than the lumen. It usually requires stenting.

Surgical. There are several surgical options depending upon the site and severity of the disease, as well as the comorbidities of the patient. These include endarterectomy, bypass (suprainguinal or infrainguinal) and primary amputation.

- Endarterectomy – this is performed for flow limiting common femoral/profunda femoris origin disease. It essentially involves removing plaque/thrombus by developing a plane in the media. Once the disease is removed, the artery is closed using a patch (vein, bovine or prosthetic).
- Bypass – options for suprainguinal (aortoiliac) disease include aortobifemoral bypass, iliofemoral bypass or femoral–femoral cross-over grafts (for unilateral iliac occlusion). For infrainguinal disease there are numerous options. These include femoropopliteal bypass (above or below knee) and femorodistal bypass (to posterior tibial, anterior tibial, dorsalis pedis or peroneal arteries). The type of graft used has an effect on patency rates; ideally reversed vein (usually the great saphenous vein), as this offers the best patency rates and the lowest risk of infection. If vein is unavailable, prosthetic material such as expanded polytetrafluoroethylene (ePTFE) may be used. They can be used in conjunction with a cuff of vein at the site of anastomosis to improve patency, i.e. Miller cuff, Taylor patch or St Mary's boot.
- Amputation – areas of tissue loss may be amputated after arterial reconstruction has been performed and nonviable tissue has become clearly demarcated. However, in some cases of chronic limb-threatening ischaemia where reconstruction is not an option and pain is uncontrolled, or the leg is not viable, the only option may be primary major amputation. Types of amputation are discussed later in this chapter.

Prognosis. The majority of patients with intermittent claudication are managed conservatively. Around 20% progress to chronic limb-threatening ischaemia over 6 years. Patients with chronic limb-threatening ischaemia have a poor prognosis, 50% dying within 5 years. Revascularisation procedures reduce the risk of mortality and limb loss.

UPPER LIMB

Causes. The upper limb is significantly less affected by peripheral disease, with most episodes of acute ischaemia being secondary to emboli. Thoracic outlet syndrome (discussed in detail later in the chapter) may be responsible for claudication or rest pain. Distal arterial disease may be due to embolisation from an area of post-stenotic dilatation beyond the site of subclavian artery compression.

Symptoms and Signs. Emboli usually lodge in one of three sites in the brachial artery: (1) proximally at the origin of the profunda brachii; (2) at the mid-arm level at the origin of the superior ulnar collateral artery; and (3) distally at the brachial bifurcation. It is rare for emboli to lodge in the subclavian or axillary arteries. Symptoms and signs are similar to those in the lower limb, as are the initial investigations.

Treatment. Analgesia. Oxygen. Intravenous heparin 5000 units. Embolectomy is required in the immediately threatened limb, but thrombolysis can be used if the ischaemia is less profound. Many ischaemic upper limbs can be managed conservatively with intravenous heparin, as the rich collateral circulation in the upper limb means that the limb is not always acutely threatened.

Cerebrovascular Disease

By far the majority of strokes are ischaemic in nature (80%) with atherosclerosis being the commonest cause. This usually affects the internal carotid artery just distal to the common carotid bifurcation. Disruption of a plaque at this point can lead to thrombus formation and secondary embolism, leading to a stroke or TIA and putting the patient at high risk of further stroke. A stroke is defined as a focal neurological deficit of >24 h of presumed vascular origin. A TIA has a similar definition but lasts <24 h. In practice, TIAs often last <30 min. Crescendo TIAs (TIAs that increase in severity and frequency over time) are a clear indication for investigation and potential surgical treatment to prevent stroke.

Symptoms and Signs. These may be classed as carotid (anterior circulation) or vertebrobasilar (posterior circulation).

- Carotid: paralysis or numbness of the contralateral arm or leg or temporary loss of vision of ipsilateral eye (amaurosis fugax). Dysphasia.
- Vertebrobasilar: bilateral motor/sensory signs, dysarthria, bilateral visual loss, balance problems, nystagmus and homonymous hemianopia.
- The presence of a carotid bruit has no real clinical relevance as it can be present with a nonsignificant stenosis and absent with a severe stenosis. Examination may reveal reduced carotid pulses or bruits over the carotid artery.

Investigations

- FBC
- U&Es
- Lipids
- Clotting screen
- HBA1c
- Thrombophilia screen (younger patient)
- Autoimmune screen (younger patient)
- ECG – arrhythmias may cause embolic strokes
- Echocardiogram – if embolic source is suspected
- CT scan – identify cerebral infarcts or haemorrhage, or rare causes of CVA, i.e. cerebral tumour or abscess
- Duplex ultrasound. Identification of significant stenosis of the internal carotid artery on the affected side (remember right-sided symptoms would be from a left carotid stenosis, and vice versa). If an internal carotid artery is occluded, surgery is pointless.
- Carotid angiography – generally only performed following CT scan for the purpose of thrombectomy
- CT/MR angiogram (Figure 16.4) – largely replaced carotid angiography in the assessment of internal carotid disease.

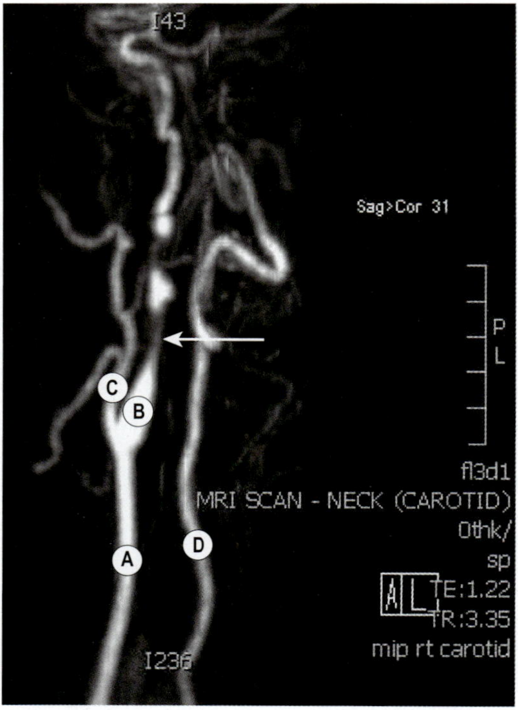

FIGURE 16.4

MRA carotid artery. (**A**) Common carotid artery. (**B**) Internal carotid artery. (**C**) External carotid artery. (**D**) Vertebral artery. There is a tight stenosis (arrow) of the internal carotid artery.

Treatment. Management depends on two factors, i.e. degree of stenosis and whether it is symptomatic or asymptomatic. Patients with a carotid stenosis of <50%, whether symptomatic or not, should be managed medically. Patients with a symptomatic stenosis >50% are generally best treated by carotid endarterectomy. Such symptomatic patients should be assessed and referred without delay, as carotid endarterectomy should be performed within 2 weeks of the index event to provide maximal stroke prevention. Asymptomatic patients with stenosis >60% and age <75 years with good surgical risk may be treated with carotid endarterectomy, but this is often not offered in the UK as 20 such operations would be required to prevent one stroke. Treatment of asymptomatic carotid stenosis in patients undergoing cardiac surgery is controversial and best considered on an individual basis.

Medical. Medical management of internal carotid artery stenosis consists of:

- Risk factor modification – control BP, control diabetes, stop smoking, treat high cholesterol.

- Statins are used to treat high cholesterol but also reduce the number of strokes and major cardiovascular events even with normal cholesterol.
- Antiplatelet drugs – treat initially with high-dose aspirin for 2 weeks following an acute event, then continue with a single antiplatelet.

Endovascular. The evidence suggests higher rates of stroke with internal carotid artery stenting following an acute event. As such, most centres would reserve its use for patients unfit for carotid endarterectomy or with contraindications to carotid endarterectomy such as previous neck radiotherapy or neck scarring around the operative site.

Surgical. Operative treatment of carotid artery stenosis is carotid endarterectomy. This involves opening the artery longitudinally and creating a subintimal plane to remove the arteriosclerotic plaque. The operation may be performed under GA or with a local anaesthetic regional cervical block with no difference in outcomes. A carotid shunt (taking blood from common carotid to internal carotid) may be used. Generally, all GA cases will use a shunt while cases performed under local anaesthetic will use a shunt selectively depending on the patient's neurological condition after the application of clamps. A bovine or prosthetic i.e. Dacron patch is used to close the arteriotomy after endarterectomy to prevent later stenosis.

Complications of carotid endarterectomy include bleeding, infection (very rare but catastrophic in the presence of a prosthetic patch), MI, stroke (in the region of 2–4% risk and may occur via embolism caused by dissection technique or postoperative thrombosis secondary to an intimal flap), temporary or permanent nerve damage (marginal mandibular nerve, hypoglossal, vagus, superior laryngeal, glossopharyngeal, spinal accessory and recurrent laryngeal). Patients should be monitored closely postoperatively, as blood pressure lability during this period (due to surgical interference to the baroreceptors within the carotid bulb) increases the risk of perioperative stroke.

Renovascular Disease

Hypertension may be caused by renal hypoperfusion, with release of renin from juxtaglomerular cells activating angiotensin. The most common causes are arteriosclerosis and fibromuscular dysplasia of the renal arteries. Arteriosclerosis usually involves the origin of the artery and occurs in the older patient. Fibromuscular dysplasia affects the middle to distal part of the artery and usually occurs in the younger patient. Renal artery stenosis has been shown to increase 5-year mortality in patients with peripheral vascular disease, and in coronary artery disease it has been shown to double the risk of death, despite coronary revascularisation.

Renal artery stenosis is an important and potentially correctable cause of renal failure in older patients. The diagnosis of renal artery stenosis is frequently made following a deterioration of renal function in patients commenced on ACE inhibitors or ARBs.

Symptoms and Signs. The major sign is hypertension – either symptomatic or picked up on routine examination, e.g. medical insurance. Of particular interest should be atypical hypertension, i.e. rapid onset or accelerated hypertension, in a young adult or child, and hypertension refractory to treatment. Other signs include a sudden deterioration in renal function, or in renal function after ACE inhibitors or ARBs. It is occasionally picked up after an incidental finding of a small kidney or arteriosclerotic disease on CT. Occasionally, it may be the cause of flash pulmonary oedema.

Investigations

- Duplex scanning
- CT/MR angiogram
- MAG3 scan with and without captopril – this can demonstrate any difference between the two kidneys and if this is exacerbated by an ACE inhibitor.

Treatment. A stenosis of >50% is considered significant. Treating the stenosis is no guarantee that either hypertension or renal failure will improve. Current indications for intervention include: ↓renal function or ↑BP despite maximum medical treatment; recurrent flash pulmonary oedema; rapid onset of severe hypertension; renal failure in patients with cardiac disease while taking ACE inhibitors or AR blockers; loss of renal mass on conservative treatment (although there is no point in offering revascularisation in a kidney measuring <7cm as there is no salvageable function); progression of stenosis.

Treatment options include medical, endovascular or surgical.

Medical. Control BP. Antiplatelet drugs. Statins. Good diabetic control. Lifestyle changes, i.e. stop smoking.

Endovascular. Options include angioplasty alone or with stenting. Offers good results, particularly with fibromuscular dysplasia.

Surgery. Occasionally indicated. Options include bypass, endarterectomy and patch, nephrectomy + bench surgery and autotransplantation. Nephrectomy (if kidney unsalvageable).

Visceral Ischaemic Disease

Visceral ischaemic disease covers a number of conditions including acute mesenteric ischaemia, chronic mesenteric ischaemia and acute mesenteric venous thrombosis.

Acute Mesenteric Ischaemia

This carries a very high mortality rate as a result of late diagnosis and due to its relative rarity. Causes are generally embolic or as a result of in situ thrombosis on an underlying stenosis. Less common causes include nonocclusive infarction (due to low flow states, i.e. hypotension and inotropes), vasculitis, radiation arteritis, fibromuscular dysplasia, aortic dissection and thrombosis of visceral arterial aneurysm. It occurs in 3% of patients following abdominal aortic aneurysm repair (10% of ruptures).

Symptoms and Signs. Embolus classically presents as acute severe abdominal pain with few, nonspecific clinical signs. There may be vomiting or diarrhoea, which may be bloody. There may be a history of atrial fibrillation, sepsis, 'mesenteric claudication' (chronic mesenteric ischaemia) or portal hypertension. The pain experienced is usually out of proportion to the early physical findings. Subsequently, the patient will develop fever, abdominal tenderness, distension and ultimately peritonitis and shock.

Investigations

- FBC (raised WCC)
- U&E
- Arterial or venous blood gas (reduced HCO_3 and raised lactate)
- Serum amylase may be raised with infarcted bowel (can be confused with acute pancreatitis).
- Triple phase CT – the portal venous phase may show signs of bowel ischaemia, and the arterial phase assesses the mesenteric arteries.
- Laparotomy (if appropriate) should not be delayed once the diagnosis is made.

Treatment. Urgent laparotomy. Venous thrombosis without infarction requires anticoagulation (see below). In the case of arterial occlusion, if there is extensive irreversible ischaemia, surgical treatment may not be possible, and terminal care may be the only option. If the length of nonviable bowel is not excessive, surgical resection with eventual stoma and mucous fistula formation may be appropriate. Following extensive resection, patients are left with a short segment of bowel and consequent metabolic problems. If CT has confirmed acute embolus in the superior mesenteric artery, an embolectomy should be performed. If a tight stenosis is found to be present at the origin of the superior mesenteric artery, bypass grafting, endarterectomy or on-table stenting should be carried out. A vein conduit should always be used if there is contamination with bowel contents. A 'second look' laparotomy is generally required to assess intestinal viability following any intervention, usually after 24–48h.

Chronic Mesenteric Ischaemia

Visceral occlusion is usually due to arteriosclerosis. In practical terms, the superior mesenteric artery is most often involved, and there generally needs to be significant disease in two neighbouring mesenteric arteries for symptoms to occur.

Symptoms and Signs. Cramping upper abdominal pain approximately 20min after a meal ('mesenteric angina'). This usually lasts 1–3h. Patients always have weight loss because of 'food fear' due to the pain caused by eating. Frequently they also have diarrhoea. An upper abdominal bruit may be audible. Occlusive vascular disease is likely elsewhere.

Investigations

- CT/MR angiogram

Treatment. Treatment is by endovascular techniques or surgery. Endovascular treatment involves angioplasty and stenting. Surgery involves endarterectomy with patching or bypass from aorta or a common iliac artery to proximal superior mesenteric artery using either reversed vein or reinforced PTFE.

HINTS AND TIPS

The diagnosis of chronic mesenteric ischaemia relies on careful and detailed history taking. Patients may appear cachetic, and there may a tendency to rush into investigations for a malignant cause. However, a thorough history elicits the diagnosis; pain, consistently 20min after meals, causing a 'food fear' (as opposed to a true 'loss of appetite') and resulting in weight loss implies chronic mesenteric ischaemia.

Acute Mesenteric Venous Thrombosis

This is less catastrophic than acute arterial occlusion. Presentation may be more prolonged over several weeks; 75% of cases are due to hypercoagulability, intra-abdominal sepsis and portal hypertension.

Symptoms and Signs. Abdominal pain which may get worse after eating and over time. Diarrhoea. Vomiting.

Investigations

- Triple-phase CT.

Treatment. Treatment depends on the clinical condition of the patient. If the patient has peritonitis, a laparotomy should be performed, any nonviable bowel resected and any source of intra-abdominal sepsis addressed. However, if the patient is stable, it may be managed conservatively with heparin and lifelong anticoagulation. If CT shows no intra-abdominal cause, a thrombophilia screen should be carried out prior to commencing anticoagulation.

Aneurysms

Definition – an aneurysm is an abnormal dilatation of an artery. Aneurysms may be true or false (see below). A true aneurysm contains all layers of the vessel wall and appears as either a fusiform or a saccular dilatation. True aneurysms are commonest in the infrarenal aorta, iliac vessels, common femoral and popliteal arteries. A false aneurysm may occur anywhere and is usually the result of trauma. (For classification of aneurysms→Table 16.2.)

Aortic Aneurysms

An aorta may be aneurysmal from the ascending aorta to the aortic bifurcation. Aortic aneurysms can be divided into thoracic (→Ch. 9), thoracoabdominal or abdominal alone. Infrarenal AAA is the most common type, affecting men > women and increasing in frequency with age.

Aetiology. Aneurysms are due to degeneration of the arterial media, particularly a reduction in elastin. The exact aetiology of aortic aneurysms is unknown, but contributing factors include: (1) elastin degradation due to increased levels of metalloproteinases; (2) flow dynamics – the infrarenal aorta is a common site as pulse pressure here is maximal due to tapering calibre and reflected waves from the bifurcation; (3) hypertension – involved in formation but also rate of expansion; (4) arteriosclerosis – not causally linked but often also present; (5) collagen defects, e.g. Marfan's disease and Ehlers–Danlos syndrome; (6) genetic association – 25% of first-degree relatives will develop an aneurysm; (7) smoking – associated with more rapid expansion; (8) association with emphysema and inguinal hernias; this may relate to a collagen defect but the exact link is unclear.

Symptoms and Signs. Abdominal aortic aneurysms are often asymptomatic and noticed abdominal examination or ultrasound scanning for other conditions. Since 2013, the UK has had a nationwide screening programme for AAA focused on males >65 years. Symptomatic AAA can cause backache by pressure on the adjacent lumbar vertebral bodies or abdominal pain (the so-called 'tender' aneurysm). Examination

TABLE 16.2

AETIOLOGY OF ANEURYSMS

True	
Congenital	Berry aneurysm of circle of Willis Aneurysmal varix associated with arteriovenous fistula
Acquired	Trauma: irradiation Infection: syphilis, mycotic aneurysm Degeneration: arteriosclerosis, cystic medial necrosis
False	Trauma

reveals a pulsatile abdominal mass just above the umbilicus. Look for other peripheral artery aneurysms (especially popliteal).

Investigations

- USS to assess the maximum diameter of the aneurysm
- CT angiogram to assess anatomy including the relationship to the renal arteries, the aortic arch and thoracic aorta
- Investigations to assess patient's fitness for surgery – FBC, U&Es, NTproBNP, clotting studies, ECG, lung function tests, cardiopulmonary exercise test, echocardiogram.

Complications. These include:

- Rupture, which may be retroperitoneal or contained, intraperitoneal or uncontained (invariably fatal) or rarely into the IVC (massive AV fistula)
- Distal emboli
- Severe back pain due to erosion of the lumbar vertebral bodies
- Thrombosis with distal ischaemia
- Compression of neighbouring structures including duodenum and IVC
- Very rarely, disseminated intravascular coagulation can occur with very large aneurysms.

Treatment. Once diagnosed, the investigations depend upon the size of the aneurysm. If <5 cm, the patient is kept under surveillance. Surveillance is yearly if <4.5 cm and 6-monthly if >4.5 cm. Once over 5 cm, the patient will undergo a CT angiogram to assess morphology and plan either open or endovascular repair. The threshold for treatment remains a diameter of >5.5 cm, but can be lowered to 5 cm in women. At this size the annual risk of rupture varies in the literature at around 3.5–10% and usually outweighs the risk of surgery. If the patient is frail with poor morbidity, no treatment may be appropriate. For those suitable for treatment, either endovascular repair (EVAR) or open repair may be undertaken. Not all aneurysms are suitable for EVAR, but it confers a much lower earlier mortality than open repair and may be attractive for high-risk cases. Open repair has better durability and is more cost-effective. Open repair involves an inlay Dacron graft or a Dacron Y graft to the iliac arteries or femoral arteries. Mortality for elective surgery should be <10%.

Ruptured Aortic Aneurysm (Figure 16.5). Classically, the patient presents with severe abdominal pain radiating to the back or iliac fossa and is associated with collapse or a hypotensive episode. A pulsatile mass may be palpable. Intraperitoneal rupture is instantly fatal; retroperitoneal rupture may tamponade the bleeding allowing the patient to reach hospital. Patients with ruptured aneurysms survive to reach hospital because of vasoconstriction, abdominal tamponade and the development of 'controlled' hypotension. The infusion of even modest amounts of crystalloid or colloid rapidly upsets that fine balance. If the patient requires significant volumes of fluids to maintain blood pressure on the way to hospital or in the emergency room, it is very unlikely that the patient will survive surgery. A patient who is conscious and talking has an adequate blood pressure for cerebral perfusion. Rarely the aneurysm may rupture to the right into the IVC causing a massive AV fistula with severe heart failure and massive lower limb oedema.

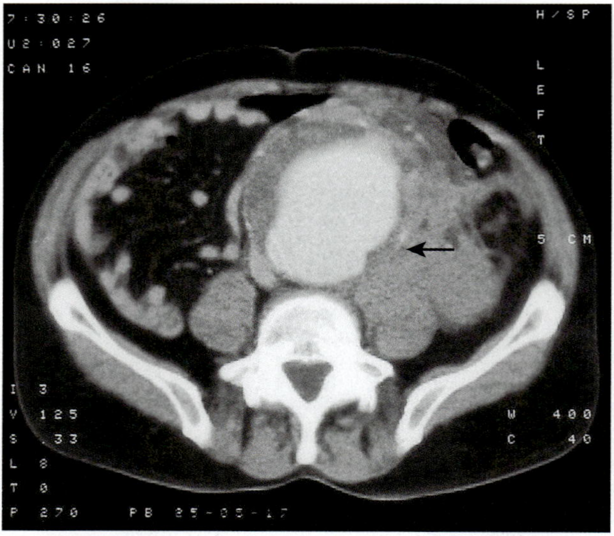

FIGURE 16.5

CT scan of the abdomen showing a large leaking abdominal aortic aneurysm. Note the areas of calcification in the wall of the aneurysm. There is evidence of leakage to the left of the aneurysm (arrow).

Investigations. If the patient is stable enough to tolerate a CT angiogram, this should be performed. It provides anatomical information that is useful for open repair and essential for endovascular repair (50% of ruptures are suitable for EVAR). Ultrasound scan (including FAST scan) will show an aneurysm but *not* a rupture.

Treatment. Emergency repair should be undertaken as soon as possible. Many centres are now using an EVAR-first strategy. Emergency EVAR has similar outcomes to open repair with shorter length of stay, improved quality of life and reduced cost. EVAR has better outcomes in women and when performed under local anaesthetic. Open repair is with an inlay Dacron graft or a Dacron Y graft. The postoperative mortality is between 30% and 50%. Postoperative morbidity is high and results from haemorrhage, ARDS, ARF, multiorgan failure, MI, stroke and colonic ischaemia. Late complications include graft infection, often with aortoduodenal fistula and life-threatening haemorrhage. This requires graft removal and reconstruction, either anatomically or extra-anatomically (axillobifemoral bypass). If the patient is fit enough, in situ replacement with vein graft (femoral vein) or bovine graft is preferred.

HINTS AND TIPS

EMERGENCY MANAGEMENT OF RUPTURED ABDOMINAL AORTIC ANEURYSM

The patient presenting with ruptured AAA requires rapid, efficient and coordinated management by emergency room physicians, anaesthetists and surgeons. This is a true surgical emergency; urgent action is required. As such, for the junior doctor on call, it is advisable to inform senior colleagues as soon as a ruptured AAA is suspected. On arrival in resus, remember A, B, C. Early anaesthetic assessment is vital. If the airway is patent and the patient is breathing independently, high-flow oxygen should be administered regardless of oxygen saturations. Wide-bore i.v. access in both antecubital fossae should be obtained. Routine bloods, along with group and save-and-crossmatch, should be requested urgently, with consideration of activating the major haemorrhage protocol, providing packed red cells, platelets and fresh frozen plasma. Heart rate and blood pressure should be continuously monitored. Do not be tempted to give fluids for a low blood pressure if the patient is conscious. In a patient surviving to hospital, the ruptured AAA bleeding will have slowed due to tamponade. Increasing the blood pressure using fluids may overcome the tamponade and cause bleeding to restart. A urinary catheter should be inserted. Once the diagnosis is confirmed, either clinically or by CT, the patient should be transferred to theatre without delay. If vascular surgery is on another site, they should be alerted as soon as possible, images transferred and a blue light transfer arranged.

Inflammatory Aneurysm

Around 5% of aneurysms are described as inflammatory. This inflammation extends through all layers of the aorta. It obscures tissue planes and makes operative dissection particularly challenging. In severe cases, the inflammation may extend into the retroperitoneum to involve the IVC and ureters, which may require preoperative stenting.

Iliac Artery Aneurysm

These may involve the common iliac and internal iliac artery. The external iliac is almost never involved. They are usually present in association with aortic aneurysm, but may occur in isolation. Aneurysms of the internal iliac are a particular challenge as operative access is difficult. Management options include:

- Surgical repair using a Dacron graft
- Endovascular stenting
- Internal iliac artery aneurysms can be safely ligated or occluded with endovascular coils/plugs if there is a patent internal iliac artery on the opposite side.

Femoral Aneurysms (Including False Aneurysms)

These usually involve the common femoral artery.

Symptoms and Signs. Usually asymptomatic pulsatile mass in the groin. May be associated with abdominal aortic aneurysms. Symptoms may include compression of local structures (common femoral vein, causing leg swelling), thrombosis and ischaemia, distal emboli and rupture. Anatomy should be investigated with CT/MR angiogram.

A false aneurysm is a pulsating haematoma, the cavity of which is in direct continuity with the lumen of an artery. It is contained by a fibrous capsule consisting of adventitia and surrounding tissues rather than the layers of the vessel wall. As flow through the defect continues, the aneurysm will slowly expand and may be extremely rapid if infection is present, e.g. in intravenous drug users. False aneurysms are common in the femoral artery and may result from:

- Percutaneous catheterisation for cardiac or other angiography; stab wounds
- Previous surgery, especially with prosthetic grafts (infection)
- Misplaced i.v. access (e.g. in IVDUs, or at femoral line placement).

Treatment. Small true aneurysms (<2.5 cm) may be kept under surveillance unless symptomatic. Rapidly expanding true aneurysms require surgery, usually with an inlay graft. Small iatrogenic false aneurysms can be treated by compression therapy with an ultrasound scan probe or left to spontaneously thrombose (<2 cm); thrombin injection can be used if compression is unsuccessful or the false aneurysm is large. If the neck of the false aneurysm is wide, precluding thrombin injection, or the overlying skin is threatened, surgical repair is required. In IVDUs, there is no role for reconstruction and generally all three femoral vessels need to be ligated, with an approximately 10% rate of limb loss and high rates of disabling claudication.

Popliteal Aneurysm

This is the commonest site for aneurysms after the aorta. Of patients with AAA, 10% have a popliteal aneurysm; 30% of patients with a popliteal aneurysm have an AAA. They are bilateral in 50% of cases.

Symptoms and Signs. Pulsatile mass in the popliteal fossa. If a medical student can palpate a popliteal pulse easily, it may be aneurysmal. Complications include thrombosis presenting as acute limb ischaemia; distal embolism; compression of local structures, e.g. popliteal vein with deep vein thrombosis (DVT), common fibular (peroneal) nerve with foot drop; and rupture (rare).

Treatment. Treatment is considered when the size is >2 cm or the aneurysm is symptomatic. Surgery is the preferred method of treatment, but endovascular stenting may be considered for patients with high risk. Endovascular repair uses a flexible covered stent to cope with the bending stresses behind the knee. Surgical repair is either by an exclusion bypass (with ligation of the popliteal artery above and below the aneurysm) or an inlay graft.

Visceral Artery Aneurysms

Aneurysms may arise from the splenic artery, hepatic artery, superior mesenteric artery or renal arteries.

Symptoms and Signs. Visceral aneurysms may produce abdominal or flank pain. Renal artery aneurysms may cause haematuria or hypertension. They are often found incidentally on CT scans or ultrasounds for other conditions.

Prognosis. Splenic artery aneurysms most commonly affect women of child-bearing age and transplant patients. They are usually asymptomatic until rupture occurs. Rupture is an uncommon but major complication. It tends to occur in the third trimester of pregnancy and is associated with a high mortality rate. In a woman of child-bearing age, treatment should be considered at any size. In other patients, consider treating at 3 cm if it remains asymptomatic. Treatment is often possible with embolisation under angiographic control. Hepatic artery aneurysms are prone to rupture. The mortality rate for surgery on visceral aneurysms is high, particularly if they rupture.

> **HINTS AND TIPS**
>
> Rupture of a splenic artery aneurysm is associated with sudden severe epigastric or left upper quadrant pain and hypovolaemia. This may be delayed, as bleeding can initially be confined to the lesser sac. In pregnancy, shock is usually immediate. The presentation of unexplained, sudden-onset hypovolaemia in the third trimester of pregnancy should raise the suspicion of splenic artery aneurysm. In this situation, clinical suspicion and USS provide the mainstay of diagnosis; rapid surgical intervention is required to save mother and baby via laparotomy, splenectomy and Caesarean section.

Other Vascular Problems

Thromboangiitis Obliterans (Buerger's Disease)

This affects small vessels of the extremities. It occurs almost exclusively in young males who are heavy cigarette smokers. It may be associated with migratory thrombophlebitis.

Symptoms and Signs. Claudication in the muscles of the foot. Digital pain, cyanosis, coldness progressing to necrosis and gangrene. Ankle and wrist pulses disappear first and the proximal pulses remain normal. Progressive digital ischaemia occurs with eventual loss of feet and hands.

Investigations. Arteriography reveals discrete foci of occlusions alternating with apparently uninvolved arterial segments in the distal circulation. Collateral vessels are classically described as 'corkscrew'.

Treatment. It is essential to stop smoking to avoid progression of the disease. Sympathectomy is only of temporary benefit – if the patient continues smoking, amputation is necessary for rest pain or gangrene. Reconstructive surgery is rarely possible because the disease involves the small distal vessels. Repeated prostacyclin infusions (iloprost) may be beneficial.

Raynaud's Phenomenon

This is a vasospastic condition of diverse aetiology. The following conditions have been implicated:

- Systemic diseases or conditions, e.g. collagen diseases (scleroderma), cryoglobulinaemia, myxoedema, macroglobulinaemia
- Compression syndromes, e.g. carpal tunnel syndrome, cervical rib, thoracic outlet syndrome
- Occupational trauma, e.g. hand–arm vibration syndrome, previously called vibration-induced white finger (pneumatic drill, chainsaw, grinders), piano playing, typing, cricket.

Symptoms and Signs. Sequential changes of pallor, cyanosis and rubor, particularly after exposure to cold. This represents vasoconstriction followed by reflex vasodilatation. In severe long-standing cases tissue necrosis may occur involving nonhealing ulcers and gangrene of the extremities. Tissue necrosis always denotes underlying pathology, i.e. the patient has secondary Raynaud's as opposed to primary Raynaud's disease.

Investigations

- FBC
- Platelets
- ESR
- Chest X-ray (CXR) (cervical rib)
- Cold agglutinins
- Serum protein electrophoresis
- Autoantibody screen
- Rheumatoid factor
- Lupus anticoagulant
- CT angiogram of aortic arch and upper limb.

Treatment

- Treatment of underlying disorder, e.g. excise cervical rib
- Avoidance of cold exposure – heated gloves and boots
- Stop smoking.
- Advice from Scleroderma & Raynaud's UK (SRUK)
- Drugs, e.g. calcium channel blockers (nifedipine), naftidrofuryl, i.v. prostaglandins (iloprost)
- Plasmapheresis in patients with Raynaud's secondary to scleroderma can temporarily improve symptoms.
- Sympathectomy (relatively ineffective)
- Very rarely, amputation may be required.

Diabetic Foot

Contributory factors include micro-angiopathy, peripheral neuropathy, impaired immunity, impaired tissue metabolism and the glucose-rich environment, which favours bacterial overgrowth.

Symptoms and Signs. The patient may present with either a neuropathic or ischaemic foot with signs of both large and small vessel disease. The neuropathic and ischaemic elements frequently coexist.

The neuropathic foot is warm, dry and has palpable pulses. Calluses may be present, as may painless penetrating ulcers at pressure points and sites of minor injury. Painless necrosis of the toes may occur. Spreading infection can occur along plantar spaces. There is usually general loss of pain and thermal sensation. In severe cases, Charcot foot may result.

The ischaemic foot is cool with absent pulses, calluses, painful ulcers, claudication and rest pain.

Investigations

- FBC
- U&Es
- HBA1c
- Blood cultures if systemically unwell
- Wound/pus swab for MC&S
- X-ray foot for osteomyelitis
- Duplex ultrasound or CT angiogram depending on availability
- TPs are more useful than ABPI in the diabetic foot.

Treatment of the Diabetic Foot

- Control hyperglycaemia with variable rate insulin infusion.
- Treat infection.
  - Give targeted iv antibiotics.
  - Drain any collection and/or remove nonviable tissue.
    - Never let the sun set on an infected diabetic foot which is making the patient unwell – always contact vascular surgery urgently in these cases.
- Revascularise if required.
  - CT/MR angiogram or duplex ultrasound
- Optimise ongoing medical management of the patient.
  - Diabetes care
    - Medical management of diabetes
    - Refer to podiatry for local debridement and wound management.
    - Refer to orthotics for offloading.
  - Manage risk factors for future disease.
    - Stop smoking.
    - Treat hypertension and hypercholesterolaemia.
    - Optimise weight and nutrition status.

HINTS AND TIPS

For optimal results, diabetic patients with foot disease should be managed by a multidisciplinary team. Only with effective management of diabetes, adequate foot care, prompt treatment of apparently minor infections and early assessment by vascular surgeons will major amputation be delayed or avoided.

Thoracic Outlet Syndrome

This represents a variety of symptoms related to arterial, venous and nerve compression as they exit from the chest. Compression usually occurs in the area bounded by the clavicle, the first rib and the scalenus anterior muscle. Causes include:

- An anatomically tight thoracic outlet, where compression occurs between first rib and clavicle
- Hypertrophy of the scalene muscles (e.g. following repetitive 'over the head' upper arm exercise, such as painting ceilings, stacking shelves, bodybuilding or swimming)
- Cervical rib (present in <1% of population)
- Fibromuscular band (from C7)
- Clavicle or first rib fractures or exostoses.

Symptoms and Signs

Neurological. More common cause. Can present with sensory and motor deficit in the distribution of C8/T1, but often symptoms are vague and nonspecific. Symptoms can be exacerbated by movement or arm position and tend to be worse at night.

Arterial. Less common. Claudication or rest pain. Distal arterial disease may be due to embolisation from an area of dilatation or frank aneurysm just beyond subclavian artery compression. Raynaud's phenomenon may be present.

Venous. Venous hypertension – compression of subclavian vein or acute upper limb DVT (Paget–Schrötter syndrome).

Investigations

- CXR: cervical rib (the CXR should include the thoracic inlet and the total number of ribs on each side counted – if there are 13, a cervical rib is present.)
- Duplex ultrasound with provocative manoeuvres, e.g. with the arm raised above the head, will give more functional information about the impingement on the subclavian artery and vein than angiography.
- CT/MR angiogram to assess vessel compression – subclavian artery stenosis or constriction by fibrous band. MR angiogram can also include provocative manoeuvres.
- Venography: compression of subclavian vein or subclavian vein thrombosis – this can be combined with thrombolysis if required.
- Nerve conduction studies to distinguish from carpal tunnel syndrome.

Treatment. With neurological symptoms, physiotherapy should be first line. Botox or local anaesthetic can be injected into scalene muscles to provide relief. For severe neurological compression, or any symptomatic arterial compression, surgical decompression of the thoracic outlet with division of fibrous bands or removal of the first rib or cervical rib if present. Aneurysms may need to be resected and repaired. For patients presenting with primary axillary vein thrombosis (Paget–Schrötter syndrome), treatment is with a combination of thrombolysis, anticoagulation and early surgical decompression of the thoracic outlet.

Arteriovenous Fistula

Two types exist:

- *Congenital* – May present as multiple small lesions. Present from birth. Clinically manifest 10–20 years. May enlarge to involve most of the limb
- *Acquired* – Due to trauma, e.g. stabbing, arteriography, iatrogenic for dialysis. Usually history of trauma and typically single communication.

Symptoms and Signs. Presentation is with pain and swelling in area of fistula, and enlarged tortuous arteries and veins. Palpation may reveal increased skin temperature. Careful examination may elicit elongation of the limb. Venous hypertension and ischaemia may be present distal to the site of the fistula. Examine for a palpable thrill and a continuous machinery bruit.

Investigations

- CXR for cardiomegaly, NTproBNP
- Limb radiograph for bone elongation
- Duplex ultrasound – noninvasive
- MRI: this will show the true extent of the lesion, which is nearly always more extensive than appears to be the case clinically.
- Arteriography: this should only be performed in a specialist unit if consideration is being given to embolisation.

Complications. Cosmetic, haemorrhage, thrombosis, distal ischaemia, venous hypertension in limb, high output cardiac failure (Branham's sign – compression of the fistula results in a fall in the heart rate).

Treatment. Not all arteriovenous fistulae require treatment. Small peripheral fistulae may be observed and frequently will never cause difficulties. Indications for intervention include haemorrhage, expansion, severe venous or arterial insufficiency, cosmetic deformity severely affecting quality of life and heart failure. Most fistulae requiring management are embolised under radiographic control. Simple ligation of feeding vessels should never be performed. Recurrence is inevitable, and when recurrence does occur, previous ligation means that it is difficult to perform angiography and embolisation. Embolisation and excision may be required for very large lesions. Management should always be carried out in a specialist unit.

Vascular Access for Haemodialysis

Vascular access may be obtained either by a dual lumen catheter placed in a central vein (internal jugular, femoral or subclavian) or the creation of an arteriovenous fistula. Dual lumen catheters are often the first-line management for patients presenting with acute renal failure (as many as 30% of patients with renal failure present in the acute stage). Central lines may be tunnelled and used long term in some patients who have no alternative route for vascular access. The preferred long-term route for haemodialysis is via an arteriovenous fistula. This is created by anastomosing a superficial vein to a nearby artery. Suitable vessels are identified using venous and arterial duplex ultrasound. Flow in the vein significantly increases and over the next 4–6 weeks the veins will dilate and become suitable for needling. The most common form of fistula is the radiocephalic fistula created between cephalic vein and radial artery either at the anatomical snuff box or at the wrist. The fistula is usually created initially in the non-dominant arm (so as to be accessible for the patient to needle). In the event of failure of a radiocephalic fistula, or lack of suitable veins to create one in the first place, fistulae may be performed at the elbow (brachiocephalic fistula, brachiobasilic fistula) or ePTFE grafts may be placed in the forearm in either straight or looped configuration or as a loop in the thigh.

Complications

- Early – bleeding causing haematoma and compression leading to thrombosis, ischaemic monomelic neuropathy (severe pain and sensorimotor symptoms requiring immediate ligation), infection
- Late – failure to mature (central vein stenosis, large tributary, inadequate artery), steal syndrome (the hand becomes ischaemic as blood is diverted into the fistula and away from the arteries supplying the hand), thrombosis, aneurysm, high output cardiac failure.

AMPUTATIONS

Indications for Amputation

- Vascular, e.g. severe rest pain with arteries unsuitable for reconstruction, gangrene
- Trauma with non-salvageable limb
- Severe infection, e.g. gas gangrene, osteomyelitis
- Tumour, e.g. osteogenic sarcoma, soft tissue sarcomas, subungual melanoma
- Useless limb, e.g. poliomyelitis, severe brachial plexus lesions associated with vascular damage.

Principles of Amputation

There are three main principles for the surgeon to consider when contemplating amputation:

- Select the appropriate level. There must be adequate circulation at that level to ensure healing. Tissues must show healthy bleeding at time of surgery.
- Amputation level must take into account the fitting of a prosthetic limb.
- Assess joints. Contractures or arthritis may influence the amputation level.

Preparation for Amputation

A major amputation is a disfiguring operation. Fully explain the operation to the patient, who may take a while to accept that it is necessary. Preoperative physiotherapy and occupational therapy should be undertaken and a visit made to the Limb Fitting Centre. Ensure that the patient is pain-free. Antibiotic prophylaxis is given with induction of anaesthesia and continued for 5 days postoperatively.

Types of Amputation

Minor. This involves simple amputation at the base of the digit, or 'ray' amputations where, e.g. in the foot, the metatarsal head and tendons are removed. This type of amputation is useful in diabetics, Buerger's disease and severe Raynaud's. Occasionally, transmetatarsal amputation may be undertaken if too many toes are missing to retain a functional foot. This requires a viable plantar flap of skin to be successful. The indications are as above.

Major

Below-Knee Amputation. This provides the patient with the best chance of mobilising with a prosthesis. Healing can be expected in 80% of patients. Contraindications include gangrene or ulceration extending to involve the planned skin flaps, fixed flexion contractures at the knee and occlusion of the profunda femoris artery. The standard tibial stump is 8–12 cm long and the fibular is transected slightly higher. A long posterior flap with muscle is fashioned and this is folded over to cushion the bone end. Function is variable, with less than half of patients being independently mobile at 2 years.

Gritti–Stokes (Through-Knee) Amputation. This amputation involves opening the knee joint, transecting the femur just above the femoral condyles and folding the anterior portion of the patella over the end of the femur. It is claimed to result in less blood loss than above-knee amputation, to provide a better lever in bed-bound patients and, in bilateral amputees, to provide a more stable sitting position.

Above-Knee Amputation. This is a common amputation in patients with arteriosclerosis. The stump of the femur is 25 cm long measured from the greater trochanter. Equal anterior and posterior myoplastic flaps are sutured over the bone end (a 'fish mouth').

Less Frequently Performed Amputations. These include Lisfranc (tarso-metatarsal disarticulation), Chopart (tarso-tarsal disarticulation) and Syme (ankle disarticulation). They are rarely used and are of historical significance only. A through-ankle amputation can be performed for immediate control of severe diabetic foot sepsis. This allows the patient to be stabilised on ICU prior to formalising a below- or above-knee amputation. Disarticulation at the hip and hindquarter amputations are usually performed for major trauma or malignancy, although they are sometimes used for vascular disease (aortoiliac).

Postoperative Care

Pain Relief. The aim is to prevent breakthrough pain rather than treating pain once it occurs. Options include epidural, PCA, nerve blocks and stump catheters (infuse local anaesthetic into the sciatic nerve).

Care of the Good Limb. This involves physiotherapy. It is important to avoid pressure ulcers by nursing on an appropriate pressure mattress.

Physiotherapy. Build up muscle power and coordination. Start as soon as the patient is comfortable and continue in gymnasium. The aim is to prevent contractures and ensure rapid mobilisation with prosthesis.

Prosthesis. Measure patient as soon as stump shrinks and volume of stump is stable.

Complications

Early. These include pain, haemorrhage, haematoma, infection, wound dehiscence, ischaemic flaps and fat embolism.

Late. These include pain, sinus formation, osteomyelitis, neuroma, phantom limb and ulceration of the skin (pressure from prosthesis or continuing ischaemia).

VENOUS DISORDERS

Varicose Veins

Definition – dilated tortuous veins. They can be divided into primary and secondary.

Primary varicose veins are the most common and are often familial. They are possibly due to weakness of the superficial vein wall that allows dilatation of the valve ring, allowing the valve to become incompetent with retrograde flow. This then leads to increased venous pressure and further valve failure, as a domino effect along the length of the vein. Other contributory factors include prolonged standing, family history, hormonal factors (more common in pregnancy – progesterone has an effect on the vein wall), ageing.

Secondary varicose veins may be classified as follows:

- Obstruction to venous outflow, e.g. pregnancy, fibroids, ovarian cysts, abdominal lymphadenopathy, pelvic cancer, iliac vein thrombosis or retroperitoneal fibrosis
- Valve destruction, e.g. DVT
- High flow and pressure, e.g. AV fistulae.

Symptoms and Signs. On inspection, there will be tortuous dilated veins of the great or small saphenous system. Patients report aching discomfort which is worse towards the end of the day and relieved by sitting with legs elevated. It is important to ask the patient about factors that may imply the presence of secondary varicose veins, such as previous DVT, previous fracture and abdominal swelling. Occasionally, initial presentation may be with complications (see below). Examine the patient standing up and assess the site and size of the veins. Check the state of the skin and subcutaneous tissue; take note of any varicose eczema, haemosiderin deposition, atrophie blanche, evidence of thrombophlebitis or ulceration. Historical tests such as Trendelenburg's and Perthe's tests are rarely used nowadays and have been replaced by duplex ultrasound. If a swelling is apparent over the saphenofemoral junction, placing the hand over the swelling and tapping the varicose veins lower down the legs may elicit a palpable thrill at the groin, confirming the presence of a saphena varix.

Investigations. Diagnosis of varicose veins is made clinically based on appearance. The extent to which superficial or deep venous incompetence contributes to their formation is assessed with duplex ultrasound. If a secondary cause is suspected, abdominal ultrasound and/or CT venogram of the abdomen and pelvis can be performed.

Complications. Superficial thrombophlebitis. Haemorrhage. Varicose eczema. Varicose pigmentation due to haemosiderin deposition. Lipodermatosclerosis. Chronic venous ulceration. Long-standing venous stasis ulcers may become malignant (Marjolin's ulcer).

Treatment. All patients with varicose veins should be encouraged to elevate their limbs as much as possible and take good care of the skin on their lower legs with emollient washes and creams. Compression hosiery can help relieve symptoms of aching and swelling. Surgical treatment should be offered if superficial venous incompetence is causing symptoms affecting activities of daily living, bleeding, skin changes or active or healed ulceration. Surgical treatment of asymptomatic varicosities for cosmetic reasons is generally only offered privately.

Surgical treatment offered depends on the venous anatomy demonstrated on duplex ultrasound. If suitable (incompetent, straight long or short saphenous vein at least 1 cm below the skin), endovenous ablation is first-line treatment. This can be done using laser, radiofrequency or glue and can be combined with foam sclerotherapy or stab avulsions of visible varicosities which are marked preoperatively with the patient standing. These procedures are generally done under local anaesthetic. Open surgery (saphenofemoral ligation and stripping) is generally reserved for recurrence following endovenous treatment or unsuitable anatomy. Saphenopopliteal disconnection can be used for varicosities involving the small saphenous system. Stripping is not performed, as this will risk damage to the sural nerve. Compression bandaging is required postoperatively and low-molecular-weight heparin given intraoperatively. Encourage early mobilisation, instructing the patient to walk for 5–10 min every hour during the day to reduce the risk of DVT. Sit with legs elevated postoperatively.

HINTS AND TIPS

MANAGEMENT OF BLEEDING FROM VARICOSE VEINS

The superficial nature of varicose veins means that they can easily be damaged due to relatively minor trauma, resulting in major bleeding. Patients should be told to apply pressure, elevate the legs and seek medical attention. Surgical intervention is rarely needed, but patients may require fluid resuscitation! Bleeding from varicose veins is an indication for urgent outpatient referral to vascular surgery for investigation and treatment of any superficial venous incompetence.

Deep Vein Thrombosis (DVT)

This is a major cause of morbidity and mortality after surgery and trauma. It may occur spontaneously with the combined oral contraceptive pill or HRT. Only about 25% of DVTs cause symptoms and signs, others being silent. Pathological features (Virchow's triad) leading to DVT include:

- Hypercoagulability (malignancy, combined oral contraceptive pill, HRT, dehydration, polycythaemia or thrombophilia)
- Stasis (trauma, surgery, prolonged bed rest, pregnancy, pelvic mass, obesity)
- Vessel wall injury (previous DVT)

In a UK study of all admissions to a district general hospital, 10% of all deaths were due to pulmonary embolism. In addition, up to 30% of patients in hospital have asymptomatic nonocclusive calf vein thrombosis.

Symptoms and Signs. Swelling of the leg, tenderness of the calf muscles, increased temperature of the leg. Homans' sign (calf pain on passive dorsiflexion of the foot) is insensitive and nonspecific. Occlusion of the iliofemoral segment produces gross swelling of the whole limb, which is painful and white (phlegmasia alba dolens). Complete blockage of the iliofemoral segment with extension of thrombosis into venules and capillaries causes extreme pain with bluish discoloration and impending venous gangrene (phlegmasia caerulea dolens).

Investigations

- D-dimer (cleavage fragment from formed thrombus – can be elevated in malignancy, infection and postoperatively)
- Duplex ultrasound
- CT venogram if iliofemoral thrombosis is suspected.

Treatment. The aims of treatment are to prevent propagation of the clot, minimise the risk of pulmonary embolism (PE) and reduce the chance of developing post-thrombotic syndrome in the future.

Prevention. General measures include adequate hydration, avoiding calf pressure and early postoperative mobilisation. Some authorities recommend stopping oral contraceptives at least 6 weeks prior to surgery, while others merely recommend heparin prophylaxis. The case for stopping HRT is controversial. Patients at special risk should be treated as follows:

- Low-molecular-weight heparin or DOAC, e.g. subcutaneous Clexane 40mg daily, or 2.5mg apixaban twice daily. This is commonly used in hospital, but in high-risk cases, such as orthopaedic operations requiring prolonged immobilisation of a limb, prophylaxis is indicated for up to 6 weeks postoperatively.
- Calf compression devices used intraoperatively
- Graduated compression stockings, or thromboembolic deterrent (TED) stockings. These should be worn preoperatively, intraoperatively and postoperatively until the patient is mobilising satisfactorily.

Therapeutic. Once the diagnosis has been confirmed, then anticoagulation is commenced. This may be with i.v. unfractionated heparin or treatment dose of low molecular weight heparin. This is then converted to a DOAC for 3–6 months. In patients for whom DOACs are unsuitable (e.g. severe CKD), warfarin can be used with a target INR of 2–2.5. Limb elevation when resting, calf exercises and compression hosiery should be encouraged. Where iliofemoral DVT is causing significant symptoms despite exemplary early conservative management, surgical treatment can be considered. A reduction in post-thrombotic syndrome has been shown following early recanalisation leading to preservation of valvular competence. However, in UK practice it is usually only used if there is an extensive iliofemoral DVT in a young patient with a mechanical cause for the DVT or with a threatened limb with impending venous gangrene. Techniques used include:

- Catheter directed thrombolysis – catheter is directed into the thrombus for local delivery of thrombolytic agents (such as tissue plasminogen activator (tPA)).
- Percutaneous mechanical thrombectomy – device used that actually breaks down the thrombus (may be combined with thrombolysis).

In addition to both these procedures, deep venous stenting may be required if a NIVL (non-thrombotic iliac vein lesion) is found following thrombus removal and thought to be a contributor to the DVT. A reduction in area of the iliac vein of at least 50% (measured using intravascular ultrasound (IVUS)) following thrombus removal is generally the threshold for a stent.

In some cases, anticoagulation may fail, be contraindicated or result in complications. In these cases, an IVC filter may be required to prevent PE. Indications for a filter include:

- Contraindication to anticoagulation, e.g. risk of bleeding
- Thromboembolic event despite adequate anticoagulation
- Complication of anticoagulation, e.g. bleeding
- Inability to achieve adequate levels of anticoagulation
- Free-floating IVC thrombus.

Chronic Venous Insufficiency

This is caused by persistent and sustained ambulatory venous hypertension. Causes include:

- Muscle pump dysfunction, e.g. fused ankle in arthritis or neurological impairment after CVA
- Abnormal valve function which may be primary (affecting both the superficial and deep veins) or secondary after DVT with destruction of deep valves (known as postphlebitic limb)
- Congenital valve absence (very rare).

Along with changes in the large veins that result in venous hypertension, there are several abnormalities at the microcirculatory level. These include:

- White blood cell (WBC) trapping. WBCs become trapped in capillaries and cause endothelial activation and release of inflammatory cytokines that increase vascular permeability and contribute to the presence of a fibrin cuff together with release of proteolytic enzymes and free radicals. In addition, they cause tissue ischaemia by blocking capillaries.
- Fibrin cuff. An increase in venous pressure is transmitted to the capillaries and opens endothelial pores resulting in molecules such as fibrinogen moving into the interstitial space. This polymerises to fibrin and may act as a barrier to oxygen diffusion causing local tissue ischaemia.

Symptoms and Signs

- Peripheral oedema. This gets worse towards the end of the day and tends to settle with elevation.
- Varicose veins

- Venous eczema and brawny induration of the skin
- Venous pigmentation associated with haemosiderin deposits in the tissues
- Venous stasis ulceration, which is common in the area of the medial malleolus
- There is often severe pain or aching associated with the swelling and ulceration.
- Venous claudication. This indicates obstruction of the deep venous system, most commonly due to an occlusive iliofemoral DVT. It is described as a 'bursting' pain that comes on with exercise and takes 10–20 min to settle.

Investigations

- Duplex ultrasound allows assessment of both superficial and venous systems.
- CT/MR venography to assess for proximal causes of insufficiency such as outflow obstruction or anatomical variants
- ABPI to indicate suitability for compression and need for further arterial investigations.

Treatment. Difficult to treat, and patient rarely gets complete relief.

Medical. Advise patient to avoid long periods of standing and to sit with legs elevated. Graduated compression stockings, four-layer bandaging or other compression adjuncts such as wraps (ensure ABPI >0.8 before using compression). Treat venous stasis ulcers by reducing swelling of the leg by bandaging, excision of necrotic tissue and control of any cellulitis with antibiotics. Clean ulcers with normal saline and emollient washes. Use emollient creams and steroid preparations for venous eczema.

Surgery. Options for surgical intervention include:

- Superficial venous surgery for management of varicose veins and includes endovenous ablation of the great saphenous vein. Useful in isolated superficial reflux or combined deep and superficial reflux. Trials have shown that treatment of superficial venous incompetence improves time to ulcer healing and reduces ulcer recurrence.
- Perforating vein surgery. Generally used following truncal endovenous ablation if an improvement in an ulcer is not seen and duplex ultrasound demonstrates reflux in a perforating vein. Can be ligated via a stab incision, ablated with laser/radiofrequency or ultrasound-guided foam sclerotherapy
- Deep venous treatment. Open operations are vanishingly rare, but venous stenting can be used where previous DVT or a NIVL is causing proximal obstruction.
- Ulcer debridement and skin grafting
- Amputation. Carried out if ulceration leads to a non-salvageable limb.

Superficial Vein Thrombosis (previously called superficial thrombophlebitis)

This is characterised by a local inflammation of a segment of superficial vein. The vein is tender, red and feels like a 'cord'. The causes are shown in Table 16.3. When close to the saphenopopliteal or saphenofemoral junctions, there is a high risk of progression to DVT. Treatment is therefore with therapeutic anticoagulation as per a DVT if the superficial vein thrombosis is within 3 cm of the junction. If it is greater than 3 cm away from the junction and >5 cm in length, 45 days of 2.5 mg fondaparinux is

TABLE 16.3

CAUSES OF SUPERFICIAL THROMBOPHLEBITIS

Varicose veins
Occult carcinoma:
- Bronchus
- Pancreas
- Stomach
- Breast

Mondor's disease – superficial thrombophlebitis on chest wall
Buerger's disease
Polycythaemia
Local bacterial infection
Polyarteritis
Iatrogenic – intravenous infusions
Drug abuse
Idiopathic

recommended. Management is generally carried out by local DVT clinics, and repeat duplex ultrasounds may be required to ensure thrombus is not propagating. Symptoms are managed with anti-inflammatories and ice packs. Following the acute event, referral should be made to the vascular surgeons for further investigation and treatment of superficial venous incompetence to prevent further episodes. Treatment should be delayed until at least 3 months after the acute event.

LYMPHOEDEMA

Definition – localised fluid retention and tissue swelling due to hypoplasia or obstruction of lymphatics. It may be primary or secondary.

Primary

Primary lymphoedema can be classified into two subsets: isolated, where the condition is not inherited; and familial, where there is a definite inherited trait. Further subdivisions can then be made according to the age of onset. Congenital hereditary lymphoedema presents at birth or within the first 2 years of life. Milroy's disease is an autosomal dominant familial form of congenital lymphoedema. Lymphoedema praecox occurs at puberty or shortly afterwards. Lymphoedema tarda occurs after the age of 30. However, lymphoedema presenting for the first time in later life should prompt a search for underlying malignancy, especially pelvic.

Secondary

Lymphatic obstruction may occur secondary to other disease processes, e.g. secondary neoplasms in lymph nodes, infection in lymph nodes, e.g. filariasis (common worldwide, rare in UK) or may occur following surgical removal of lymph glands, i.e. block dissection or radiotherapy.

Symptoms and Signs. There is progressive swelling of one or both extremities, usually beginning around the ankle but often involving the whole extremity. The scrotum may be involved. Oedema is nonpitting and does not settle with elevation. Often the leg aches and feels tight but there is no pain. Minor trauma will cause cellulitis. Need to differentiate from other causes of leg swelling (→Table 16.4).

TABLE 16.4
CAUSES OF SWELLING OF THE LEG

Local	
Acute swelling	Trauma DVT Cellulitis Allergy Rheumatoid arthritis Ruptured Baker's cyst

Chronic swelling	Venous:
	• Chronic venous insufficiency
	  • Superficial venous incompetence
	  • Deep venous incompetence
	  • Deep venous obstruction (pregnancy, pelvic tumours, absent IVC, previous DVT (postphlebitic limb))
	  • Congenital malformations, e.g. arteriovenous fistulae
	  • Failure of calf muscle pump (paralysis, immobility, ankle fusion)
	  • Dependency

General	
	Congestive cardiac failure Hypoalbuminaemia, e.g. liver failure, malnutrition Lymphoedema Renal failure Fluid overload Chemotherapy Myxoedema Nephrotic syndrome

Investigations. Lymphoedema is essentially a clinical diagnosis, and no further investigations are required in the great majority of patients. Where investigations are necessary, the following may be used:

- Lymphoscintigraphy – isotope lymphoscintigraphy is easy to perform and less traumatic for patients than lymphangiography.
- Lymphangiography (used rarely)
- CT scan to exclude pelvic malignancy.

Treatment. It is important that lymphoedema is differentiated from other causes of lower limb swelling. Treatment is either medical or surgical. The aim of treatment is to control the oedema and to prevent infection. Compression hosiery or devices (Flowtron therapy) are the mainstay of treatment. Check ABPIs before applying compression. Compliance is essential. Diuretics are contraindicated in lymphoedema. Avoid prolonged standing. Massage. Exercise. If any breaks in the skin occur, e.g. insect bites or minor trauma, antibiotics should be prescribed. Cellulitis and fungal infections should be treated promptly. Occasionally, surgical treatment is helpful but does very little to improve the cosmetic appearance. Surgery is only suitable for a minority of patients. The choices include reduction procedures (excess tissue is removed and the defect either closed directly or skin grafted) or bypass (via omental pedicles, anastomosing lymph nodes to veins or direct lymphovenous anastomosis). Complications include recurrent cellulitis and lymphangitis usually caused by *Streptococci*, which respond to penicillin. Lymphangiosarcoma may occur. The tendency is for steady progression of the swelling and recurrent infections.

VASCULAR TRAUMA

This includes penetrating trauma (90%), blunt trauma and iatrogenic trauma. In penetrating trauma, the vessel may be partially or completely transected. High-velocity gunshot wounds cause massive tissue loss and extensive vascular damage. With blunt trauma, vessels can be injured directly, e.g. crush injury or indirectly by distraction, e.g. fractures and dislocations. Iatrogenic trauma may occur during surgery, interventional radiology procedures or while obtaining access to the circulation, e.g. arterial lines and CVP lines. It may also occur with accidental intra-arterial injection, e.g. intravenous drug users. Prompt diagnosis and treatment are essential to save life and limb. Complete transection of an artery because of penetrating trauma may stop the bleeding, owing to vessel retraction. Partial transection is more serious as the remaining intact wall holds the vessel open, resulting in torrential haemorrhage. Blunt injury usually leads to an intimal tear with a resulting intimal dissection flap, which may compromise the distal circulation. Arteriovenous fistula may occur when an artery and a vein close to each other are injured. Venous injuries are usually due to penetrating trauma. Haemorrhage and/or thrombosis may result.

Symptoms and Signs. It is important to establish the mechanism of injury, degree of violence, type of weapon, time of incident. Hypotension and hypovolaemic shock require urgent management. Clinical signs can be divided into HARD signs (distal ischaemia, expanding and/or pulsatile haematoma, palpable thrill or audible bruit and active bleeding) and SOFT signs (history of bleeding from wound, injury close to the course of a major vessel, haematoma, distal nerve deficit, unexplained tachycardia or hypotension). Make note of associated injuries, e.g. nerve injuries, fractures, head injury.

Investigations. There may be no time for investigations, as urgent transfer to theatre may be required.

- Trauma CT, including arterial phases of any area of concern
- Plain radiographs, if time permits, e.g. fractures, position of bullets or foreign bodies
- Pulse oximetry can assess oxygen saturation in both limbs – a decrease may indicate injury.
- ABPIs – compare injured to uninjured limb – a ratio of <0.9 in a healthy limb indicates vascular compromise.
- Duplex ultrasound
- Angiography – this is both diagnostic and therapeutic, with the ability to place covered stents for bleeding and uncovered stents for intimal flaps, and gain proximal control of an artery with a balloon.

Treatment. Principles of treatment include:

- Management of airway
- Arrest of haemorrhage

- Correction of hypovolaemia
- Diagnosis of type and degree of injury
- Repair of vessels
- Management of associated injuries
- Rehabilitation.

Emergency Measures. Initial management should be guided by ATLS principles with attention to airway and breathing first. Circulation is addressed with insertion of two large-bore i.v. lines and assessment of any haemorrhage with vital signs and thorough examination. Litres of blood can be held in abdominal, thoracic and long bone compartments with minimal or no external bleeding. Compression should be applied to external haemorrhage. In major thoracic penetrating injuries, emergency thoracotomy is occasionally necessary to control the bleeding. In exsanguinating penetrating abdominal trauma, it may be necessary to perform a thoracotomy or laparotomy to cross clamp the aorta. Fracture/dislocations with obvious deformity and distal ischaemia need reduction and splinting. If no vascular injuries are obvious (i.e. no hard signs), then any investigations are carried out after the primary survey is completed and the patient is stable.

Principles of surgical management include:

- Fractures should be stabilised before vascular repair. A shunt can be inserted during orthopaedic repairs if necessary (suitable for large and medium-sized arteries).
- Simple lacerations with no intimal damage may be closed by direct suture.
- Lacerations in smaller arteries can be closed by a vein patch.
- In vessels that are transected, end-to-end anastomosis can be performed. If the ends are far apart, an interposition graft using either reversed autologous vein (from the opposite leg if a lower limb injury) or PTFE may be used.
- In complex injuries, bypass procedures may be required after ligation of major arteries. These may need to be extra-anatomic (i.e. running in a different course to the bypassed artery), to provide tissue coverage in major injuries.
- In some cases, the patient may be too unstable for complex vascular reconstruction. In these cases, vessels may be simply ligated (external carotid, subclavian artery, internal iliac artery may be ligated with little sequelae and virtually all veins other than the suprarenal IVC portal vein and superior mesenteric vein can be ligated).
- Packing can be used for venous bleeding, but it is unlikely to stop arterial bleeding.
- Fasciotomy should be performed in prolonged ischaemia to prevent compartment syndrome. Rarely, amputation may be required for the unsalvageable limb – this can be predicted using the Mangled Extremity Severity Score (MESS).

Complications. Thrombosis. Secondary haemorrhage. False aneurysm. AV fistulae. Compartment syndrome. Lymphatic leaks or lymphocele due to damage of lymphatic vessels. Distal vascular insufficiency. Ischaemic muscular contractures.

PROCEDURE

FEMORAL EMBOLECTOMY

The stages of a femoral embolectomy are as follows:

- A longitudinal incision is made in the groin over the femoral artery at the mid-inguinal point, i.e. halfway between the anterior superior iliac spine and the pubic symphysis. This is the surface marking of the femoral artery that will not be palpable due to the embolism.
- The incision is extended through the subcutaneous fat to the femoral vessels. The common femoral, superficial femoral and the profunda femoris arteries are dissected free and controlled with vascular slings.
- An arteriotomy is made in the artery directly over the origin of the profunda femoris artery. This may be a transverse incision, which is less likely to lead to subsequent stenosis, or longitudinal, which is easier to extend if a bypass operation becomes necessary.
- A 5F embolectomy catheter is passed up the common femoral into the iliac vessels. The balloon is inflated and gently withdrawn.
- Once the clot is retrieved, an assistant will need to control the inflow with the vascular sling and a vascular clamp (return of inflow with clot withdrawal will lead to a sudden gush of blood). This is repeated until no further clot is retrieved and the surgeon is happy with the inflow. The common femoral artery is then flushed with heparinised saline and clamped.
- A 4F embolectomy catheter is now passed down the profunda femoris artery and the superficial femoral artery. Once no more clot is retrieved and the surgeon is happy with the degree of back bleeding, the vessels are flushed with heparinised saline and clamped.
- The arteriotomy is closed with interrupted or continuous 6/0 Prolene sutures.
- Fascia and subcutaneous fat is closed with 3/0 Vicryl and clips are used for skin closure.

Chapter 17

Urology

Manar Malki • Elizabeth Chandra

CHAPTER OUTLINE

TAKING A UROLOGICAL HISTORY

Conditions of the urinary tract may present with very nonspecific symptoms; this is particularly true of the upper urinary tract. Symptoms can include: malaise, pyrexia, night sweats, vague back or abdominal pain and weight loss. However, there are a number of very specific urological symptoms to be aware of.

Symptoms

Haematuria. (For causes →Table 17.1) This is the passage of red blood cells in the urine and may be either visible (microscopic) or nonvisible (macroscopic). It may be associated with pain: dysuria or suprapubic pain suggests UTI or possibly a bladder stone; colicky loin pain would suggest an underlying ureteric stone or ureteric blood clot. Painless haematuria is of more concern and may suggest a urological malignancy. Care must be taken to avoid menstrual bleeding being mistaken for haematuria. Other causes of red urine include excessive beetroot ingestion, rifampicin, porphyria, haemoglobinuria and myoglobinuria.

Lower Urinary Tract Symptoms (LUTS). A group of symptoms which can be separated into storage symptoms and voiding symptoms.

Storage Symptoms. Frequency, urgency, urge urinary incontinence, nocturia.

Voiding Symptoms. Dysuria, hesitancy, poor stream, terminal dribbling, sensation of incomplete bladder emptying.

Pain. Type and site of pain suggest different pathologies. Dull flank pain is related to kidney pathology; colicky 'loin to groin' pain is ureteric, commonly stone related; suprapubic suggests bladder problems; prostate pain with be felt in the perineum or penis tip and testicles, and dysuria suggests infection.

Urinary Incontinence. This is classified as: stress, urge, mixed and overflow urinary incontinence.

Stress urinary incontinence occurs with increased abdominal pressure: coughing, lifting, etc.

TABLE 17.1

CAUSES OF HAEMATURIA

Kidney	Glomerular disease Polycystic kidneys Carcinoma Stone Trauma (including renal biopsy) Tuberculosis Embolism Renal vein thrombosis Vascular malformation
Ureter	Stone Neoplasm
Bladder	Carcinoma Stone Trauma Inflammatory – cystitis, tuberculosis, bilharzia
Prostate	Benign prostatic hypertrophy Neoplasm
Urethra	Trauma Stone Urethritis Neoplasm
General	Anticoagulants Thrombocytopenia Haemophilia Sickle cell disease Malaria

Urge urinary incontinence occurs immediately following a strong sensation of the desire to void.

Mixed urinary incontinence occurs when a patient has both urge and stress urinary incontinence.

Overflow urinary incontinence occurs when the urinary bladder is abnormally distended with large post-void residual volume. It typically happens to patients with chronic urinary retention.

Past Medical History

Previous episodes and their timescale are essential to elicit. Some medical conditions predispose to urological disease; for example, high-output stomas increase the chance of stone disease due to dehydration.

Drug History

Remember that some drugs may require stopping or altering if renal function is impaired. Furthermore, drugs may be causative in pathology, e.g. diuretics lead to dehydration and increased incidence of stones.

Social History

Smoking is a risk factor for all urological malignancies. A detailed occupational history is required; in particular bladder cancer has strong occupational risk factors; people working in the dye industry, painters and hairdressers all have increased risk due to occupational chemical exposure. Travel history: exposure to schistosomiasis may lead to urinary involvement.

Family History

There are familial links in prostate cancer, kidney cancer and bladder cancer in young patients. Certain benign and malignant urological conditions can be linked to inherited diseases such as tuberous sclerosis, von Hippel-Lindau (VHL) syndrome and Lynch syndrome. Kidney stones can also be hereditary, particularly in patients with metabolic disorders.

UROLOGICAL INVESTIGATIONS

Assessment of a urological patient is not complete without a number of simple tests. Urinalysis and a basic U&E plus FBC are required in all patients with addition of other tests according to their presentation.

Essential

- Urinalysis or 'dipstick' testing: this will show if there is microscopic haematuria, a possible urine infection or intrinsic renal disease.
- U&E and creatinine: these give an indication of renal function.
- FBC: can give an indication of infection, or anaemia secondary to malignancy or renal disease.

If Appropriate to Presentation

- Midstream urine: MC&S can confirm infection. Urine cytology can show abnormal or malignant cells.
- PSA: this has age-specific ranges and will be elevated in BPH, prostate cancer, prostatitis and acute urinary retention.
- Creatinine clearance: this is rarely done as it requires a 24-h urine collection which patients are poorly compliant with. It gives a more accurate estimation of renal function than serum creatinine alone.
- Paired serum and urine biochemistry investigations.

Imaging

- X-ray KUB: rarely used in the UK now, as it has been superseded by computerised tomography (CT). Can be useful for identifying radio-opaque calculi and monitoring their progress.
- Intravenous urogram: this gives information about renal function and clear images of the ureters allowing outline of calculi but again has been mainly replaced by CT.
- USS: this is very useful in investigating urological disease, much of which can affect young people, which means radiation doses should be limited:
  - Renal USS shows hydronephrosis and cysts or masses within the kidney parenchyma or calyceal system. USS can also demonstrate significant kidney stones (>4mm).
  - Ureters can be visualised to assess dilatation, flow and contents such as stones and tumours.
  - Bladder USS shows stones and bladder tumours, bladder filling and residual volumes.

- Transrectal USS is used to measure the size of the prostate and take prostate biopsies.
- USS of testis and scrotum can show tumours, and if Doppler is used, may indicate testicular torsion.

- CT: different CT modalities are used to evaluate various urological conditions. The specific type of CT scan used mainly depends on the clinical indication.
  - Noncontrast CT scan: It is the gold standard for investigating kidney and ureteric stones.
  - Contrast-enhanced CT scan: It involves the administration of a contrast agent intravenously. Different phases of scanning are used to evaluate different urological conditions such as renal tumours, urothelial tumours and filling defects in ureters.
- Magentic resonance imaging (MRI): is the gold-standard imaging for investigating prostate cancer. It can also be helpful in further evaluating some complex renal lesions.
- Isotope bone scan: used to screen for bone metastasis from prostate cancer.
- DMSA: a radioisotope static scan which identifies functioning renal tissue by virtue of uptake of a radioactive substance within functioning renal tissue. DMSA provides an accurate evaluation of the split function of the kidneys. It demonstrates areas of renal scarring and is commonly used in paediatric patients.
- MAG3: a radioisotope dynamic scan which identifies functioning renal tissue similarly to DMSA. MAG3 provides information about renal blood flow, tubular filtration and urinary excretion. It is usually used to assess renal perfusion and obstructive uropathy, and to evaluate a renal transplant function.

PROCEDURE

FLEXIBLE CYSTOSCOPY

Flexible cystoscopy can be performed under local or general anaesthetic to view the inside of the urinary bladder.

Flexible cystoscopy lists are a large part of the urologist's workload. In the UK lists are normally dedicated, fast moving, local anaesthetic day case lists. Few people are unable to tolerate a local anaesthetic flexible cystoscopy.

1. Clean and drape patient.
2. Insert lignocaine 2% gel.
3. Introduce scope to the urethra with the water running.
4. Proceed along the urethra swiftly always maintaining the view of the lumen. Do not progress if resistance is felt and the lumen is not visible.
5. Once within the bladder, stop the flow of water when filling is adequate, and then use a systematic approach to visualising all areas.
   a. Visualise the trigone and identify both ureteral orifices.
   b. Move on to visualise the base and posterior bladder wall.
   c. Visualise air bubble in bladder dome.
   d. Examine both lateral walls.
   e. Perform a J manoeuvre to visualise internal bladder neck, prostate in men and trigone from alternative view.
   f. Restart the water flow, examine bladder neck and urethra on withdrawal.
6. Clean patient and cover them, giving the patient some privacy to redress themselves before leaving.

CONGENITAL DISORDERS OF THE URINARY TRACT

Kidney and Ureter

Congenital Absence of One Kidney. Incidence is 1:1000.

Pelvic Kidney. Incidence is 1:800. Often associated with reflux or pelvi-ureteric junction obstruction (PUJO). Large pelvic kidney may interfere with childbirth.

Horseshoe Kidney. Incidence is 1:400 to 1:600. The kidneys lie vertically and lower than normal. Renal pelvis rotated anteriorly and the lower poles joined medially. This condition is often associated with reflux, PUJO, renal tumour and undescended testes.

Pelvi-ureteric Junction Obstruction (PUJO). Aetiology can be congenital or acquired. Lower pole aberrant vessel may aggravate but rarely responsible for condition. Patients can present with history of loin pain, failure to thrive, recurrent UTI, mass, hypertension. Often discovered on prenatal USS.

Infantile Polycystic Disease. Incidence is 1:10,000. Rare, autosomal recessive.

Adult Polycystic Disease. Incidence is 1:1500. Autosomal dominant, involving both kidneys. Patients usually present aged 30–40 years with hypertension, mass, haematuria, renal failure. May be associated with extrarenal disease such as cysts in the liver, and berry aneurysms (6–16%). Family screening and genetic counselling.

Medullary Sponge Kidney. Incidence is between 1:5000 and 1:20,000. Characterised by congenital dilatation or cysts of the distal collecting ducts. May be associated with hypercalciuria, impaired urinary concentration.

Ureteric Duplication. Often bilateral. The ureter from the upper pole moiety lies medial and inferior to the lower pole ureter at the bladder (Weigert–Meyer rule).

Ureterocele. Dilatation of the submucosal portion of the ureter. It is often detected as a filling defect on IVU.

Megaureter. Secondary to either dysplastic (nonobstructed) or obstructed ureter. May be associated with stones, UTI, reflux.

Vesicoureteric Reflux. Reflux is the abnormal passage of urine from bladder to the ureter. Primary reflux (1%) is due to a defect of the vesicoureteric junction. Usually resolving spontaneously in 70% of cases. Secondary reflux is usually due to outflow obstruction – causes include posterior urethral valve, urethral stenosis, neuropathic bladder and detrusor sphincter dyssynergia (DSD) 20% of children presenting with recurrent UTI have reflux.

Diagnosis. Urinary tract USS, Voiding cystourethrogram (VCUG), urodynamic study if suspicious of voiding dysfunction.

Treatment. Conservative management for low-grade reflux including low-dose antibiotic prophylaxis and regular voiding.

Endoscopic ureteric injection of Deflux, or ureteric reimplantation.

Bladder

Ectopia Vesica (Exstrophy of the Bladder). This occurs in 1:20,000–40,000. It is more common in the male. The anterior wall of the bladder fails to close. The posterior bladder wall, the trigone and posterior urethra are exposed and urine leaks onto the skin.

Complications. Ureteric dilatation and pyelonephritis.

Treatment. Bladder closure, pelvic osteotomy and abdominal wall closure can be achieved if performed early. Alternatively, reimplantation of the ureters into an ileal loop conduit with excision of the bladder and repair of the abdominal wall defect may be required.

Urachal Abnormalities. Defects may result from the primitive urachal connections between bladder and umbilicus. If the tract persists, urine may discharge from the umbilicus. An urachal cyst may occur if part of the urachus persists but is closed off above and below. Infection may occur in a urachal cyst. Treatment is by excision.

Urethra

The urethra may terminate on the ventral aspect of the penis (hypospadias) or on its dorsal aspect (epispadias). Hypospadias may result in difficulty with intercourse. Plastic reconstruction of the urethra may be required. Epispadias is rare and more disabling and difficult to correct than hypospadias. It may be associated with incontinence. Plastic reconstruction or urinary diversions are possible treatments. In the female, the urethra may open onto the anterior vaginal wall.

Urethral valves may occur in the posterior urethra. The condition is rare, occurring with an incidence of 1:5000, 50% of cases being diagnosed in children under 1 year of age. They cause dilatation of the prostatic urethra, bladder, ureters and renal pelvis. It is often diagnosed on prenatal USS. Rarely, there may be uraemia with palpable bladder and kidneys at birth. Milder cases present later in childhood with difficulty in voiding, recurrent UTIs and uraemia. Treatment is by transurethral resection of the valves. With early presentation, the prognosis is good. With extensive renal damage, dialysis and transplantation may be required.

STONE DISEASE

Urinary tract stones account for a large proportion of the urological work. When covering urological acute admissions, it would be normal to see several patients with new-onset or recurrent symptoms from stone disease. In the UK and developed countries, upper urinary tract calculi are more common, whereas in developing countries bladder calculi predominate (these are discussed at the end of this section). In most developed countries incidence of ureteric stones is 1–2% of the population; however, many remain asymptomatic. Men are more commonly affected than women and they most commonly occur in people between 20–50 years of age. Calculi can form anywhere along the urinary tract from the kidney to the bladder. Bladder stones are often related to incomplete bladder emptying.

Aetiology

Dehydration is the most common cause for developing renal stones. There is an increased incidence during the summer months. However, underlying causes such as infection, anatomical malformations and metabolic disorders can be responsible. Infection is a common precipitating factor as is urinary stasis. There are several metabolic conditions that can result in urinary stones (Table 17.2).

Types of Stones

Composition of stones can vary depending on the underlying cause. Ninety percent of urinary stones are radio-opaque, which is important to remember when investigating patients. There is some international geographical variation in the most likely composition of stones. The figures below apply to UK stone composition.

Calcium Oxalate (75%). 'Mulberry' stones covered with sharp projections. They cause bleeding and are often black owing to altered blood on their surface. Because of their sharp surface they give symptoms when comparatively small.

TABLE 17.2

METABOLIC CAUSES OF UROLITHIASIS
Hyperparathyroidism
Idiopathic hypercalciuria
Disseminated malignancy
Hypervitaminosis D
Sarcoidosis
Hyperthyroidism
Cystinuria
Hyperoxaluria
Xanthinuria
Hyperuricosuria

Phosphate (15%). These stones occur in patients with renal tubular acidosis (RTA), a defect of renal tubular H^+ secretion resulting in impaired ability of the kidney to acidify urine.

Struvite (2–20%). Usually 'triple phosphate': a compound of calcium, magnesium and ammonium phosphate. Known as 'struvite' stones. They are smooth and dirty white and can enlarge rapidly in the kidney to fill the calyces forming a staghorn calculus. Often a result of repeated or chronic urinary tract infection, especially if caused by *Proteus* spp.

Urate (5%). Arise due to high uric acid in the urine. Hard, smooth, faceted and light brown in colour. Pure uric acid stones are radiolucent.

Cystine (2%). Usually multiple, white and translucent and very hard. Secondary to metabolic disorder causing decreased reabsorption of cystine from the renal tubules.

Xanthine and Pyruvate Stones. Rare. Due to an inborn error of metabolism.

Symptoms and Signs. Stones will cause different symptoms dependent on their position in the renal tract:

- Renal stones: occasional loin pain and discomfort but may have colic if stone becomes lodged at the pelvi-ureteric junction (PUJ)
- Ureteric stones: colicky pain radiating from loin to groin; patients are sweaty, restless, nauseous and may vomit.

All renal tract calculi can result in haematuria that is normally microscopic. If infection is present, patients will be pyrexial, tachycardic, have dysuria and an underlying constant pain between colic attacks.

Infected obstructed kidney is a urological emergency. Patients often deteriorates rapidly. Patients requires prompt treatment with intravenous antibiotics and de-obstruction of the kidney (stent or nephrostomy tube).

Investigations. Must include:

- Urine dipstick: will show microscopic haematuria and indicate possible infection
- MSSU sent for MC&S: aid with treating any infection present
- U&E: possible renal impairment if obstruction present
- FBC: supports diagnosis of infection.

A urine dipstick and an MSSU must be done prior to any antibiotics being given. Following this, imaging is required, and the choice of modality will depend on the patient's presentation and local facilities.

- CT KUB (noncontrast): now the most used imaging investigation in the UK and considered gold standard. A noncontrast study is performed. Stone size, position and degree of obstruction can be assessed.
- KUB radiograph: 90% of calculi are radio-opaque, and thus this can show the presence of a stone but is more commonly used in a serial manner to follow the passage of the stone over a few days rather than for initial diagnosis.
- USS: can show hydronephrosis and allow placement of nephrostomy tube. It is useful if the patient is known to have a renal stone on a recent CT KUB.
- IVU: rarely used in the UK but still valuable in identifying stones and confirming obstruction if CT is not available.

Following the initial management, the following should be performed:

- Blood tests for: calcium, phosphate, uric acid
- 24-h urine for calcium, phosphate, oxalate, urate, cystine and xanthine.

Treatment

Acute Episode

- Analgesia: diclofenac is most effective given per rectum. Opiates are necessary if patients cannot have NSAID or pain is effectively controlled.
- Antiemetic
- Increased fluids – oral if possible; i.v. if necessary
- Collect and sieve all urine to retrieve calculus for analysis.
- i.v. antibiotics if infection is present
- Decompression if obstruction is present; this can be done by:
  - Percutaneous nephrostomy (USS guided under local anaesthesia)
  - Ureteral stent insertion in theatre (under general anaesthesia).

If pain persists and the patient is not improving, serial radiographs can assess progress of the stone; majority of stones <4mm will usually pass spontaneously; 50% of stones between 4mm and 7mm will pass spontaneously. Stones >7mm usually require intervention.

Stone Treatment. Choosing the appropriate treatment is dependent on the size, number and location of the stones. This may be carried out by ureteroscopy and fragmentation of the stone; fragmentation is typically performed with laser. Alternatively, fragmentation with extracorporeal shock wave lithotripter (ESWL) is performed. Large kidney stones can be treated with percutaneous nephrolithotomy (PCNL). Removal of a calculus by open surgical technique is now rare.

Bladder Stones

These can occur in men with prostatic outflow obstruction but are more common in developing countries secondary to infections with bilharzia and other worms. Symptoms include dull suprapubic discomfort, dysuria, difficulty initiating urination, strangury. Terminal haematuria may occur.

Treatment. Small stones may be removed cystoscopically after crushing with a Maeurmayer stone punch, laser or disintegration using an ultrasound and pneumatic lithotripter. Large stones >5cm are removed by suprapubic cystostomy. Patients should be investigated for an underlying bladder outflow obstruction and treated appropriately if required.

Prevention of Recurrence. Up to 50% of patients may have recurrence within 5 years. Depending on the cause, preventative measures involve:

- High fluid intake especially in hot weather – good fluid intake 2–3L per day
- Moderate milk and dairy intake
- Prompt treatment of UTIs
- Calcium stones: low-calcium diet, thiazide diuretics acidify urine
- Oxalate stones: reduce oxalate intake – exclude rhubarb, spinach, tomatoes, strawberries, tea and chocolate
- Urate stones: allopurinol, urinary alkalinisation
- Urinary alkalisation with sodium bicarbonate or potassium citrate can be helpful for patients with cystine and urate stones.

PROCEDURE

PERCUTANEOUS NEPHROSTOMY

In this procedure a small catheter / drainage tube is passed into the calyceal system of the obstructed kidney to allow urine to pass out. It is performed via a modified Seldinger technique under radiological guidance.

1. Needle passed through skin at point of posterior axillary line 2–3cm below 12th rib
2. Radiological guidance used to ensure entry into the calyceal system
3. Wire passed through needle and needle removed
4. Appropriate dilatation of tract to allow placement of catheter
5. Dressed to maintain sterility and attached to drainage bag.

PROCEDURE

CYSTOSCOPY AND STENT INSERTION

This can be used to overcome an obstruction of the ureter and provide a patent lumen for urine to drain:

1. Enter bladder as per cystoscopy.
2. Identify ureteric orifice and insert a guidewire under radiological screening.
3. A contrast study (retrograde ureteropyelogram) is usually performed via a ureteric catheter to delineate the anatomy of the renal pelvis.
4. A double J ureteric stent is passed over the guidewire and positioned correctly with radiological assistance; remove wire.
5. Empty bladder and remove the scope.

OBSTRUCTIVE UROPATHY

Obstruction of the urinary system below the level of the calyceal system will lead to hydronephrosis. There is distension of the calyces and pelvis of the kidney owing to obstruction to the outflow of urine. Depending on the level or cause of obstruction, it may be bilateral or unilateral. (For causes of hydronephrosis →Table 17.3.)

TABLE 17.3

CAUSES OF HYDRONEPHROSIS

Unilateral	Pelvi-ureteric junction obstruction: • Congenital pelvi-ureteric junction obstruction • Aberrant renal vessels • Calculus • Tumours of the renal pelvis or PUJ Ureteric obstruction: • Calculus • Ureteric invasion, e.g. cervical, rectal or colonic tumour • Ureteric tumour • Iatrogenic – damage at surgery
Bilateral	Urethral valves Urethral or meatal stenosis Chronic urinary retention Advanced prostate cancer Extensive bladder tumours Direct extension of cervical/rectal cancer Retroperitoneal fibrosis

HINTS AND TIPS

When questioned on a ward round, it is always helpful to have a system to help you answer succinctly and avoid forgetting important causes; when considering causes of obstruction, the following system can be used:

- Within the lumen (calculus)
- Within the wall (TCC of the ureter)
- Outside the wall (retroperitoneal fibrosis, advanced colonic tumour).

Symptoms and Signs. The symptoms of obstructive uropathy can vary depending on the location and severity of obstruction. Some patients with obstructive uropathy might not experience any symptoms, especially in the early stages of the condition.

Some patients might present with loin pain and possibly fever with rigours if infection is present. Symptoms of renal failure if obstruction is long-standing or bilateral. In extreme cases, the kidney may be palpable or ballotable on examination. Palpable prostate PR.

Investigations. Initial investigations should include:

- FBC, clotting profile
- U&Es
- LFTs
- MSSU (if urine sample obtainable).

Imaging

- USS: this is the most useful initial imaging. It confirms the diagnosis and may identify the cause; it can also be used therapeutically to place a nephrostomy if required.
- KUB: not very useful but may show enlarged renal outline or opaque calculi.

- IVU (Figure 17.1): there will be pelvic dilatation with clubbing of the calyces, the site of obstruction will be identified; there may be trabeculation of bladder if obstruction is distal. IVUs are rarely used to make a diagnosis of hydronephrosis. It has been largely replaced with CT urogram.
- CT urogram: contrast-enhanced CT scan confirms diagnosis and is likely to identify cause. It aids in determining if the cause of hydronephrosis is intraluminal or extraluminal.
- Cystoscopy: identifies cause of bladder outlet obstruction or bladder tumour.
- Retrograde uretero-pyelogram study: defines exact site of obstruction.
- Isotope renography: if significant renal damage suspected, to establish percentage of renal function remaining.

Treatment. Treatment will be directed at the underlying cause. The presence of acute infection or marked renal impairment requires urgent decompression of the urinary tract under antibiotic cover. This may be achieved by percutaneous

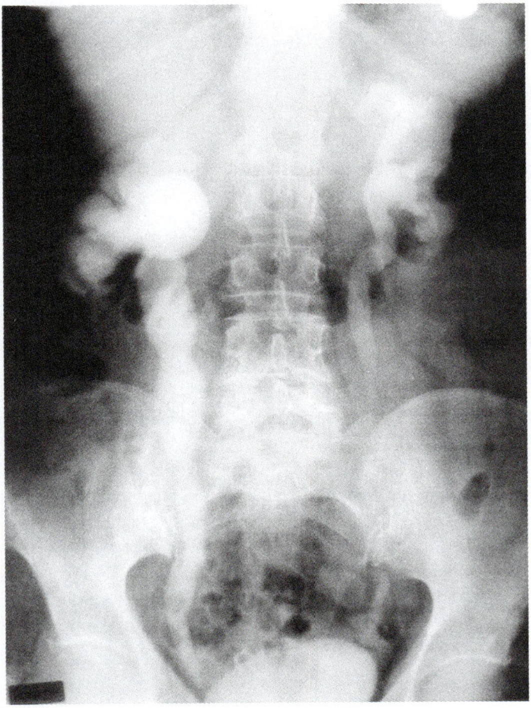

FIGURE 17.1

Intravenous urogram.There is a right-sided hydronephrosis and hydroureter. Note the dilatation of the pelvis with clubbing of the calyces and dilatation of the ureter down to its entry into the bladder.

nephrostomy or ureteric (JJ) stent insertion for ureteric obstruction. For prostate and urethral obstruction, options include indwelling urethral catheter or suprapubic catheter or cystostomy. A nonfunctioning kidney, especially if infected, should be removed.

Complications. These include: infection leading to pyelonephritis and urosepsis; stone formation in stagnant urine; hypertension due to renal ischaemia; traumatic rupture of a hydronephrotic kidney; and uraemia.

URINARY TRACT INFECTIONS (UTI)

These may be divided into those affecting the kidney (pyelonephritis) and those affecting the bladder (cystitis). UTIs are more common in women – most women will have a UTI sometime during their life. Risk factors include urinary tract malformations, urinary tract obstruction, calculus, prostatic obstruction, bladder diverticulum, spinal injury, trauma, urinary tract tumour, diabetes mellitus, immunosuppression.

Symptoms and Signs

Acute Pyelonephritis. Patients will complain of loin pain, dysuria, frequency, fever, rigours, cloudy or bloodstained urine. Tenderness in the loin and flank.

Cystitis. Frequency, urgency, dysuria, haematuria, often no fever. May have tenderness suprapubically.

Investigations

- Urinalysis: presence of leukocytes and nitrites together strongly suggests UTI. Haematuria and proteinuria may also be present.
- MSSU for MC&S (**before** antibiotics are given): colony count of >100,000 organisms/mL of a fresh MSSU is significant. Microscopy shows pus cells and organisms (usually Gram-negative rods).
- FBC
- U&Es.

Common organisms include *Escherichia coli, Proteus mirabilis, Klebsiella pneumoniae, Pseudomonas aeruginosa* and *Enterococcus faecalis*.

Treatment. Make sure the patient is well hydrated. Give antibiotics; co-amoxiclav or trimethoprim are appropriate initial treatments, although checking with the local microbiology department for local sensitivities will be valuable, as resistance is increasing. Change antibiotic according to organism and sensitivities. Avoid sexual intercourse while infected.

If the infection fails to settle on appropriate antibiotics or recurs rapidly after stopping antibiotics, further investigation is required. Any man with history of confirmed UTI should undergo investigation. In females, recurrent episodes of UTIs that have been appropriately treated also warrant further investigation. Failure to respond to treatment suggests inappropriate antibiotics, failure to complete the course of antibiotics, resistant organisms, underlying obstruction, calculus, tumour, urinary retention or specific infection, e.g. TB. Further investigation of recurrent attacks includes ultrasound, flexible cystoscopy.

Sterile Pyuria

This means pus cells are apparent on microscopy but there is no growth on culture. Causes include inadequately treated UTI, TB, tumour, stone, prostatitis, polycystic kidneys, appendicitis, diverticulitis or analgesic abuse.

Urinary Tract Tuberculosis

Genitourinary tuberculosis is always secondary to TB elsewhere. The urinary tract is involved by haematogenous spread. The kidney is affected most frequently, the lower urinary tract being secondarily infected by descending infection, giving rise to cystitis or infection of the epididymis or seminal vesicles.

The renal lesion is often silent, but patients may have repeated UTIs with frequency, dysuria and haematuria. Importantly the patient will also have systemic symptoms: weight loss, fever and night sweats. Men may get epididymitis and scrotal sinuses.

Diagnosis requires at least three early morning urines. Microscopy shows sterile pyuria; however, Ziehl–Neelsen staining of early morning specimen of urine may demonstrate acid-fast bacilli. Culture of tubercle bacilli takes up to 6 weeks.

Treatment in the UK is by specialist TB services. Combined therapy with two to three antituberculosis drugs. Surgery may be needed to remove a totally destroyed kidney or to deal with complications, e.g. repair of ureteric stricture or enlargement of small fibrotic bladder.

URETHRAL STRICTURES

Causes include idiopathic origin, infection, trauma, foreign bodies, stones, tumours and iatrogenic, i.e. post catheterisation or instrumentation.

Symptoms and Signs. Weak stream, dribbling, acute or chronic retention leading to recurrent UTIs.

Investigations

- Flexible cystoscopy under local anaesthetic
- Retrograde or antegrade cystourethrogram.

Treatment. Intermittent self-catheterisation helps with bladder emptying and can be used to a certain extent to promote dilatation of the stricture. Optical urethrotomy during rigid cystoscopy can be performed. Recurrent urethral strictures can be treated endoscopically with Optilume Drug Coated Balloon (DCB).

Short segment strictures can also be excised and primary anastomosis performed: alternatively surgical reconstruction (urethroplasty) with skin flaps from buccal mucosa can be performed. Patients often end up requiring repeated or regular procedures to treat difficult strictures.

URINARY RETENTION

The retention of urine may be acute, chronic or acute-on-chronic. Patients with acute retention present as urological emergencies. Chronic retention has an insidious onset and may present in the late stages. (For causes →Table 17.4).

Acute Urinary Retention

Symptoms and Signs. Patients present with a few-hour history of being unable to pass urine despite trying. They are uncomfortable, restless and complain of suprapubic pain. On examination, an enlarged prostate. Causes include enlarged prostate, UTI, constipation and underlying neurological disease.

Treatment. Urgent catheterisation after administration of analgesia. Where prostatic obstruction is present, bigger catheters (16Ch catheter) are often easier to pass than smaller sizes and are less likely to cause trauma. If this is not possible, either suprapubic catheterisation or cystoscopically guided urethral catheterisation is required. A sample of the first passed urine should be sent for MC&S and the residual volume recorded.

TABLE 17.4

CAUSES OF URINARY RETENTION

Local	
Intraluminal cause	Urethral valves Prostatic enlargement Tumours Stones Blood clot Meatal ulcer or stenosis
Luminal cause	Urethral trauma Urethral stricture Urethral tumour
Extraluminal cause	Faecal impaction Pelvic tumour Pregnant uterus Phimosis
General	
Postoperative Neurogenic	Spinal cord injuries Spinal cord disease, e.g. tabes dorsalis, spinal tumour, multiple sclerosis, diabetic autonomic neuropathy
Drugs	Anticholinergics, antidepressants, alcohol

Postoperative retention may be due to anxiety, supine posture, pain, drugs, fluid overload, unrecognised enlarged prostate with minimal symptoms. After urological procedures, it may be due to blood clot in the bladder. Before catheterising a patient in the postoperative period, other attempts should be made to allow the patient to pass urine, e.g. standing up in a warm room relaxed, running tap or bathing in warm water. Full recovery of bladder function and normal voiding usually occur within a few days.

Medical treatment of the underlying cause, such as infection and constipation, is mandatory before removing the catheter. In cases where benign prostate enlargement is the cause, a trial of alfa blocker (like Tamsulosin) may be considered before removing the catheter.

Surgical treatments offer various minimally invasive options, such as Urolift, Rezum, prostatic artery embolisation or more definitive surgical options: bipolar transurethral resection of the prostate (TURP), holmium laser enucleation of the prostate (HoLEP), green light laser prostatectomy and Aquablation utilising the AquaBeam system.

Chronic Urinary Retention

This may be low pressure or high pressure. There is usually >1 L urine in the bladder. In high-pressure chronic urinary retention there is reflux of urine up the ureters causing unilateral or bilateral hydronephrosis and renal impairment.

Symptoms and Signs. Chronic urinary retention is painless. History of long-standing LUTS and repeated UTIs. Overflow and nocturnal urinary incontinence can leave a smell of urine on the patient and their clothes. They may have an underlying neurological condition; this may be undiagnosed and signs should be sought. Palpable bladder and prostatic enlargement. Signs of uraemia.

Investigations

- MSSU: send for MC&S.
- FBC: infection may be present.
- U&Es: renal function may have been impaired.
- USS: to check upper urinary tract for hydronephrosis, may also show causative bladder tumour or stone.

Treatment. As with acute retention, attempt catheterisation after giving analgesia. If the catheter will not pass, carry out a suprapubic catheterisation. Secondary diuresis may occur. Patients often need fluid replacement in the first 48h after decompression.

Long-term treatment is by treating the cause of bladder outlet obstruction or, if that is not possible, urethral, suprapubic or intermittent self-catheterisation.

The surgical treatment options for chronic urinary retention encompass various surgical approaches. These include bipolar TURP, HoLEP, green light laser prostatectomy, and Aquablation with the AquaBeam system.

TUMOURS OF THE RENAL TRACT

Kidney

Benign tumours are rare. Renal cell cancer for 90% of renal tumours. Transitional cell tumours occur in the renal pelvis.

Renal Cell Carcinoma

This arises from renal tubular epithelium. There are around 13,300 new kidney cancer cases in the UK every year. Males are affected almost twice as commonly as females. It usually occurs over the age of 40 years. Risk factors include: smoking, obesity, analgesic phenacetin use and exposure to asbestos. Spread is by direct extension into perinephric tissues; intravascular invasion of the renal vein causing haematological spread to lung, bone, liver, brain; and lymphatic spread to the para-aortic nodes.

Symptoms and Signs. The most common presentation of renal cell carcinoma is now an incidental finding (60%) on imaging of the abdomen (USS, CT, etc.) performed for unrelated conditions.

Traditionally, it is thought to present with a triad of: haematuria, loin pain and a flank mass; this is now a rare presentation (8%) and is likely representative of advanced disease. Paraneoplastic syndromes can occur due to factors secreted by the tumour, resulting in: PUO, anaemia, polycythaemia, hypertension and hypercalcaemia. Symptoms and signs due to metastases include hepatomegaly, breathlessness and pathological fractures.

Investigations

- Blood tests: FBC, ESR, U&Es, calcium, LFTs
- Urinalysis: likely to show haematuria ± proteinuria
- USS: identifies tumour quickly and accurately
- CT thorax and abdomen with contrast (Figure 17.2): now the standard investigation; provides diagnosis and details of primary tumour, and possible organ metastases
- Isotope bone scan: shows bone metastases.

Treatment. Small renal tumours (≤4cm) are typically managed with nephron sparing treatment options, which include robotic assisted partial nephrectomy, cryoablation or

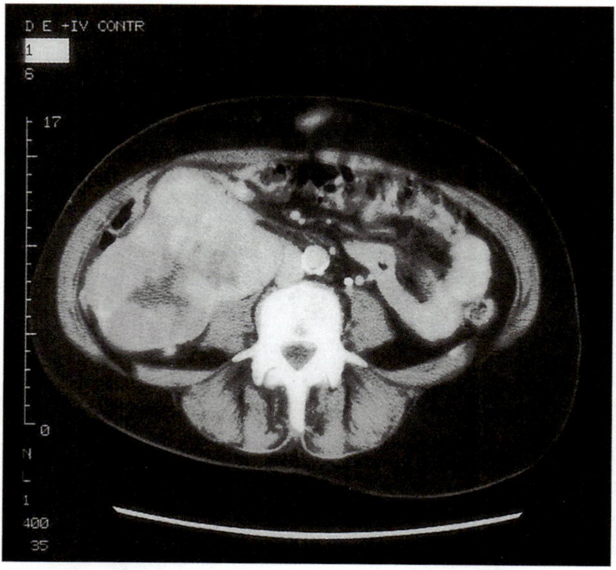

FIGURE 17.2
Abdominal CT scan. There is a renal cell carcinoma of the right kidney.

radiofrequency ablation. Larger tumours are treated with laparoscopic or open radical nephrectomy. In some cases, solitary metastases may be treated by surgery. Unfortunately, many renal tumours are discovered at advanced stage. In these cases, the treatment is systematic with immunotherapy and TKI's (tyrosine kinase inhibitors).

TKIs and immunotherapy have revolutionised the treatment landscape for patients with kidney cancer. Several trials have demonstrated significant clinical benefits in patients with metastatic renal cancer, leading to improved overall survival. These treatments are also being used as adjutant treatment for nonmetastatic patients with aggressive cancer.

Radiotherapy is used to treat pain from metastases in selected palliative patients.

Prognosis. If the tumour is localised to the kidney, nephrectomy offers a 5-year survival of 70–90%.

Renal Pelvis and Ureter

TCC of the renal pelvis is uncommon, accounting for 10% of all renal tumours and 4% of all urinary cancers. TCC of the ureter is rare, accounting for 1% of all newly presenting urinary cancer.

Symptoms and Signs. Haematuria and loin pain are common: a dull ache due to pressure from the tumour or colic due to obstruction from tumour or clot.

Investigations

- Urinalysis
- IVU/ CT urogram: IVU is rarely used. CT urogram typically demonstrates a filling defect or enhancing soft tissue in the ureter or renal pelvis. It also gives an idea on the severity of the hydronephrosis and any associated lymphadenopathy.

- CT chest: for staging
- Cystoscopy, retrograde ureteropyelogram ± ureteroscopy and biopsy.

Treatment. Nephroureterectomy with excision of a cuff of bladder wall is the gold standard treatment for TCC of the renal pelvis or ureter. However, for low-grade small volume TCC, endoscopic management with ureteroscopy and laser ablation may be a viable option.

Bladder

Some 95% of tumours in the bladder are TCCs. Chronic irritation from stones or infection may result in keratinising squamous cell metaplasia, giving rise to SCCs. Adenocarcinomas are rare. Incidence of bladder cancers is 16.4 per 100,000 population in the UK and are more common in men than women, with a ratio of 5:2. Aetiological factors for TCCs include smoking, aromatic hydrocarbons (rubber and dye industry), polycyclic aromatic hydrocarbons (painters). When TCCs occur, it is a result of field change in the transitional epithelium, thus synchronous and metachronous tumours are common. Patients should have their upper tracts and bladder examined regularly. Four percent of patients with a bladder TCC will be found to have an upper tract TCC (renal pelvis or ureter) in the 5 years following their bladder TCC diagnosis and up to 35% of patients with an upper tract TCC will be found to have or go on to have a bladder TCC. Most are superficial (nonmuscle invasive tumours) at presentation. Spread occurs by direct invasion into the prostate, urethra, sigmoid colon, rectum or, in the female, to the uterus and vagina. The ureteric orifices may be occluded giving rise to hydronephrosis and renal failure. Lymphatic spread is to the iliac and para-aortic nodes and haematological spread occurs late to the liver and lungs.

Symptoms and Signs. Most commonly presents with painless haematuria. Dysuria, frequency and urgency can occur. Hydronephrosis is a result of ureter or ureteric orifice involvement and subsequent blockage; it can result in CRF. It usually indicates muscle invasive disease. Advanced disease may cause pain from pelvic invasion. Examination is usually negative in the early stages. Grading is as follows:

- CIS: very early; high-grade cancer cells are only in the superficial mucosal layer.
- Ta: completely confined to mucosa
- T1: confined to submucosa/lamina propria
- T2: superficial muscle involved – localised rubbery thickening if anterior
  T2a: cancer has grown into the superficial muscle
  T2b: cancer has grown into the deeper muscle
- T3: tumour invades the perivesical tissue – mobile mass
  T3a: microscopically
  T3b: macroscopically (extravesical mass)
- T4: invasion beyond bladder to adjacent structures – fixed mass
  T4a: cancer has spread to the prostate, uterus or vagina
  T4b: tumour invades pelvic or abdominal wall.

Investigations

- FBC
- U&Es
- Urine cytology in selected patients
- IVU: will show filling defects and hydronephrosis but is largely historical

- USS: most common first line investigation will show tumours > 1 cm
- Flexible cystoscopy: usually under local anaesthetic ± biopsy and histological examination
- MRI: for staging of invasive bladder cancer
- CT: for staging
- Positron emission tomography (PET) scan: can be used to check if bladder cancer has spread to lymph nodes or other areas.

Treatment

- T1: transurethral resection or cystodiathermy via rigid cystoscopy (see procedure box). Resection is preferable, as histological samples can be sent. Tumour base biopsies should be sent separately to allow assessment for muscular invasion. For multiple small tumours, intravesical chemotherapy with mitomycin is given. Intravesical BCG therapy is reserved for high-grade superficial bladder cancer or carcinoma in situ. Check cystoscopy should be carried out at 3 months and then at regular intervals (6 months to a year). Further follow-up protocols are controversial and vary from place to place.
- T2: T2 tumours and above invade the detrusor muscle by definition and should not be managed by transurethral resection alone. A radical cystectomy is the 'gold standard' treatment, but radical radiotherapy may be effective in those not fit for surgery. Cystectomy requires urinary diversion by implantation of the ureters into an ileal conduit or formation of a 'neobladder'. The latter can be drained by self-catheterisation through a continent stoma, or anastomosed to the urethra to allow normal voiding per urethra.
- T3: this may be treated by radical radiotherapy, cystectomy or a combination of both.
- T4: palliative radiotherapy, systemic chemotherapy with cisplatin and gemcitabine may produce remissions.

Prognosis. Early tumours are curable, but recurrence is common; T1 tumours have a 70% chance of recurrence at 5 years and an 85% 5-year survival rate, falling to 60% with T2 and 40% with T3. Patients with T4 tumours rarely survive for more than 1 year.

HINTS AND TIPS

Microscopic / nonvisible haematuria is a common finding by GPs performing urinalysis for numerous reasons; it is also a common presentation of TCC in otherwise well patients. As such many urology departments will have a 'straight to test, one stop haematuria service'. Patients attend to a day unit where they have bloods and urine samples taken. They will undergo a renal tract USS and local anaesthetic flexible cystoscopy to look for evidence of disease.

CT urogram is the gold standard test to assess upper tracts in patients with history of visible haematuria. If this is negative, the patient can be discharged back to the GP with reassurance that there is nothing serious causing the haematuria. In such cases, it will often resolve spontaneously and may have been the result of undiagnosed infection, contamination in menstruating women or leakage from dilated bladder neck veins due to prostatic enlargement in men. This service also accommodates the follow-up of patients with previous TCC.

PROCEDURE

RIGID CYSTOSCOPY

This is a sterile procedure performed in an operating theatre under general or spinal anaesthetic. Introducing infection into the urinary tract causes significant morbidity and mortality even amongst young fit patients. Rigid cystoscopy is used for observation and investigation, and, by way of different adjuncts to the scope, can also be used therapeutically.

- Patients should be cleaned and covered with surgical drapes.
- The cystoscope is assembled.
- Fluid is connected and flows through the scope.
- The scope is inserted under direct vision and advanced only when the urethral lumen is in clear view until the bladder is reached.
- The flow of fluid is stopped once optimal filling is achieved.
- All areas of the bladder are viewed systematically by turning the scope and advancing and retracting it within the bladder.
- Fluid should be emptied from the bladder through the scope before removal.
- To exit the bladder, the fluid is restarted and the scope slowly removed. The urethra should be examined on removal of the scope.

PROSTATE

The three commonest conditions of the prostate are: bladder outflow obstruction due to benign prostatic enlargement (over 50s), prostatic cancer (over 65s) and prostatitis in young adults.

Benign Prostatic Hyperplasia

You may hear this being referred to as benign prostatic hypertrophy; however, this is incorrect, as the condition is the result of increased **numbers** of prostatic cells rather than an increase in the **size** of the cells (which would be hypertrophy). All of the prostatic cells, glandular and stromal cells, are affected. It occurs most commonly in the central and transitional zone of the prostate, surrounding the prostatic urethra. Most men over the age of 50 years are affected, and it is the commonest cause of LUTS in middle-aged and elderly men. As BPH progresses, obstruction to bladder outflow occurs and the bladder hypertrophies. Diverticula of the bladder, urinary infection, hydronephrosis and renal failure may ensue.

Symptoms and Signs. Patients may present acutely or routinely to the outpatient clinic. Acutely, BPH can result in acute urinary retention. In clinic, patients present with one or more LUTS. Chronic retention can cause overflow incontinence resulting in a stale urine smell and increasing the chances of UTI and bladder stones. Hydronephrosis is possible if the ureteric orifices are incompetent. Haematuria may occur as bladder neck veins dilate due to constriction from the prostate. On PR there will be a smooth enlarged prostate with a palpable median sulcus.

Investigations

- FBC
- U&Es: obstruction can cause renal impairment
- Urinalysis ± MSSU
- PSA: has age-specific levels and may be slightly elevated

- USS: assess upper urinary tract (hydronephrosis), bladder, residual urine
- Flowmetry and residual volume assessment
- Cystoscopy: to rule out the presence of urethral stricture or large bladder tumour
- Transrectal USS: assess the size of the prostate.

Treatment. If patients present with acute retention, a timely placed catheter will result in instant relief and the most grateful patient you may come across in practice! If this is not possible, a catheter placed under cystoscopic guidance or suprapubic catheter may be necessary.

Medical treatment is usually suitable for patients presenting with acute urinary retention. Medical therapy includes alpha adrenergic antagonists, which relax prostatic smooth muscle, and 5-alpha-reductase inhibitors, which over time can reduce prostate volume.

If medical treatment fails to settle symptoms and the patient is surgically fit, surgical treatment should be considered.

Prostate procedures can be broadly classified into two main categories: minimally invasive techniques (MIST) and decavitating procedures.

1. MIST: These approaches are designed to cause less disruption to the body. MIST generally carry a lower risk of causing sexual dysfunction. MIST offer shorter recovery times compared with traditional open surgeries. Examples of MIST include:
   - UroLift: utilises small implants/ clips to alleviate prostate obstruction.
   - Rezum: Steam is employed to reduce the size of the prostate tissue.
   - iTind: expands and applies gentle pressure on the prostate, causing remodelling the tissue and creating a wider channel.
   - PAE (Prostatic Artery Embolisation): Blood flow to the prostate is blocked to decrease its size.
2. Decavitating Procedures: These are conventional surgical approaches that involve creating a cavity or space within the prostate to relieve obstruction. Typically, a portion of the prostate tissue is removed or resected. Examples of decavitating procedures include:
   - TURP: Electricity is issued to remove excess prostate tissue.
   - Green Light Laser Therapy: Laser energy is applied to vaporise excess prostate tissue.
   - HoLEP: A laser is used to remove obstructive prostate tissue.
   - Aquablation: A high-velocity waterjet is employed to remove prostate tissue.

The choice between these categories depends on factors such as the prostate size, symptom severity, overall health and individual preferences. While MIST offer quicker recovery and less discomfort, some of these treatments might not be suitable for patients with high-pressure chronic urinary retention.

Prostatic Carcinoma

This is the commonest cancer in men in developed countries. One in six men will be diagnosed with prostate cancer in their lifetime. It is rare below the age of 50 years with incidence peaking in the eighth decade. In the UK, 25% of patients present with advanced disease, when potentially curative treatment is not possible. Early asymptomatic disease can be detected by PSA testing or if a hard prostatic nodule is felt on PR. This may prompt multiparametric MRI scan of the prostate. If an abnormal area is identified, histological confirmation is required through transperineal template biopsies of the prostate or less frequently employed transrectal prostate biopsy. It is also common for foci of carcinoma to be found incidentally in specimens resected at TURP for bladder outflow obstruction.

Prostate cancer spreads to adjacent organs, e.g. bladder, urethra and seminal vesicles; spread to the rectum is rare. Lymphatic spread is to iliac and para-aortic nodes. Haematogenous spread occurs early, especially to the pelvis, spine and skull causing osteosclerotic metastases.

Symptoms and Signs. Many patients are asymptomatic. No formal screening programme is in place in the UK, but men may be picked up on a 'well man screen' via a PR or PSA. LUTS may be present, but as prostate cancer normally occurs in the peripheral zone, some patients might be asymptomatic.

Systemic symptoms include malaise, weight loss and symptoms of anaemia. Symptoms secondary to metastases include bone pain, pathological fractures and sciatica.

Investigations

- FBC
- U&Es
- LFTs (including ALP)
- PSA: to facilitate early detection and evaluate response to treatment
- Multiparametric MRI scan of the prostate (mp MRI)
- Transperineal biopsies of the prostate.

If prostate cancer is found, further investigations include:

- CT: staging
- Isotope bone scan: sensitive indicator of early bone metastases
- USS: shows residual urine, upper urinary tract obstruction
- PET scan: specifics tracers can be used to detect prostate cancer such as 18F Choline and 18F PSMA.

Gleason Grade and Scoring. Prostate cancers are currently graded according to the Gleason grade and a score calculated. The histological specimens are graded from 0–5 with 0 being benign and 5 being the most poorly differentiated cancer cells. The Gleason score is calculated by adding the scores of the two most frequent grades found in the specimen.

Treatment. Treatment depends on stage and grade of the disease and overall life expectancy of the patient.

- Watchful waiting: monitoring prostate cancer that isn't causing any problems. The aim is to avoid treatment unless patients get symptoms. This is suitable for patients with prostate cancer which is not likely to cause any problems during their lifetimes.
- Active surveillance: patients with low-grade, low-stage cancers have regular PSAs and only receive treatment if progression is suspected secondary to a rise in PSA.
- Androgen deprivation therapy (ADT). This treatment is suitable for patients with progressing disease or locally advanced and metastatic disease. Growth of prostate cancer is stimulated by testosterone; this can be targeted for treatment. However, all cancers will eventually become hormone resistant. Antiandrogens such as bicalutamide stop testosterone acting on the prostate directly and can be

used as treatment or given as a short course prior to luteinising hormone – releasing hormone (LHRH) agonist treatment. LHRH agonists cause an initial increase in testosterone but downregulate the pituitary receptors in the long term, thus reducing testosterone secretion.

- Medical advancements in hormone therapy and oncology treatments for prostate cancer have made significant progress over the recent years.
  - LHRH agonists: Leuprolide and goserelin are used to reduce testosterone production by the testes.
  - LHRH antagonists: Degarelix reduces testosterone production without the initial testosterone flare.
  - Chemotherapy: Docetaxel and cabazitaxel used in advanced hormone-resistant prostate cancer cases.
  - Novel Androgen Receptor Inhibitors: like enzalutamide and apalutamide targeting androgen receptors on cancer cells.
  - Androgen Biosynthesis Inhibitors: Abiraterone acetate inhibits androgen production in testes and adrenal glands.
- Radiotherapy: this can be done by external beam or brachytherapy. Used for localised disease in patients with life expectancy of >10 years where cure is desired. Also used to manage pain from bony metastases in palliative patients. Potential side effects include long-term urinary and bowels symptoms (bleeding, irritation), erectile dysfunction, small risks of developing secondary cancer (bladder, bowel).
- Robotic-assisted laparoscopic radical prostatectomy: performed for patients with >10 years' life expectancy and localised disease. Complications include incontinence (5–10%), erectile dysfunction (up to 50%) and anastomotic urethral strictures.

Prognosis. This is dependent on stage at presentation. Patients with clinically localised tumours treated radically may expect a normal life expectancy. Half of the patients diagnosed with metastatic disease at presentation will survive their cancer for 5 years or more from diagnosis.

Prostatitis

This occurs most commonly in young adults. It can be acute or chronic in nature. Acute bacterial prostatitis usually presents as an acute febrile illness. Chronic prostatitis presents with recurrent UTIs or pain radiating to tip of the penis, testes and perineum. The commonest causative microbes are *E. coli, Staphylococcus aureus* and *Neisseria gonorrhoeae*; chlamydia is also possible, as is TB.

Symptoms and Signs

Acute Bacterial Prostatitis. Patients will complain of fever, malaise, low back pain, perineal pain and urinary symptoms (frequency, urgency, dysuria and reduced urinary flow). Examination will reveal an enlarged tender prostate.

Chronic Prostatitis. Patients will have symptoms of UTI, either continually or repeatedly, and may have a dull perineal ache. On examination they may have an indurated irregular prostate.

Investigations. In acute prostatitis:

- FBC: raised WCC
- MSSU for MC&S: usually shows bacterial growth
- Blood culture.

In chronic prostatitis:

- MSSU and urethral swabs post prostatic massage may yield secretions containing white cells and occasionally organisms.
- If initial culture is negative, consider culture for TB (takes 6 weeks).

Treatment. Acute prostatitis is treated with bed rest, antibiotics (often i.v. initially) and analgesia. Prostatic abscess or chronic prostatitis may occur as a complication or if inadequate treatment is given.

Prostatic abscess is usually drained transurethrally or aspirated transperineally. Chronic prostatitis is treated with long-term antibiotics, e.g. ciprofloxacin for 6–8 weeks.

TESTES AND EPIDIDYMIS

Imperfectly Descended Testes

About 5% of full-term babies do not have one or both testes in the scrotum at birth. In the first year of life many descend, leaving only 0.3% undescended at 1 year. When the testes cannot be found in the scrotum, it may be because they are:

- Retractile
- Ectopic
- Incompletely descended.

A retractile testis is a normal testis associated with an active cremasteric reflex, the testis being drawn up to the superficial inguinal ring. An ectopic testis is one that has descended to an abnormal site and may be found in the superficial inguinal pouch, the perineum, the femoral triangle or at the root of the penis. An incompletely descended testis lies in the normal course of descent – lying anywhere from the posterior abdominal wall to the top of the scrotum.

Symptoms and Signs. The mother may have noticed that the testes are absent from the scrotum. In later life, it may be noticed at a routine medical examination. A retractile testis may be brought down into the scrotum by applying gentle traction with the child relaxed in a warm room. The mother may have noticed that the testes are only present when the child is warm and relaxed, e.g. in the bath. The parents can be reassured that the testes are normal and will eventually take up permanent scrotal residence. An incompletely descended testis cannot be palpated in the inguinal canal because of the tough overlying external oblique aponeurosis. If the testis is palpable easily along the line of the inguinal canal, it is almost certainly superficial to the external oblique aponeurosis and therefore ectopic. Absence of both testicles from the scrotum is called cryptorchidism. Some 90% of imperfectly descended testes have an associated inguinal hernia.

Treatment. Retractile testes are normal. Parental reassurance is all that is required. An ectopic or incompletely descended testis must be placed in the scrotum. Treatment of an undescended testis should be carried out as early as possible. The testis is mobilised on the cord, any coexisting hernia repaired and the testis fixed in the scrotum. This is usually done by placing it in a pouch fashioned between the dartos muscle and the skin, i.e. orchidopexy. The Fowler-Stephens technique (one or two staged procedure) is usually used to fix intra-abdominal testes.

Complications of Imperfect Descent. Defective spermatogenesis with infertility in bilateral cases, risk of torsion, risk of tumour or trauma.

Hydrocele

A hydrocele is a collection of fluid in the tunica vaginalis. A primary or idiopathic hydrocele develops slowly and becomes large and tense. It usually occurs in those over 40 years. A secondary hydrocele tends to be small and lax and occurs secondary to inflammation or tumour of the underlying testes. Hydroceles usually transilluminate if flashlight is directed to the side or underneath the hydrocele. It tends to occur in the younger age group. Primary hydroceles may be classified as follows:

Vaginal Hydrocele. This surrounds the testes in the layers of the tunica vaginalis and does not connect with the peritoneal cavity.

Congenital Hydrocele. This is associated with a hernial sac. It connects with the peritoneal cavity via patent processus vaginalis.

Infantile Hydrocele. This extends from the testes to the deep inguinal ring. It does not connect with the peritoneal cavity.

Hydrocele of the Cord. This lies along the cord anywhere from the deep inguinal ring to the upper scrotum. It does not connect with either the peritoneal cavity or the tunica vaginalis. A similar swelling may develop in the female and is known as a hydrocele of the canal of Nuck.

Symptoms and Signs. Scrotal swelling. Testes cannot be felt separately. Fluctuant. Transilluminates. Can 'get above it'. Congenital hydrocele in infants may fill during the day and empty while lying down at night. A hydrocele of the cord moves downwards when traction is applied to the testis.

Treatment. A congenital hydrocele may be associated with a hernia. Treatment is by surgical excision of the peritoneal remnant as in herniotomy. An infantile, noncommunicating hydrocele usually resolves spontaneously or needle aspiration may be required. A symptomatic vaginal hydrocele in an adult may be treated by surgical excision. A primary hydrocele in an elderly and unfit patient may be treated by aspiration. This may need to be done every few months. Surgery involves opening the tunica vaginalis longitudinally, emptying the hydrocele, everting the sac after excising the redundant sac and suturing the sac behind the cord – thus obliterating the potential space. Secondary hydroceles require treatment of the underlying condition.

Epididymal Cyst

They may be small, large, multiple, unilateral or bilateral. If they contain opalescent milky fluid demonstrated on aspiration, they are called spermatoceles.

Symptoms and Signs. Usually occur over 40 years of age. Scrotal swelling. Slowly enlarges. Painless. Lie above and slightly behind the testes. Testis can be felt separately. Can 'get above it'. Usually smooth and lobulated. Fluctuant.

Treatment. None unless large – where they may show through the trousers and interfere with walking. Aspiration may help, but most cysts are multiloculated. Large cysts require excision. Surgical excision might result in epididymal scarring and infertility up to 2%.

Varicocele

These are varicosities of the pampiniform plexus. More common on the left side.

Symptoms and Signs. Varicose veins in the scrotum appear on standing. Disappear on lying down. Heavy or dragging sensation in scrotum. The patient must be examined standing or the diagnosis will be missed. The veins in the scrotum are often described as feeling like a 'bag of worms', but feeling like a 'plate of lukewarm spaghetti' is probably a better comparison. Bilateral varicoceles may cause subfertility. The affected testis may be smaller. Sudden onset of a left varicocele which does not disappear on lying down in the older patient may be caused by obstruction of the left renal vein by a renal carcinoma – USS of the kidney is appropriate.

Treatment. In the asymptomatic patient, no treatment is required – especially if the condition is unilateral. Scrotal support for aching and discomfort. Failure of symptoms to settle with scrotal support or evidence of subfertility are indications for intervention. Most varicoceles can be treated by embolisation and obliteration under radiological control. If surgery is indicated, it is via an inguinal approach, all testicular veins bar one being ligated at the deep inguinal ring. Alternatively, the gonadal vein can be clipped laparoscopically.

Infections of the Testis and Epididymis

Inflammation of the testis and epididymis may be acute or chronic. It is often viral but may be due to sexually transmitted infections such as chlamydia and gonorrhoea or secondary to UTI. Chronic epididymo-orchitis may be due to TB. In the young patient, the differentiation from torsion is often impossible and the scrotum should be explored.

Symptoms and Signs. Patients present with a painful, exquisitely tender testicle that is swollen and may have overlying erythema. There is normally systemic illness with associated pyrexia. MSSU is the essential investigation and should be sent for MC&S.

Treatment

Acute. Bed rest with adequate analgesia and antibiotics. Antibiotic choice should be driven by local resistance patterns and adjusted once results of culture are known. The swelling may take as long as 2 months to resolve.

Chronic. TB – antituberculosis drugs. Long-term antibiotic therapy for nontuberculous epididymo-orchitis. Rarely, orchidectomy is performed if improvement does not occur after prolonged antibiotic treatment.

Testicular Torsion

In some circumstances the testis is able to twist within the scrotum causing structures within the cord to become compressed. This compromises the venous drainage and, eventually, the arterial supply leading to necrosis of the testis. It is thought to occur in patients with congenital abnormalities such as high investment of the tunica vaginalis or when the epididymis and testis are separated by a mesorchium. Incidence is highest between 10 and 20 years.

Testicular torsion is a urological emergency; to be sure of testicular salvage, untwisting should be carried out within 6h of symptoms.

Testicular torsion is difficult to differentiate from epididymo-orchitis or torsion of a testicular appendage. The latter is associated with the 'blue dot sign' on the inferior pole of the testis, but this may only be visible in young boys. There is no investigation that satisfactorily confirms the diagnosis meaning the scrotum must be explored in most cases.

Symptoms and Signs. Patients report sudden onset of severe pain in the scrotum and groin and radiating to the lower abdomen associated with vomiting. It may follow strain, lifting, exercise or masturbation. Examination reveals a swollen, exquisitely tender testis that may be drawn up to the groin and have a horizontal lie.

Treatment. Explore the scrotum as soon as possible. Untwist the testis if torsion is present. If the testis is not irreversibly infarcted, fix it to the scrotum with nondissolvable sutures. If the testis is infarcted, it should be removed, as should an infarcted testicular appendage. Controversy surrounds the practice of fixing the contralateral testis at the same time. Opening the contralateral hemiscrotum puts the testis at risk of iatrogenic torsion or damage and infection. However, leaving it may result in subsequent torsion and testicular loss.

> **HINTS AND TIPS**
>
> A young male who presents with sudden-onset abdominal pain should always undergo testicular examination. It is not uncommon, especially in teenagers, for the testicular pain to be mistaken for abdominal pain by the patient or doctor taking the history. In the case of torsion, even if the pain is felt in the abdomen, the testis will be exquisitely tender, and the patient is likely to be unwilling for you to handle the scrotum even gently. It is difficult, if not impossible, to distinguish between torsion and epididymo-orchitis. There is rarely time to carry out investigations. If there is any doubt about the diagnosis, assume that it is torsion and explore the scrotum surgically.

Testicular Trauma

This usually results from sports injuries or violence. Trauma may result in bleeding into the layers of the tunica vaginalis resulting in haematocele. Surgical repair should be performed if a rupture to the tunica albuginea is identified.

Symptoms and Signs. Severe pain, scrotal swelling, bruising, tender enlarged testicle.

Investigations. Scrotal ultrasound, this should be repeated 6 weeks after the trauma to ensure there is not an underlying testicular malignancy.

Treatment. This should be treated conservatively with bed rest and scrotal support if possible. Surgical exploration may be required to evacuate the haematocele and repair a split in the tunica albuginea. If swelling and irregularity of the testis persists after allowing adequate time for recovery, suspect a testicular tumour. Unsuspected pre-existing testicular tumours may be unmasked following trauma.

Testicular Tumours

This is the commonest malignancy (7 cases per 100,000 population in the UK) in young men (20–40 years); 90% arise from germ cells and are either seminomas or nonseminomas germ cell tumours (NSGCT previously teratomas). The other 10% are lymphomas, Sertoli cell tumours or Leydig cell tumours. NSGCT most commonly occur between 20 and 30 years; seminomas between 30 and 40 years. Imperfectly descended testes have a 4–10 times increased incidence of malignancy.

Symptoms and Signs. Usually presents as a painless swelling of the testis. Some may have heaviness in the scrotum and a small lax hydrocele. Occasionally they may have a palpable abdominal mass due to para-aortic node spread. It is important to examine the neck as a lump in left side of neck can be an involved left supraclavicular node. Patients may even present with chest symptoms due to lung metastases.

Investigations

- USS testis
- CXR: crude test for lung metastases
- Tumour markers: AFP, β-HCG (elevated in some NSGCT), LDH
- CT scan: thorax, abdomen and pelvis for lymph node and visceral metastases.

Treatment. Orchidectomy for likely malignancy should be performed via an inguinal incision. Clamp the spermatic cord with a soft clamp prior to palpation or mobilisation of the testis to prevent tumour dissemination. If malignancy is doubted, the testis is split ('bivalved'), examined and frozen sections sent. If tumour markers remain elevated following orchidectomy, metastases are likely.
In the case of metastasis, adjuvant therapy is required:

- Seminomas are very radiosensitive. Radiotherapy to iliac and para-aortic nodes plus chemotherapy as for teratoma. Survival is 90–95% at 5 years.
- NSGCT require combination chemotherapy. Agents used include etoposide, vinblastine, methotrexate, bleomycin, cisplatin, in various combinations of three. Survival is between 60% and 90% at 5 years. Surgery may be used for tumour debulking of retroperitoneal nodes.

PENIS

The majority of surgical conditions of the penis relate to problems with the foreskin and glans and the need for circumcision. Carcinoma of the penis and Peyronie's disease are rare.

Conditions of the Foreskin

BALANOPOSTHITIS. This is inflammation of the glans and foreskin. In children, it may be due to faecal organisms or *Staphylococci* and result in phimosis from scarring. Recurrent attacks may occur in adults, associated with poor hygiene. If *Candida* is the infecting organism, exclude diabetes. Treatment is by antibiotics or topical application of antifungal agents. Circumcision may be required for patients with recurrent episodes of balanoposthitis.

PHIMOSIS. It is usually congenital. The foreskin is normally nonretractile at birth, and separation occurs within a wide age range up to early teens. Ballooning may occur on voiding, but true phimosis is rare in children unless it is acquired as a result of chronic inflammation of the prepuce or from balanitis xerotica obliterans (BXO; see below). In the extreme case, retention of urine with hydroureters and hydronephrosis may rarely occur. However, this is more often due to meatal stenosis, which may be hidden by the phimosis. In adults, phimosis may interfere with sexual intercourse.

TREATMENT. Steroid cream and gentle daily retraction if recurrent balanitis in children. Circumcision for acquired causes of phimosis or failed conservative treatment.

PARAPHIMOSIS. This occurs when the foreskin retracts over the corona of the glans and cannot be reduced. It forms a tight constriction around the glans interfering with venous return causing swelling of the glans and foreskin, further exacerbating the difficulty of reduction. It may occur after masturbation, sexual intercourse, bathing glans or following catheterisation if the foreskin is not properly replaced (iatrogenic).

Treatment. Prompt reduction is essential to prevent glans necrosis. Apply local anaesthetic jelly and give analgesia before attempting manual reduction. If severe oedema is present, consider a penile ring block with injected local anaesthetic in the first instance. If unsuccessful, reduction under general anaesthetic can be attempted with or without a 'dorsal slit' if required. This divides the tight constriction ring and allows the foreskin to reduce. Formal circumcision should be carried out when the oedema has subsided.

Balanitis Xerotica Obliterans (BXO). It is also known as lichen sclerosis of the foreskin. This is a condition of the foreskin characterised by loss of skin elasticity and fibrosis, resulting in phimosis. Steroid treatment can be trialled first. Circumcision is often required for persistent BXO cases.

Circumcision. The indications for circumcision are shown in Table 17.5.

Carcinoma of the Penis

This is rare. It occurs in older men >60 years and does not occur in men circumcised at birth. Poor hygiene and accumulation of smegma may be etiological factors. Most are SCC. The tumour starts in the sulcus between the glans and the foreskin. Spread is to the inguinal nodes. Blood spread to the lungs or bone is rare.

Symptoms and Signs. There is a firm ulcerated painless lesion on the glans and offensive bloodstained discharge from under the foreskin. Late presenters have a large fungating mass and inguinal lymphadenopathy which can be reactive not metastatic. A red velvety lesion on the glans (erythroplasia of Queyrat) is a premalignant condition.

Treatment. Glans resurfacing, cryotherapy and laser therapy can be used for localised superficial cancer. If the urethra is involved, amputation of the penis is required; depending on spread, this may be a glansectomy, partial penectomy or total penectomy. Radiotherapy can be used as primary or in combination with surgery. If lymph nodes are involved, sentinel lymph node or formal lymph nodes dissection of the groin should be carried out or radiotherapy may be given as a palliative measure. Early presenters do well and are often cured.

Peyronie's Disease

Fibrotic plaques occur in the corpora cavernosa preventing normal elasticity and causing angulation on erection associated with discomfort and pain. This idiopathic condition occurs in men of 40–60 years. Spontaneous resolution occasionally occurs. Oral, topical and injected intralesional therapies have been tried but are largely unsuccessful. Surgery, such as Nesbit's procedure, most commonly involves excising a wedge of corpora at the most extreme external curvature to straighten the penis, but shortening will occur and there may be recurrence. Surgery could be considered for patients whose sexual function is impacted or experiencing pain during sexual intercourse.

TABLE 17.5

INDICATIONS FOR CIRCUMCISION
Phimosis
Paraphimosis
Recurrent balanoposthitis
Diagnosis of underlying penile tumours
Trauma and tumour of foreskin

Priapism

This is persistent, painful erection unassociated with sexual desire. Prompt treatment is required to avoid necrosis. Causes include idiopathic, leukaemia, sickle cell disease, disseminated and pelvic malignancy.

Treatment

- Aspiration of blood from the corpora cavernosa with a wide-bore needle and irrigation with heparinised saline
- Anastomosis of the great saphenous vein to the engorged corpora cavernosa, thus establishing venous drainage of the corpora.

Chapter 18

Orthopaedics

Akshdeep Bawa • James Hahnel

CHAPTER OUTLINE

FRACTURES

A fracture is a complete or partial break in the continuity of a bone. There are several ways of describing fractures. Usually this is according to pattern/configuration of fracture stating whether there is a laceration associated with it (open) or not (closed). Fractures are classified to enable standardised treatment methods to be used. Fractures may occur due to diseased bone (pathological). An internationally accepted abbreviation for fracture is the symbol '#'.

HINTS AND TIPS

The following would be a typical way to describe a fracture:

'There is a closed extra-articular fracture of the distal one-third radius with a 30° dorsal inclination and slight shortening. There is an associated ulna styloid fracture with minimal displacement'.

Causation

Trauma. The fracture occurs in a normal bone as a result of trauma. The pattern depends upon the direction of the force. Direct force usually results in a transverse fracture. Indirect force, e.g. a twisting injury, usually results in a spiral or oblique fracture. Axial compression results in a comminuted, crush or burst fracture. An avulsion fracture is caused by traction, usually a tendon or ligament tearing off a bony fragment, e.g. a base of fifth metatarsal fracture caused by peroneus brevis avulsion.

Stress Fractures. The bone is fatigued by repetitive stress like a metal spoon that is bent multiple times. This type of fracture occurs in individuals undertaking increased amounts of often unaccustomed exercise, e.g. 'march' metatarsal fractures in soldiers.

Pathological Fractures. These occur in bones already compromised by underlying disease. The trauma may be quite minimal or even nonexistent. Common underlying causes include osteoporosis and metastases.

Pattern (Figure 18.1)

Transverse Fracture. This is caused by direct force.

Spiral or Oblique Fracture. This is caused by force transmitted from a distance often in a twisting motion.

Segmental Fracture. Two separate fractures in the same bone.

Crush Fracture. This is caused by direct compression in cancellous bone.

Burst Fracture. This is caused by strong axial compression, e.g. vertebrae.

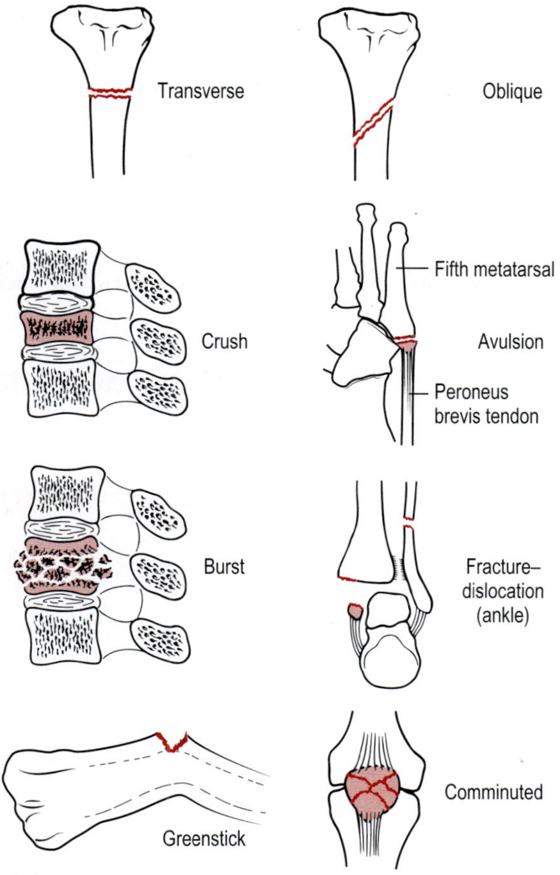

FIGURE 18.1
Types of fracture.

Avulsion Fracture. This is caused by sudden, strong traction by a tendon or ligament avulsing a bony fragment.

Fracture–Dislocation. This occurs when there is fracture of a bone involved in a joint with complete loss of congruity of the joint surfaces. Partial loss of congruity is a fracture subluxation.

Greenstick Fracture. An incomplete paediatric fracture in which cortical continuity is lost only on one side of the bone.

Buckle Fracture. Another incomplete paediatric fracture where bone buckles (defined as a plastic deformity) due to the trauma.

Comminuted Fracture. One in which the bone is broken into more than two fragments.

Relation to Surrounding Structures

Closed Fracture. There is no skin or body cavity wound communicating with the site of fracture.

Open Fracture. There is communication between the site of fracture and the skin or body cavity wound, e.g. fractured tibial shaft protruding through the skin.

Intra-Articular Fracture. The fracture involves an articular surface.

Extra-Articular Fracture. The fracture does not extend into the joint surface.

Assessment of Fractures

Symptoms and Signs. History to assess mechanism of injury. Pain. Loss of function. Loss of sensation or paralysis. Tenderness. Deformity. Swelling. Crepitus. Abnormal mobility. Discrepancy in length of limbs, associated nerve and vascular injuries. Examine for any associated injuries. Is it an open fracture?

HINTS AND TIPS

When in the emergency department – important questions to ask:

- Name, age, handedness, job and main hobbies
- Mechanism of injury
- Past medical history, medications, allergies
- When did they last eat or drink? (in case they require surgery)
- Does anything else hurt?

Examine:

- The bone to confirm fracture (be gentle!)
- Sensation/power/pulses
- The joint/bone above and below the fracture
- Is the pain disproportionate to injury with passive movement (may indicate compartment syndrome)? – EMERGENCY.

To do:

- Pain relief (including titrated morphine) and immobilisation of fracture (usually in a splint or cast)
- Keep starved if for emergency theatre. Talk to senior doctor if not sure whether for emergency theatre before letting eat and drink.
- If open fracture, photograph, irrigate externally if dirty, dress with saline soaked gauze, immobilise. Give antibiotics (BOA/BAPRAS guidelines recommend co-amoxiclav 1.2 g i.v. t.d.s. or clindamycin 600 mg i.v. q.d.s. until surgery) ± tetanus immunoglobulins if appropriate. Reduce and immobilise fracture.

HINTS AND TIPS—Cont'd

- Remember to get a check X-ray in cast to show current position of fracture.
- Indications for emergency theatre:
- Grossly contaminated/marine, agricultural or sewage-exposed open wounds
- Neurovascularly compromised limb including compartment syndrome
- An open wound, not grossly contaminated and not neurovascularly compromised, may be operated on by a senior doctor on the next available trauma list.
- Keep 'NIL BY MOUTH' and let everyone know this including the patient.

INVESTIGATIONS. Radiographs: in two planes at right angles. With long bones, include joints at either end. Radiograph – practice describing it (as if you were describing to your boss over the telephone): classify it, if possible, including pre-existing disease (e.g. pathological fracture through a metastasis) or foreign body in open fracture. Occasionally a fracture may not be apparent on initial radiograph (e.g. stress fracture, scaphoid fracture), and further radiographs may be required later when callus or late radiolucent line associated with healing is apparent. Commonly, further imaging may be required (e.g. computerised tomography (CT) scan/ magnetic resonance imaging (MRI) scan).

HINTS AND TIPS

Look for a straight line in a joint effusion, e.g. lateral of knee. This may be a fat/ blood interface line representing a lipohaemarthrosis confirming a fracture even if not initially obvious.

Principles of Fracture Treatment

First Aid

Follow Advanced Trauma Life Support (ATLS) principles (→ Ch. 4). Ensure clear airway with C-spine control, ensure adequate breathing with oxygen. Stop bleeding, maintaining adequate balanced resuscitation with i.v. fluid/blood. Splintage and treatment of open fractures as above. Patients with multiple injuries (polytrauma) may need to be transferred to a major trauma centre following initial stabilisation and before definitive treatment.

Treatment of Shock

Considerable blood loss can occur with fractures; >1.5L blood can be lost with a femoral shaft fracture alone. Ensure that the patient is haemodynamically stable if going for CT. Consider direct transfer to theatre, if not stable, for definitive haemostasis.

Definitive Fracture Management

1. Reduction, i.e. the restoration of the displaced fragments to their anatomical position
2. Stabilisation, i.e. keeping the bony fragments in the reduced position until union occurs

3. Rehabilitation starts as soon as possible after the injury. It is aimed initially at maintaining the function of the uninjured parts, and once the fracture is sufficiently united, restoring function of the injured parts.

REDUCTION. This means aligning the fragments of bone back to their anatomical alignment and position. Small displacements in extra-articular fractures may be acceptable, although joint surfaces should be anatomically reduced. Emergency reduction should be performed in the presence of nerve or vessel compromise.

How Should It Be Done? Reduction may be either closed or open.

Closed Reduction. This may be by manipulation or traction; the latter being applied via the skin or skeleton. Perfect anatomical reduction is less commonly achieved.

Open Reduction. This is performed when accurate alignment of fragments is needed; internal fixation is required to maintain the reduction and when early mobilisation is required. This carries the risk of infection, nerve damage and wound healing problems.

How Is Reduction Held? Some fractures are intrinsically stable and require no additional stabilisation. Others require external or internal fixation.

Types of Stability

Absolute Stability. Fracture fragments are held rigidly together by compression, allowing bone healing by remodelling. Little or no external callus forms, e.g. ankle fracture fixation.

Relative Stability. Fracture fragments are held approximately opposed without compression. Micromovement occurs at the fracture site and abundant bridging callus forms, e.g. forearm fracture stabilised with a cast.

METHODS OF STABILISING A FRACTURE

External

Plaster of Paris or Synthetic Material Casts. Usually applied over a layer of wool. Where there is excessive swelling, a slab may be used initially, a full cast being applied later. This allows the cast to expand with the expanding limb. The position of the bone should be checked by radiograph after the cast has been applied. The distal circulation should be observed because a tight plaster may interfere with blood flow. This may be with advice to the patient and advice leaflet or healthcare professional observation if on the ward. Cast bracing involves the use of hinged/jointed casts. This allows joint mobility and fracture stability, as well as patient mobility.

Traction. This is now most commonly used as temporary stabilisation of femoral fractures below the lesser trochanter. It is rarely used in modern practice as definitive treatment, except in exceptional circumstances. This is used to overcome the powerful pull of muscles, which may cause shortening or angulation. Traction may be fixed, e.g. a Thomas splint for femoral shaft fractures or sliding (balanced) where the patient's weight is balanced against an applied load. The patient's weight and friction forces counter the applied traction. The patient can move the limb or can move about the bed while traction continues to act in the desired direction. Traction may be applied to the skin via adhesive tape or to bone (skeletal traction) via Steinmann or Denham pins. Skull traction for cervical fractures/dislocations should ONLY be performed by a doctor experienced in this field with the patient being awake because of the risk of cord compression from herniated intervertebral discs.

Internal Fixation

Wires. Kirschner (K) wires may be used to internally splint a fracture fragment in two separate planes, e.g. distal radial fracture, or used with a figure-of-eight tension band wire, e.g. fractures of the olecranon.

Screws. Stainless steel, titanium alloy or cobalt chrome screws are used typically to provide compression across a fracture site (e.g. fibula fracture) and are often held by a 'neutralisation' plate. The screws may be used in isolation, e.g. fractures of the medial malleolus.

Plating. A plate is fastened to both fragments by screws (Figure 18.2). Plates can be designed to compress a fracture, neutralise (support) a fracture compressed by lag screws or bridge a comminuted fracture.

Intramedullary Nail. A nail is passed within the medullary cavity of a long bone across the fracture and locked with transverse locking screws. It is commonly used for long bone fractures, e.g. femoral shaft fractures.

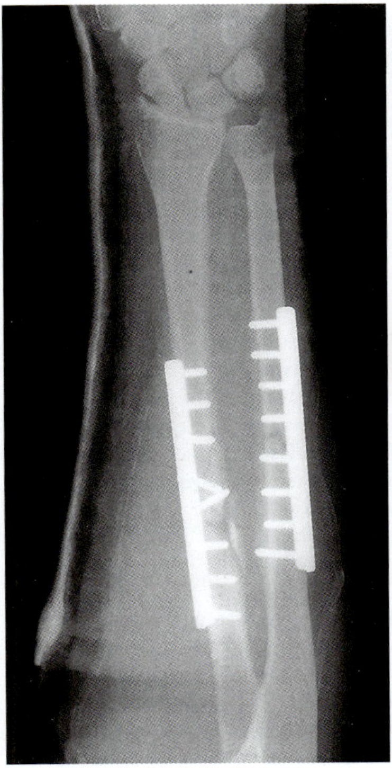

FIGURE 18.2

A fracture of the radius and ulna fixed with plates and screws. The radial fracture is comminuted.

External Fixation Devices. The fragments are transfixed by pins or wires, which are then held in an external fixation device to immobilise the fragments. Complex, comminuted fractures can be reduced and immobilised by this method. The fracture can be held while surgery for associated injuries, e.g. skin, vascular or nerve, is carried out.

Indications for Internal Fixation

- Failure to maintain adequate reduction by external methods
- Intra-articular fractures to secure good alignment of joint surfaces and prevent later osteoarthritis (OA)
- Polytrauma – patients with multiple injuries where internal fixation may facilitate nursing and patient mobility
- Where damage to other structures, e.g. vessels and nerves, requires stability for good results following repair
- Pathological fractures.

OPEN FRACTURES. Principles of management of open fractures include:

- ATLS: identify and treat life-threatening injuries first. This includes treatment of haemorrhagic shock.
- In the emergency department – photograph the wound, remove contaminants, dress with saline soaked gauze and immobilise. Give antibiotics (BOA/BAPRAS guidelines recommend co-amoxiclav 1.2 g i.v. t.d.s. or clindamycin 600 mg i.v. q.d.s. until surgery) ± tetanus immunoglobulins if appropriate. Reduce and immobilise fracture.
- In the operating theatre – fracture – extend the laceration to allow exploration of the wound and to deliver the bone for irrigation. Debride and irrigate the wound removing any foreign bodies and all devitalised tissue. A minimum of 6 L of saline washout should be used. Repair any damage to blood vessels or nerves (rarely required). External or internal fracture stabilisation as above. For dirty wounds, marine or farmyard, external fixation with a 48-h second look, debridement and washout is appropriate. However, if adequate debridement is carried out, clean wounds may be closed primarily with internal fixation. If plastic surgery is required, internal fixation facilitates easier skin cover. Massive wounds may require early free tissue flap coverage. If plaster of Paris is applied, a window may be cut in it so the wound can be observed and infection excluded.
- Plastic surgeons should be involved early.

REHABILITATION. The aims should be restoration of function of the injured part and rehabilitation of the patient as a whole. Specific advice includes suitable exercises, active use as much as compatible with fracture healing, active exercises, physiotherapy, occupational therapy, advice from social worker, employment advice.

Complications of Fractures

Immediate (at Time of Fracture)

- Haemorrhage: may be internal or external. Internal haemorrhage can be considerable at the fracture site, e.g. up to 1.5 L with a fractured femoral shaft.
- Injury to nerves and vessels
- Injury to underlying structures, e.g. brain damage with skull fractures, splenic rupture with left lower rib fractures, urethral trauma with pelvic fractures.

Early (During the Period of Initial Treatment)

Local

- Compartment syndrome due to high-energy trauma, muscle/vessel damage or tight plaster casts
- Nerve palsies from tight plaster casts, or involved in callus or iatrogenic injury
- Wound infection or wound dehiscence
- Loss of reduction of fracture
- Pressure sores.

General

Venous Thromboembolism (VTE) (for Deep Vein Thrombosis (DVT) and Pulmonary Embolism (PE)→ Ch. 5). This is relatively common and a potentially serious complication. Risk factors include previous VTE, increased severity of injuries, prolonged surgery, age >60 years, obesity, immobility, malignancy, thrombophilia and pregnancy. Chemical (LMWH) and mechanical prophylaxis (foot/calf pumps/TED stockings) should be considered in all patients. Patients present with painful swelling in their legs, shortness of breath or chest pain typically around 4–10 days post surgical intervention. Investigation or at least treatment should be an emergency pending investigation. Early senior review is advised due to the potential bleeding risks in surgical patients with treatment dose LMWH.

Compartment Syndrome. This is elevation of interstitial pressure in a closed fascial compartment that results in microvascular compromise. It may occur with or without arterial injury. Muscle swells and compartment pressure rises. Ischaemia results from pressure on surrounding small arteries. Distal pulses may still be palpable and the diagnosis therefore missed. Awareness of the possibility of the diagnosis is vital, particularly when the pain is out of proportion to the injury. The leg is most commonly involved (anterior and deep flexor compartments most frequently), although it can occur in any muscle compartment. Treatment is by prompt fasciotomy, which allows the muscle to expand and relieves the pressure on the vessels.

HINTS AND TIPS

Venous thromboembolism and compartment syndrome are relatively common and life-threatening conditions where early identification and treatment are key. Make sure that you know what to look out for and involve senior doctor early.

Acute Urinary Retention. Always exclude the possibility of bladder or urethral injury.

Pneumonia

Fat Embolism. This usually complicates fractures of a major long bone at 3–10 days postinjury. Embolisation of the pulmonary and systemic microvasculature with lipid globules occurs. The main effects are on the brain and lung. The patient may suddenly become drowsy, pyrexial and tachycardic. A petechial rash may appear on the upper trunk. Coma and death may occur. With lung involvement, the patient develops confusion, breathing difficulties and cyanosis. PO_2 will be reduced. Radiograph appearance is similar to that of acute respiratory distress syndrome (ARDS). Renal problems may occur with excretion of lipid droplets. Diagnosis may be confirmed by finding lipid globules in urine or sputum. Treatment is by oxygen therapy, ventilation and renal support. Early operative immobilisation of fractured long bones may reduce incidence.

Crush Syndrome. This is due to extensive crushing of muscle or extensive muscle necrosis, e.g. with ischaemia due to arterial injury. Myoglobin is released into the circulation. Myoglobinuria and renal failure may ensue. Oliguria with dark brownish-red urine should suggest the diagnosis. Prompt treatment with fluids and an osmotic diuretic may prevent renal failure. Dialysis may be required. HDU/ICU is commonly required. Removal of all dead muscle, possibly by amputation of the limb, may be required. Especially important in patients presenting after a long lie, such as elderly after a fall or intravenous drug use (IVDU) due to drug affects.

Late (After the Period of Initial Treatment)

Delayed Union. The fracture does not heal in the expected time. Absence of callus and mobility at the fracture site are features.

Nonunion. The fracture remains un-united. Nonunion may be hypertrophic (due to excessive movement) or atrophic due to poor blood supply, infection or pathological fracture. A pseudarthrosis (false joint) may result. Hypertrophic produces nonbridging callus. Atrophic produces no callus. Treatment options include more rigid stabilisation, bone grafting, intramedullary bone reaming or pulsed electromagnetic stimulation.

Malunion. Healing has resulted in a deformed position. This may be because of shortening, malrotation or angulation. Treatment depends on the degree of deformity and age of the patient. In children, considerable remodelling may occur resulting in correction of the deformity. In recent fractures manipulation or wedging of the plaster cast may suffice. In older fractures osteotomy may be required. Deformity may put strain on adjacent joints, resulting in OA.

Complex Regional Pain Syndrome (Causalgia, Reflex Sympathetic Osteodystrophy, Sudeck's Atrophy). The limb becomes painful, swollen and stiff with a reddened, smooth, shiny appearance to the skin. Radiograph shows patchy porosis of the bone. Most commonly seen after a distal radial fracture, in which case the symptoms affect the hand and wrist. Physiotherapy is required over a prolonged period of weeks or months. The prognosis is usually good.

Avascular Necrosis of Bone. Part of a bone necrotises when its blood supply is interrupted by the fracture. Common sites are:

- The head of the femur with intracapsular fractures where retinacular and intramedullary vessels supplying the femoral head are disrupted
- The proximal part of the scaphoid bone in fractures across the waist; the blood supply enters from the distal end.

Diagnosis is by radiograph, MRI or three-phase bone scan. OA and collapse of bone may result.

Myositis Ossificans. Calcification with subsequent ossification occurs in a haematoma associated with either stripping of the periosteum or reactive proliferation in soft tissues causing ectopic calcification. It is most common in injuries around the elbow and those involving quadriceps femoris. Initially treatment involves strict rest, NSAIDs and avoidance of passive movements. When radiographs show that the shadow of calcification has been replaced by a clear outline of ossification, exercise may be reinstituted. Occasionally surgical excision of the ossification is necessary, but only when the bone is mature. Recurrence is common.

Osteoarthritis (OA). This may result from mal-aligned fractures putting strain on joints or after intra-articular fractures (e.g. femoral or tibial malunions affecting the weight-bearing line between the femoral head and ankle result in excessive strain on either the medial or lateral side of the knee).

Post-Traumatic Stress Disorder. Compensation neurosis and malingering should also be considered.

SPINAL TRAUMA

The incidence in the UK of spinal injuries is about 15 per million of the population per year. RTAs account for over 50%, the remainder being due to accidents at home, industrial accidents, sports injuries and assault. Spinal fractures are commonly part of a polytrauma presentation and are frequently identified despite distracting injuries by trauma CT of neck, chest, abdomen and pelvis. Correct management reduces the risk of spinal cord injury. Ideal management includes immobilisation, imaging the injury early for identification and classification with early involvement from spinal surgeons. All unconscious patients and those with distracting injuries elsewhere must be assumed to have a spinal injury until proved otherwise.

Management of Spinal Injuries

1. Follow ATLS principles for emergency management. Do not remove a helmet unless trained to do so and with help.
2. During the primary survey, maintain C-spine immobilisation with manual inline stabilisation or collar, sandbags and tape, and log roll the patient. Concentrate on the life-threatening injuries (ABCDE). Start thinking about the spine in more detail during D (assessment of neurological status) and E (exposure to identify injuries).
3. At the start of the secondary survey while removing the spinal board, assess the spine. 'Log roll' for a proper and safe examination of the back. Look for localised bruising and tenderness. Spinal deformity.
4. Full neurological examination to assess the level and the extent of cord damage. Record pin-prick sensation (spinothalamic tracts); fine touch and joint position sense (posterior columns); power of muscle groups according to Medical Research Council Scale (corticospinal tracts); reflexes – limbs, abdominal, anal and bulbocavernous. Cranial nerves. Priapism indicates a high lesion. A neurological examination should be repeated following the period of potential spinal shock.

HINTS AND TIPS

Perform the formal neurological examination once the patient is on the ward. It is a lot quieter, and the patient is normally more cooperative.

5. Radiological investigation: a lateral C-spine radiograph will reveal 85% of cervical spine fractures. However, this is no longer an essential part of the primary ATLS survey, especially if the C-spine is scanned during a trauma CT scan. A CT neck should be requested if the C7/T1 junction is not easily visualised on a lateral radiograph. A C-spine radiograph series comprises an AP, lateral and odontoid peg view. Unstable fractures include fracture–dislocations, Chance fractures, burst fractures, fractures of atlas and axis. CT scan may give clearer 3D view of the damage. MRI shows cord compression and soft tissue damage more clearly.

6. Initial assessment should define two aspects. First, is there a cord injury and is it complete or incomplete (distal sparing easiest to demonstrate as motor activity)? Second, is there a significant spinal injury and is it stable or unstable? Note that these two aspects of the injury can be quite independent (e.g. central cord syndrome after a forced extension injury in a spondylitic patient with no spinal fracture).

Whiplash-Associated Disorder

Car struck from behind. Neck extends with sudden acceleration and then flexes forward with sudden deceleration. Usually ligamentous and soft tissue damage only, although there may be pain and paraesthesia in the arms and hands. Radiographs are normal or show mild pre-existing degenerative changes.

Treatment. Rest followed by physiotherapy. Prognosis is variable, with some patients recovering while others have prolonged symptoms that may be permanent and require a collar. (In some patients, symptoms settle miraculously after awards of compensation!)

Fractures and Dislocations of the Spine

Classification by Mechanism of Injury

- Compression: burst fracture (potentially unstable)
- Flexion compression: anterior wedge fracture. Possible disruption of posterior ligaments.
- Flexion rotation: shearing of all restraining ligaments. Unifacet or bifacet dislocations. These fractures are the commonest cause of neurological damage.
- Hyperextension: disruption of the anterior structures. These fractures may cause momentary cord compression leading to 'central cord syndrome'.

Cervical Spine Fractures and Dislocations

Injuries most often occur because of RTAs or sport. A fall on the head with the neck forcibly bent, e.g. flexion and rotation. Subluxation or dislocation occurs with possible disruption of disc. Forced extension, e.g. a fall on the face or forehead, may occur, resulting in cervical spine injury. If a cervical spine injury is suspected, the first move should be to safeguard the cord by controlling neck movements. Do not allow the head to flex forward, and do not hyperextend the neck. Keep in a neutral position.

Symptoms and Signs. Often associated head injury, so patient may be unconscious. Assume cervical spine injury. Conscious patient may have pain, muscle spasm and localised tenderness. Pain may radiate down the arms. Look for neurological signs. The patient with damage above C4 is unlikely to survive because of paralysis of all respiratory muscles. Transection above sympathetic outflow causes bradycardia and hypotension.

Investigations

Radiographs

- Lateral to show C1–T1
- AP and AP through open mouth to show odontoid
- Flexion and extension views to assess stability (this should only be performed by trained senior doctors on neurosurgical request)
- CT scan – should be performed if high-energy injury or radiographs are inadequate.

Treatment

Fractures of the Atlas. These are usually fractured as a result of vertical compression force breaking the ring into four pieces. Inherently unstable, requiring halo jacket immobilisation and fusion if nonunion occurs.

C1–C2 Subluxation. This is due to failure of the transverse ligament. Neurosurgical treatment is by initial traction in extension, then posterior fusion.

Odontoid Peg Fracture. It is uncommon and easily missed. All but the rare apical avulsion type require traction followed by a halo jacket with posterior fusion for nonunion.

Burst Fractures. These may be stable, in which case treatment is by halo jacket. If unstable, traction followed by a halo jacket is required. Decompression of the cord and fusion may be necessary.

Anterior Wedge Fractures. These may be stable (treatment in a collar) or unstable with opening of the posterior elements (halo jacket or posterior fusion).

Facet Joint Dislocations. These are always unstable. Treatment is by awake reduction and posterior fusion following MRI to check for sequestrated disc.

Isolated Spinous Process Avulsion. These are stable and require treatment in a collar.

Thoracic Spine

Flexion injuries result in crush or wedge fractures, which are usually stable. Such fractures may occur with minimal trauma if the vertebral body is weakened, e.g. osteoporosis or secondary metastatic deposits. Fracture–dislocations tend to occur at the thoracolumbar junction and are caused by flexion and rotation injuries, e.g. a fall from a height on to the shoulders. If the disc and posterior ligaments are disrupted, the injury is unstable. Paraplegia is common in fracture–dislocations.

Symptoms and Signs. History of fall from height on shoulder or heavy weight falling on flexed back. Pain over spine. Palpable gap along spinous processes with unstable fracture–dislocations. Associated injuries. Neurological deficit.

Investigations. Preferably trauma CT or if not available AP and lateral spine radiographs.

Treatment. Simple flexion injuries with crush or wedge fractures are treated by bed rest and analgesia followed by mobilisation when pain allows, occasionally in a thoracolumbar sacral orthosis (TLSO) brace. If trauma is minimal, an underlying pathological cause should be sought such as osteoporosis or less commonly myeloma, metastases, osteomalacia. Fracture-dislocations may be treated conservatively or operatively. Conservative management includes careful nursing with regular turning on a special spinal bed until core stability returns followed by TLSO brace for 3 months. Spontaneous interbody fusion usually occurs. If there is paraplegia, care is as for the paraplegic patient. To offset the problem of long-term bed rest, operative treatment may be undertaken. The fracture may be stabilised by internal fixation.

Lumbar Spine

Compression fractures are the most common and may result from a fall from a height on to the heels. With a burst fracture, a fragment of bone may be displaced posteriorly and cause damage to the cord or cauda equina syndrome.

Symptoms and Signs. History of fall from height on to heels. Pain over lumbar spine. Pain and spasm in paravertebral muscles. Look for associated calcaneal fractures or hip injury. Paraplegia.

Investigations. AP and lateral radiograph of lumbar spine (Figure 18.3) or trauma CT.

Treatment. Where there is no neurological damage and the fracture is not comminuted, immobilisation in a TLSO brace will suffice until union occurs. Pathological fractures will require fixation. Unstable fractures may require fixation.

Fractures of the Transverse Processes

The most common are in the lumbar region. They may result from direct violence in a crushing injury or violent muscular contraction. Treatment is symptomatic. There is often severe soft tissue trauma and associated haematoma; prolonged pain may occur. Fractures of L5 transverse processes are suggestive of pelvic trauma.

Fractures of Sacrum and Coccyx

This may accompany fractures of the pelvis or occur as isolated fractures due to direct violence. Undisplaced fractures of the sacrum in isolation require non-weight-bearing for 3 months on that side and are treated symptomatically. Displaced fractures may injure sacral nerves with consequent neurological deficit.

Coccydynia

This causes chronic pain in the coccygeal region. It may follow a fall on the buttocks. The pain interferes with sitting. Treatment is by injection of local anaesthetic and depot

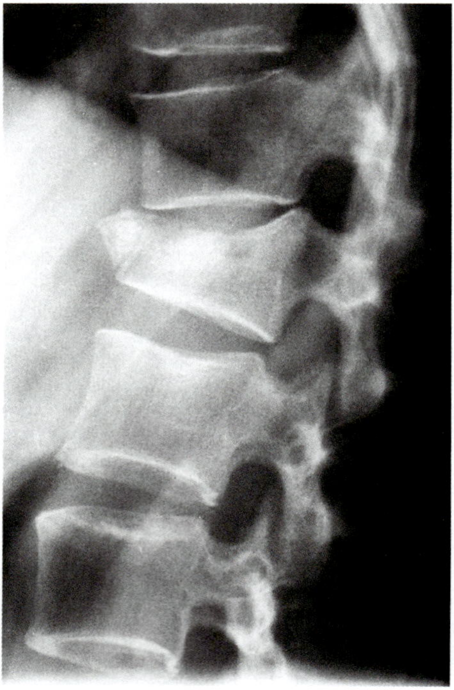

FIGURE 18.3
Lateral radiograph of the thoracolumbar spine. There is an anterior wedge fracture of the body of the first lumbar vertebra.

steroid or manipulation under anaesthesia (if fracture–dislocation). If conservative management fails, excision of the coccyx may be required.

Spinal Cord Injury

Types of Spinal Cord Injury

The extent and level of cord damage is very important in determining recovery and final prognosis. Thoracic cord injuries tend to be complete. Incomplete injuries can be identified by the sparing of some tracts, and these injuries tend to show much better recovery. The early picture is obscured by 'spinal shock' where all cord function ceases for 24–48h.

Anterior Cord Syndrome. The posterior column still functions (proprioception, vibration sensation).

Central Cord Syndrome – Common in Elderly. Relative sparing of motor supply to legs. Sacral sparing (sensation, anal tone).

Brown-Séquard Syndrome – Rare. Hemitransection of the cord. Preserved contralateral motor function, position and vibration sense. Preserved ipsilateral pain and temperature sensation.

Mixed Syndromes. These are combinations of the above.

Management and Complications of Cord Injury

Respiratory. Impairment of respiratory function is common after injury to the cervical spine. This may relate to partial phrenic nerve palsy, intercostal paralysis, inability to expectorate and a ventilation–perfusion disorder. Associated chest injuries may be present. Monitor by chest X-ray (CXR) and ABG. Ventilation and bronchoscopy may be needed.

Cardiovascular. Bradycardia and hypotension may occur owing to damage to sympathetic outflow. Excessive i.v. fluids to attempt to correct hypotension may cause pulmonary oedema. Avoid pharyngeal suction, as it may potentiate bradycardia via a vagal reflex and lead to cardiac arrest.

Urinary Tract. Insert catheter to avoid overdistension of an atonic bladder. If potential urethral injury (perineal bruising or pelvic fracture), perform retrograde urethrogram. Suprapubic or intermittent self-catheterisation may be required later. Stasis in the urinary tract combined with hypercalciuria due to immobilisation may lead to repeated urinary tract infections and stone formation. Urinary catheter should be changed frequently.

Gastrointestinal. Paralytic ileus follows a few days after injury. Avoid oral fluids; i.v. fluids and nasogastric (NG) suction will be required until bowel sounds return. Beware stress ulceration with perforation. Signs may be lacking. Shoulder tip referred pain may be the only clinical indication.

Hypothermia. Hypothermia may occur owing to paralysis of the sympathetic nervous system. The patient should be kept warm.

Thromboembolism. The incidence of DVT and PE is high. Start subcutaneous LMWH 6h after injury. Continue until the patient is mobile in a wheelchair.

Pressure Sores. These form as a result of pressure ischaemia, particularly over bony prominences. Regularly turning in bed every 2h is essential. The patient's bottom should be lifted off a wheelchair seat every 15min for a similar reason. Established sores require aggressive treatment with plastic reconstruction if necessary.

Long-Term Management of Spinal Trauma

Nursing Care

Good nursing care is essential and should always be in a specialised spinal unit. Objectives include: prevention of secondary complications; facilitation of maximum functional recovery; support for patients and family in adaptation to changed physical status; education of patients and relatives in all aspects of long-term care.

Physiotherapy

This involves care of both the chest and paralysed limbs initially. Later care involves help with strengthening nonparalysed muscles; adaptation to a wheelchair; relearning ability to balance; transfer from wheelchair to bed, toilet, etc.; bracing and gait training.

Occupational Therapy

This helps adjustment to a lifetime of disability. Help is given to reach the highest levels of physical and psychological independence at home and at work. Help is provided with the activities of daily living, home alterations, recreation and work.

Social Services

This provides help with finance, adaptation of home and employment.

Others

Long-term help with bladder problems, chronic pain and sexual problems will be required.

Prognosis

It is important to indicate the probable degree of recovery at an early stage to both patients and relatives. Recovery after a complete cord lesion is unlikely. It is, however, difficult to forecast the degree of recovery in an incomplete lesion as improvement may occur after resolution of oedema and contusion. The most encouraging signs are those of incompleteness of paralysis or early return of cord function. Patients with early recovery usually achieve the most recovery. In incomplete lesions, improvement may continue for several years. Death in the first days after injury is likely to be due to respiratory failure with high tetraplegia.

The level of cervical transection is crucial to long-term prognosis. Above C4, the patient usually dies of respiratory failure. At C4, patients are able to use their mouth to control a wheelchair. At C5 with special aids they can feed, wash and move their chair. However, they cannot transfer in and out of the chair or dress themselves. At C6 they can drive a special car and dress the upper body but are unable to transfer themselves from a chair. At C7 their ability is intermediate between that of C6 and C8, the latter being the ability to lead an independent wheelchair life. The other causes of morbidity and mortality include PE, pressure sores and chronic renal failure (CRF) (late).

PELVIC FRACTURES

The pelvis is a ring of bone and ligaments, which includes the innominate bone, sacrum, sacroiliac joints and pubic symphysis. When fractures occur, the ring tends to break in two places (like breaking a polo mint). If only one fracture is visible on radiograph, the possibility of sacroiliac joint disruption should be considered. Pelvic fractures occur in younger patients in RTAs. Elderly patients may sustain isolated pubic ramus fractures, which respond to analgesics and mobilisation. Mortality for closed pelvic fractures varies between 5% and 15% with a mortality of 50% for open fractures. The pelvis is very vascular, and injuries are associated with considerable blood loss. Pelvic visceral and urethral damage may occur.

Symptoms and Signs. Pelvic pain. Abrasions. Bruising. Haemodynamic shock. Inability to pass urine. Bleeding per urethra. Bleeding per rectum (PR). Bleeding per vaginal (PV). Perineal bruising. High 'floating' prostate on examination PR.

Investigations

- Pelvic radiograph (AP centred on the sacrum)
- Trauma CT scan (Inlet and outlet pelvic radiographs if CT not available)
- Intravenous urography (IVU)
- Urethrogram.

Treatment

Shock – Balanced Fluid Resuscitation. Initial fluid bolus dose resuscitation is usually 1–2 L of warmed crystalloid dependent on haemodynamic status. 'The first clot is the best clot' is a concept introduced to ensure that the first clot the patient makes following their injury is not blown off with aggressive fluid resuscitation. The ideal blood pressure during resuscitation is normally below that of day-to-day life. The amount of fluid and blood required for resuscitation is difficult to predict on initial evaluation of the patient and should be titrated according to the response of the bolus dose of fluid. The aim is to ensure continuation of adequate end organ perfusion and oxygenation (i.e. via urinary output, level of consciousness and peripheral perfusion). In the emergency department, pelvic binders may be used to control haemorrhage from pelvic fractures. In the operating room with 'open book' types of fracture, emergency stabilisation with an external fixator reduces bleeding. For other fractures, radiological intra-arterial embolisation is the best option to slow bleeding.

The Fracture Itself. Acetabular fractures require accurate reduction and fixation. A CT scan is required to assess for loose bodies and articular congruity. A tertiary referral service should be involved to assess the patient and provide definitive care. A variety of internal fixation methods is available followed by ipsilateral non-weight-bearing for 3 months.

Urethral Trauma. Avoid catheterisation. If the patient can pass urine and it is clear, all is well. Otherwise, consider suprapubic catheterisation or cystotomy. Retrograde urethrogram and IVU may be required.

Complications. Haemorrhage and shock, urethral or bladder injury, rectal injury, paralytic ileus, DVT, damage to hip joint. Late post-traumatic OA may occur in acetabular injuries. Vaginal injury, sciatic nerve injury, malunion may lead to obstetric difficulties. Sexual dysfunction.

INJURIES TO THE LOWER LIMB

Hip and Thigh

Traumatic Dislocation of the Hip

The majority are posterior and follow impact directed along the femoral shaft when the hip is flexed and adducted, e.g. RTA when the knee strikes the dashboard. Anterior, inferior and central dislocations are rare, the latter being caused by the head of the femur being driven into the acetabulum.

Symptoms and Signs. Often other severe injuries. Shock. Thigh is flexed, adducted and internally rotated with posterior dislocations. May be associated injury to femur or patella. Sciatic nerve injury should be assessed prior to reduction.

Investigations

- Good-quality radiograph of hip with lateral film
- Judet views (45° oblique views of hip)
- Radiograph of femur and patella.

Treatment. Reduction under general anaesthesia (GA) with muscle relaxation. If the hip is stable and there is no associated fracture, patient is mobilised with weight-bearing as tolerated. If a bone fragment is displaced from the posterior acetabulum, open reduction and internal fixation of the fragment may be required.

Complications. Associated fractures. Sciatic nerve damage. Avascular necrosis of femoral head. Late OA of hip.

Fractures of the Proximal Femur

The blood supply to the head of the femur comes from three sources:

- Retinacular vessels in the capsule
- Medullary vessels in the femoral neck
- Via the ligamentum teres.

The main source is via the retinacular vessels, and these may be damaged in fractures of the femoral neck. Fractures may be classified as intracapsular (subcapital, transcervical) or extracapsular (basal, intertrochanteric→Figure 18.4). Extracapsular fractures do not damage the blood supply to the femoral head, and therefore there are no risks of avascular necrosis of the femoral head and nonunion. They are most common in the elderly, especially females with osteoporotic bones when the traumatic cause is relatively trivial, e.g. a fall in the house. In the young patient they result from major trauma.

Symptoms and Signs. Elderly female. Minor trauma. Tripped over carpet. Tripped over pavement. Pain in the hip. Adduction of limb. Shortening and external rotation only if the fracture is displaced. Movements painful. Weight-bearing usually impossible. Beware hypothermia.

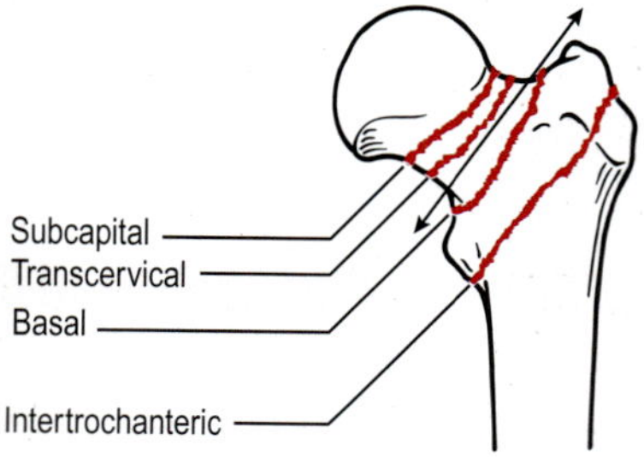

FIGURE 18.4

Fractures of the femoral neck. The arrowed line separates intracapsular (to the left) and extracapsular (to the right) fracture sites. Intracapsular fractures are associated with avascular necrosis of the femoral head.

Investigations

- Radiographs in two planes (→Figure 18.5 AP view)
- FBC
- U&Es
- Coagulation screen
- Blood sugar
- CXR
- ECG. In the elderly patient there is the possibility of intercurrent disease.

Complications. These are of the elderly undergoing surgery, e.g. pneumonia, MI, CVA, DVT and PE; 30% of elderly patients die within 12 months of the injury. Avascular necrosis of the femoral head. Nonunion. Malunion with varus angulation and shortening.

Treatment

General. Pain relief. DVT prophylaxis. Further investigation if pathological fracture suspected (calcium, CXR, bone scan, long films to include joints above and below, myeloma screen).

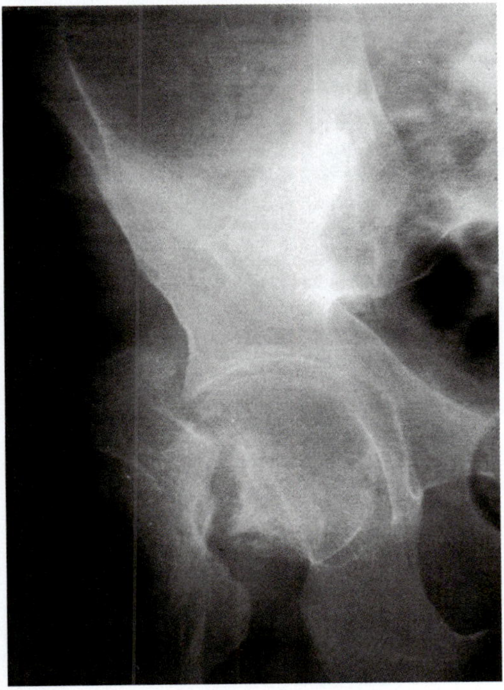

FIGURE 18.5

A subcapital fracture of the neck of the femur.

Fracture. Planned trauma list <36 h after injury. The aim is to allow full weight-bearing mobilisation as soon as possible following surgery. The aim of early surgery is to allow nursing, mobilisation and rehabilitation:

- Intracapsular: undisplaced (fixed with screws if able to non-weight-bear); displaced – femoral head replacement, i.e. hemiarthroplasty (most common treatment), e.g. Exeter trauma stem or primary total hip replacement if cognitively intact (abbreviated mental test score (AMTS) >6), mobile out of home without walking aid and anaesthetically fit.
- Extracapsular: cantilever device, e.g. dynamic hip screw; load sharing device, e.g. cephalomedullary nail, gamma nail.

Fractures of the Femoral Shaft

Common in younger people and usually result from severe trauma in RTAs. They may occur at any site and be of variable pattern. Treatment is either conservative (traction – rarely used) or more commonly operative (intramedullary nail or temporary external fixator device). There are frequently associated injuries, especially ipsilateral femoral neck fractures.

Symptoms and Signs. Severe pain in thigh. Deformity. Haemodynamic shock. Potential complications: Vascular injury to femoral vessels. Injury to sciatic nerve.

Investigations

- Radiographs in two planes
- Femoral angiography may be required if vascular injury is suspected.

Treatment. ATLS protocol. Splint leg (preferably traction splint). Pain relief (titrated opiates as required). Balanced fluid resuscitation using crystalloid or blood as required. FBC, U&Es. Crossmatch (blood loss can be 2–4 units). Check if fracture is open. Give tetanus prophylaxis and antibiotics if open fracture.

Conservative. Useful in children under the age of 4 years and those for whom surgical treatment is contraindicated (e.g. skin condition, pre-existing infection, etc.). In those over the age of skeletal maturity, long-term conservative treatment is not recommended due to the risk of pressure sores and fracture malunion. This is also a more expensive form of treatment.

Skin traction and temporary stabilisation in Thomas splint. *Conservative definitive treatment* – pre-toddler (<2 years) – gallows traction followed by hip spica. Toddler – balanced traction until moves comfortably on bed and callus evidence on radiographs, then hip spica. In adults, skeletal traction with a Steinmann pin and balanced traction applied through the skeletal pin with the knee flexed on a special knee flexion attachment. Fractures heal quickly in children. In adults cast bracing may be used after 6–8 weeks.

Surgical

- Internal fixation: *Open physes* – elastic stable intramedullary nails (ESIN) aged 4–13 years to avoid the growth plate. *Closed physes* – achieved by a locked intramedullary nail. This allows accurate reduction and compression and ensures early mobilisation of the patient. There is a risk of infection and osteomyelitis. This form of treatment is useful for multiple fractures, pathological fractures and when there is associated vascular injury.

- External fixation: used especially for open fractures where there is soft tissue damage. Pins are inserted above and below the fracture site and reduction and alignment maintained by an external fixator device.

Complications. DVT. PE. Fat embolism. Infection. Shortening. Angulation. Nonunion.

Fractures and Dislocations Around the Knee

Fractures are usually intra-articular causing haemarthrosis, which should be aspirated to decrease pain. They can be caused by a direct blow (car bumper, car dashboard), vertical compression (fall from a height) or excessive strain (forced abduction at the knee). Associated ligamentous and neurovascular injuries are common. Conservative treatment for these injuries involves a long leg cylinder plaster, then a hinged cast brace. This type of treatment is also used after open reduction/internal fixation. The knee joint needs accurate repair of the articular surfaces to reduce the risk of post-traumatic OA.

Supracondylar Fractures (→ Figure 18.6)

These are intra-articular or extra-articular. The distal fragment is pulled backwards by the gastrocnemius. The popliteal artery may be damaged by the distal fragment. Conservative treatment is by skeletal traction via the proximal tibia with the knee in about 30° of flexion. Internal fixation is required for all displaced intra-articular fractures (polyaxial/fixed angle locking plates, retrograde intramedullary nails).

Isolated Femoral Condylar Fractures

These are usually displaced so internal fixation is advised with lag screw or headless compression screw.

Tibial Plateau Fractures

In these fractures, vertical compression forces or strains drive the femoral condyle through the tibial plateau. Fragments of tibial plateau/condyle may be cleaved off, depressed or both. Both condyles may be damaged. Displaced or depressed fragments should be reduced and internally fixed, often with support from a bone graft and a buttress plate.

Dislocation of the Knee

This is an uncommon injury. It is usually associated with damage to the popliteal artery or local nerves. After reduction under anaesthesia any ruptured ligaments should be repaired. Immobilisation in plaster, then cast brace is required for several months.

Injuries to the Extensor Mechanism

These involve the following:

- Tear of quadriceps insertion into the patella
- Transverse fracture of patella with separation
- Rupture of the patellar tendon, avulsion of tibial tuberosity.
- Forced flexion of the knee against a contracting quadriceps causes the extensor mechanism to give way.

Symptoms and Signs. Pain. Knee cannot be fully actively extended against gravity producing extensor lag. Palpable gap and point of maximum tenderness at site of lesion.

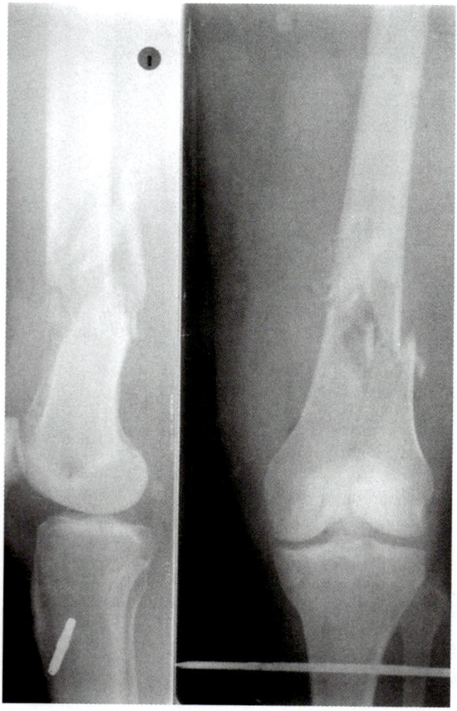

FIGURE 18.6

A supracondylar fracture of the femur. In the lateral view, the distal fragment is tilted backwards and may damage the popliteal artery.

Investigations. Radiograph: patella 'high' if patellar tendon ruptured; patella 'low' with upper part tilted forward with quadriceps tear. Ultrasound scan (USS) confirms diagnosis.

Treatment. Operative repair of defect in the extensor mechanism. Immobilisation. Exact regimen varies dependent on strength of fixation. Suggested: 0–30° for first 3 weeks, 0–60° between weeks 3 and 6, 0–90° from weeks 6 to 9. Full range of movement thereafter.

Fractures and Dislocations of the Patella

Fractures

An avulsion or transverse fracture is caused by a violent contraction of quadriceps against resistance. A comminuted fracture is caused by direct violence, e.g. a blow from a bat or in an RTA.

Treatment. This depends on whether the extensor mechanism is intact and on the degree of comminution. If the extensor mechanism is intact and there is no severe comminution, treatment in a plaster cylinder for 3–4 weeks will suffice. Transverse fractures with separation are held with a tension band wire or two longitudinal screws. Mobilisation is possible after 3 weeks in a plaster cylinder. If the extensor mechanism is ruptured, surgical repair is required. A long-term complication is OA of the patellofemoral compartment.

Dislocation of the Patella

This may be acute or recurrent and occurs laterally.

Acute or Traumatic. This results from a blow on the side of the knee. The patella is visibly displaced. The knee remains flexed until the patella is reduced by medial directed pressure. There may be a tear in the medial patellofemoral ligament and capsule or avulsion of the medial side of the patella. May be associated with haemarthrosis. Treatment involves quadriceps exercises as pain allows.

Recurrent. Usually affects adolescent girls. Associated with flattening of lateral condyle, small high-riding patella or genu valgum. Dislocation occurs spontaneously or with minor trauma. The knee locks in semiflexion. Spontaneous reduction usually occurs. After a single incident, intensive physiotherapy to strengthen vastus medialis. Surgery is indicated in recurrent cases.

Fractures of the Tibial Shaft

These are common fractures occurring as a result of RTAs, sports injuries and industrial accidents. They are often open. Oblique and spiral fractures are commonly unstable when reduced. Up to 20% of cases develop nonunion.

Treatment. Numerous methods are available depending on fracture.

Stable Fractures. Undisplaced fractures are treated with above-knee cast immobilisation and reviewed on a weekly basis for first 2–4 weeks. When callus forms on the X-ray, conversion to weight-bearing is encouraged. Commonly displaced tibial fractures in skeletally mature patients are treated with either intramedullary fixation or a fine-wire external fixator (Ilizarov frame). This enables earlier weight-bearing mobilisation and less frequent follow-up. For some patients, unsuitable for invasive surgery or where fixation is not possible, closed reduction under GA is still a very good way of treating particularly a transverse fracture. The leg hangs over the end of the operating table, gravity maintaining position of the fragments. The ankle is dorsiflexed to a right angle and an above-knee plaster applied with the knee in slight flexion. Position should be checked with radiographs immediately after plastering and at weekly intervals until callus forms, and then the patient may be treated in a tibial tuberosity weight-bearing Sarmiento-type cast.

Unstable Fractures. With spiral, oblique or comminuted fractures, a long leg plaster is insufficient. Closed injuries should be fixed with an intramedullary nail. Where the fracture is very proximal, very distal, segmental or there is substantial bone loss, a fine-wire external fixator (Ilizarov) makes an ideal choice of reduction and fixation and allows for bone transport osteogenesis. The treatment of severe open injuries is controversial and may be with a fine-wire external fixator or an intramedullary nail at the preference of the surgeon. Either method can be used for open fractures with minimal soft tissue damage.

Open Wounds. All open wounds must be explored, irrigated and treated in conjunction with a plastic surgeon if bone is exposed at the base of the wound. It is recommended that unless the wound is heavily contaminated or exposed to marine or farmyard debris, early stabilisation and plastic surgery soft tissue coverage of exposed bone is achieved on the next available trauma list with senior surgeons. The 6-h rule of injury to theatre no longer applies.

Complications. Delayed union. Nonunion. Infection. Nerve damage. Stiffness of knee, ankle, foot. Compartment syndrome.

Isolated Fractures of the Fibula

These are uncommon. They are usually associated with tibial fractures and with direct violence. Beware common peroneal (common fibular) nerve injury in fractures of neck of the fibula. Treatment is symptomatic until pain settles. Exclude Maisonneuve ankle injury, i.e. diastasis (see below).

Fractures Around the Ankle

These are due to indirect forces transmitted from the foot (e.g. twisted ankle). The ligaments and malleoli may be injured in various combinations. Severe force may cause associated dislocation.

Classification (Figure 18.7)

There are two main classification systems used. The Weber classification is used in everyday practice and describes the X-ray appearance of the fracture. The Lauge-Hansen classification describes the starting point and deforming force and generally is more useful for research purposes but is actually remarkably similar to the Weber classification. The Weber classification is based on the level of the fracture in relation to the joint syndesmosis of the distal fibula. Three malleoli are described – medial, lateral (distal fibular) and posterior, which is the posterior most distal tip of the tibia.

- Weber Type A fractures are horizontal avulsion fractures found below the syndesmosis. They are stable fractures and are amenable to conservative treatment with a full weight-bearing cast for 6 weeks.

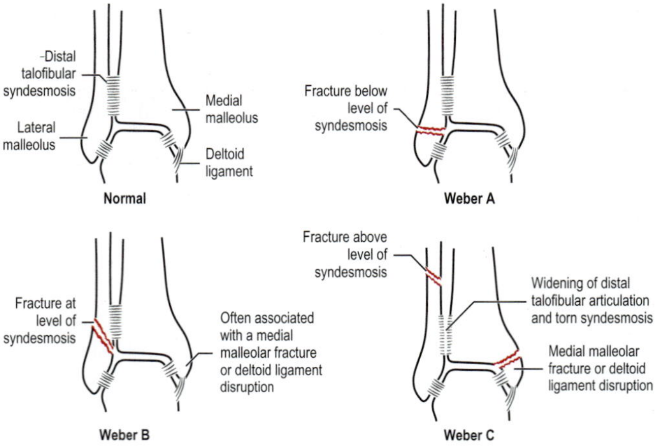

FIGURE 18.7
Weber classification of ankle injuries.

- Weber Type B fracture is a spiral fibular fracture that starts at the level of the syndesmosis. This fracture may be bimalleolar/trimalleolar. The importance is the presence of articular congruity in the cast and whether the medial side is tender or not. If nontender, there will be no medial malleolar fracture or disruption of the deltoid medial ligament. Therefore, there will be lesser possibility of talar shift. This is a stable fracture and may be treated as a type A but with X-ray checks at 1 and 2 weeks. Otherwise, open reduction and internal fixation are required.
- Weber Type C fracture is above the level of the syndesmosis and disrupts and ligamentous attachment between the fibular and the tibia distal to the fracture. These fractures are unstable and require open reduction and internal fixation with non-weight-bearing for 12 weeks.

AXIAL COMPRESSION FRACTURES (PLAFOND FRACTURE). These account for <10% of lower limb fractures. These are caused by a fall on the foot from a height. The talus is driven into the articular surface of the tibia, which is comminuted. This is a severe injury and is difficult to treat. Massive soft tissue swelling occurs.

Investigations

- AP and lateral films
- Note site of fractures and talus shift or tilt.
- CT scan helps delineate fracture anatomy – almost mandatory.

Treatment. This is difficult to treat. Initial treatment requires reduction of the ankle joint, immobilisation and minimisation of swelling with elevation. Consider using a hinged external fixator from tibia to tarsal bones or an Ilizarov external fixator.

MAISONNEUVE FRACTURE (→ FIGURE 18.8). A twisting injury causes a high fibular fracture with a radiological normal ankle joint. The syndesmosis is often disrupted, however, along with rupture of the deltoid ligament. There is disruption of the interosseous tibiofibular ligament. Treatment involves syndesmosis screws and non-weight-bearing for 6 weeks with protected (in immobilisation) weight-bearing for further 6 weeks.

HINTS AND TIPS

Fracture–dislocation of the ankle – this high-energy injury may pose risk of damage to skin, nerves or blood vessels. In the event of vascular compromise, it is recommended that reduction of the dislocation is achieved at the earliest opportunity either at the scene of the accident, in the emergency department or, if irreducible (due to the deltoid ligament being stuck in the medial gutter), in theatre. Prereduction X-rays should not be carried out so as not to delay reduction of the ankle joint. Definitive fixation should be delayed until the swelling settles to avoid wound healing problems.

Fractures and Dislocations in the Foot

Talus Fracture

This is rare, accounting for <1% of all foot fractures. The blood supply is from distal to proximal, and therefore fractures across the neck may result in avascular necrosis. It is

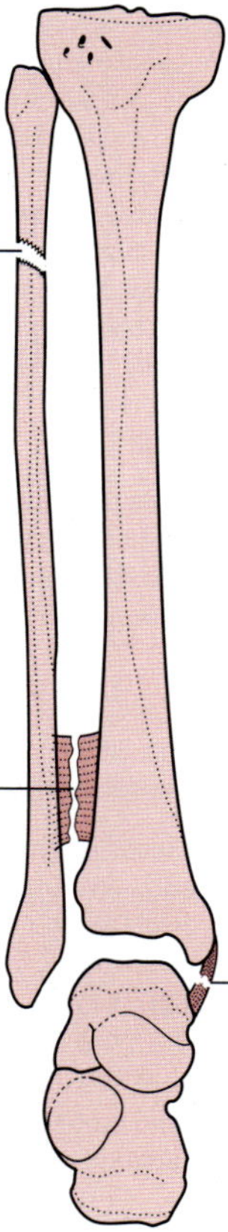

FIGURE 18.8

Diastasis of the inferior tibiofibular joint with rupture of the interosseous membrane. There is an associated high fibular fracture (Maisonneuve fracture).

usually caused by forced dorsiflexion. Undisplaced fractures are treated in plaster. The foot should be maintained in plantar flexion following closed reduction of displaced fractures; 8–12 weeks' immobilisation is required. Avascular necrosis leads to OA. Displaced fractures require internal fixation after reduction. CT scan is required to determine degree of displacement due to risk of avascular necrosis. Generally associated with a poor outcome and high risk of post-traumatic arthritis.

Calcaneal Fracture

This is caused by a fall from height onto the heel. It may be bilateral. Look for fractures elsewhere, especially burst fractures of the spine. Conservative treatment is by bed rest and elevation of the legs to reduce swelling. Operative treatment is now less favoured as a result of the publication (July BMJ 2014) of the UK heel trial (151 patients) which showed no advantage in pain and function of operative versus surgical treatment for displaced calcaneal fractures. Early subtalar fusion is often beneficial. Ankle exercises are required. Initial non-weight-bearing for 6–8 weeks. Partial weight-bearing on crutches is then permitted. Healing takes up to 10 weeks. Complications include pain, stiffness at the subtalar joint, and local nerve and tendon entrapment.

Metatarsal Fractures

Avulsion fracture of the base of the fifth metatarsal is common and is caused by an inversion injury combined with forced plantar flexion, e.g. misstepping on a stair. The peroneus brevis tendon avulses the styloid process at the base of the fifth metatarsal. Treatment is full weight-bearing in a metatarsal shoe walking plaster for 4–6 weeks. Fracture of the proximal (rather than base) fifth metatarsal (Jones fracture) is due to forefoot adduction trauma and may require open reduction and fixation along with non-weight-bearing for 6–8 weeks.

Shaft Fractures

These occur with crushing injuries and are often multiple. Elevation of the foot followed by mobilisation in a plaster slipper non-weight-bearing cast for 6 weeks is required. If displacement is gross, manipulation or internal fixation may be required.

Stress Fracture ('March' Fracture)

This usually affects the second metatarsal neck and is caused by the stress of long hours of walking, e.g. new army recruits. It may not be apparent on an early radiograph but only show on a repeated radiograph when callus is forming. Treatment is a below-knee walking plaster for 6 weeks. In mild cases, rest only is required.

Lisfranc Fracture

This is principally a dislocation of some or all of the tarsometatarsal joints of the foot, particularly the second metatarsal head fitting into the keystone of the cuneiform bones. Clinical suspicion is aroused due to massive swelling and potentially normal X-rays. X-rays should be repeated weight-bearing, AP, oblique and lateral, and the dislocation may be emphasised. CT scan may confirm the diagnosis. Open reduction and internal fixation are required.

Fractures of the Toes

These are common injuries. Fracture occasionally interferes with circulation requiring surgery. Otherwise splintage by strapping to the adjacent toe will suffice. Great toe fractures may require fixation often simply with K-wire fixation.

INJURIES TO THE UPPER LIMB

Fractures and Dislocations Around the Shoulder

Clavicular Fracture

This is caused by falls on the outstretched hand or point of the shoulder. The bone usually breaks between the middle and outer third. Fractures of the outer end may be associated with fractures of the coracoid and damage to the coracoclavicular ligament.

Symptoms and Signs. Pain in shoulder region. Supports weight of arm with other hand. The proximal portion is drawn upwards by sternomastoid. The distal portion droops owing to the weight of the arm. Tenderness over the site.

Investigations. Radiograph (AP). Check position and deformity.

Treatment. Support the arm in a triangular sling. With displaced fractures 3 weeks of support is usually sufficient. Rarely, displacement may be sufficient to warrant internal fixation, especially if the skin over the fracture is in danger of necrosis.

Complications. Rare. Occasionally injury to brachial plexus or axillary artery may occur.

Dislocation of the Sternoclavicular Joint

This is rare and involves subluxation or dislocation of the joint surface. Usually the medial end of the clavicle dislocates forward and the deformity is obvious. Posterior dislocation is rare and may lead to tracheal pressure. This requires open reduction to relieve tracheal compression. Otherwise treatment is usually symptomatic.

Acromioclavicular Joint

Subluxation. Not uncommon in rugby players who present with a lump over the joint. Treatment is by rest in a sling until symptoms subside. The lump over the joint often persists.

Dislocation. Complete dislocation occurs only when the coracoclavicular ligament is disrupted. The clavicle is elevated and the point of the shoulder lowered. Bruising and tenderness occur. Radiographs show a gap between coracoid process and clavicle. Treatment is usually conservative with a sling, but reconstruction may be required depending on the degree of displacement.

Scapular Fracture

This is usually caused by direct violence. There may be extensive bruising. Treatment is by rest, analgesia, collar and cuff. Mobilise when pain allows. CT if suspicion of glenoid involvement.

Dislocation of the Shoulder

The commonest form is anterior (95%) and is caused by a fall on the outstretched hand. In the younger patient the capsule is strong and does not tear. The glenoid labrum and capsule are avulsed from the bone, allowing recurrent dislocations to occur. In the older patient the capsule is torn – this heals after reduction. Recurrent dislocation is less common in the older patient. Dislocations may also occur posteriorly (commonly epileptics) and inferiorly (squash players).

Symptoms and Signs. Fall on outstretched hand. Pain. Patient supports arm, which is abducted. The normal contour of the shoulder is lost. Check for axillary nerve damage – anaesthesia over skin at insertion of deltoid.

Investigations. Radiograph (Figure 18.9): humeral head not in contact with the glenoid; check for associated fractures of the humeral head and neck.

Treatment. Reduction under GA or intravenous sedation. Two methods are available:

Kocher's Method. Flex the elbow to a right angle and apply slow gentle traction in the line of the humerus. Rotate the humerus externally using the forearm as a lever. Adduct the humerus across the trunk. Then internally rotate the humerus. Avoid this method in the elderly owing to risk of iatrogenic fracture.

Hippocratic Method. Wrap a towel around the axilla with assistant pulling cranially and pull downwards on the arm. Confirm the position with radiograph. Immobilise the arm in a sling for 3 weeks.

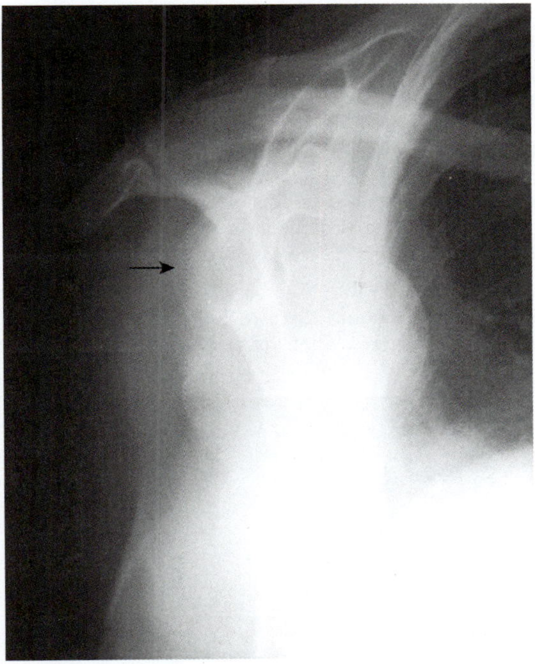

FIGURE 18.9

Anterior dislocation of the shoulder joint. The humeral head lies below and medial to the glenoid (arrow).

Complications. Early complications include axillary nerve damage and associated fractures. Late complications include stiffness and recurrent dislocation. Complete rotator cuff tear in the elderly.

Recurrent Dislocation

This usually follows damage to the glenoid labrum (Bankart lesion) or humeral head (Hill–Sachs's lesion) at the time of original dislocation. Dislocation occurs on movement of the arm, especially if raised and externally rotated. Radiograph may reveal a depression on the humeral head (Hill–Sachs's lesion).

Treatment. Operative: the operation of choice is Bankart's operation, where the torn glenoid labrum is reattached to the bone. Reconstruction of the anterior labrum is the gold standard and should be carried out arthroscopically. Open reconstruction is becoming rarer. Results of surgery are good.

Posterior dislocation is uncommon. An axillary radiograph is essential for diagnosis.

Fractures of the Humerus

Proximal Humerus (Figure 18.10)

This is usually due to indirect violence, i.e. a fall on the shoulder, often in the elderly.

Treatment. Undisplaced fractures are treated with a collar and cuff (for gravitational traction), then physiotherapy. Hanging casts have gone out of fashion. Significantly displaced avulsion (>1 cm) of the tuberosities or anatomical neck fractures should be internally fixed with repair of the rotator cuff. Surgical neck fractures are usually treated in a collar and cuff for 3–6 weeks and then physiotherapy starting with pendulum arm exercises followed by active assisted movements.

Complications. Axillary nerve damage. Shoulder stiffness.

Shaft of the Humerus

This is caused by a direct blow or a fall on the outstretched hand. The fracture is usually oblique and may be displaced. Check for radial nerve damage (wrist drop and

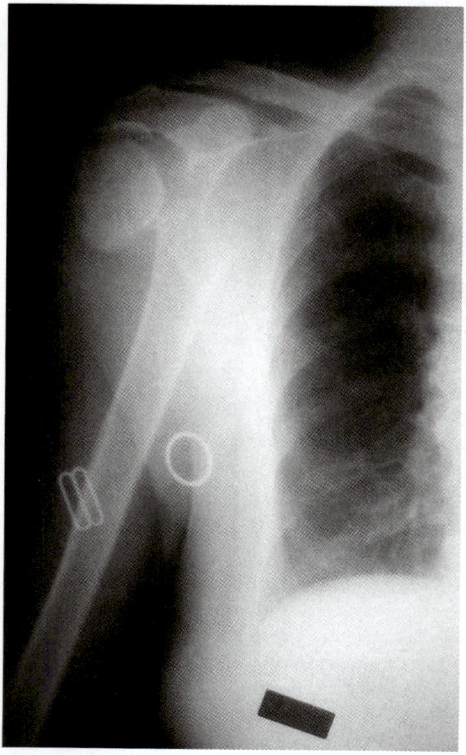

FIGURE 18.10

A fracture of the neck of the humerus. This shows severe displacement. The axillary nerve is in danger with such a fracture.

anaesthesia in the first web space on the dorsal aspect). These are typically due to fractures at the distal two-thirds junction as the radial nerve crosses from the posterior to anterior muscle compartments.

Treatment. The weight of the arm effects reduction. A 'U' slab is applied to the upper arm and the wrist supported with a collar and cuff initially. The 'U' slab extends over the shoulder and under the elbow. 'U' slabs are rarely used after the initial 2 weeks when they are replaced with a humeral brace (a thermoplastic moulded splint). Occasionally, open reduction and internal fixation may be required using a plate or an intramedullary nail especially in neurologically compromised patients. Internal fixation is appropriate in polytrauma patients.

Complications. Radial nerve damage and nonunion.

Fractures and Dislocations Around the Elbow

Supracondylar Fracture

This is chiefly a fracture of childhood but may occur in adults. There is a history of a fall on the outstretched hand followed by pain and swelling around the elbow. The lower fragment is usually displaced, rotated and in extension. The brachial artery and median nerve are vulnerable to injury.

Treatment. Reduction under anaesthesia. Longitudinal traction is inserted on the forearm, medial and lateral displacement is corrected along with rotation. Fractures are held with flexion and forearm pronation and stabilised if required with cross K-wires (lateral side first) and medial side under direct vision due to the proximity of the ulnar nerve to the medial epicondyle. Check radiograph for position. Check that the radial pulse does not disappear through overflexing the swollen elbow. Admission is necessary to observe the circulation for 24h. If all is well, the patient is discharged after 24h, the fracture being immobilised for 4–5 weeks, after which active exercise is commenced.

Problems may occur after this type of treatment. The pulse may not return after manipulation, but provided the hand remains pink with good capillary return, there is no cause for alarm. Pallor, poor capillary return, excessive pain and inability to bring about full passive extension of the fingers are signs for alarm. Reduce the degree of flexion. If the pulse does not return, extend the arm vertically. If the circulation is not restored, the forearm needs surgical decompression with exploration of the brachial artery. If the pulse was present prior to reduction and lost after reduction, surgical exploration of the artery is mandatory.

Complications. This fracture is prone to several complications, particularly in children. Damage to brachial artery. Nerve injury (median). Stiffness. Malunion causing cubitus varus or gunstock deformity. Epiphyseal damage with later deformity. Myositis ossificans. OA. Volkmann's ischaemic contracture. Chronic regional pain syndrome may occur in adults.

Lateral Condyle/Epicondyle

Lateral condylar fractures occurring in young children are injuries of the capitellar epiphysis. Displaced lateral condyles should be fixed to prevent valgus deformity and tardy ulnar nerve palsy due to traction. Lateral epicondylar avulsions are very rare and should be fixed if displaced.

Medial Condyle/Epicondyle

Medial condylar fractures are rare and should be fixed if displaced. Medial epicondylar fractures are more common and are associated with elbow dislocations (50%). They should be fixed if displaced by >0.5–1cm or fragments need washing out of the joint.

Dislocation of the Elbow

It is caused by a fall on the hand with the elbow partly flexed. Dislocation is almost always posterior. Occasionally there are fractures of adjacent bones. Median or ulnar nerve palsy may occur. Damage to the brachial artery is rare.

Treatment. Reduction is usually easy. The elbow is held in slight flexion and then pressure is applied to the olecranon posteriorly until reduction occurs. The elbow is immobilised for 1–3 weeks in a collar and cuff, after which active exercises are encouraged.

Fracture–dislocation of the elbow is a more serious injury involving fractures of the humeral condyles, radial head or coronoid. Manipulative reduction and internal fixation may be necessary. A stiff elbow is the usual outcome. Vascular injury and myositis ossificans may also occur.

Fractures of the Radius and Ulna

These are common and caused by either indirect violence from a fall on the outstretched hand, with or without rotation, or direct violence, which usually causes fracture of a single bone.

Fracture of the Radial Head

This varies from a fine vertical crack to severe comminution. There is localised tenderness over the radial head with minor injury. With comminution the elbow is painful and swollen with restriction of all movement. Minor cracks and undisplaced fractures may be rested in a collar and cuff sling for 2 weeks. Displaced large fragments may be internally fixed. Comminuted fractures may require excision or replacement of the radial head.

Fracture of the Olecranon

This is caused by direct violence as an isolated injury or as part of a fracture–dislocation of the elbow. Displaced fractures are internally fixed with tension band wires, periarticular locking plates or lag screws for coronoid fractures.

Fractures of the Radial and Ulnar Shafts

These injuries are common and are often open. They are usually caused by direct violence. An injury to the forearm usually affects the two bones, or one bone plus one radioulnar joint. A displaced fracture of the midshaft of either bone alone can occur if the radial head dislocates with an ulnar fracture (Monteggia's fracture) or the distal radioulnar joint dislocates with a fracture of the radius (Galeazzi fracture). Radiographs of the forearm must therefore include both wrist and elbow joints. Occasionally direct violence fractures only one bone, e.g. the ulnar, as when lifting the flexed arm to ward off a blow. In children, fractures are of the greenstick type with angulation. In adults, the fractures are transverse or oblique.

Treatment

Children. Manipulative reduction is usually successful. Position (<10° angulation and <50% displacement acceptable) is maintained in an above-elbow plaster cast from axilla to metacarpal heads with the elbow at a right angle. Off-ended fractures or unstable fractures may need open reduction and stabilisation with ESIN (e.g. Nancy nails).

Adults. Accurate alignment is essential to allow pronation and supination. Open reduction and plating is usually undertaken followed by 2–4 weeks in plaster.

Fractures of the Distal Radius

COLLES' FRACTURE (FIGURE 18.11). This is a dorsally displaced and angulated fracture of the distal radius with associated ulnar styloid fracture 2.5 cm from the wrist joint. It is common in elderly osteoporotic women following a low-energy fall.

DISTAL RADIAL FRACTURE. A similar fracture is found in younger adults. While there is not the same degree of dorsal cancellous bone collapse as with the osteoporotic Colles' fracture, the high-energy nature of the injury often leads to comminution or intra-articular extension of the fracture. These are more aggressively treated by surgery due to higher patient demand.

Symptoms and Signs. Fall on outstretched hand. Pain. Limitation of wrist movement. 'Dinner fork' deformity. Check for distal neurovascular deficit.

Investigations. Radiograph in two planes (Figure 18.12): distal fragment is displaced dorsally, radially (with pull-off of the ulnar styloid) and supinated; check for intra-articular fracture lines and associated scaphoid fracture.

Treatment. Undisplaced or greenstick fractures require immobilisation in a below-elbow plaster for 3–4 weeks. Significant displacement requires manipulation under general or regional anaesthesia.

More minor corrections or emergency reduction to relieve pressure on a compromised median nerve may be achieved under a haematoma block in the emergency department. This technique is best demonstrated by a more senior colleague in the first instance. 10 mL of 1% lignocaine or 0.5% bupivacaine is introduced into the fracture site via a dorsal approach, left to take effect, and with the assistance of nitrous oxide, reduction of the fracture into a more acceptable position is achieved. Alternatively, the procedure may be carried out under a Bier's block.

The fracture is disimpacted by traction and increasing the deformity. The distal fragment is levered over the proximal, the wrist flexed, ulnar deviated and pronated. A dorsal plaster slab is applied to hold this position. A check radiograph is taken and

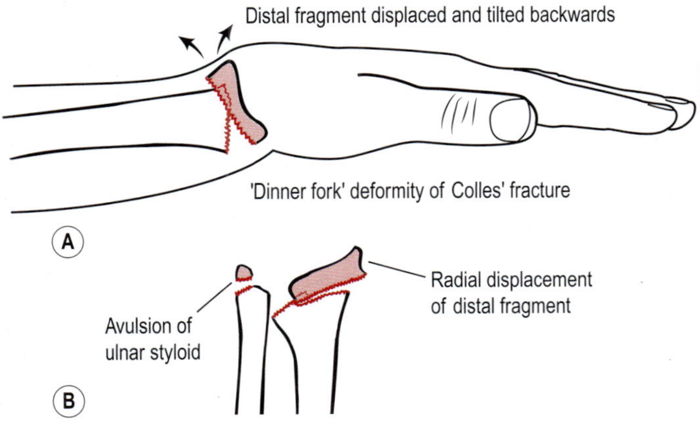

FIGURE 18.11
Colles' fracture. (**A**) Lateral view. (**B**) AP view.

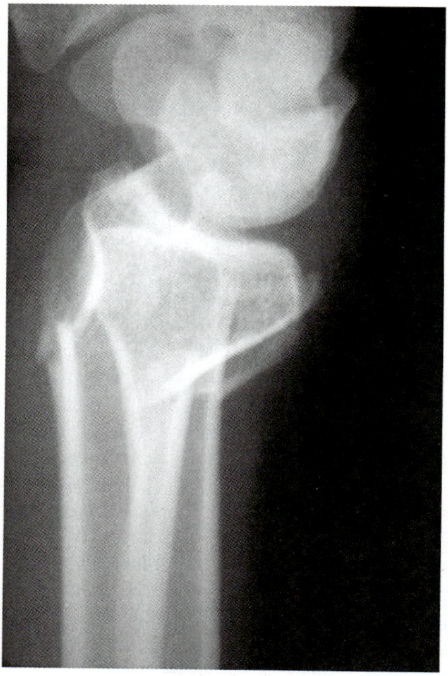

FIGURE 18.12
A radiograph of the wrist (lateral view) showing a typical Colles' fracture. There is dorsal inclination, displacement and impaction.

the arm supported in a sling. Further radiographs are taken at 1 and 2 weeks to check reduction. Swelling has usually subsided by this time and the plaster is completed and the sling abandoned. The plaster is removed at 6 weeks and exercises commenced. Operative treatment is required for intra-articular fractures (especially in the young) and failed reduction or failed plaster immobilisation.

Complications. Stiffness and oedema of the hand. Malunion with angulation. This may be associated with pain from subluxation of the inferior radioulnar joint. Median nerve symptoms occur but usually subside spontaneously. Later rupture of the tendon of extensor pollicis longus may occur where it crosses the fracture. Complex regional pain syndrome.

SMITH'S FRACTURE. This is a fracture of the lower end of the radius with forward (volar) angulation. It is the reverse of a Colles' fracture. Conservative treatment is manipulation using the reverse procedure for Colles' fracture. An above-elbow plaster is applied for 6 weeks with the wrist dorsiflexed and the forearm fully supinated. Operative treatment (volar plating) is often required owing to instability of the fracture in plaster.

BARTON'S FRACTURE. This is an intra-articular fracture–dislocation of the radiocarpal joints in the coronal plane. Internal fixation is required.

Fractures and Dislocations of the Carpal Bones

Fracture of the Scaphoid

This accounts for 15% of wrist injuries and is the most commonly fractured carpal bone. Caused by a fall on the outstretched hand or a blow to the palm of the hand. The blood supply to the bone comes from distal to proximal, and hence there is a risk of avascular necrosis of the proximal fragment (up to 100% with proximal one-fifth fracture). The scaphoid spans both rows of carpal bones hence the high risk of nonunion.

Symptoms and Signs. Fall on outstretched hand. Painful swollen wrist with tenderness in the anatomical snuffbox, scaphoid tubercle and on AP compression of the scaphoid.

Investigations

- Radiograph: scaphoid views
- Bone scan
- CT/MRI.

Treatment. If this fracture is suspected clinically but is not confirmed on radiograph, treat on clinical grounds as a fracture to scaphoid. Re-radiograph in 2 weeks when the fracture may show. A bone scan/MRI may be helpful. The wrist is immobilised in a scaphoid or Colles' cast. The plaster is worn for 6 weeks initially when radiological evidence of union should be apparent. Union may be delayed and a plaster may need to be worn for 3 months. Fixation of fractures with more than 1 mm displacement is advised.

Complications. Avascular necrosis of the proximal segment. Delayed union and nonunion requiring bone grafting and internal fixation. OA of the wrist (scaphoid nonunion advanced collapse) is a long-term sequel.

Dislocation of the Carpus

Commonly missed. Caused by a fall on an extended hand. If the radiograph looks unusual, especially the lateral view, obtain specialist advice. Volar (anterior) dislocation of the lunate is the commonest and may cause acute median nerve compression. Check for associated scaphoid fracture. Closed or open reduction is performed. Methods of immobilisation are controversial, but application of a plaster ± K-wires for 6–8 weeks may be required.

Fractures and Dislocations of the Metacarpals and Phalanges

When assessing fractures of the metacarpals or phalanges, beware of rotational displacement. This may not be obvious until the fingers are flexed, when they cross over each other abnormally.

Fractures at the Base of the Thumb

Extra-articular fractures can usually be treated conservatively by manipulation and plaster casting. Intra-articular fractures of the thumb may produce late OA. Bennett's fracture is oblique, and the small fragment is on the ulnar side of the base of the first metacarpal where the deep oblique ligament attaches. Most are treated with closed reduction and K-wires under GA, but occasionally open reduction and internal fixation are required. Late OA is rarely seen.

Fractures of the Metacarpal Bones

These are caused by direct violence or by punching with a closed fist. Very important to identify the 'fight bite' injury where a tooth penetrates the metacarpophalangeal joint (MCPJ). Condition often missed. Requires wash-out.

Treatment. Undisplaced fractures are treated in a back slab or by strapping the injured finger to its neighbour. Displaced or multiple fractures require reduction and/or internal fixation. Active movements are encouraged.

Fractures and Dislocations of the Phalanges

These are often serious injuries and may be associated with tendon and nerve damage.

Treatment. Dislocation can usually be reduced under local anaesthetic. Undisplaced fractures may be treated by strapping the injured finger to its neighbour leaving the joints free. Active movements are encouraged. Unstable or displaced fractures may need open reduction and internal fixation with crossed Kirschner wires or miniscrews.

Fractures of the Terminal Phalanges

These are usually crush injuries and may be open. There may be subungual haematoma that contributes to the pain. The latter can be drained by piercing the nail with a hot wire, giving instant relief. Open fractures are treated with wound toilet, leaving the wound open, Tetanus toxoid and broad-spectrum antibiotics. Occasionally, partial amputation of the finger is required.

Mallet Finger

This injury is caused by 'stubbing' a finger when it is actively extended. Forced passive flexion leads to avulsion of the extensor tendon from the base of the terminal phalanx often with a flake of bone. Examination reveals 'extensor lag' in which the distal phalanx is flexed and cannot be actively extended. Treatment is by immobilisation of the distal interphalangeal joint in a 'mallet finger' splint, which hyperextends the terminal interphalangeal joint while allowing flexion of the proximal interphalangeal joint. The splint is worn for 6 weeks. Occasionally healing does not occur, but the disability is usually slight, although it may be more pronounced and require fusion of the distal interphalangeal joint.

CONDITIONS OF JOINTS

Arthritis

The term is used to describe both inflammatory and degenerative disease.

Osteoarthritis (Osteoarthrosis, OA)

This is a term applied to degenerative disease of a joint caused by wear and tear that affects the articular cartilage and subchondral bone. At first, the synovial membrane is normal, but later thickening and fibrosis occur. OA may be primary or secondary. In the former there is no underlying cause. It may arise as a result of senile changes and may affect more than one joint. Secondary OA occurs if there has been previous damage to the joint, e.g. congenital deformity, trauma, infection, avascular necrosis, gout, haemophilia.

Symptoms and Signs. Pain. Stiffness. Deformity. Pain increases in severity as the disease progresses. Sleep is often disturbed. Synovial thickening and bony enlargement of joint because of osteophytes. Effusions. Tenderness. Loss of movement. Crepitus. Fixed deformities. Disturbances of gait.

Investigations. Radiographs (Figure 18.13): narrowing of joint space, subchondral bone sclerosis, subchondral cysts, osteophytes, evidence of other underlying pathology. Symptoms do not necessarily correlate with the severity of radiological changes.

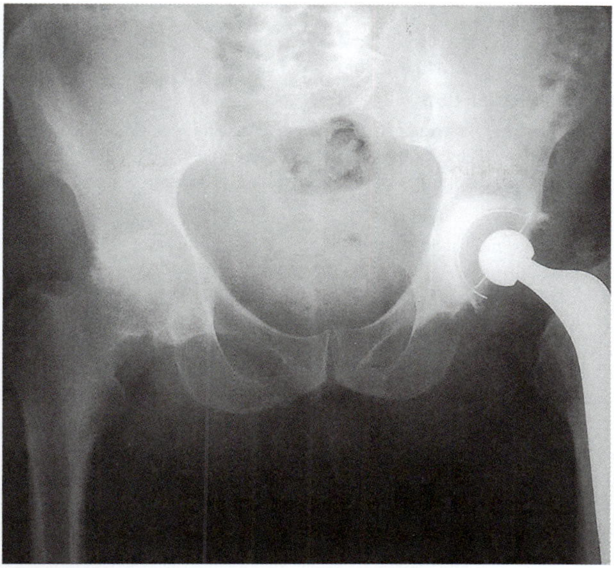

FIGURE 18.13

A radiograph of the pelvis. There is osteoarthritis of the right hip joint. The joint space is diminished and there is sclerosis of the surrounding bone. On the left side, the patient has had an arthroplasty (hip replacement).

Treatment. Principles of treatment involve pain relief, improvement of mobility and correction of deformity. Management may be conservative or surgical.

Conservative. Analgesia: start with mild analgesia, e.g. paracetamol; NSAIDs are usually required eventually.

- Lose weight
- Walking stick
- Physiotherapy
- Steroid or hyaluronic acid injections
- Changing occupation to a lighter job.

Surgical. Disturbance of sleep, severe uncontrolled pain and gross lack of mobility are indications for surgery. The following procedures may be undertaken depending upon the level of symptoms and joint involved:

- Arthroscopy or open debridement: occasionally synovectomy and removal of osteophytes can give temporary relief.
- Replacement arthroplasty (→Figure 18.13): most joints can be replaced by artificial joints, e.g. hip and knee.
- Osteotomy: weight-bearing axis redistributes weight to the least worn side. Pain relief is often dramatic and failure of the procedure is slow.

- Excision arthroplasty: for small joints, e.g. small toes
- Arthrodesis: surgical fusion of the joint, relieves pain, e.g. first metatarsophalangeal joint (MTPJ) joint in hallux rigidus.

Rheumatoid Arthritis (RA)

Only surgical aspects of management will be dealt with here. (The reader is referred to a textbook of medicine for the details of the symptoms and medical management of this disease.) Surgery is undertaken for pain relief, not for cosmetic effect. Procedures include:

- Synovectomy: gives good pain relief. The knees and finger joints are most suitable for this treatment.
- Repair or reconstruction of ruptured tendons
- Joint fusion, e.g. painful wrist; atlantoaxial subluxation
- Arthroplasty: the same prostheses and procedures are used as for OA. However, hand deformities are often most trouble in RA, and various arthroplasties of the finger joints are indicated. Flexible silastic implants giving stability whilst allowing movement are the most popular. Infection can be a problem, as the patients have often been on long-term steroids.

Other Conditions of Joints

Loose Bodies

These may occur in any joint, but the knee is by far the commonest site. Causes include osteochondritis dissecans (see below), detached osteophytes in OA, osteochondral fractures, torn menisci and synovial chondromatosis, where cartilaginous nodules form in the synovium and may become detached.

Symptoms and Signs. Pain and swelling. 'Locking' (inability to fully extend the knee). Giving way. Occasionally, the loose body may be palpable.

Investigations

- Radiograph
- Arthroscopy.

Treatment. Arthroscopic or occasionally open removal.

Osteochondritis Dissecans

In this, an area of bone with its overlying articular cartilage becomes necrotic, separates and drops into the joint cavity as a loose body. It is associated with local trauma (50%).

Symptoms and Signs. Late childhood or young adults. Commonly affects the knee. Occasionally multiple joints. Knee – usually medial femoral condyle. Pain and swelling. Loose body may cause locking or giving way.

Investigations

- Radiographs
- MRI – high signal on T_2 images deep to the fragment in situ supports diagnosis of loose fragments.

Treatment. In the early stages before separation, rest in a plaster cast or bandage may allow healing. If separation is incomplete, pinning may help revascularisation. A loose body needs removal. Drilling the defect may help healing.

Neuropathic Joints (Charcot's Joints)

A diffuse destructing deformity and dislocation often found in diabetes. A joint which has lost pain and proprioception appreciation is subject to harmful stresses and strains. Destruction of the joint results. The patient usually presents with a painless, deformed joint. Causes include diabetic neuropathy, tabes dorsalis, syringomyelia and leprosy. Vibration sense, position sense and deep pain sensation are absent or reduced. Treatment requires non-weight-bearing immobilisation followed by a graduated return to ankle–foot orthoses. Arthrodesis and arthroplasty are usually unsuccessful. Supporting appliances may be the most appropriate treatment.

Haemophilia and Related Disorders

The main orthopaedic problems relate to acute haemarthroses and bleeding into muscles. They may occur spontaneously or as a result of injury, which may be minor. Recurrent bleeding into the same joint results in degenerative changes, capsular fibrosis, contracture and deformity. The knee, elbow and ankle are the joints most frequently affected.

Symptoms and Signs. Pain, muscular spasm, swelling over joint. Local tenderness. Bruising. Long-standing cases show deformity of joint. Muscle wasting and synovial thickening. Patients presenting for the first time with a haemarthrosis need detailed haematological investigation.

TREATMENT. Analgesia, splintage, possible factor VIII replacement. Large haemarthroses require aspiration under factor VIII cover. The chronically damaged joint is prone to repeated bleeds, and an orthosis (a caliper in case of a knee joint) may be necessary for long-term protection. Synovectomy and soft tissue release for severe contractures.

ARTHROPLASTY

This is surgical refashioning of a joint, the aims being to relieve pain, restore mobility and provide stability. There are basically four types of arthroplasty:

- *Total* (→Figure 18.13). Both articular surfaces are replaced, e.g. Exeter's hip replacement system replacing both ball and socket.
- *Partial arthroplasty*, e.g. medial unicompartmental knee replacement where one compartment of the knee is affected with arthritis with the other compartments remaining normal, e.g. Oxford knee replacement.
- *Hemiarthroplasty*. This is used where one surface of the joint is in good condition, e.g. a Stryker Exeter trauma stem (ETS) hip hemiarthroplasty prosthesis in fractured neck of femur where the acetabulum is normal and therefore only the ball of the ball-and-socket joint is replaced. It is rarely suitable for OA.
- *Excision (Girdlestone procedure)*. The joint surfaces are excised. Fibrous tissue forms across the gap. There is often residual instability and considerable shortening. This method is usually regarded as an end stage/salvage procedure following repeated infection of a joint replacement. Following first-time revisions for infection, antibiotic-loaded cement spacers or temporary joints are now more commonly used.

Design of Joint Replacements

- Bearing surface – most commonly metal on plastic (UHMWPE), ceramic on polythene and ceramic on ceramic. Occasionally metal on metal (cobalt – chrome; recently fallen out of favour for some brands due to metal debris hypersensitivity reaction termed 'aseptic lymphocyte-dominated vasculitis associated lesion' (ALVAL)). Ceramic heads have less wear than metal but are more expensive.
- Fixation method – implants are either cemented, uncemented or a hybrid combination of both. Cemented prostheses use cement (polymethyl methacrylate) as grout. Under load the prosthesis will slowly move in the cement over time (creep). Uncemented prostheses osseointegrate by either ingrowth or ongrowth by the bone bonding to the hydroxyapatite coating which is plasma sprayed to the metal material or by growing into the porous coating or porous material (trabecular metal). Initial stability of the implant is required in compacted cancellous bone to allow this bone growth.
- Implant design:
- Cemented stem – modern polished tapered design allows the implant to subside maintaining congruity of the implant shape in the cement mantle, ensuring axial compression of the cement mantle (hoop stresses).
- Uncemented stem – often constructed of titanium to allow closer elasticity of the implant to the surrounding bone.
- Cemented cup – contemporary materials use highly cross-linked UHMWPE.
- Uncemented cup – either hemispherical or rim fit design. Allow for either polyethylene or ceramic line.
- Head size – large head reduces risk of dislocation at the expense of increased wear.
- Degree of constraint – constraint is defined as the effect of the elements of knee implant design that provide the stability needed to counteract forces about the knee after arthroplasty, in the presence of a deficient soft tissue envelope. Most knee replacements are merely held together by the natural ligament tension of the collateral ligaments and the posterior cruciate ligament. They are not connected by any link and therefore have the least amount of constraint. Working through the range of available knee replacements, it is possible to gradually increase the linkage between components resorting finally to a fully hinge-linked knee. This is the maximum degree of constraint in knee replacements. Generally higher degree of constraint results in earlier failure of the implant, usually at the implant/bone interface.

Practice of Joint Replacement

Indications. Walking distance less than half a mile, pain limiting activity (e.g. golf) despite adequate analgesia and especially pain disturbing sleep.

Preoperative Preparation (Good Practice). Discussion with patient of conservative vs operative options. Make patient aware of risks and rewards of surgery.

Intraoperative Preparation (Enhanced Recovery). X-ray templating to plan operation. Team brief. DVT prophylaxis. Prophylactic antibiotics and tranexamic acid. Opiate free spinal anaesthetic. Ultraclean air with unidirectional laminar flow ventilation. Strict aseptic technique. Inclusion of antibiotics in bone cement. Meticulous dissection, positioning of prosthesis, soft tissue reconstruction. Early mobilisation with mechanical and chemical thromboprophylaxis.

HINTS AND TIPS

CONSENTING FOR A TOTAL HIP REPLACEMENT

At 1 year postsurgery >90% of patients forget day-to-day that they have a hip replacement in situ. At 20 years, less than 15% of hip replacements need revision (UK National Joint registry).

Specific risks of total hip replacement surgery: infection (1 in 400 hips need revision due to deep infection), nerve/vessel damage (<1%), leg length discrepancy, dislocation (3%). Future revision surgery.

Generic risks of major surgery: DVT (symptomatic 2%)/PE (<0.1%), chest infection, heart attack, stroke, 1 in 200 risk of death within 90 days.

Follow-up: 2 months, 1 year (then 7 years and every 3 years for under-75-year-olds)

CONSENTING FOR TOTAL KNEE REPLACEMENT

Same as hip except can replace leg length discrepancy and dislocation with stiffness.

Complications

Early. As for any major operation, but especially bleeding, DVT, PE. Neurovascular injury. Dislocation. Wound infection.

Intermediate. Recurrent dislocation. Heterotopic ossification.

Late. Septic or aseptic loosening (failure of the interface to bone). Implant wear or failure.

CONDITIONS OF MENISCI, LIGAMENTS, TENDONS, CAPSULES AND BURSAE

Knee

Meniscal Tears

This is a common knee injury. The medial is affected more often than the lateral. Commonly associated with a twisting injury

Symptoms and Signs. Two groups:

1. Young male. Twists the knee. Usually knee is flexed and weight is on injured leg. Commonly occurs with anterior cruciate injury. Bucket handle tear may occur causing acute true locking (inability to straighten knee).
2. Patient over 40 years old. Trivial twisting injury to knee causes degenerate meniscal tear.

Pain on side of knee where meniscus is torn. Knee may catch, click and 'lock'. Knee swells slowly over 24h (immediate swelling indicates anterior cruciate ligament injury). Settles with resting. Symptoms may then recur with 'recurrent locking'. In the chronic phase – wasted quadriceps, effusion, tenderness over meniscus in joint line. McMurray's test is positive if the tear is posterior. Diagnosis is usually made on classical history and signs.

Investigations

- Plain radiographs normal
- Exclude other conditions, e.g. radio-opaque loose bodies.
- MRI scan
- Arthroscopy (for treatment rather than diagnosis).

Treatment. Tears in the periphery of the meniscus in physiologically younger patients can be repaired. Otherwise, partial meniscal resection.

Ligamentous Damage

Damage to the collateral ligaments and cruciate ligaments occurs frequently in sports people. Generally classed as grade 1 – tenderness at ligament attachment and on stressing but no laxity (up to 5mm freedom); grade 2 – 5–10mm freedom; grade 3 – 10mm+ freedom.

COLLATERAL LIGAMENTS

Medial. An abduction strain on the tibia ruptures the medial ligament. Valgus straining with 10° of flexion will demonstrate opening of the joint. If a cruciate ligament is also damaged, the joint will open even in full extension. Clinical diagnosis with confirmation via MRI.

Lateral. Rarely occurs in isolation. Instability is rarer because the biceps femoris tendon helps stabilise the lateral side of the knee.

CRUCIATE LIGAMENT TEARS

Anterior. Usually caused by noncontact hyperextension or forward movement of the tibia on the femur with the knee flexed. There may be associated meniscal tears or damage to collateral ligaments. Examination reveals an effusion and a positive 'anterior drawer sign' – the tibia can be pulled forwards on the femur with the knee flexed. Lachman's test with knee flexed at 20° and tibia drawn forward is more sensitive than 'anterior drawer' test. Pivot shift test is most specific.

Posterior. Usually torn by a force drawing the tibia backwards on the femur with the knee flexed. There is almost always other ligamentous injury. Examination reveals 'posterior sag', i.e. the tibia moves backwards on the femur when eliciting the 'posterior drawer sign'.

Treatment of Ligamentous Injuries. Isolated collateral ligament injuries are initially treated in a brace. Multiple or complex injuries are best treated surgically. Chronic injuries with symptomatic instability benefit from surgery. Acute posterior cruciate ligament or posterolateral corner injuries require surgery within 5–12 days. Others may be treated when chronic.

Bursae Around the Knee

HOUSEMAID'S KNEE (PREPATELLAR BURSITIS). Commonly seen in carpet fitters or those working on their knees (originally described when housemaids used to scrub floors). Leaning forward on the knees brings the prepatellar bursa in contact with the floor. Treatment is by modification of work pattern (wear pads), aspiration or, rarely, excision.

CLERGYMAN'S KNEE (INFRAPATELLAR BURSITIS). Rarely seen. Caused by frequent kneeling on the floor and sitting back on the heels which brings the infrapatellar bursa in contact with the floor (originally described in clergymen who prayed in this position). Treatment is by work modification, aspiration or, rarely, excision.

Semimembranosus Bursa. It occurs between the tendon of semimembranosus and deeper structures. Cystic swelling on medial aspect of popliteal fossa. Usually occurs in children and young adults. Most resolve spontaneously. Conservative treatment, aspiration and injection of steroid or very rarely excision is required.

Baker's Cyst. This is included here for convenience but is not a bursa. It is a cystic lesion of the knee joint most commonly due to a one-way valve forming from a meniscal tear in the knee. It presents as a swelling in the popliteal fossa. The cyst usually communicates with the back of the joint through a small defect in the capsule. Surgery is rarely required unless the cyst becomes tense and very painful. If there is any doubt about the diagnosis, MRI should be carried out. The cyst may rupture and cause pain behind the knee and in the calf. It may be difficult to distinguish from a DVT (ultrasound will confirm or exclude the diagnosis of DVT). A thrombosed popliteal aneurysm enters into the differential diagnosis of a painful Baker's cyst. Check the other limb (popliteal aneurysms may be bilateral) and the distal circulation.

Ankle

Sprained Ankle

The anterior talofibular ligament is the most common ankle ligament that may be torn during an inversion injury. Pain, swelling and tenderness occur below and in front of the lateral malleolus. Treatment is by analgesia, physiotherapy and occasionally an ankle–foot orthosis.

Rupture of the Achilles Tendon

This usually occurs during sport, e.g. tennis or due to a missed step. The patient feels 'something give' and feels like 'being kicked in the back of the heel'. Examination usually reveals a gap in the tendon. The calf squeeze test is positive. Conservative treatment is by plaster immobilisation in full plantar flexion followed by progressive immobilisation up to the neutral position. Full weight-bearing is possible when in a boot with heel wedges. Surgical repair may be necessary in the young, active patient and is followed by immobilisation in plaster to reduce the risk of re-rupture. Immobilisation is required in both cases for 12 weeks. Operative repair is required for re-rupture and delay in diagnosis of >1 week.

Plantar Fasciitis

This occurs in late middle age. The pain is under the heel. In the younger patient it may be associated with Reiter's disease. The pain is often worse on standing after a period of rest and improves somewhat with walking. Examination reveals tenderness at the attachment of the plantar fascia to the undersurface of os calcis. A lateral radiograph may show an associated calcaneal spur. Treatment is by a soft heel pad or local injection of steroid and local anaesthetic or both. The condition is self-limiting.

Shoulder

A variety of conditions may occur in middle life at the shoulder girdle. They probably represent a spectrum of related conditions of low-grade inflammatory or degenerative aetiology. They include conditions variously known as impingement syndrome, rotator cuff tears, frozen shoulder, rupture of the long head of biceps and acromioclavicular arthritis. Conditions previously known as supraspinatus tendinitis, subacromial bursitis and painful arc syndrome are now grouped together under the title impingement syndrome.

Impingement Syndrome

Mechanical impingement of the rotator cuff muscles on the undersurface of the acromion can cause inflammation and pain with overhead activities. The insertion of supraspinatus is a relatively avascular area susceptible to repeated trauma and degeneration. Pain may be felt in the mid-arc of abduction with positive impingement tests – shoulder forward flexed 90° and internal rotation impacts supraspinatus tendon between acromion and greater tuberosity.

Investigations

- Radiographs to exclude arthritis; sclerosis of acromion and tuberosity
- USS – cuff inflammation or tendinosis
- MRI.

Treatment. Modification of activity. NSAIDs. Physiotherapy. Subacromial steroid injection. If symptoms persist, arthroscopic subacromial decompression may be required.

Frozen Shoulder

Now thought to be due to fibrosis of the capsule of the shoulder joint. Often no predisposing cause is found. Stiffness and pain predominate with loss of external rotation. May be primary (of unknown aetiology) or secondary, e.g. trauma. More common in diabetics.

Treatment. Spontaneous resolution usually occurs over 2 years. Manipulation under anaesthetic is often carried out early with good pain relief and improved function. Physiotherapy helps. Some patients require open or arthroscopic capsule release.

Rotator Cuff Tears

Most commonly affects supraspinatus but can involve subscapularis and infraspinatus. Usually occurs in a tendon that is already degenerate. It follows trivial trauma or normal everyday activity. There is a sudden pain in the shoulder and an inability to initiate abduction. If initial abduction can be started passively (e.g. by tilting the body to the side to initiate abduction by gravity), deltoid can continue abduction. Diagnosis may be confirmed by USS or MRI. Surgical treatment may be required for large tears.

Rupture of the Long Head of Biceps

This usually occurs in a previously diseased tendon. There is acute pain, tenderness and 'bunching up' of the muscle in the lower part of the upper arm when the elbow is flexed. There is little residual functional disability.

Elbow

Tennis Elbow (Lateral Epicondylitis)

This is chronic inflammation or degeneration of the extensor carpi radialis brevis at its origin on the lateral epicondyle. It affects anyone whose work involves extending and twisting the forearm. In some cases there is no obvious cause. There is pain on the outer side of the elbow radiating down the back of the forearm. It becomes worse on gripping. Tenderness is localised to the lateral epicondyle. Resisted supination exacerbates the pain. Treatment is by rest, tennis elbow brace and injection of local anaesthetic and hydrocortisone. Surgery is rarely indicated but involves release of the common tendon origin.

Golfer's Elbow (Medial Epicondylitis)

This is similar to tennis elbow but affects the medial epicondyle. Pain occurs on hyper-extending the fingers and wrist. Treatment is by rest and injection of local anaesthetic and steroid. If the latter treatment is given, remember the close proximity of the ulnar nerve.

Student's Elbow (Olecranon Bursitis)

This occurs owing to prolonged pressure over the olecranon bursa, e.g. a student studying long into the night and resting the head in the hand with the elbow on the table. For obvious reasons, the condition is uncommon in present-day students. Examination reveals a swelling over the olecranon, which may be acutely inflamed. In the acute phase, aspiration (occasionally pus is obtained) ± antibiotics (only if infected) are required. NSAIDs are usually given for pain relief. In the chronic phase, straw-coloured fluid is aspirated. Surgical excision is rarely required.

Wrist

Tenosynovitis

This is inflammation of a tendon sheath. It is caused by the trauma of repetitive movements and affects the tendons of the fingers and thumb, especially dorsally, where they cross the wrist within their synovial sheath. There is localised tenderness and crepitation on movement of digits. Treatment is by rest, local splinting and NSAIDs. A specific form affects the tendon sheaths of abductor pollicis longus and extensor pollicis brevis as they cross the radial styloid (de Quervain's tenosynovitis). Pain occurs at the site and is exacerbated by gripping and by extending the thumb. Forced flexion of the thumb with ulnar deviation of the wrist exacerbates the pain. Treatment in the acute phase involves splints and local injection of hydrocortisone. Chronic cases require surgical division of the tendon sheath.

Hand

Ganglion

A ganglion is a cystic swelling in relation to a joint or tendon sheath. It may represent cystic-myxomatous degeneration of fibrous tissue. It is common on the dorsum of the hand and also occurs in relation to the wrist and ankle. It is a painless, cystic swelling that is fluctuant and transilluminates and is filled with a crystal-clear gel. Treatment is aspiration with injection of steroid or surgical excision. The latter should be done under GA or brachial block using a tourniquet, as they often extend down inside the underlying joints. Recurrence is less common when treated surgically.

Trigger Finger

The fibrous flexor sheath thickens and the lumen narrows. The narrowed area causes friction against the tendon, creating a localised nodule in the tendon. The condition occurs at the level of the metacarpal head or neck. As the nodule passes through the area of stenosis, a click or snap is felt and the digit 'triggers'. Sometimes, the digit frankly locks in flexion and cannot be extended. If the finger is fully flexed the patient may have to extend it passively. A nodule may be palpable at the site of thickening.

Spontaneous resolution may occur. Around 70% will respond to steroid injection to the entrance of the tendon sheath. Surgical treatment may be required and is by longitudinal division of the A1 pulley at the opening. Multiple 'triggering' digits should arouse the suspicion of RA.

Dupuytren's Contracture

This is a condition of the palmar fascia involving nodules and contractures. Aetiology is unknown but it is associated with family history, diabetes, alcoholism, liver disease and antiepileptic drugs. It may be associated with Peyronie's disease and retroperitoneal fibrosis.

Symptoms and Signs. Mainly elderly males, but can occur in females. Nodular thickening of the palmar fascia. Contracture of the proximal interphalangeal joint and the metacarpophalangeal joint usually affecting the ring or little finger.

Treatment. If the patient cannot place the hand flat on the table, surgery is often required. This involves careful dissection of the palmar fascia, fasciotomy and/or local fasciectomy. Recurrence may occur. If the deformity is great and involves a single digit, amputation may be appropriate.

MISCELLANEOUS CONDITIONS OF THE LIMBS

Upper Limb

Ulnar Neuritis

The ulnar nerve lies in a groove behind the medial epicondyle. Pressure or chronic friction may occur in the groove. Cubitus valgus (increased carrying angle) may stretch the nerve. Symptoms include pain in the forearm, paraesthesia in the ulnar one and a half fingers and wasting of the small muscles of the hand supplied by the ulnar nerve. Electromyography (EMG) studies confirm the diagnosis. Treatment is by decompression or by transposition of the ulnar nerve anterior to the medial epicondyle.

Carpal Tunnel Syndrome

In this condition the median nerve is compressed in the carpal tunnel. It may be associated with pregnancy, RA, myxoedema, OA, anterior dislocation of the lunate and arteriovenous fistula at the wrist for dialysis. Middle-aged women are most affected.

Symptoms and Signs. Pain and paraesthesia in the thumb, index and middle fingers. Worse in bed at night. Relieved by hanging arm out of bed. Clumsiness when carrying out fine movements. Wasting of thenar muscles and reduction of sensation in distribution of median nerve in hand occur in advanced cases. No objective findings in early cases. Pressure over the carpal tunnel may reproduce symptoms.

Investigations. Nerve conduction studies may help.

Differential Diagnosis. Thoracic outlet syndrome, cervical spondylosis, peripheral neuritis.

Treatment. Mild cases may be treated by splintage at night. Injection of the carpal tunnel with steroid may be appropriate. Carpal tunnel decompression by operative division of the flexor retinaculum. Cases presenting in pregnancy often settle spontaneously after delivery.

Lower Limb

Metatarsalgia

This is pain under the metatarsal heads. It is caused by a dropped transverse arch, often in elderly obese ladies. It is tender over the second and third metatarsal heads with callosities. Treatment is with a medial arch support or metatarsal dome. Morton's metatarsalgia is due to a plantar digital neuroma, probably due to chronic trauma at the confluence of the medial and lateral plantar nerves against the metatarsal transverse ligament. It also affects middle-aged women. Usually it affects the cleft between the third and fourth toes. Treatment includes toe spacers and wide toe box shoes or division of the metatarsal ligament. If symptoms do not settle, steroid and local anaesthetic infiltration or exploration and excision of neuroma may be necessary. Other causes include stress fracture, plantar warts, inflammatory conditions (e.g. RA), Freiberg's disease.

Hallux Valgus

This is common in females. The first metatarsal deviates medially and the great toe laterally creating a bulge often covered with a 'bunion' due to a thickened overlying bursa. The great toe may overlap or under-ride the second toe. It may be a result of wearing unsuitable footwear, especially in adolescence. It is often familial. Metatarsalgia may coexist.

Treatment. Mild cases require accommodating wide shoe footwear. Surgery is necessary for gross deformity or associated arthritis. If there is no arthritis, realignment operations are appropriate, e.g. chevron, scarf osteotomy or Lapidus procedure should be carried out. Arthrodesis or resection arthroplasty is required if there is secondary OA.

Hallux Rigidus

This is OA of the first metatarsophalangeal joint. It is a common condition that occurs in young adults, but the cause is unknown. There is pain on walking, especially 'pushing off' and a stiff, painful, enlarged joint. Radiographs show OA. Treatment in mild cases is by a carbon fibre insole to stiffen the gait cycle where forefoot dorsiflexion occurs. Severe cases require arthrodesis.

Hammer Toes

This is a toe (usually the second) with a fixed flexion deformity of the proximal interphalangeal joint and compensatory hyperextension of the adjacent joints. Painful overlying corns occur. Treatment is by arthrodesis or excision of the proximal interphalangeal joints with extensor tenotomy.

Mallet Toe

This is a toe with flexion deformity of the distal interphalangeal joint with a corn at the tip of the toe or over the joint. Distal interphalangeal joint fusion is indicated.

INFECTION OF BONES AND JOINTS

Acute Infection of Bones and Joints

Acute Osteomyelitis

This is a disease of growing bones or immunosuppressed or diabetic adults. It is usually due to *Staphylococcus aureus* and rarely due to *Streptococcus, Pneumococcus, Haemophilus* or *Salmonella*. The infection usually starts at the relative avascular metaphysis of a long bone or centre of a short bone. Common sites include the lower end of the femur, upper end of the tibia, humerus, radius, ulna and vertebral bodies. Suppuration occurs, and pus under tension causes bone necrosis. Pus breaks out under the periosteum, strips it and penetrates through, forming a sinus. Alternatively, the pus can decompress into the joint causing septic arthritis. Necrotic bone is called a 'sequestrum'. New subperiosteal bone forms around the dead bone forming a shell (involucrum).

Symptoms and Signs. Young patients. Recent history of infection (e.g. respiratory) or trauma. Pain in limb. Severely aggravated by movement. Swelling and redness of affected area – usually localised to metaphyseal area. Loss of function. Malaise. Pyrexia. Tenderness and heat over site of infection. Oedema. Pus with fluctuation is a late sign. Sympathetic effusion in nearby joint.

Investigations

- WCC↑
- CRP↑
- Blood cultures
- Joint aspirate early if septic arthritis suspected
- MRI scan.

Treatment. After obtaining blood cultures ± drainage of pus, start antibiotics preferably once cultures known from microbiology, e.g. fusidic acid and flucloxacillin i.v. Splint the limb to relieve pain. Prolonged intravenous antibiotic therapy up to 6 weeks may be necessary. Resolving temperature and falling CRP are good guides to recovery.

Acute Pyogenic Arthritis

This is a blood-borne infection, especially in infants. Staphylococci, streptococci and gonococci may be causative organisms. It may arise following osteomyelitis, where the metaphysis is intracapsular, e.g. hip joint. It is a complication of RA in patients on steroids. Occasionally it follows penetrating injuries of joints.

Symptoms and Signs. Hot, tender, painful, swollen joint. All movements are painful and there is surrounding muscle spasm. High fever. Rigours.

Investigations

- WCC↑
- CRP↑
- Blood culture
- USS
- Joint aspiration with Gram film
- Culture and sensitivity
- Radiographs are of little value in early stages; later, subperiosteal new bone with periarticular porosis.

Differential Diagnosis. Osteomyelitis with sympathetic effusion. RA. Reiter's disease. Gout. Rheumatic fever.

Treatment. Washout of joint. Antibiotic. Fusidic acid and flucloxacillin initially and then according to culture. Splintage. Analgesia. Surgical drainage may be necessary.

Chronic Infections of Bones and Joints

Chronic Osteomyelitis

This may follow acute osteomyelitis but is more common following surgery for an open fracture, especially when foreign material is implanted. It may be chronic from the outset, e.g. tuberculosis.

SECONDARY TO ACUTE OSTEOMYELITIS. In this condition, the bone becomes sclerotic and thickened. Sequestra are present and involucrum and sinuses may be present.

Symptoms and Signs. Flare-ups with pain, swelling, discharging sinus and abscess formation. Spontaneous recovery may occur.

Investigations

- Radiographs: show thickening of bone and cavity formation, sequestra (denser than normal bone) may be present
- CRP↑
- WCC↑
- MRI/CT scan to define sequestrum/abscess
- Culture and sensitivity. Drainage if discharge present.

Treatment. Treat acute episodes with appropriate antibiotic. Surgery is indicated if discharge is marked, sequestra or large cavities are present, or attacks of pain and pyrexia are frequent. Open the cavity, debride and vac pac (negative pressure dressing), allow the superficial wound to granulate, excise sequestra. Rarely, amputation may be necessary.

Complications. Amyloid. Pathological fracture. Squamous carcinoma in a sinus track.

Chronic osteomyelitis may occur secondary to trauma or secondary to insertion of a joint replacement or internal fixation device. Chronic osteomyelitis secondary to trauma is treated as above, but fracture stabilisation needs an external fixation device. If an internal fixation device or joint replacement is associated with chronic osteomyelitis, it must be removed.

Chronic Osteomyelitis Due to Specific Chronic Infections. This may arise as a result of tuberculosis, syphilis (tertiary) or mycotic infections. Tuberculosis is the most common.

Tuberculosis of Bones and Joints. This occurs worldwide, especially in developing countries. In Europe it is more common in the immigrant population and in the elderly and is on the increase. It is usually blood-borne. The primary site is usually in the lung. Destruction of bone and articular cartilage occurs. The synovial membrane is studded with tubercles, which extend under the articular cartilage, destroying it. Abscess formation occurs, especially in spinal tuberculosis. This may discharge into the psoas sheath and present under the inguinal ligament of the groin as a psoas abscess. Joints are often destroyed and undergo fibrosis or bony ankylosis.

Symptoms and Signs. History of tuberculosis (TB) contact. Infection of bone alone unusual. Usually involves both bone and joint. Malaise, weight loss, night sweats. Local pain, stiffness or limping. Local tenderness, soft tissue swelling, joint effusion. Local muscle atrophy. Discharge of cold abscess with sinus formation. Backache with TB of spine (Pott's disease). Wasting of back muscles, spasm, movement restricted. Localised kyphosis or 'gibbus' due to vertebral collapse. Paraplegia may occur.

Investigations

- WCC↑ with lymphocytosis
- CRP↑
- Mantoux test/QuantiFERON test
- Joint aspiration with Ziehl–Neelsen staining and culture
- Biopsy: needle or open
- Sputum and urine culture

- Radiographs show: osteoporosis around joint; erosion of joint surfaces; destruction of bone and intervertebral discs; soft tissue shadows, e.g. psoas abscess
- CXR: initial pulmonary infection.

Treatment. Antituberculous drugs. Rest. Splintage. Traction, e.g. TB hip. Surgery – drainage of abscess, excision of affected bone with grafting, synovectomy, arthrodesis of diseased joints. Spinal tuberculosis is treated initially by immobilisation in a spinal support until stability achieved, usually by bony fusion of the vertebral bodies. Drainage of cold abscesses and removal of necrotic bone may be necessary, with surgical fusion of adjacent vertebrae.

BONE TUMOURS

These may be benign or malignant. Secondary tumours are much more common than primary. Secondaries occur from the lung, breast, prostate, thyroid and kidney. Primary malignant tumours are rare but they have a bad prognosis and affect patients in a younger age group. The management of suspected primary bone tumours is a specialist multidisciplinary task and may involve discussion with National Tumour Centres.

Investigations. Diagnosis of primary bone tumours is very difficult. Staging CT scan of thorax, abdomen and pelvis is often sought along with biopsy of the secondary lesion. Various imaging techniques can be used to determine the extent of the lesion. Pulmonary and cerebral metastases should be sought.

Biopsy. Careful surgery reduces dissemination of the tumour and may allow limb-conserving surgery. Histology may be very difficult to interpret.

Treatment. Some combination of surgery (curettage and bone grafting, wide local excision, amputation) and for malignant tumours, radiotherapy or chemotherapy. The margin for resection is determined by staging the involvement of adjacent muscles and joints.

Benign Tumours

Osteoma ('Ivory' Osteoma)

This is a growth from the surface of bone. It is common on the surface of the vault of the skull. A smooth, nontender mound, it rarely causes symptoms. If symptomatic, it can be cured by excision.

Osteoid Osteoma

It usually occurs in long bones or spine in young males. There is severe continuous boring pain – usually worse at night and with characteristic marked relief by aspirin. It is probably not a true neoplasm. Radiographs show dense sclerosis surrounding a small central lucent nidus (osteoid). Treatment is by radioablation (90% successful), which gives dramatic relief of pain. 50% burn out.

Chondroma

A cartilaginous tumour, common in the phalanges and metacarpals. An enchondroma is a chondroma growing in the centre of a bone. A periosteal chondroma is a chondroma growing on the surface of a bone. Osteochondroma is a cartilage-capped bony outgrowth (commonest bone tumour, malignant potential, especially if >2 cm cartilage cap or multiple). Treatment is indicated only when the swelling is large, when excision should be undertaken. Occasionally multiple enchondromatosis occurs (Ollier's disease) associated with arteriovenous (AV) malformations (Maffucci's syndrome). These have significant future malignant potential.

Fibroma and Fibrous Dysplasia

This is a spectrum of conditions with failure or partial failure of ossification replaced by fibrous tissue. These are usually asymptomatic and often regress at puberty or after a fracture.

Bone Cysts

These are fluid- or blood-filled cavities. They vary from multiloculated cysts containing clear fluid in children and adolescents to large aneurysmal bone cysts that may cause 'bulging out' of one side of a bone. Pathological fractures are common. Treatment is by excision and bone grafting.

Malignant Tumours

Primary

Osteosarcoma (Osteogenic Sarcoma). This is the most common primary tumour of bone. It occurs under the age of 30 years and is more common in males. It occurs in long bones. In older patients it is usually associated with Paget's disease; in the young it commonly affects the lower end of the femur or upper end of the tibia. It usually affects the metaphysis. Spread is via the bloodstream to the lungs; 10–20% have metastases at presentation.

Symptoms and Signs. Bone pain. Swelling. Limp. Cough due to lung metastases. Tumour grows rapidly. Hot, tender swelling on examination.

Investigations. Radiograph (Figure 18.14): bone destruction, grows out of cortex elevating periosteum with deposition of subperiosteal bone (Codman's triangle), radiating spicules of bone ('sunray' spicules), soft tissue invasion:

- ESR↑
- Alkaline phosphatase↑
- CT scan: shows invasion of the tumour, lung secondaries
- Biopsy.

Treatment. Classically, amputation was carried out as soon as diagnosis was made. Current treatment involves pre-adjuvant chemotherapy, restaging and then wide excision. If multiple pulmonary metastases at time of presentation, treatment is by chemotherapy alone. Solitary pulmonary metastases may be resected.

Prognosis. The 5-year survival is 60–70%, with pre-adjuvant chemotherapy followed by surgery.

Osteoclastoma (Giant Cell Tumour). This occurs in young adults, at the ends of long bones. It has a low malignant potential (2%) but is locally recurrent and aggressive. Metastases are uncommon, occur late and are to the lungs.

Symptoms and Signs. Pain. Swelling. Pathological fractures.

Investigations

- Radiograph: multilocular cystic lesion expanding the cortex extending into epiphyses
- Biopsy.

Treatment. Various treatments have been advocated, i.e. curettage, curettage and bone grafting, curettage and injection of Denosumab, insertion of, polymethylmethacrylate

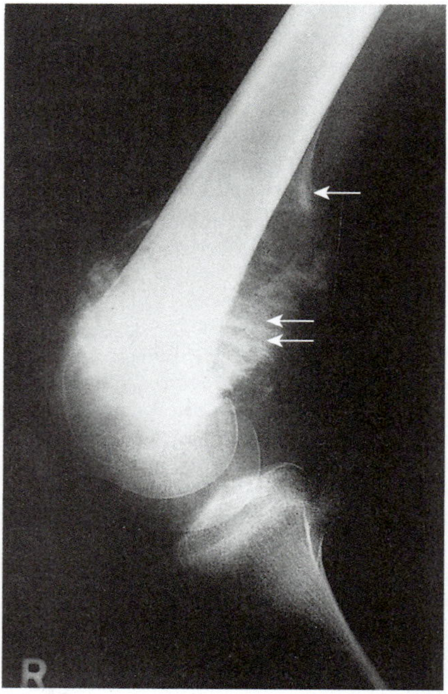

FIGURE 18.14

Osteogenic sarcoma of the lower end of the femur showing 'Codman's triangle' (top arrow) and 'sunray spicules' (bottom two arrows).

cement, primary resection, radiotherapy and embolisation of feeding vessels. The success rate is around 85%.

Ewing's Tumour (Primitive Peripheral Neuroectodermal Tumour). It is highly malignant and arises from the marrow. Common sites are the pelvis, knee, femoral diaphysis, proximal humerus. It affects children and young adults and spreads rapidly via the bloodstream to lungs, liver and other bones.

Symptoms and Signs. Pain. Tenderness. Swelling. Pyrexia.

Investigations

- WCC↑
- Radiographs: bone destruction, intense periosteal reaction, soft tissue swelling, 'onion-skin' layers of new bone around lesion
- Biopsy.

Treatment. Aim is wide surgical excision and limb salvage. Chemotherapy and radiotherapy. Amputation may be required for very large lesions.

Prognosis. The 5-year survival rate is approximately 60–70%.

CHONDROSARCOMA. This is a slow-growing tumour arising from chondroblasts. It occurs between 30 and 50 years and may arise *de novo* or in a pre-existing osteochondroma (Ollier's or Maffucci's). It occurs in the shoulder/pelvic girdles, knee and spine. Radiographs reveal a diffuse swelling with 'popcorn' calcification. Metastases occur to the lungs. Treatment is by wide excision or amputation. Survival dependent on grade – 50% of patients survive 5 years.

FIBROSARCOMA. This is more common in soft tissues (malignant fibrous histiocytoma) and much less aggressive in bone.

MYELOMA (PLASMA CELL DYSCRASIA). The commonest primary bone malignancy, it arises from marrow plasma cells. It is rare before 50 years. There is very early dissemination with widespread marrow replacement (multiple myelomatosis).

Symptoms and Signs. Anaemia. Malaise. Bone pain (backache). Pathological fracture.

Investigations

- ESR (>100)
- Anaemia
- Hypercalcaemia
- Increased gamma globulins
- Urinary Bence–Jones protein
- Bone marrow aspirate
- Radiographs: multiple punched-out lesions.

Treatment. Chemotherapy with radiotherapy for localised pain. Surgery for compression symptoms; prophylactic nailing of long bones.

Secondary

Secondary deposits occur in bone from the lung, thyroid, breast, prostate and kidney.

Symptoms and Signs. Bone pain. May be past history of primary tumour or primary may not be apparent. Pathological fracture. Full clinical examination of likely primary sites is required.

Investigations

- Radiograph individual bone: osteolytic, mixed or osteosclerotic (prostate) lesions
- Bone scan (Figure 18.15)
- Alkaline phosphatase ↑
- PSA ↑
- CA125
- TFTs
- Calcium ↑
- Staging CT scan of chest, abdomen and pelvis to locate primary.

Treatment. Severe bone pain at one site may be treated by local radiotherapy or systemic irradiation (thyroid with radio-iodine).

- Pathological fractures are treated by internal fixation and radiotherapy.
- Hormonal manipulation. Breast responds to oophorectomy. Prostate responds to hormone manipulation.

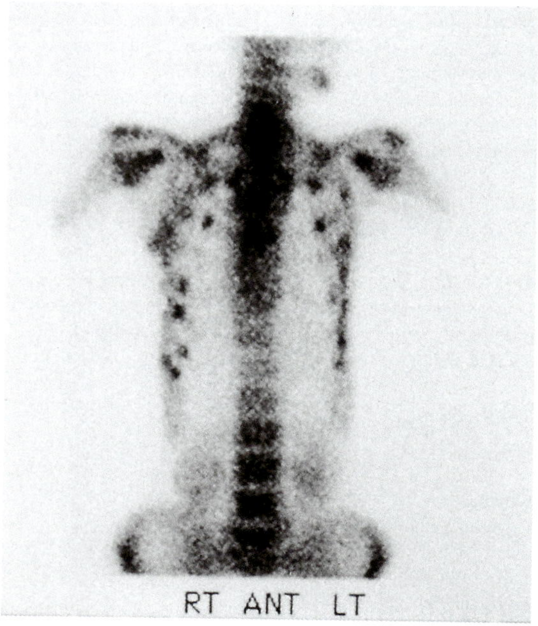

FIGURE 18.15

A bone scan showing secondary deposits (hot spots) in the bony skeleton, especially in the ribs.

BACKACHE

This is an extremely common complaint accounting for about 20% of musculoskeletal triage referrals. Most cases are either traumatic or degenerative, but other causes are numerous (Table 18.1). The more common causes will be described in this section.

Osteoarthritis (OA) of the Spine

In this condition, disc degeneration causes narrowing of the space between vertebral bodies. The posterior intervertebral facet joints may become osteoarthritic. Osteophytes form and may encroach on nerve roots.

Symptoms and Signs. Back pain radiating to buttock or thigh but not beyond. Usually cyclical in nature, associated with overuse or episodes of abnormal movement.

Investigations. Radiographs: disc space narrowing, osteophyte formation.

Treatment. Simple analgesia. NSAIDs. Physiotherapy, heat, exercises, manipulation. Spinal support. Facet joint injections. General advice re: posture, weight loss, lifting, etc. In severe cases, decompression and surgical fusion may be required.

Prolapsed Intervertebral Disc

This is a common cause of low back pain and sciatica. There is often a history of pain or mild injury, e.g. while lifting. Backache and radicular pain occur. Most disc prolapses

TABLE 18.1

CAUSES OF BACKACHE

Congenital	
	Kyphoscoliosis Spina bifida Spondylolisthesis
Acquired	
Traumatic	Vertebral fractures Ligamentous injury Joint strain Muscle tears
Infective	Osteomyelitis – acute and chronic, TB
Inflammatory	Ankylosing spondylitis Discitis Rheumatology disorders
Neoplastic	Primary tumours (rare) Metastases (common)
Degenerative	Osteoarthritis Intervertebral disc lesions
Metabolic	Osteoporosis Osteomalacia
Endocrine	Cushing's disease (osteoporosis)
Idiopathic	Paget's disease Scheuermann's disease
Psychogenic	Psychosomatic backache is common.
Visceral	Penetrating peptic ulcer Carcinoma of the pancreas Carcinoma of the rectum
Vascular	Aortic aneurysm Acute aortic dissection
Renal	Carcinoma of the kidney Renal calculus Inflammatory disease
Gynaecological	Uterine tumours Pelvic inflammatory disease Endometriosis

are posterior and pass lateral to the posterior longitudinal ligament (paracentral disc) causing compression of the transiting nerve root. Far lateral discs may compress the exiting nerve root also (Figure 18.16). Central disc prolapses may compress the cord (cord compression) or more commonly, as discs herniated at the level of the cauda equina, cause cauda equina syndrome.

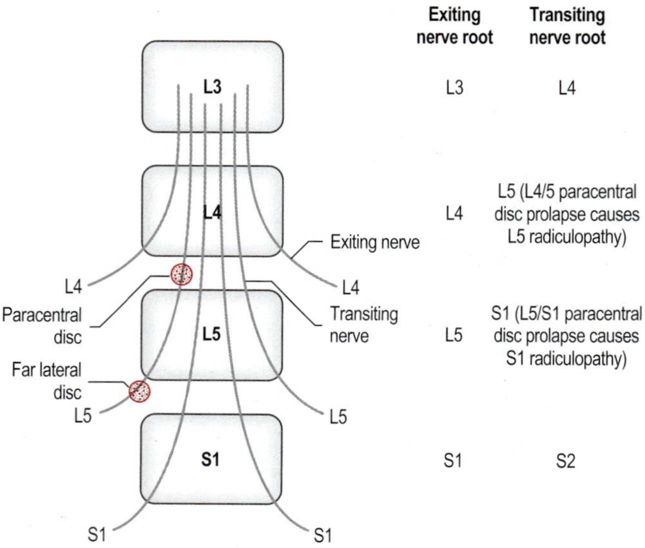

FIGURE 18.16

Prolapsed intervertebral disc. Radiculopathy in relation to transiting and exiting nerve roots. Paracentral disc lesions compress the transiting nerve. Far lateral disc lesions compress the exiting nerve.

Symptoms and Signs

Back Pain. Worse on movement, coughing, straining. May radiate to buttock and thigh without nerve root entrapment. Associated spasm and loss of lordosis. Restricted movements.

Nerve Root Compression. Most commonly L5 or S1. Dermatomal distribution of pain and anaesthesia. Segmental weakness (L5 – big toe extensor, S1 – foot evertors). Sciatic stretch test (reproduction of radicular leg pain on passive straight leg elevation and foot dorsiflexion). Depressed reflexes, e.g. L3/4 – depressed knee jerk, L5/S1 – depressed ankle jerk.

Cauda Equina Syndrome. **Absolute surgical emergency**. Compression of sacral outflow, saddle paraesthesia. Reduced anal sphincter tone. Reduced bladder coordination, painless retention and overflow. Loss of anal reflex. Bilateral leg symptoms.

Investigations

- Radiograph: often of little help, mild scoliosis, loss of lumbar lordosis, may be loss of disc spacing in chronic cases
- MRI (Figure 18.17).

Treatment of Disc Prolapse. Need correlation of symptoms with MRI.

Conservative. **Conservative treatment is not appropriate for cauda equina syndrome**. Reassurance. Analgesia. Physiotherapy. Avoid prolonged bed rest. Mobilisation.

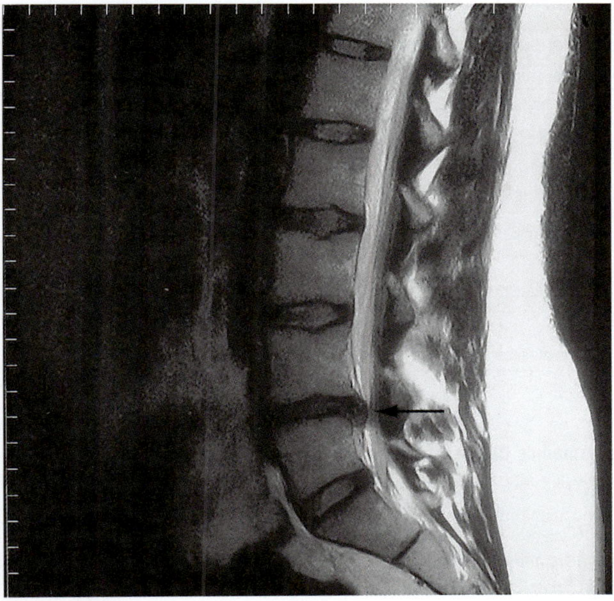

FIGURE 18.17
MRI showing a prolapsed intervertebral disc (arrow).

Surgical. **An absolute indication for urgent surgery is cauda equina syndrome**. Muscle weakness is also an indication for urgent surgical assessment. Other indications include failed conservative management for 6 weeks to 3 months; repeated occurrence of radiculopathy. Operative treatment involves surgical removal of the sequestrated part of the disc. This may be carried out by the open method, i.e. discectomy, partial laminectomy and removal of the disc material pressing on the nerve root, or by microdiscectomy, a minimally invasive technique using a special microscope to view the disc and nerves.

Spondylolisthesis

In this condition, one vertebra slips forward relative to the one below, usually L5 on S1 or less commonly L4 on L5. A classification of spondylolisthesis is shown in Table 18.2.

Symptoms and Signs. Chronic backache, worse on standing. May present in late childhood or early adult life. Sciatica. Neurological symptoms in lower limbs. 'Step' palpable in the line of the spinous processes with marked skin creases below the ribs.

Investigations. Radiographs: oblique views show defect in pars interarticularis ('Scottie dog' decapitation sign).

Treatment. Mild slips require conservative treatment with physiotherapy. With severe slips, decompression and spinal fusion are indicated.

TABLE 18.2

CLASSIFICATION OF SPONDYLOLISTHESIS

Type	Classification	Age	Description
I	Congenital (dysplastic)	Child	Congenital dysplasia of superior facet
II	Isthmic (most common defect in pars interarticularis)	5–50 years	Predisposition leading to elongation/stress fracture of pars interarticularis (L5–S1)
III	Degenerative	Older age	Facet arthrosis leading to subluxation (L4–L5)
IV	Traumatic	Younger age	Acute fractures in posterior elements (other than pars)
V	Pathological	Any age	Incompetence of posterior elements due to bone disease
VI	Postsurgical	Adult	Excessive resection of neural arches/facets

Scheuermann's Disease (Adolescent Kyphosis)

The ring epiphyses of the vertebral bodies are affected by osteochondritis. The vertebral bodies grow abnormally and become wedge-shaped. The condition occurs between 12 and 18 years.

Symptoms and Signs. Mild backache or no pain at all. A gradual curve or kyphosis develops.

Investigations. Radiographs: wedging of vertebrae and irregularity of vertebral end-plates.

Treatment. Other than postural exercises, treatment is rarely necessary. Occasionally bracing or spinal fusion may be necessary.

Ankylosing Spondylitis

This affects young adults, males more commonly than females. It usually starts in the sacroiliac joints and extends to involve the whole spine. Ossification occurs in the ligaments of the spine and intervertebral discs, and the spine is converted to a solid column of bone with an increasing kyphosis (bamboo spine). There is an association with HLA-B27.

Symptoms and Signs. Young adult males. First sign is often reduced chest expansion. Low back pain, stiffness in the lumbar region. Most marked on rising in the morning and improving with activity initially. Eventually deformity occurs with flexion in the spine and hips and the patient may have difficulty raising the head to look forwards. Iritis and plantar fasciitis may occur.

Investigations

- ESR↑
- Radiographs: special views of sacroiliac joints, irregularity, sclerosis, fusion. Later changes of ossification in spinal ligaments and discs (bamboo spine).

Treatment. The progress of the disease is rarely influenced. Analgesics. Physiotherapy. Joint replacements may be necessary to deal with deformities. Osteotomy of the spine may be required.

Complications. In the past, this condition was treated with radiotherapy. Leukaemia may develop as a complication of this. Excessive use of analgesia may cause CRF.

Cervical Spondylosis

This is a degenerative condition of the cervical spine with narrowing of the intervertebral discs and osteophyte formation of the adjacent vertebral bodies. OA develops in the synovial intervertebral joints. The condition is common in the middle-aged and elderly. It may cause pressure on the nerve roots or the cord itself.

Symptoms and Signs. Painful, tender cervical spine with reduced neck movement. Pain may radiate over the occiput and to the shoulders. When nerve roots are involved, pain radiates into the arm and hand. Stiff neck, limited movement of neck. Diminished reflexes in the arm, dermatomal sensory loss, signs of lower motor neuron weakness. Rarely bladder involvement from cord compression. Rarely spasticity of legs.

Investigations

- AP and lateral radiographs of cervical spine (Figure 18.18): narrowing of disc space, lipping of vertebrae, osteophytes, sclerosis of posterolateral joints with encroachment on foramina
- If neurological symptoms, MRI.

Differential Diagnosis. Thoracic outlet syndrome, shoulder disorders, carpal tunnel syndrome, peripheral neuropathy, spinal cord tumour, syringomyelia.

Treatment. Reassurance and symptomatic treatment in mild cases. NSAIDs, collar, short-wave diathermy. Gentle traction. The need for surgery is rare but may be required to decompress the nerve roots or cord.

Cervical Disc Prolapse

This should be distinguished from cervical spondylosis. It usually occurs in a young adult.

Symptoms and Signs

Lateral Cervical Protrusion. Acute neck pain often with severe pain radiating into the arm or hand with paraesthesia and weakness. Restricted neck movement, spasm in neck muscles, paraesthesia in dermatomal pattern in arm and hand. Weakness of muscle supplied by affected nerve root. Diminished reflexes.

Midline Protrusion. If massive, may cause no root pain but may produce a spastic quadriplegia by interfering with the anterior and lateral columns of the spinal cord. There may also be bladder symptoms. Milder degrees of midline protrusion may cause a spastic gait with reduced fine movements in the hand and associated bladder involvement.

Investigations

- AP and lateral radiographs of cervical spine
- MRI is the investigation of choice.

Treatment. In mild cases, analgesia, collar, heat treatment. Acute onset of neurological signs or progressive appearance of neurological signs is an indication for surgery. Surgery involves removal of the disc material by an anterior approach with or without intervertebral fusion.

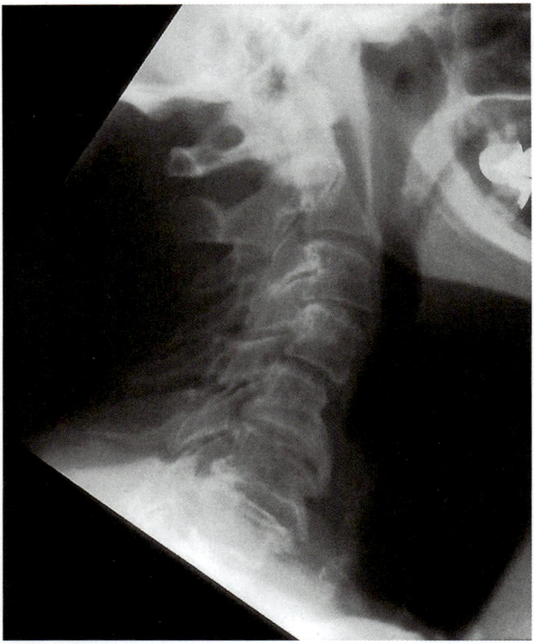

FIGURE 18.18

A lateral radiograph of the cervical spine showing cervical spondylosis. There is gross anterior lipping of C5, 6 and 7. There is marked narrowing of the disc spaces.

HINTS AND TIPS

Backache is a common symptom, and the majority of cases are mechanical, of which 90% resolve within 6 weeks. Any patient with acute back pain associated with bilateral sciatica, saddle anaesthesia and disturbance of bladder or bowel function should be considered to have cauda equina syndrome until proven otherwise. They require an acute MRI scan within 12 h and, if the diagnosis is confirmed, immediate referral to a spinal surgeon/neurosurgeon.

In men over the age of 55 years with low back pain the diagnosis of metastatic prostatic cancer should be considered. Perform a digital rectal examination.

Back pain without any restriction of spinal movement or which is not exacerbated by spinal movement is unlikely to be related to the vertebral column – consider renal problems, pancreatic disease and aortic aneurysm in such cases.

METABOLIC BONE DISEASE

Osteomalacia and Rickets

Vitamin D deficiency causes the failure of osteoid to ossify. Rickets is the childhood form of osteomalacia. In children, classical deformities occur, i.e. bowing of the femur and tibia, large head, chest deformity with thickening of the costochondral junctions (rickety rosary), enlarged epiphyses. In adults, bone pain and pathological fractures occur (especially in the elderly with associated osteoporosis). Treatment is with vitamin D and calcium. Orthopaedic correction may be required for severe deformities in children.

Osteoporosis

This is a reduction in bone mass per unit volume. The causes are multifactorial. It is common in postmenopausal women. Pathological fractures are common (hip, wedge fractures of vertebrae, Colles' fracture). Radiograph shows osteopenia, i.e. loss of bone density and cortical widening to increase bending stiffness, when 30–40% of bone mass has been lost. Treatment is difficult but should correct any underlying cause. Calcium and vitamin D should be given if the diet is deficient. Bisphosphonates inhibit bone resorption. Hormone replacement therapy (HRT) helps prevent postmenopausal osteoporosis at the expense of a small risk of endometrial carcinoma.

Hyperparathyroidism (→ Ch. 12)

Pathological fractures may occur.

Paget's Disease of Bone

This is a difficult disease to categorise but is included here for convenience. The aetiology is unknown. Disorderly bone resorption and replacement leads to softening, increased vascularity, painful enlargement and bowing of bones. It occurs in middle to old age and is more common in males. The skull, vertebrae, pelvis and long bones are affected. Some cases are symptomless, being picked up on routine radiograph (Figure 18.19). Complications include compressive symptoms due to skull enlargement (e.g. blindness, deafness, cranial nerve entrapment), paraplegia, pathological fractures, high-output cardiac failure due to vascularity of bone. Osteogenic sarcoma may develop after many years. In mild cases no treatment is required. In severe cases, calcitonin and bisphosphonates may help.

PAEDIATRIC ORTHOPAEDICS

Scoliosis

This is a lateral curvature of the spine in the coronal plane. Untreated, the condition may progress to obvious deformities, embarrassment of respiratory function and neurological lesions. Scoliosis may be postural or structural. Postural scoliosis is usually mild and disappears on recumbency. It may be due to a short lower limb, hip deformity or spasm of the paravertebral muscles, e.g. associated with a prolapsed intervertebral disc. In structural scoliosis, in addition to the lateral curve, the vertebral bodies are also rotated. In the thoracic region this leads to rib asymmetry with flatness on the concave side and a hump on the convex side, which produces the hunchback deformity initially best seen on flexion. Structural scoliosis may be:

- Idiopathic (98%)
- Congenital – failure of segmentation or formation of vertebrae

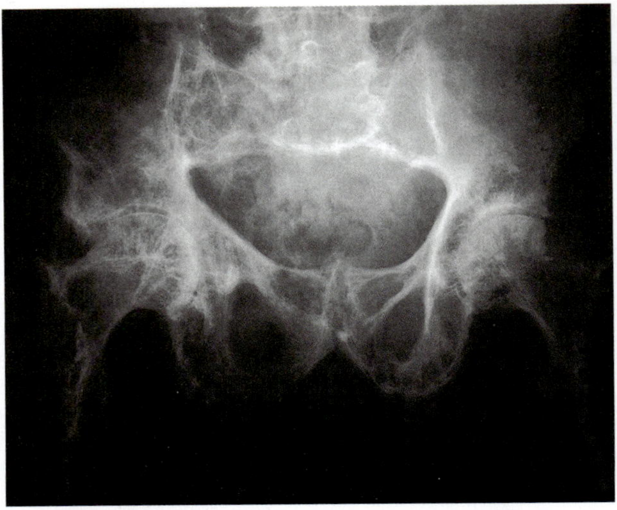

FIGURE 18.19
Paget's disease of bone. The pelvic bones are thickened and patchily sclerotic.

- Neuromuscular disorders
- Connective tissue disease, e.g. Marfan's, Ehlers–Danlos
- Trauma
- Infection, e.g. TB
- Tumour.

The management of idiopathic scoliosis is described below.

Adolescent Idiopathic Scoliosis

This is more common in girls aged 10 years onwards. It is usually convex to the right and thoracic curves are most common.

Symptoms and Signs. Usually noticed by parents. One shoulder higher than other. Development of rib hump. More obvious on flexion.

Investigations. Radiograph in two planes: used to measure the degree of deformity and to assess progress.

Treatment. Many cases progress. If the scoliosis is minor and not progressing, it can be watched. Curves >30–40° or progressive curves require bracing. More severe curves at presentation and those that progress rapidly require surgery. Internal fixation is carried out following discectomy using various implants to hold the correction until fusion occurs.

Conditions of the Hip

Developmental Dysplasia of the Hip (DDH)

This describes a wide spectrum of hip abnormalities ranging from mild acetabular dysplasia to complete dislocation of the hip secondary to capsular laxity and mechanical factors. This condition was formerly known as congenital dislocation of the hip

(CDH). The incidence is 1.5:1000 live births and girls are affected more than boys (85% girls). The left hip is more commonly affected than the right. There are hereditary factors – an increased risk if one parent has DDH. There is also an association with breech delivery and the first-born child.

Symptoms and Signs. Routine examination in the neonate. Asymmetric groin fold, limited hip abduction in 90° flexion. Hip and knee are flexed to a right angle and the thigh is then abducted. There is a jerk or 'clunk' as the head slips into the joint over the acetabulum (positive Ortolani's test – Ortolani's test relocates a dislocated hip). Barlow's test dislocates the hip with the hip at 90° flexion and in adduction. When reassessed at 3 weeks after the initial test only 1:10 of hips will remain unstable. Currently, if risk factors are present or the hip is felt to be unstable, then a USS will be carried out between 2 and 4 weeks postpartum. If the diagnosis is missed at routine testing, the child may present in later life with a limp or a typical waddling Trendelenburg's gait (if the condition is bilateral). Association with torticollis, metatarsus adductus, club foot.

Investigations

- USS <6–8 months old – α-angle – line drawn down lateral edge of ileum and acetabular roof from triradiate cartilage (normal >60°)
- Radiographs >10 months old – Shenton's line; positioning of the limb in 45° abduction shows a break in continuity of a line drawn around the margins of the obturator foramen and carried down on to the femoral neck.

Treatment. Ideally, all cases should be diagnosed at birth and treatment started immediately. In early infancy, Pavlik harness for 3 months or less. The hip is held in the 'frog' position. Check USS should be carried out to assess acetabular development. If the condition is diagnosed between 6 and 18 months, it is necessary to reduce the hip and maintain reduction until the acetabulum develops enough to hold the femoral head. This may be achieved by hip spica plaster or open reduction. In older children, acetabuloplasty or osteotomies may be required to correct the deformity.

Prognosis. The earlier the treatment, the better the result. Delayed diagnosis, especially beyond 18 months, makes it difficult to achieve a good result. OA may develop in later life.

Irritable Hip

This usually occurs under the age of 10 years and is more common in boys. The aetiology is unknown and the condition is self-limiting, the diagnosis being made after exclusion of other conditions.

Symptoms and Signs. Pain in hip. Limp. Occasionally mild constitutional upset. Mild spasm and restriction of movement.

Investigations

- Radiographs are normal but important to exclude Perthes' disease
- FBC/CRP to exclude sepsis
- USS ± aspiration
- MRI in refractory cases to exclude osteomyelitis.

Treatment. Bed rest plus analgesia. Usually settles within 2 weeks.

Differential Diagnosis. It is important to distinguish the condition from Perthes' disease, TB and septic arthritis. The patient must be carefully followed up with physical examination and radiographs to exclude other conditions, e.g. developing Perthes'.

Perthes' Disease

This is a noninflammatory deformity of the proximal femur secondary to vascular insult leading to osteonecrosis of the proximal femoral epiphysis. It is bilateral in 10%, is commoner in boys and usually occurs between 4–8 years, being maximum around 7–8 years.

Symptoms and Signs. Pain in the groin or referred to the knee. Otherwise well. Decreased range of joint movements.

Investigations

- Hip radiographs: early changes include increased joint space and flattening of the epiphyses; later changes show collapse and deformity of the femoral head with new bone formation. Severe deformity of the femoral head risks early arthritis.
- Arthrogram or MRI – assesses congruency throughout the full range of movement.

Treatment. Physiotherapy using muscle strengthening and stretching exercises produces significant improvement in articular range of motion, muscular strength and articular dysfunction. Surgery may be indicated for children >6 years. Surgery involves various forms of osteotomy. The aim is to produce a congruent joint with maximum contact between immature femoral head and acetabulum. Paediatric orthopaedic referral is strongly recommended.

Prognosis. Prognosis is dependent on age. Less than 6 years of age, outcome is good regardless of treatment. Between 6 and 8 years of age, the results are not always satisfactory with containment of the femoral epiphysis within the confines of the acetabulum. Children older than 8–9 years at initial onset will have a poor prognosis and may be expected to have a restricted range of movements.

Slipped Upper Femoral Epiphysis

This occurs from ages 10–18 years and boys are more affected than girls. The child may be overweight and may have delayed sexual development in some cases. The capital femoral epiphyses appear slipped downwards and backwards (in actual fact, the neck is the segment displaced); 25% are bilateral, of which 15–30% occur simultaneously.

Symptoms and Signs. Pain in hip. Limp. Pain may be referred to knee. Leg lies in external rotation and passive internal rotation is diminished. Classified as stable or unstable depending on whether patient can weight-bear (Loder's classification).

Investigations. Radiographs: AP and frog leg lateral views; both hips should be radiographed. Early slipped upper femoral epiphysis may be identified by Klein's line, i.e. a line drawn along the upper border of the femoral neck should intersect some part of the femoral head on AP X-ray. If not, displacement has occurred.

Treatment. If the patient presents acutely, the head is fixed in situ with a single screw to prevent further slipping. Reduction is rarely performed as it increases the risk of avascular necrosis. In the chronic case, pinning should be carried out if feasible, i.e. if the slip is not too great to allow this. Osteotomies may be necessary either as a primary or secondary procedure. Prophylactic fixation of the other side is controversial.

Complications. Avascular necrosis of the femoral head, chondrolysis and OA may occur almost exclusively in the unstable group.

Club Foot (Talipes Equinovarus)

The aetiology of this is unknown, but there may be a neurological defect in some cases, and in others intrauterine factors, e.g. pressure or position may be involved. It is more common in boys and may be bilateral. There are three elements of the deformity:

- Equinus – the hind foot is drawn up with a tight Achilles tendon
- Varus – the sole faces inwards
- Adduction of the forefoot – the inner border of the forefoot is concave.

Symptoms and Signs. The deformity is as described above. Can be identified by USS *in utero*. Usually picked up at routine postnatal examination. Exclude associated DDH and spina bifida.

Treatment. Commenced at birth. Usually nonsurgical (85%). The 'Ponseti regime' corrects the deformity with weekly serial casts for 3 months. Often, percutaneous tenotomy of the Achilles tendon is needed. Posteromedial soft tissue release is now rarely carried out, if ever. After serial casts, Denis Browne's splint (boots and bars) is used for up to 3 years.

Prognosis. Usually good, but relapses may occur. Follow-up for several years is required. Further surgery may be required if relapse occurs.

Osteochondritides

A group of conditions in which developing epiphyseal areas, in children and adolescents, are affected. The underlying pathology may be avascular necrosis, but trauma and stress injuries have been implicated. Several epiphyses may be involved, and there are a number of eponyms in common usage to describe the various conditions: vertebral epiphyseal plates (Scheuermann's disease); femoral capital epiphyses (Perthes' disease); tibial tuberosity (Osgood–Schlatter disease); carpal lunate (Kienböck's disease), os calcis (Sever's disease); tarsal navicular (Köhler's disease); metatarsal heads (Freiberg's disease – usually second metatarsal).

Symptoms and Signs. Local pain and muscle spasm.

Investigations. Radiographs: dense and fragmented bone. Progress of the disease is followed by radiograph.

Treatment. These conditions are usually self-limiting. Treatment of the various conditions involves rest, splinting or excision of bone fragments. The three most common of the conditions are Scheuermann's disease, Perthes' disease and Osgood–Schlatter disease. The former two conditions are described elsewhere in the chapter. The latter is described below.

Osteochondritis of the Tibial Tubercle (Osgood–Schlatter Disease)

This is a common condition affecting adolescent boys in which the epiphyses of the tibial tubercle are involved (strictly speaking it is an apophysis). (An apophysis is an insertion of a tendon and does not contribute to longitudinal growth of a bone like an epiphysis.)

Symptoms and Signs. Boys of 10–14 years. Often related to physical activity, e.g. football. Pain and swelling accurately localised to the tibial tubercle. Examination reveals a tender swelling. Knee joint is normal.

Investigations. Radiographs: fragmentation of the tubercle.

Treatment. Restriction of physical activity. In severe cases, rest in a plaster cylinder or rarely surgery to remove fragments of bone may be necessary. Most cases settle spontaneously, but it may take up to 2 years.

Chapter 19

Neurosurgery

Charbel Moussallem • Tarek P. Sunna

CHAPTER OUTLINE

HEAD INJURY

In the UK, head injuries account for annual attendance rates at A&E departments of almost 1 million people. Head injury is the commonest cause of death and disability in people aged 1–40 years in the UK. Some 20% of all patients attending A&E departments with head injuries are admitted, and over 25% of these have alcohol-related head injuries. More than 50% of patients admitted with head injuries are discharged within 24h. Head injuries, therefore, cause a considerable workload and bed occupancy. It is therefore necessary to have a protocol to decide which patients need admission and which patients need further investigation. The challenge is identifying the smaller group of patients who have sustained a more significant head injury and/or at risk of deterioration. For this specific group, the approach should be in the realm of a multidisciplinary team, especially those with associated injuries. Teams to be included are trauma teams and intensive care units.

Assessment

All patients with head injury should be assessed within 15min of arrival in A&E. Assessment should always follow Advanced Trauma Life Support (ATLS) principles, even for apparent minor head injuries. All patients are monitored using the Glasgow Coma Scale after initial resuscitation (→Table 4.1, Ch. 4). In all cases, the diagnosis and initial treatment of serious extracranial injuries takes priority over investigations of head injury or transfer to a neurosurgical unit. There should be a low threshold to consider the possibility of a coexisting cervical spine injury, and extreme care should be taken during the need for urgent intubation of such patients.

Criteria for Urgent Computerised Tomography (CT) Scan and Consultation With a Neurosurgical Unit

The presence of one or more of the following:

- Glasgow Coma Scale (GCS) <13 on initial assessment in the A&E department
- GCS <15, 2h after the injury on assessment in the A&E department

- Suspected open or depressed skull fracture
- Any sign of basal skull fracture (hemotympanum), 'panda' eyes/ raccoon eyes, cerebrospinal fluid (CSF) leakage from the ear or nose, Battle's sign)
- Post-traumatic seizure
- Focal neurological deficit
- More than one episode of vomiting
- Age 65 years or over
- Any history of bleeding or clotting disorders
- Dangerous mechanism of injury, e.g. a pedestrian or cyclist struck by a motor vehicle
- More than 30 min retrograde amnesia of events immediately before the head injury
- In addition, in the case of children:
  - Children under the age of 1 year with craniofacial bruising, swelling or a significant scalp laceration (>5 cm)
  - Any suspicion of nonaccidental injury and other associated injuries that points towards child abuse (a comprehensive physical exam required to uncover these injuries).

Criteria for Hospital Admission After Recent Head Injury

The presence of one or more of the following:

- Confusion or any other depression of the level of consciousness at the time of examination
- Skull fracture
- Neurological signs; persistent or worsening headache or vomiting
- Signs suggesting skull base fracture, e.g. hemotympanum, panda eyes, Battle's sign
- Difficulty in assessing the patient, e.g. alcohol, the young, epilepsy
- Other medical conditions, e.g. haemophilia
- The patient's social conditions or lack of responsible adult/relative if discharged
- Patient under the effect of alcohol or other drugs of abuse.

Criteria for Involving the Neurosurgical Department

All patients with a nonminor head injury should be discussed with a neurosurgeon but only following CT scan of the head. Regardless of imaging, other reasons for discussing a patient's care plan with a neurosurgeon include:

- Persisting coma (GCS 8 or less) after initial resuscitation
- Unexplained confusion which persists for more than 4 h
- Deterioration in GCS score after admission (greater attention should be paid to motor response deterioration)
- Progressive focal neurological signs
- A seizure without full recovery
- Definite or suspected penetrating injury
- A CSF leak.

The reader is referred to the UK's National Institute for Health and Care Excellence (NICE) Guidelines for up-to-date advice on head injury management.

Severe head injuries should always be managed in specialist centres with immediate access to neurosurgery.

HINTS AND TIPS

When making a referral to the neurosurgeon:

1. Make sure you have seen the patient, read the notes and have the CT head scan results to hand.
2. Make sure you have requested the CT radiographer to have images available for the neurosurgical centre, including all reconstructed views with axial, coronal and sagittal cuts for the CT brain (in most cases this can be 'linked' via the electronic imaging system).
3. Know the mechanism of injury, estimated time of injury and relevant background history details.
4. Know the patient's current vital signs.
5. Be able to give the current mini-neurologic examination findings (GCS, lateralising signs, pupils), or if patient is intubated/ventilated, be able to give the immediate pre-intubation mini-neurologic examination findings (GCS, lateralising signs and pupils) and the current pupillary status.
6. Be able to list any other injuries identified, any resuscitative interventions and also what imaging over and above CT head has been done, e.g. CT abdomen, neck imaging.
7. Know if the patient is taking any form of anticoagulation or antiplatelet.
8. Aware of any lab abnormality including thrombocytopenia or elevated INR.

The neurosurgeon will not accept a patient with a head injury who is not safe to transfer, i.e. the patient should have normal range vital signs (no tachycardia, hypotension, tachypnoea or hypoxia). Scalp lacerations should be sutured. Limb fractures should be splinted.

Types of Brain Injury

Primary

This is the damage caused as an immediate result of trauma. It results in contusions, lacerations or diffuse brain damage. Treatment cannot reverse primary brain injury.

Secondary

This develops as a result of complications such as intracranial bleeding, cerebral hypoxia, cerebral oedema and infection. A lot of research today is done trying to mitigate all the mechanisms that lead to the exacerbation of these secondary injuries at any step in the cascade. The prevention, recognition and treatment of these secondary complications are the mainstay of treatment of the patient with head injuries. In any trauma situation where a head injury is suspected, it is important to deal with any systemic cause of brain injury before the primary brain injury. Hence, A for airway, B for breathing, C for circulation before D for disability. A patient will die or suffer irreversible neurological deficit from prolonged hypoxia associated with an upper airway obstruction or chest injury; or prolonged hypotension associated with blood loss, before they will die, or suffer irreversible neurological deficit from a brain problem such as an extradural hematoma. This is why a neurosurgeon will always ask about vital signs and will not accept a patient for transfer to the neurosurgical unit if the key trauma vital signs (pulse, BP, respiratory rate, O_2 saturation) are not within normal range.

Assessment of Head Injury

Emergency

- Establish an airway.
- Ensure adequate breathing.
- Maintain the circulation.
- Make a thorough but rapid examination of the patient and exclude significant extracranial injuries.
- Evaluate neurologic status with mini-neurologic examination (GCS (→Table 4.1), lateralising signs and pupils) making sure the patient is not under the effects of any sedative medication.
- Look for open skull wounds with significant underlying deformity or apparent soiling.
- Splint long bone fractures.
- Assume cervical spine injury until proved otherwise.

Evaluate Central Nervous System (CNS) Injury

Assess the level of consciousness as this is the most significant factor after head injury. Use GCS (→Table 4.1) and check pupillary reactions. Pupillary changes may indicate brain swelling or compression. Pressure on a cerebral hemisphere causes the third nerve on that side to be stretched over the edge of the tentorium. The resultant paralysis of the nerve allows unopposed action of the dilator pupillae under the control of the sympathetic nervous system, and the pupils dilate. There is also loss of light reaction of the pupil on the affected side. If compression continues, the contralateral third nerve is compressed and the opposite pupil also dilates and is fixed to light. Bilateral fixed dilated pupils in a patient with a head injury are a grave prognostic sign and recovery is rare. Pupillary changes are always late signs ('undertaker signs') and are always preceded by an alteration in conscious level caused by raised intracranial pressure. Direct blows to the eyes can cause dilated pupils in patients without severe brain injury.

Pulse, Respiration and Blood Pressure. As intracranial pressure rises, the pulse slows, the respirations become slow/irregular and eventually of the Cheyne–Stokes type. The BP rises. These are signs of midbrain compression and, properly managed, are avoidable in those with salvageable head injuries.

Check for CSF Rhinorrhoea or Otorrhoea

Check for these signs. Periorbital bruising and retromastoid bruising imply basal skull fracture.

Patients with apparent otorrhea or rhinorrhoea should be evaluated by the ENT team assessing the need for further investigations or interventions including endoscopy, packing of the nose or the ears, thin-cut CT with dedicated views for the temporal bone and the anterior and middle skull base.

Scalp Lacerations or Depressed Fractures

Check these using a gloved finger. If in doubt, perform a CT scan. Lacerations with no underlying bony injuries should be promptly closed in the emergency department using skin staplers or suturing.

Assess Amnesia

Post-traumatic amnesia (loss from time of the injury) gives an assessment of the severity of the injury. Retrograde amnesia correlates poorly with the severity of the injury. Patients seen initially may appear fully conscious and oriented. Do not make allowances when assessing. They are often amnesic of events in A&E when asked at a later date.

CT and Magnetic Resonance Imaging (MRI) Brain Scanning

CT is the optimal initial examination in acute situations, as scan time is short and blood, in particular, is well demonstrated. CT also provides excellent bone detail and should be performed if a significant brain injury is suspected. Axial, coronal and sagittal reconstructions are required for detailed assessment of the cranial vaults and their contents. Resuscitation must always precede any form of imaging, however sophisticated. A cervical spine X-ray or CT scan of the cervical spine is mandatory for all significant head injuries and must include C7/T1.

Assessing a CT Scan of the Head

Soft Tissue Window

- Is there an intracranial mass?
- Is there hydrocephalus?
- Is there intracranial blood? (Blood is white on a 'soft tissue window'.) Note, however, that the appearance of blood over about a 10-day period evolves, becoming lower in attenuation, goes from white to grey to black on a 'soft tissue window', hence the particular scan appearance of a chronic subdural haematoma (→Figure 19.1A).

Bone Window

- Is there a skull fracture, soft tissue swelling or fluid levels in the paranasal sinuses?
- Look for pneumocephaly pointing towards any dural breaches or underlying fractures.
- A selection of CT images of the head covering a variety of conditions is shown in Figure 19.1.

Assessing an MRI Scan

- Keep in mind that MR imaging has a minor role in assessment of the brain in trauma setting due to the paucity of data it can give compared to the time required to perform the study.
- The role of MR becomes significant especially in stroke patients and in patients with spinal cord injury to assess the degree of cord injury/compression and the ligamentous complex disruptions.
- Two key questions to ask when requesting an MRI:
  - Does the patient have any metal or implants that may preclude MRI?
  - Could the patient be claustrophobic?
- Unlike CT, which is usually presented in only an axial plane, MRI is often in three planes (axial, coronal, sagittal).

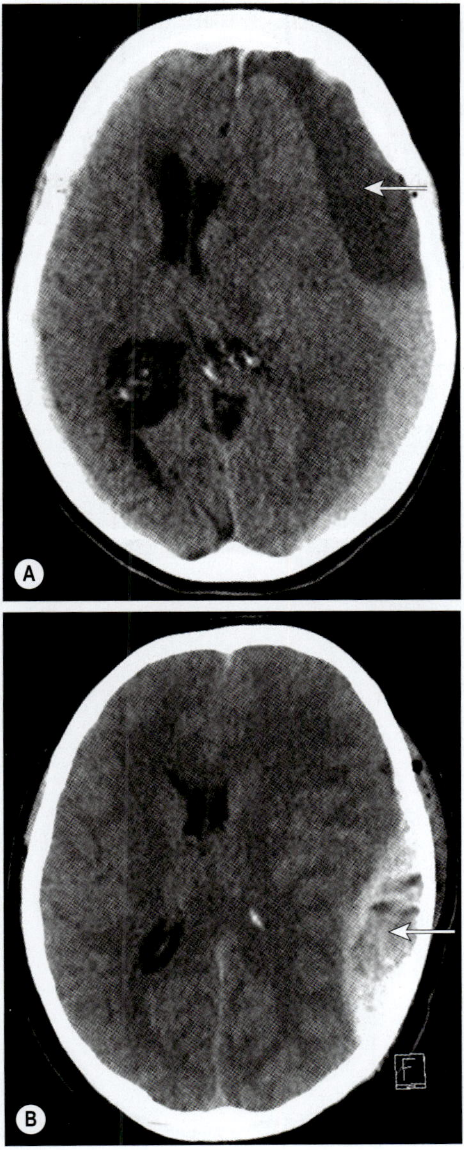

FIGURE 19.1

A selection of CT images of the head. (**A**) Chronic subdural haematoma (arrow). (**B**) Extradural haematoma (arrow).

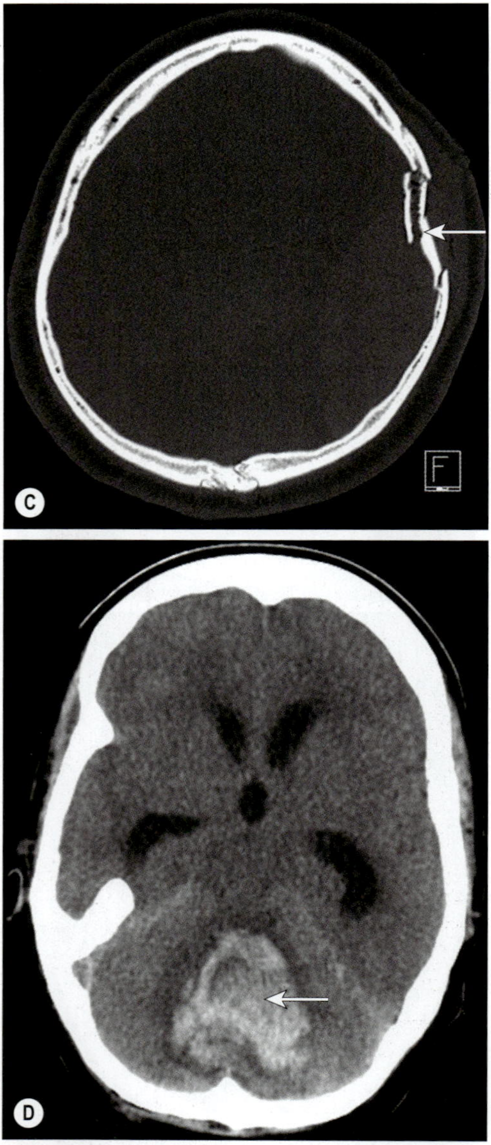

FIGURE 19.1, Cont'd

(**C**) A depressed skull fracture (arrow). Bone windows. (**D**) Cerebellar haematoma with oedema (arrow); there is also secondary hydrocephalus.

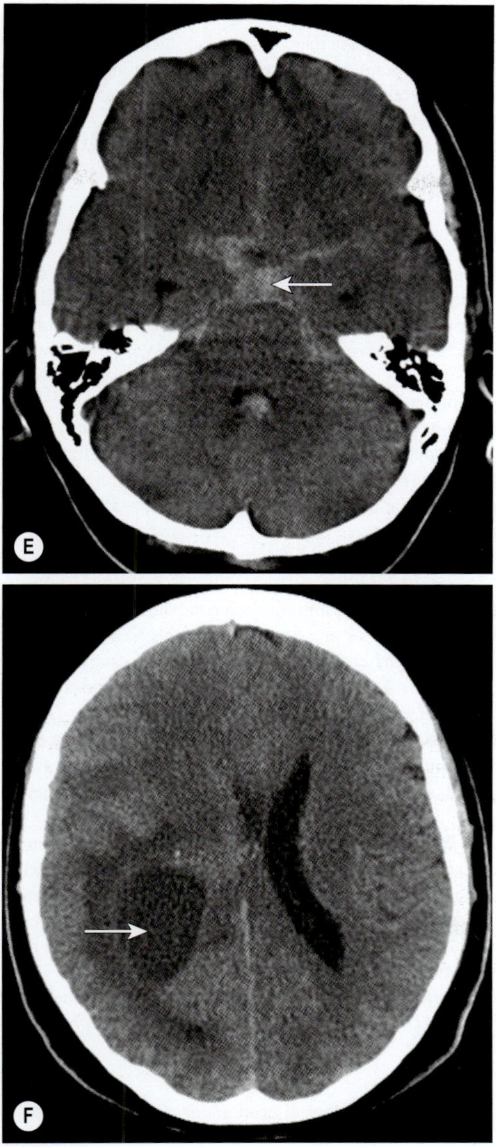

FIGURE 19.1, Cont'd

(**E**) SAH. The central pattern of blood resembles a 'man with outstretched arms and legs' (arrow). (**F**) There is a cystic mass in the right cerebral hemisphere (arrow). It is potentially a tumour, but an abscess would have to be excluded.

Incidental Findings on MRI Cranial Imaging

- Incidental findings are where there is an unexpected or unrelated finding on a scan separate to the context in which the scan was arranged.
- Incidental findings on average are identified in 10% of patients undergoing cranial MRI imaging.
- Incidental findings increase with age and include: arachnoid cyst – 1%; intracranial berry aneurysm-associated – 1%; meningioma – 1%; Chiari malformation – 1%; demyelination – 1%.

Skull Fractures

A skull fracture is an indication for hospital admission. Patients with skull fractures are more likely to suffer secondary brain damage. Skull fractures are classified as closed, i.e. the skin over the underlying fracture is intact, or open (compound) where the skin overlying the fracture is broken, or the fracture connects with an air sinus or the external auditory canal.

They may be further classified as follows:

Linear, Stellate or Comminuted Nondepressed. These fractures are serious if they cross major vascular channels, e.g. the groove for the middle meningeal artery.

Depressed Fracture (→ Figure 19.1C). A portion of the vault of the skull is depressed inwards. Surgery may be required to elevate the fracture. Depending on the degree of depression, fractures that are depressed more than the thickness of the skull need to be elevated, removing any bone fragments and repairing any underlying dural injury.

Compound Fracture. Organisms enter via compound skull fractures. Prophylactic antibiotics should be used for all compound fractures. Current prophylaxis includes cefuroxime given for a minimum of 1 week. It is not necessary for the drug to cross the blood–brain barrier if given for prophylaxis, but it is necessary for it to cross the blood–brain barrier if given for specific treatment of meningitis.

Compound Comminuted Fractures With Damage to the Underlying Brain. These are treated by removing all bony fragments, debridement and closure. Failure to remove all bony fragments may lead to development of cerebral abscess. They are associated with epilepsy.

Fractures of the Base of the Skull. They usually involve the anterior or middle cranial fossa. Those affecting the anterior fossa may cause nasal bleeding, periorbital haematoma, subconjunctival haemorrhage, CSF rhinorrhoea and cranial nerve injuries (I–V). Middle cranial fossa fractures involving the petrous temporal bone may cause bleeding from the ear, CSF otorrhoea, bruising over the ear and over the mastoid and cranial nerve injuries (VII and VIII).

Skull base fractures in close proximity to major vascular channels like the internal carotid artery should be assessed with a dedicated CT angiography of the brain to rule out any vascular injury.

Summary

The emphasis in the management of head injuries is on damage to the underlying structures rather than on any skull fracture per se. CT scanning is the investigation of choice for patients with head injury, and no patient with a significant head injury should be admitted to a hospital A&E department that does not have immediate 24-h access to CT scanning.

Management of CSF Leakage. It may be difficult to distinguish bleeding from blood mixed with CSF. Place a drop of the blood-stained discharge on a clean white gauze. If CSF is present, there will be a spreading yellowish ring around a central stain of blood (halo sign). CSF leakage implies that the dura and arachnoid are torn and therefore there is a potential pathway allowing infection to spread to the meninges and brain. The head of the bed should be elevated 30°. The patient should be advised not to blow their nose. In many cases, the leakage settles spontaneously, but all CSF leaks should be referred for a neurosurgical opinion. Where CSF rhinorrhoea occurs, do not pass a nasogastric tube. Do not pack the nose or ears.

CSF leaks that do not resolve spontaneously may need to be managed by CSF drainage using a lumbar drain or even surgical intervention through endoscopic or open techniques.

Intracranial Bleeding

This may be extradural, subdural (acute or chronic) or intracerebral. Subarachnoid haemorrhage (SAH) commonly follows trauma.

Extradural

This results from bleeding between the bone and the dura. It is most likely to occur when a fracture occurs in the temporal region crossing the middle meningeal artery. It may occasionally occur without a fracture. Usually low-speed injury.

Symptoms and Signs. History of head injury (may be relatively minor). Temporary concussion. Recovery ('lucid interval'), then increasing headache, decreased conscious level, coma. There may be no lucid period or the patient may have the signs when admitted unconscious. Falling pulse rate. Rising BP. Reduced and irregular respiration (Cushing triad). Dilated ipsilateral pupil. Contralateral hemiparesis or focal fits. May be boggy swelling overlying the site of the fracture as extradural blood may track through the fracture and into the subcutaneous tissues.

Investigations. CT scan (→Figure 19.1B). This should *always* be done immediately, before surgery is contemplated. Blood in the epidural space takes a biconvex shape (Lens Shape) which is pathognomonic for such a finding.

Treatment. This is a true emergency and requires neurosurgical assistance. If none is immediately available and the patient's condition is critical despite resuscitation, i.v. mannitol should be given and ventilation commenced. A burr hole (p. XXX) should be made over the suspected site of clot. Enlarge the hole with bone-nibbling forceps. Gently evacuate the clot. Clip or diathermy the bleeding vessel.

Subdural

ACUTE. This results from tearing small bridging veins that bleed into the subdural space and is usually associated with a lacerated brain resulting from high-speed injuries. The haematoma spreads over a large area. The patient usually has marked brain injury at the outset and is comatose, but the condition deteriorates further. Can rarely be caused by a ruptured aneurysm, which can cause the patient's collapse and a secondary head injury. The history of the event should be distinguished from primary trauma.

Symptoms and Signs. Severe head injury. Maybe rapid deterioration. Signs of raised intracranial pressure (ICP). Localising signs. Pupillary inequality.

Investigations. CT scan – crescent shaped haematoma on the brain convexity.

Treatment. Craniotomy. Evacuation of clot. Recovery depends on the degree of underlying brain damage.

A craniectomy rather than a craniotomy can be performed without returning the bone flap in cases where severe brain oedema is suspected to develop postoperatively keeping space for the brain to expand without causing further damage.

CHRONIC. Usually in the elderly. Brain shrinkage makes the bridging veins between cortex and venous sinuses vulnerable. May have only been a trivial and forgotten head injury. It may occur weeks or months after the injury, presenting with neurological signs, headache or coma, confusion or personality change. There may be fluctuating level of consciousness.

Investigations. CT scan (→Figure 19.1A). Different blood ages can be noted on imaging including acute, subacute and chronic blood that has the same signal as CSF.

Treatment. Evacuation of clot via burr holes and short course of dexamethasone. Re-accumulation may occur.

A subdural drain with an external drainage system can be kept for a few days to evacuate as much as possible of the subdural material and decrease the recurrence rates.

Intracerebral

This occurs as a result of primary brain injury but may expand causing secondary brain damage. It may extend into the ventricles. A discrete haematoma may require craniotomy if the patient's condition deteriorates. Always consider other primary causes for the intracerebral haematoma causing collapse and secondary head injury.

Cerebral Hypoxia

This is a major and preventable cause of secondary brain injury. Respiratory failure after head injury may be peripheral or central. Peripheral causes include upper airway obstruction, e.g. tongue, vomit, chest injuries, pneumothorax, pneumonitis, shock lung. Central causes include primary brainstem injury or depressant drugs, e.g. alcohol. Hypertension may also contribute.

Management of Head Injuries

HINTS AND TIPS

Always consider – is this only a head injury or was it caused by something else, e.g. myocardial infarction, fit, intracranial bleed? A good history is vital.

Minor

The most important question is: does the patient need a CT scan and/or admission? The patient should be monitored for 24h. The majority of complications will occur during this time. If no problems occur after 24h, the patient can be discharged into the care of a responsible adult. Patients should be given an information sheet detailing *symptoms and signs* for which they should be on the look-out, with instructions to return to the hospital should any of these symptoms occur. They should be advised about post-concussion symptoms and be referred to a head injury clinic for further management.

Observations During Admission. The primary observations are for the GCS (→Table 4.1). In addition, pulse, BP, respiratory rate, limb weakness and pupillary size and reaction are monitored. These are carried out by the nursing staff on the ward, the frequency depending on the severity of the symptoms. Hourly observations are usually the norm. Signs of deterioration include falling coma score, falling pulse rate, raised BP, reduced or irregular respirations, dilatation of the pupils, loss of light reflex and asymmetrical pupils. An alteration of conscious level occurs before signs of brainstem compression.

Major

Does the patient need a neurosurgical referral? As indicated earlier in the chapter, all major head injuries require discussion with a neurosurgeon. If the patient deteriorates rapidly and an extradural haemorrhage is suspected, burr holes may be required, but if appropriately diagnosed, it is usually preferable to transfer the patient immediately to a neurosurgical unit. In many patients with head injury, no surgical intervention is warranted. These patients may be in a coma with diffuse cerebral injury and oedema and may require ventilation. Other injuries may be present. Intensive care will be required. The following may be required in management:

- Monitoring of vital signs and neurological status
- Assisted ventilation
- i.v. fluids and nasogastric aspiration
- Avoidance of fluid overload
- Maintain electrolyte balance, avoid hyponatraemia (which exacerbates cerebral oedema)
- Control raised ICP, e.g. i.v. mannitol (osmotic effect reduces cerebral oedema); furosemide; controlled ventilation assists management of cerebral oedema; dexamethasone is not effective in head injuries in the control of cerebral oedema.

Other Complications of Head Injury

Epilepsy. Post-traumatic epilepsy may occur, particularly after prolonged post-traumatic amnesia, depressed fractures and intracerebral haematoma. It is associated with cortical damage and subsequent scarring. Long-term anticonvulsive therapy is usually required. Prophylactic anticonvulsants are given to patients in high-risk categories, although efficacy is uncertain.

Postconcussion Syndrome. Headache, dizziness, fatigue and poor memory are common after head injury. Loss of ability to concentrate and a labile emotional state are often sequelae. Management includes reassurance and symptomatic treatment. Often strong reassurance is necessary to explain that the condition is usually self-limiting within a few weeks or months. In most patients, symptoms cease within 12 months. Imipramine may be helpful. Strong codeine-based analgesics should be avoided. Failing to recognise and treat the syndrome can cause significant morbidity and psychiatric disturbance (depression). This may be helped by cognitive behavioural therapy.

Brainstem Death. Regrettably, some patients do not recover from head injury and are dependent on life-support systems. The brain stem death criteria were drawn up to allow a way of determining which patients had sustained irreversible brain damage so that they were not kept on life-support systems to no avail and to the distress of relatives and the nursing staff. The diagnosis of brain death depends on the demonstration of permanent and irreversible destruction of brainstem function (p. 463).

Management of Raised Intracranial Pressure (ICP)

Causes of raised ICP include head injury, meningoencephalitis, haemorrhage (extradural, subdural, subarachnoid, intracerebral), tumour, infection, hydrocephalus.

Symptoms and Signs. Headache, drowsiness, vomiting, fits, irritability, listlessness, slowing pulse, rising BP. Irregular respiration. As the pressure increases, the cerebral hemisphere is pushed through the tentorial hiatus alongside the brainstem. The third nerve is compressed against the edge of the tentorium and the brainstem is compressed by the herniating cerebral hemisphere – symptoms and signs: deepening coma, irregular slow breathing progressing to Cheyne–Stokes respiration and apnoea. Pressure on the third nerve causes ipsilateral and then bilateral pupillary dilatation. Eventually, the patient exhibits the decerebrate posture.

A sixth nerve palsy may be an early false localising sign. The long intracranial course of this nerve makes it susceptible to stretching.

Investigations

- CT scan

HINTS AND TIPS

Lumbar puncture should not be carried out in the presence of raised ICP. If the spinal CSF pressure is reduced by removing CSF, the high ICP may force the brainstem and cerebellar tonsils through the foramen magnum (coning) with fatal results.

Treatment

- Monitor conscious level with GCS (→Table 4.1).
- Ensure adequate oxygenation.
- Avoid fluid overload.
- Nurse with head elevated at 15–20° to promote cerebral venous drainage.
- Controlled ventilation
- Hyperosmolar agents, e.g. mannitol – osmotic diuretic that reduces oedema in the relatively normal parts of the brain
- Dexamethasone is very valuable in some forms of cerebral oedema, e.g. that associated with cerebral tumours, but not head injury.
- ICP monitoring may be helpful in some patients.
- Neurosurgical intervention may be required. This must be carried out before signs of midbrain compression become established.

INTRACRANIAL TUMOURS

These are classified as primary and secondary. Primary tumours are further classified as either parenchymal/intrinsic or extra-axial/extrinsic. Metastatic brain cancer is considered to be the most common among intracranial tumours. Primary cancer sites include lung, breast, bowel and skin (melanoma). Surgery, radiosurgery and/or radiotherapy may be offered depending on number of metastases, extent of extracranial disease and estimated prognosis by the primary site oncologist. Staging, doing a whole-body CT and histological diagnosis of primary tumour are usually required before neurosurgery involvement.

Symptoms and Signs. One, or a combination of: new-onset seizures, signs of increased ICP (headache, drowsiness, vomiting), intracranial localising syndromes (lobe syndromes, cerebellar syndrome, parasellar syndrome). Patients may also present with dementia, confusion or stroke (e.g. reflecting a bleed into a tumour) and one or more cranial neuropathies (e.g. unilateral sensorineural hearing loss or any nerve palsy depending on the location of the tumour). Thus, any patient with any of the above presentations should undergo cranial imaging. On many occasions, benign intracranial tumours are identified when cranial imaging is performed for an unrelated indication, e.g. in the context of a head injury. When an asymptomatic tumour is identified on imaging, it is termed 'incidental' but, of course, is still clinically significant. Headaches are very common in the population. The majority of patients with headaches have no worrisome underlying disease process. Most patients with intracranial tumours do not present with headaches. However, most patients suffering from new-onset headaches will always be worried about having a brain tumour. Thus, a head scan is always of value in reassuring patients presenting with new onset of headaches. These patients will likely go on to ultimately get a scan somewhere, and with the prevalence of incidental findings on, for example, MRI, a small but significant proportion will be found to have an incidental benign tumour unrelated to their headaches, although not necessarily in the patient's eyes.

Investigation. Cranial imaging, CT head acutely, subsequently MRI head.

Parenchymal/Intrinsic Tumours

- Account for two-thirds of primary tumours
- These tumours arise from within the brain substance or parenchyma and generally merge in an indistinct manner with normal brain tissue
- The usual tumour type are **gliomas** (derived from cells of glial origin: astrocytes, oligodendrocytes), and they are classified as low-grade and high-grade gliomas.
- High-grade gliomas are classified as the following:
    - WHO grade III and IV diffuse astrocytic
    - Anaplastic astrocytoma IDH-mutant (grade III)
    - Anaplastic oligodendroglioma, IDH-mutant and 1p/19q-codeleted (grade III)
    - Anaplastic pleomorphic xanthoastrocytoma (grade III)
    - Glioblastoma, IDH-wildtype (grade IV)
    - Glioblastoma, IDH-mutant (grade IV) and diffuse midline glioma, H3 K27M-mutant (grade IV).
- **Two-thirds of gliomas are glioblastoma multiforme (GBMs)**. GBMs can occur at any age, have generally a grim prognosis irrespective of treatment (median survival of about 1 year, 10% alive at 2 years). These are considered as malignant tumours but do not metastasise outside the CNS. The Stupp protocol (radiotherapy and temozolomide) is the treatment modality involved in treating GBMs.
- Gliomas, as well as being identified by the cell of origin, e.g. astrocytoma, oligodendroglioma, are further categorised by WHO grade on the basis of a range of histologic features such as cellularity, presence of mitotic figures, vascular endothelial proliferation and necrosis. Grading is from 1 to 4, with 1 also being considered 'benign', 2 'low grade', 3 'intermediate grade' or anaplastic and 4 as per

GBMs above. These histologic subtypes are important for deciding treatment and for providing a prognosis.

Extra-Axial/Extrinsic Tumours

- Account for one-third of primary tumours (although likely to be a higher proportion and with an apparent increasing incidence due to greater access to MR imaging and identification of smaller asymptomatic incidental tumours) and are generally benign.
- These tumours arise from a structure outside the brain parenchyma itself, indent and are surgically separable from the brain at most times.
- Metastatic lesions enter the CNS after spreading through the bloodstream and entering through a breakdown in the blood–brain barrier.
- Up to 50% of such tumours identified in an incidental context appear 'burnt out' and do not grow.
- The remainder have a growth rate of about a 2–3mm increase in cross-sectional diameter per year (still significant considering volume is a cube of diameter), with a minority having more significant growth rates.
- All patients with benign brain tumours are subject to long-term surveillance scanning, even in those who receive surgical intervention, as a small proportion of patients will develop local recurrent disease. The importance of identifying this early recurrent disease is that it can be generally treated by radiosurgery before the advent of further symptoms and avoid open surgery.
- The decision to undergo radiosurgery versus surgical intervention for metastatic lesions depends on several factors including the size of the lesion, the location of the lesion and whether it occupies an eloquent area or not, the mass effect caused by the lesion and the neurological deficits forming the clinical status of the patient.

Major Categories of Extra-Axial/Extrinsic Tumours

- Meningiomas (arising from meninges) make up more than one-third of all primary CNS tumours. WHO (2016) classified meningiomas into 15 subtypes across 3 grades based on histologic criteria. This grading system has major implications on treatment modalities, since it correlates with the risk of recurrence and overall survival. WHO grade I makes up 80.5% of all meningiomas and has benign histology and behaviour. WHO grades II and III make up 17.7% and 1.7% of meningiomas. Those have more aggressive course with atypical to malignant histology. Meningiomas that have high proliferation index have greater risk of recurrence and are more associated with WHO grades II and III.
- Pituitary adenomas (arising from pituitary gland).
- Nerve sheath tumours, most commonly vestibular schwannomas (more popularly known as 'acoustic neuromas' (dealt with separately below) – derived from Schwann cells, supporting cells within a cranial nerve.

Management. Treatment decisions are usually made in the context of a specialist multidisciplinary team, e.g. neuro-oncologic, skull base, pituitary or paediatric.

1. Interval imaging, usually MRI:
   a. Interval imaging is generally advised where an imaging finding is likely to represent a low-grade or benign tumour which is incidental, small,

asymptomatic, causing minimal symptoms or symptoms that are unlikely to be benefitted by surgery, or where the balance of risks is against surgery.

   b. Note that difficulties arranging surveillance MR imaging might include (1) patient claustrophobia, (2) presence of an MR incompatible implant (or implant where compatibility is uncertain) and (3) financial constraints in third-world countries. If this is the case, consider CT scanning instead.

2. Surgery:
   a. The indications for surgery include (1) symptom management, (2) prevent likely function- or life-threatening deterioration, (3) where there is diagnostic uncertainty or (4) where progression is demonstrated on surveillance imaging.
   b. Tumour size and rate of growth are important considerations.
   c. Posterior fossa masses have a particularly critical significance considering their location being present in a smaller space in the posterior fossa (bounded by the suboccipital bone and tentorium), the contained structures at risk from compression (especially brainstem) and the potential for development of hydrocephalus.
   d. Surgical access for tumour removal is by craniotomy or endoscopy.
   e. Tumour removal may be incomplete. This is done to maximise preservation of vital neurovascular structures or where the boundaries of the tumour are indistinct from the surrounding brain.
   f. Sometimes surgical tumour removal is not considered appropriate, but a histologic diagnosis is still required. A burr hole biopsy is then performed with the tumour target identified using neuronavigation/stereotactic techniques.
3. Radiation:
   a. Whole brain radiotherapy and stereotactic radiosurgery are used for secondary brain tumours.
   b. Whole brain radiotherapy and intensity modulated radiotherapy are used for primary malignant brain tumours.
   c. Stereotactic radiosurgery is the usual modality for smaller benign extrinsic tumours or postsurgical remnants. It is also increasingly used to treat brain metastases.
4. Chemotherapy: temozolomide which is an alkylating agent, given orally, is the most frequently used agent especially involved in treatment of GBMs.

Acoustic Neuroma (Vestibular Schwannoma)

This arises from Schwann cells of the nerve sheath of the eighth cranial nerve at the internal auditory meatus. As the tumour grows, it can expand the internal auditory canal and extend into the cerebellopontine angle compressing the pons, cerebellum and adjacent cranial nerves. It may be a feature of neurofibromatosis type 2 (NF2).

Symptoms and Signs. An acoustic neuroma should always be considered in a patient with unilateral sensorineural deafness, especially with tinnitus. Facial weakness with unilateral taste loss is a later manifestation. Facial numbness with loss of corneal reflex may occur when the trigeminal nerve is stretched by the tumour. Dysphagia, hoarseness and dysarthria may arise owing to involvement of nerves IX, X, XII. Ultimately cerebellar signs and features of raised ICP may also occur.

Investigations

- CT
- MRI.

Treatment. Surgical excision. Stereotactic radiosurgery is commonly used depending on the size of the lesion, particularly for small tumours. Small tumours are generally observed with surveillance scans initially as >50% remain static.

PITUITARY TUMOURS

These cause symptoms due to their endocrine capacity or due to their effects on the optic chiasma.

- Secretory tumours (e.g. prolactinoma). Many tumours contain a mixture of secretory cells. Presentation is influenced by the hormonal production and size of the tumour. These tumours are usually small.
- Nonsecretory tumours. Null cell adenomas – usually grow to a larger size and present because of local mass effects.

Symptoms and Signs. These depend on whether the symptoms are due to the endocrine capacity or local pressure effects. Bitemporal hemianopia results from compression of the optic chiasma. Compression of secretory cells by nonsecretory tumours may result in hypopituitarism. Symptoms include reduced libido, infertility, amenorrhoea, myxoedema, depression, loss of sexual characteristics and hypoadrenalism. In children, growth arrest may occur. Hormonally active tumours may result in the following:

- Overproduction of growth hormone: before fusion of the epiphyses this will cause gigantism; in adult life, acromegaly results
- Hyperprolactinaemia: this is characterised by amenorrhoea, infertility, galactorrhoea and impotence
- Cushing's disease (→Ch. 12).

Investigations

- MRI
- Visual field assessment
- Hormonal analysis.

Treatment. Surgery or medical therapy in selected cases. Tumour removal may be carried out by the transnasal endoscopic route. Some pituitary tumours are radiosensitive, and radiotherapy may be used as an adjunct to surgery or rarely as primary therapy in those with large tumours or in poor general health. Radiotherapy may be administered by external beam or stereotactic radiosurgery. Hormonally responsive tumours, e.g. prolactinoma, acromegaly, should be treated with hormonal antagonists. If prolactinomas are refractory to medical treatment or in cases of progression of the lesion causing neurological impairment, surgery is then sought.

Craniopharyngioma

This is a cystic benign tumour arising in a remnant of Rathke's pouch. It may be present in childhood or adult life. Symptoms are those of hypopituitarism due to compression, visual defects or raised ICP. The treatment of choice is surgical intervention with findings of'oil machinery fluid'. Studies have shown that total excision of the lesion caused more neurological deficits and clinical impairment when compared with fenestration or limited surgical resection followed by radiation therapy.

TABLE 19.1

CLASSIFICATION OF SPINAL TUMOURS

Extradural	Secondary spinal deposits are most common
	Primary bone tumours, e.g. osteoblastoma and myeloma
Intradural–extramedullary	Meningioma
	Neurofibroma
Intramedullary	Rare and include astrocytomas and ependymomas

SPINAL TUMOURS

Spinal tumours are classified in Table 19.1.

Symptoms and Signs. Pain, especially nocturnal. Radiation in dermatomal patterns. Progressive symptoms. Symptoms and signs of cord compression. Sensory changes below level of involvement. Motor weakness with spasticity. Bowel or bladder sphincter impairment. Cord compression causes spasticity with increased reflexes and extensor plantar response, together with retention of urine, overflow and constipation. Cauda equina lesions cause signs of lower motor neuron lesion with flaccidity, diminished reflexes and paralysis of the anal and bladder sphincters resulting in incontinence. Spinal tenderness, especially in the thoracic region, suggests malignant deposits.

Differential Diagnosis. Intervertebral disc pathologies, especially central disc protrusions. Cord infarction. Syringomyelia. Motor neuron disease. Osteoporosis. Fractures. Extradural abscess. Haematoma. Myelitis. Subacute combined degeneration.

Investigations

- MRI is the investigation of choice.
- Spinal radiographs: erosion, vertebral collapse, enlarged intervertebral foramina, intralesional calcifications which might point-out to certain tumours such as meningiomas
- CT myelography if MRI is not available.

Treatment

Primary Tumours. Laminectomy. Surgical intervention is aimed at obtaining tissue diagnosis, removal of tumour and cord decompression. Microsurgery has improved outcomes. Meningiomas and neurofibromas could be completely excised, as could ependymomas.

Metastatic Lesions. Radiotherapy and chemotherapy may be helpful in palliation. The prognosis is poor. Surgical biopsy and decompression with stabilisation may be required.

INTRACRANIAL VASCULAR LESIONS

HINTS AND TIPS

A patient presenting with sudden onset of severe headache associated with vomiting and/or neurologic deficits should always have subarachnoid haemorrhage excluded by CT and, if suspicion remains high despite a negative CT, by a lumbar puncture.

These include:

- Intracranial berry or saccular aneurysms (of the circle of Willis). Fifty percent of patients die, 25% survive with long-term complications and neurologic deficits, and 25% survive with good outcomes. Risk factors for aneurysms include a positive family history, hypertension, smoking and alcohol. Some aneurysms are associated with adult polycystic kidney disease, Ehlers–Danlos syndrome and other connective tissue disorders, coarctation of the aorta and aortic aneurysms.
- Arteriovenous malformations (AVM)
- Arteriovenous fistula (AVF)
- Cavernous malformations
- Unknown cause, i.e. angiogram negative

Symptoms and Signs. A spectrum of signs and symptoms include:

- Sudden death
- Classic history of sudden severe ('thunderclap') headache that reaches maximal intensity in 1 min, associated with nausea, vomiting, collapse and often coma
- Symptoms and signs of meningismus, e.g. neck stiffness
- Cranial neuropathies and/or focal neurologic deficits
- Seizures
- Incidental finding on imaging.

Investigations

- CT head without contrast (→Figure 19.1E) → initial diagnostic method
- Lumbar puncture (LP) if CT scan negative (10%), looking for blood, xanthochromia or increased bilirubin on spectrophotometry
- Cerebral catheter angiography or CT angiography if SAH is proven to investigate its aetiology, with cerebral catheter angiography being the gold-standard method for evaluation of cerebral aneurysms.

Treatment. Early consultation with a neurosurgeon is required. Treatment involves securing the aneurysm either by craniotomy with application of a spring titanium clip to the neck of the aneurysm or endovascular placement of platinum coils with or without stents within the aneurysm. In general, endovascular treatment is associated with better short-term outcomes, whereas open surgical clipping is associated with less re-bleeding risk and a permanent occlusion of the aneurysm. For complex aneurysms, a combination of both surgical techniques can be used.

AVMs can be surgically excised, treated by embolisation or stereotactic radiosurgery, depending on their grade, location and complexity.

HYDROCEPHALUS

Hydrocephalus is the result of a disruption in cerebrospinal fluid (CSF) dynamics resulting in the accumulation of CSF, build-up of elevated ICP and enlargement of the ventricular system. Clinically, hydrocephalus may be divided into two categories; congenital and acquired. Congenital hydrocephalus results from a defect in brain development that restricts CSF flow. Some examples of associated congenital defects include Dandy–Walker malformation, aqueductal stenosis, myelomeningocele, arachnoid cysts, among others.

Acquired hydrocephalus usually presents with signs of increased ICP, unless it occurs before the age of 3 years when the skull vault may expand as in congenital hydrocephalus. Causes of acquired hydrocephalus include trauma, meningitis, cerebral tumours and SAH. Elderly patients may develop normal-pressure hydrocephalus characterised by ventriculomegaly without elevated ICP, as its name implies. Its aetiology and pathophysiology remain poorly understood.

Symptoms and Signs

Congenital

- Failure to thrive
- Abnormal skull development with enlarged head circumference, especially if crossing percentiles on head circumference plotting charts
- Bulging fontanelles which fail to close at the appropriate time
- Failure of upward gaze ('setting sun' sign) and sixth cranial nerve palsy
- Inconsolable irritability and intractable vomiting not attributable to other causes.

Acquired

- Features of raised ICP
- Associated clinical signs of the cause (head trauma, SAH, tumour, meningitis, etc.). In acquired hydrocephalus occurring before the age of 3 years, the skull may expand as in congenital hydrocephalus because the suture lines have not closed yet.

In the Elderly. Normal-pressure hydrocephalus may occur in old age, presenting with a triad known as the Hakim-Adams triad of confusion/dementia, ataxia and urinary incontinence. The symptoms of the triad may not necessarily occur simultaneously, and they may overlap with those seen in other common neurological disorders.

Investigations

- Brain ultrasound scan (USS) if fontanelles are still open (infants)
- CT/MRI confirms ventricular dilatation and may identify the cause. MRI allows better visualisation of the posterior fossa which may be the site of obstruction.
- CSF analysis; to exclude infection if a shunt is in situ
- Shunt series; to exclude shunt malfunction if ventriculoperitoneal shunt is in situ.

Treatment. The management of hydrocephalus is surgical. It constitutes of CSF diversion procedures, that can be temporary such as external ventricular drain (EVD) placement, or permanent such as intracranial CSF shunting system insertion (usually ventriculoperitoneal shunt) and endoscopic third ventriculostomy (ETV) in selected cases – a fenestration is made endoscopically in the floor of the third ventricle to create an alternative communication between ventricular system and subarachnoid space. The isolated use of choroid plexus coagulation is obsolete, however, its combination with ETV has shown variable results and is under scrutiny by the neurosurgical society.

CNS BACTERIAL INFECTIONS

HINTS AND TIPS

Brain abscess, empyema and meningitis are potentially life-threatening conditions and considered neurological emergencies. Any patient who is suspected of having a CNS bacterial infection or who already has an established diagnosis should be managed in an emergency manner, and delays should be avoided. The mortality rate is high, e.g. 20% of patients with brain abscesses.

Most commonly occurs as a complication of ear infections or paranasal sinus infections.

Clinical Syndrome Presentation. Symptoms of elevated ICP. Meningeal irritation. Focal neurologic deficits. Seizures. Acute mental status changes.

Investigations. CT, pre- and postcontrast. Enhanced MRI if empyema needs to be excluded or if there is suspicion of cerebellar abscess. LP to rule out meningitis but only after obtaining CT head (risk of brain herniation secondary to LP). Always send peripheral blood cultures.

Management. Intracranial pus (empyema/brain abscess) always requires burr hole surgical evacuation. Antibiotic therapy is administered over 3 months (6 weeks i.v. and 6 weeks orally). The patient is followed up with weekly CT scans and inflammatory markers in blood. Occasionally further pus drainage is required. The patient is at high risk for epilepsy. Screen for any unidentified risk factors, e.g. diabetes mellitus, AIDS, heart disease, etc.

POSTOPERATIVE COMPLICATIONS IN NEUROSURGERY

HINTS AND TIPS

Complications in neurosurgery can be precipitous in time and severe in outcome, i.e. permanent neurological deficit or even death. The consultant neurosurgeon should always be immediately involved when a complication is suspected or identified.

Complications Following Cranial Surgery

The following are the important causes of postoperative deterioration in patients who have undergone recent cranial surgery. They can be identified based on neuro-assessment and by performing three quick and easily executed investigations: (1) U&E, (2) ABG and (3) CT head.

Complications include:

- Haemorrhage/intracranial haematoma (CT scan)
- Hydrocephalus (CT scan)
- Hypercapnia (ABG). Hypercapnia may represent either a brain problem (which can be identified on CT scan) or the persisting effect of sedation or centrally acting analgesic agents such as opiates.
- Hypoxia (ABG). Hypoxia usually represents the development of a lower respiratory tract infection. Pulmonary embolism cannot be ruled out.
- Hyponatraemia (U&E). It may reflect undergoing syndrome of inappropriate antidiuretic hormone secretion (SIADH), cerebral salt wasting, corticosteroid deficiency in the context of hypopituitarism or prolonged dexamethasone administration resulting in iatrogenic adrenal suppression.
- Infarct (CT scan). A diagnosis is made on the basis of the development of a sudden or rapidly progressive neurological deficit. Early CT can be normal, and thus early identification of an infarct is a diagnosis of exclusion.

- Infection. Due to bone flap infection. CSF infection, i.e. meningitis or ventriculitis associated with intraoperative breach of a paranasal air sinus or placement of an EVD, lumbar drain or ventriculoperitoneal shunt should also be considered.
- Seizures
- Swelling of the brain (CT scan). Management is multifactorial and can include intubation/ventilation, dexamethasone, mannitol and ultimately removal of a craniotomy bone flap or decompressive craniectomy.

NEUROSURGICAL PROCEDURES FOR PAIN RELIEF

Destructive operations of the nervous system for the treatment of pain should only be used when other, simpler measures have been used and failed. These should be undertaken in specialist neurosurgical centres. They are mainly used for relieving severe neuralgias and the pain of malignant disease.

Procedures include cordotomy (division of the anterolateral spinothalamic tracts that transmit pain to the brain); dorsal root entry zone destruction (for pain resulting from nerve injury, e.g. phantom limb pain, postherpetic neuralgia); sacral neurectomy (section of nerve roots below S3 for pain of pelvic cancer); neurovascular decompression for trigeminal neuralgia that can be treated by open surgery or via percutaneous ganglion injection (trigeminal neuralgia is thought to be due to distortion of the nerve by blood vessels). In addition, intrathecal baclofen pumps that might be used for spasticity and resulting pain.

BRAINSTEM DEATH

The nature of some neurosurgical diseases is such that a patient may have an irreversible and catastrophic brain insult that is not compatible with survival, but systemic organs are able to remain functioning for a period of time. In such circumstances, a comatose patient may be declared 'brain(stem) dead' using specific criteria and may be a candidate for organ donation. The specific criteria vary from country to country but all unite in a common basis, are irreversible and calamitous, and are associated with absent brainstem reflexes in totality.

- The diagnosis of death by neurological criteria should be made by at least two medical practitioners who have been registered for more than 5 years and are competent in the conduct and interpretation of brainstem testing. At least one of the doctors must be a consultant. Neither must be potentially involved in the care of patients who might be in receipt of organs donated by the patient.
- Testing should be performed completely and successfully on two occasions with both doctors present.
- There should a confirmed severe irreversible brain damage of known aetiology.
- There is a set of criteria for the diagnosis of brainstem death:
  - The patient must not be medicated with any CNS depressant drugs or neuromuscular blocking agents.
  - The core temperature must be >34°C.
  - There should be no metabolic disturbance.
  - The cause of the brain damage must be known.
- Prior to testing, body temperature should be >34°C, the mean arterial pressure should be consistently >60mmHg with maintenance of normocarbia and

avoidance of hypoxia, acidaemia or alkalemia ($PaCO_2$ <6.0 KPa, PaO_2 >10 KPa and pH 7.35–7.45). Serum Na^+ should be between 115 and 160 mmol/L; serum K^+ should be >2 mmol/L; serum PO_4 and Mg^{2+} should not be profoundly elevated (>3.0 mmol/L) or lowered (<0.5 mmol/L) from normal. Blood glucose should be between 3.0 and 20.0 mmol/L. If endocrinological disturbances are expected, it is obligatory to ensure appropriate hormonal assays are undertaken.

Clinical Testing

1. The pupils are fixed and dilated and do not respond to sharp changes in light intensity.
2. There is no corneal reflex.
3. The oculovestibular reflexes are absent. No eye movements are seen during or following the slow injection of at least 50 mL of ice-cold water over 1 min into each external auditory meatus in turn. Clear access to the tympanic membrane must be established by direct inspection.
4. No motor responses within the cranial nerve distribution can be elicited by adequate stimulation of any somatic area or vice versa, e.g. by supraorbital pressure and pressure applied to the nail bed of a finger. Care must be taken to distinguish central response from primitive spinally mediated reflexes that can be confused in this context.
5. There is no cough reflex response to bronchial stimulation by a suction catheter placed down the trachea to the carina or gag response to stimulation of the posterior pharynx with a spatula.
6. There is no evidence of spontaneous respiration or respiratory effort during the apnoea test.

Once two sets of brainstem death criteria are satisfied, the decision to discontinue ventilation is made. The official time of death is that of the timing of the first set of tests. The possibility of a patient becoming an organ donor should be discussed sensitively with the next of kin. Many relatives gain some consolation out of death of their loved ones knowing that their organs are giving life to others.

NEUROSURGICAL PROCEDURES

PROCEDURE

BURR HOLES

- Burr holes are performed in many circumstances in neurosurgery, e.g. drainage of a chronic subdural haematoma, drainage of an extradural haematoma, insertion of an EVD for hydrocephalus and aspiration of a brain abscess, as well as for performing endoscopic surgeries such as stereotactic biopsies and ETV. The procedure for an exploratory burr hole for an extradural haematoma is described below. Normally the procedure would be carried out in a specialised neurosurgical centre, the exact site of the haematoma having been confirmed by CT scan. However, in many parts of the world, especially remote areas, specialist neurosurgical care and imaging are not always available, and the risks of delay associated with secondary transfer to a neurosurgical unit have to be balanced with the risks of the procedure being performed by a nonspecialist surgeon. In such a situation where an extradural haematoma is suspected and imaging is not available, exploratory burr holes are required.
- Shave and prepare the skull over the temporal region between the ear and the external limit of the orbit on the side of the suspected compression.
- Under general or local anaesthetic (with adrenaline) appropriate to the clinical situation, make a 3 cm incision down to the periosteum.
- Push the periosteum off the bone with a scalpel and insert a self-retaining retractor.
- Control bleeding from the scalp with haemostats applied to the aponeurosis.
- Make the burr hole 2 cm above and behind the orbital process of the frontal bone over the course of the middle meningeal artery.
- Make a burr hole with a power tool or alternatively with a hand-held Hudson Brace drill, initially with a perforator burr (until the drill is felt to 'wobble', reflecting penetration of the skull inner table) and then a conical burr until the burr 'sticks'.
- Stop bleeding from diploe with bone wax.
- If extradural haematoma is located, it may be necessary to enlarge the opening further with a rongeur.
- Remove clot carefully and wash with saline.
- Control bleeding from middle meningeal artery using bipolar cautery or ligature.
- Control venous bleeding with piece of crushed muscle or gelfoam.
- If no extradural haematoma is found, incise dura and check for subdural haematoma.
- Meticulous haemostasis.
- Close the scalp in two layers (Galea and skin).

PROCEDURE

CRANIOTOMY

There are multiple ways a craniotomy (making a 'trapdoor' in the skull to access the cranial cavity) can be made depending on circumstances, including anatomic location, whether the bone flap has a blood supply maintained by pedicling to scalp soft tissue or not and combining with other techniques such as facial bone osteotomies. A series of simple steps is presented below:

- Under a general anaesthetic, the patient's head is placed on a horseshoe support or alternatively fixed in a surgical clamp (e.g. Mayfield clamp and pins) attached to the operating table.
- The scalp incision is marked out, the area prepped (e.g. hair parted or 'strip' shaved), painted with antiseptic and sterile draped.
- The scalp is incised and raised off the skull in a subpericranial (subperiosteal) manner. Plastic scalp Raney clips are then applied full thickness to scalp, or alternatively traditional artery clips are applied to the galeal layer to evert the scalp, to control scalp bleeding.
- One or more burr holes are made at the margin of the planned exposure using the perforator attachment of a power tool/drill. Saline irrigation is required during drilling.
- Dura is then separated as much as possible from the overlying bone via the burr holes using a dental tool or number 1 or number 3 Penfield.
- Using the craniotome attachment of the neurosurgical power tool, the craniotomy is completed. Saline irrigation is required during drilling.
- The bone flap is lifted off the dura separating any remaining dural adherence from the undersurface of the bone (this might be more difficult in elderly due to adhesions).
- If the dura is to be opened, the dura is then tented up with a 'dural hook' instrument and cut with a fine blade. The dura is then further opened with e.g. dural scissors, and the brain exposed.
- The remaining part of the procedure is determined by the purpose of the surgery.
- Following closure of any opened dura with a dissolvable suture, the bone flap is fixed in place in at least three points using titanium miniplates/screws or clamps or if not available, with Tevdek sutures. Note, if the bone flap is left out (e.g. because of brain swelling or infection), this is termed a 'craniectomy'.
- Subsequent closure is with dissolvable sutures to galea, and steel staples or nylon sutures to scalp.

Chapter 20

Plastic Surgery and Skin

Marcus J.D. Wagstaff • Diaa Othman

CHAPTER OUTLINE

Plastic surgery has evolved from the need and technical possibility to reconstruct larger and more complex soft tissue defects. Knowledge of anatomy, vascularity, wound healing and vessel, bone, nerve and tendon reconstructive techniques are applied. The specialty encompasses multiple subspecialist interests.

Injuries and infections of the upper limb and soft tissues, burn injuries and facial soft tissue trauma and associated fractures form the trauma workload. Plastic surgeons often work with other specialties to reconstruct defects that cannot close directly, e.g. orthopaedics (compound upper and lower limb fractures), general surgeons and gynaecologists (abdominal wall reconstruction, sarcoma surgery, perineal defects), cardiothoracic surgeons (sternal dehiscence and chest wall defects), neurosurgeons (craniofacial and spinal defects) and head and neck surgeons (facial reconstruction following tumour excision and trauma, facial palsy correction). The importance of aesthetics in these reconstructions has led to the evolution of cosmetic surgery.

Encapsulating plastic surgery in one chapter is challenging; however, the principles most relevant to the surgeon-in-training are outlined here, namely the reconstructive ladder, burns management, hand injuries and infections, common cosmetic surgery procedures and cleft lip and palate. Other elements of plastic surgery described elsewhere in this book include: wounds and necrotising fasciitis (Ch. 6), head and neck surgery (Ch. 8), breast surgery (Ch. 11) and orthopaedic hand surgery (Ch. 18).

THE RECONSTRUCTIVE LADDER (FIGURE 20.1)

This algorithm is commonly applied when addressing soft tissue defects, either post-surgery or traumatic. If the wound cannot be closed using the first rung of the ladder, then the second is considered, and so on. As the techniques increase in complexity, they increase in risk. In some circumstances, cosmetic or functional considerations indicate a more complex technique (and accordingly the term commonly used is the reconstructive elevator).

1. Direct closure
2. Healing by secondary intention
3. Free skin graft

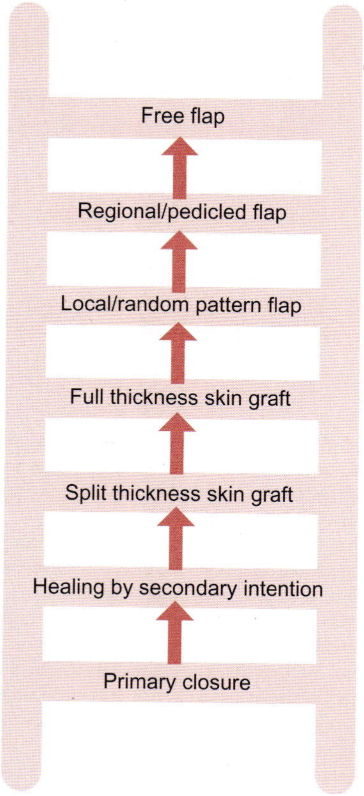

FIGURE 20.1
The reconstructive ladder.

4. Free composite graft
5. Local flap
6. Regional flap
7. Tissue expansion
8. Bioengineered tissue
9. Free flap
10. Tissue transplantation.

PROVIDING SKIN COVER

Direct Closure

Following excision of simple skin lesions or debridement of necrotic tissue in small wounds, the edges may approximate without tension and without deforming neighbouring structures such as the eyebrow, nose, lip or eyelid. Direct closure with simple interrupted or continuous suturing techniques is usually the best approach. Eversion of skin edges is essential with the choice of suture and timing of removal related to the anatomical site. Planned excisions are best performed along relaxed skin tension lines to orientate scars into natural skin creases to improve the cosmetic result.

Healing by Secondary Intention

Defects with a vascularised bed that are too large to directly close can be allowed to heal by secondary intention using appropriate dressings. Exposed bone, tendon or prosthesis negates this possibility. It is considered, however, that such wounds will heal slowly with contraction, which may distort local structures and limit motion if near a joint. Such scars can become hypertrophic and therefore problematic. Good results from secondary intention can be seen after excision of small skin cancers in the inner canthal region and may be the most appropriate choice in lower limb ulcers compromised by venous insufficiency where skin grafts are less likely to survive.

An important development in this field of secondary healing is negative pressure wound therapy (NPWT), which accelerates the healing process by increasing vascularisation and preparing the wound bed for better graft take.

Skin Graft

A graft is tissue removed completely from one part of the body and inset onto another site. It is separated from its blood supply and therefore depends on being placed on a healthy vascular bed for its revascularisation. Skin grafts revascularise or 'take' over a period of several days. Vascularisation commences over the first 2–3 days and is overlapped by a subsequent phase of remodelling and graft maturation lasting several weeks/months. Grafts need to be secured to the tissue bed by sutures or dressings to protect against shear stresses whilst revascularising.

Split-Skin Graft (Figure 20.2)

This consists of the epidermis and upper papillary dermis. This may be shaved with either a freehand Watson knife or a power dermatome. A thin split-skin graft is approximately 0.25 mm thick. The usual donor site is the thigh. The donor site heals by re-epithelialisation under dressings over 10 days.

Split-skin grafts are used in the resurfacing of burns and to cover defects after removal of larger skin tumours. The skin graft takes over 3–5 days. Disadvantages include post-graft contracture, lack of resistance to trauma and absence of normal skin properties, e.g. suppleness, hair growth. The graft can be passed through a 'mesher', which creates multiple holes so that the graft looks like a string vest. Wide meshing allows large areas to be covered and enables easier contouring and egress of underlying blood. A disadvantage is that the mesh pattern can still be visible once the scar has matured.

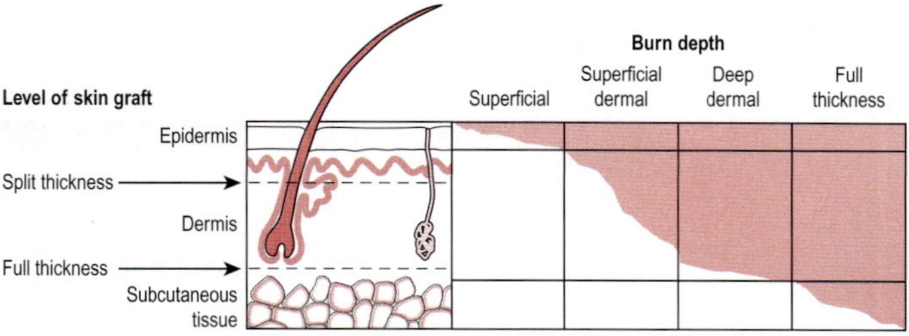

FIGURE 20.2

Cross-section of skin showing depth of burn and levels of skin graft.

Full-Thickness Graft (→ Figure 20.2)

This consists of the epidermis and dermis and therefore includes all skin elements, e.g. hair follicles, sweat glands. Main uses are for facial areas and hands. Usual donor sites include supraclavicular, postauricular, medial arm and inguinal areas. The donor area requires direct closure.

Advantages include the fact that full-thickness grafts are more robust and undergo less contraction than a split-skin graft, and produce a better cosmetic result. Disadvantages include limited donor site area and increased failure of take (compared with split-skin). Successful take depends on the same factors as split-skin grafting. A tie-over dressing can be used to fix the graft onto the bed, often with added sutures 'quilting' the graft to the bed.

Composite Skin Graft

A composite graft contains more than one layer of tissues, most commonly a skin layer along with another tissue such as fat, cartilage or other attached tissues depending on the need of the recipient site. This functions to provide a combination of function and structural support to the reconstructed defect. The downside of this graft is its high metabolic demand, increasing its risk of graft failure in comparison to simple skin grafts. A common example of such grafts is using ear helical rim skin and cartilage composite graft in reconstruction of nasal alar defect, especially in paediatric nasal aloe burns.

HINTS AND TIPS

ENSURING SKIN GRAFT TAKE

Factors which have a negative effect on graft take that may be ameliorated include:

- Patient factors:
  - Diabetes mellitus
  - Peripheral vascular disease
  - Peripheral vasoconstriction from inotrope infusion
- Wound factors:
  - Presence of necrotic tissue
  - Infection with *Pseudomonas aeruginosa* and group A *Streptococcus* spp.
- Operative factors:
  - Inadequate debridement
  - Inadequate haemostasis (presence of haematoma underneath the graft)
  - Poor wound bed for revascularisation (bare bone or cartilage).
  - Thicker skin grafts have a higher metabolic demand during revascularisation.
- Postoperative Factors
  - Postoperative shear stress preventing establishment of revascularisation
  - Poor handling of the graft during first graft check

Flaps

A flap is a piece of vascularised tissue used for reconstruction. It can be defined by its composition, e.g. skin (cutaneous), fasciocutaneous, adipofascial or muscle with or without skin or bone. It can be local (raised from an area sharing a border with the defect) and move by advancement, rotation or transposition. It can be geometrically designed to rely on the unnamed vasculature from the base of the flap (random pattern→Figure 20.3); based on a named or identified vessel – the pedicle, e.g. groin flap, deltopectoral flap; or based on a vessel perforating from the deeper tissues. These 'pedicled' flaps do not necessarily share a border with the defect (regional) and can be moved into the defect around a pivot point, related to the axis around the pedicle. General indications for flap cover include: avascular areas, e.g. exposed bone, tendon or major blood vessels, irradiated areas or areas to undergo radiotherapy. (For a selection of pedicled flaps→Figure 20.4.)

Free Flaps

The pedicle to the flap is completely divided and the flap transferred to another area of the body where revascularisation is achieved by microvascular anastomosis. Free flaps may be composed of muscle, fasciocutaneous tissue, bone (e.g. fibula, scapula, iliac crest, radius) or a combination of these. Advantages include a single-stage reconstruction, a wide choice of donor sites allowing better tailoring and choice of a flap to suit the defect without the constraint of a fixed pedicle and a good success rate (around 95%). Disadvantages include long operating time and the need for specialised equipment and expertise. (For a selection of free flaps→Figure 20.5.)

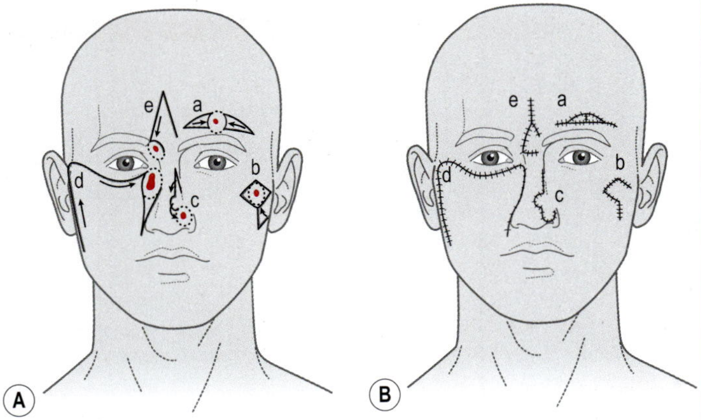

FIGURE 20.3

(**A**) Some random pattern flap designs used for facial defects and (**B**) their resultant scars. (a) Bilateral V–Y advancement flaps, move together to complete the primary (excised) defect, without raising eyebrow. The secondary (flap) defects can be closed directly. (b) Rhomboid flap recruits adjacent mobile skin as a transposition flap to cover the primary defect, yet allows direct closure of the secondary defect. (c) Bilobed flap utilises two transposition flaps recruiting mobile tissue from dorsum of bridge of nose to cover the secondary defect of the transposition flap used to cover the primary defect. (d) Cheek rotation flap utilises skin laterally via a cheek–lid margin incision extending in the preauricular line. (e) Glabellar 'hatchet' flap rotates and advances mobile skin between the brows to cover the primary defect. The secondary defect is closed in a V–Y fashion.

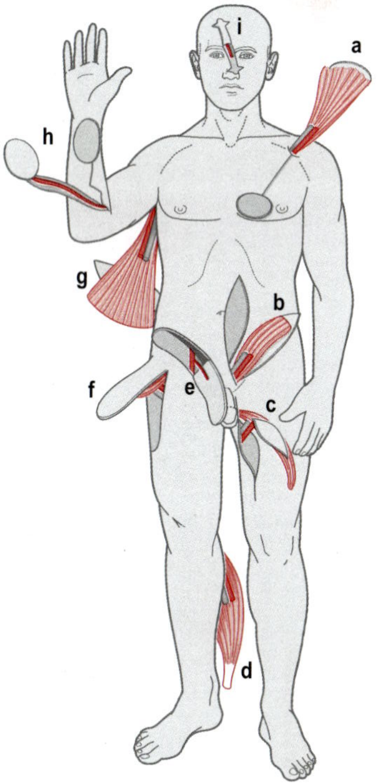

FIGURE 20.4
Some of the more commonly used pedicled flaps (a–i):

	Name of Flap	Composition	Blood Supply of Flap	Indications
a	Pectoralis major	Muscle ± skin	Thoracoacromial vessels	Head, neck, shoulder defects
b	Rectus abdominis	Muscle ± skin (Vertical skin paddle = VRAM) (Transverse = TRAM)	Deep inferior epigastric vessels or superior epigastric vessels	Perineum, groin, sternum defects; TRAM – breast reconstruction
c	Gracilis	Muscle ± skin	Medial circumflex femoral vessels	Groin, perineum, vaginal reconstruction
d	Medial gastrocnemius	Muscle	Medial sural vessels	Knee and upper third leg defects
e	Groin	Fasciocutaneous	Superficial circumflex iliac vessels	Hand, wrist, groin, perineum, abdomen defects
f	Tensor fascia lata (TFL)	Musculocutaneous	Ascending branch lateral circumflex femoral vessels	Groin, lower abdomen, ischium, trochanteric defects
g	Latissimus dorsi	Muscle ± skin	Thoracodorsal vessels	Breast reconstruction, upper arm, thoracic defects
h	Radial forearm	Fasciocutaneous	Radial vessels	Elbow, forearm defects
i	Forehead	Cutaneous	Supratrochlear vessels	Nasal reconstruction

TRAM, transverse rectus abdominis musculocutaneous; VRAM, vertical rectus abdominis musculocutaneous.

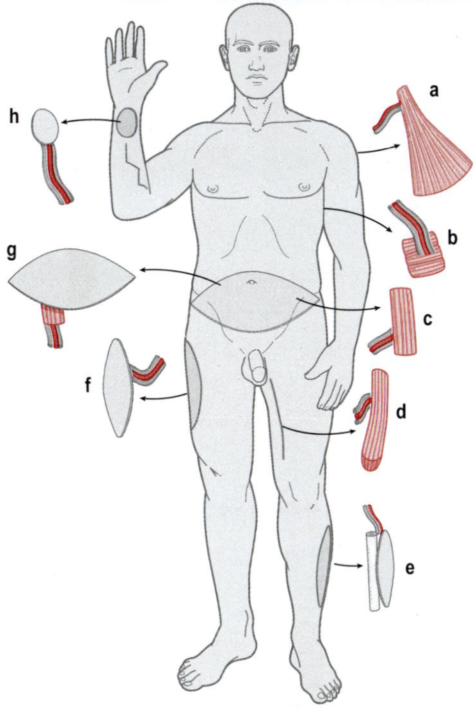

FIGURE 20.5
Some of the more commonly used free flaps (a–h):

	Name	Composition	Blood Supply	Indications
a	Latissimus dorsi	Muscle ± skin	Thoracodorsal or subscapular vessels	Lower limb, large defects, scalp
b	Serratus anterior	Muscle	Thoracodorsal or subscapular vessels	Lower limb, small defects
c	Rectus abdominis	Muscle	Deep inferior epigastric vessels	Head and neck, tongue, maxilla, skull base, calvarium, lower limb
d	Gracilis	Muscle ± skin	Medial circumflex femoral vessels	Lower limb, midsized defects, facial reanimation; with skin paddle – breast reconstruction
e	Fibula	Bone ± skin	Peroneal vessels	Bony defects of mandible, lower limb
f	ALT	Fasciocutaneous	Descending branch of lateral circumflex femoral vessels	Lower limb, head and neck, general soft tissue defects
g	TRAM	Muscle and skin = TRAM flap Fasciocutaneous based on perforators = DIEP flap	Deep inferior epigastric vessels	Breast reconstruction
h	Radial forearm	Fasciocutaneous ± bone	Radial vessels	Head and neck, floor of mouth, mandible, tongue, larynx, lower limb

DIEP, deep inferior epigastric perforators; TRAM, transverse rectus abdominis musculocutaneous.

Tissue Expansion

Creation of new skin adjacent to a proposed defect can be achieved using an inflatable silicone implant, which is implanted underneath the nearby normal skin. The implant is inflated through a remote port (either internally buried under the skin or pulled out externally), by injecting normal saline every few days over weeks and months. The skin responds by growing to meet the demands of the tension. Once sufficient skin expansion has been produced, the defect is created, the silicone expander is removed after a period of skin relaxation (usually 2–3 weeks), the excess skin flap is mobilised, and the defect is closed. The time required to inflate the balloon to produce more skin may take 4 weeks to 6 months and depends on the site, amount of skin required and the age of the patient.

Such expanders are available in different sizes and shapes, such as circular, rectangular, crescentic and some being custom made for challenging defects. Compliance is the main issue with these expanders, especially in paediatrics, and complications include haematoma, infection, leakage/collapse and extrusion of the device through the skin. Indications include:

- To replace hair-bearing scalp where there has been extensive hair loss from trauma or burns, adjacent hair-bearing skin being expanded to replace the defect
- To allow expansion of skin following mastectomy prior to insertion of a permanent prosthesis.

Bioengineered Tissues

Using human tissues in reconstructive surgery is not without drawbacks. This includes increased operative times, complexity, cost, limited tissue availability, tissue failure and donor sites complications. Tissue engineering refers to a field of biomaterials combining scaffolds, cells and biologically active molecules and integrating these into structural and functional tissue development as essential constructs for restoring damaged tissues. These include a wide spectrum of skin tissues, cartilage tissues and bone tissues, all derived from human, animal or synthetic materials to aid the goal of the reconstructive technique.

ALPHABETICAL CLASSIFICATION OF IDEAL PROPERTIES OF DRESSINGS.

"ABCDEFGHI"

Available, absorptive
Barrier (protective)
Cost effective, conformable, comfortable
Dead or necrotic material removal
Epithelialisation encouraged
Granulation encouraged
Healing promoted, hydration
Flexible
Irritation-free

BURNS

A burn is the destruction of tissue due to external stress. Burns may be caused by heat, cold, ultraviolet (UV) light, irradiation, electricity, chemicals and friction. In the UK there are about 300 hospital deaths annually from burns, with approximately 250,000 injuries each year. Domestic burns and scalds, especially in children and the elderly, form a large proportion of the 175,000 patients presenting to A&E units.

Classification of Skin Types and Tanning Response (Fitzpatrick scale)

Fitzpatrick scale (also known as Fitzpatrick skin typing test or Fitzpatrick phototyping scale) is a numerical classification schema for human skin colour, as a way to estimate the response of different types of skin to UV light. It was initially developed on the basis of skin colour to measure the correct dose of ultraviolet A (UVA) for PUVA therapy (combination treatment which consists of Psoralens (P) and then exposing the skin to UVA).The initial testing was based only on hair and eye colour and resulted in too high UVA doses for some patients; hence, it was altered to be based on the patients' reports of how their skin responds to the sun. Fitzpatrick scale remains a recognised tool for dermatological research into human skin pigmentation.

FITZPATRICK SKIN TYPE CLASSIFICATION

Skin type	Tanning response	Skin colour
I	Always burns, never tans	White, freckled
II	Burns easily, tans with difficulty; Mild burn, average tan	White
III	Mild burn, average tan	White to olive
IV	Rarely burns, tans easily	Brown
V	Very rarely burns, tans very easily	Dark brown
VI	Never burns, tans easily	Black

Classification of Zones of Injury (Jackson's Model)

Inner zone: Coagulative necrosis resulting in irreversible tissue loss.

Intermediate zone: Stasis, decreased tissue perfusion; potentially salvageable with adequate resuscitation.

Outer zone: Hyperaemia.

Classification of Pathophysiology

Local Effects

1. Release of inflammatory mediators: by capillary wall, white blood cells and platelets
2. Vessel: vasodilatation and increased permeability
3. Oedema: resulting from fluid (protein and trace elements) leak from the circulation into the interstitial space.

Systemic Effects (>20–30%)

CVS – Hypovolaemia, RBC destruction, flame haemorrhages of myocardium

RS – Pulmonary oedema, tracheobronchitis, pneumonia

GI – Loss of protective function, bacterial translocation, curling ulcers therefore prophylaxis

Liver – Peroxidation of hepatocytes

Immunosuppression – Decrease in the mechanical barrier, decrease in nonspecific and specific (humoral and cellular) immunity, Glucose intolerance – Massive catecholamine release

Clotting deranged – pulmonary embolism/ deep vein thrombosis, therefore prophylaxis required

Classification of Depth (→ Figure 20.2)

Superficial

This involves the superficial epidermis only. The underlying germinal layer is intact. It presents with a blanching erythema and pain which resolves over the first 24h. Analgesia is usually all that is required.

Superficial Partial Thickness

Damage penetrates to the depth of the superficial dermis. Patients present with blanching erythema, with blistering and pain. Healing occurs from epithelial elements within the skin appendages (hair follicles, sweat glands, sebaceous glands), taking approximately 3 weeks using appropriate dressings.

Deep Dermal

Tissue damage may extend into the remaining dermis, damaging sources of epithelial growth, such as sweat glands and hair follicles. Blistering occurs. The underlying dermis may be nonblanching and white or pink with fixed staining. There may be some surviving skin appendages, and a second look at 48h and later will demonstrate any progression of the depth of the burn and potential for healing without the need for skin grafting. Those that are not anticipated to heal by 3 weeks are proceeded to skin grafting to prevent wound contracture and hypertrophic scarring.

Full Thickness

All layers of the skin are destroyed, presenting with a white, insensate, nonblanching or brown and leathery appearance or eschar. If left, the wound heals by separation of the eschar and healing by secondary intention with subsequent contraction of fibrous tissue and centripetal growth of the peripheral epithelium. In all but the smallest full-thickness burns, skin grafting is required to prevent dense scarring, contractures and deformity.

Classification of Burn Type

Thermal
Chemical
Electrical
Inhalational
Frictional

Classification of Thermal Burns

Scald
Flame
Flash
Contact

Classification of Chemical Burns

Alkalis (cause a liquefactive necrosis)
Acids (cause a coagulative necrosis)
Organic compounds
Phosphorus

Classification of Electrical Burns

Low voltage <1,000V
High voltage >1,000V

Extremely high voltage

Lightning:

a) Direct (fatal)
b) Sideflash (hits a tree and discharges current through the air or ground to victim)

Classification of Inhalational Burn

Supraglottic
Subglottic
Systemic

Management of Burns

First Aid

1. Follow basic life support guidelines regarding airway, breathing and circulation management.
2. Stop the burning process, remove associated clothing and jewellery. Dousing with tepid water for 20 min within 3 h of the burn has both a quenching and analgesic affect. Beware of copious cold water irrigation in the young scalded infant, as this may induce hypothermia and increase the depth of the burn.
3. If a chemical burn, perform copious irrigation with cool water.
4. Cover the burn in cling film. Avoid tight circumferential cover, as the wound will swell.
5. Get the patient to hospital.

Assessment and Immediate Management of the Patient With Significant Burns

1. Initial assessment is made using Advanced Trauma Life Support (ATLS) principles: airway, breathing, circulation, disability and exposure. Do not forget to assess for associated injuries that may be a greater threat to life than the burn itself.
2. Airway – apply 100% oxygen. Look for signs of inhalation injury, hoarse voice, brassy cough, soot around mouth or nostrils, singed nasal hair, oromucosal oedema and ulceration. Supraglottic thermal burns can swell and obstruct the airway, and therefore any evidence of airway injury is assessed by a senior anaesthetist for consideration of early endotracheal intubation to protect against later obstruction.
3. Breathing – inhalation of smoke causes injury to the subglottic airway, and systemic toxicity of carbon monoxide, hydrogen cyanide and other toxins may present in an unconscious or confused patient.
4. Ensure an adequate circulation. Obtain i.v. access with two large-bore cannulae in burns >15% total body surface area (TBSA) in adults or 10% in children and resuscitate according to the Parkland formula (see below). If resuscitating, pass a urinary catheter.
5. Assess the site, depth and TBSA of the burns. Use the 'rule of nines' to calculate TBSA (→Figure 20.6). Alternatively, the palm and finger surface of the patient's hand may be used as representing 1% of the TBSA. It may be difficult to determine the depth of a burn clinically. Frequently there are areas of partial and full thickness burns. Partial thickness burns may show erythema. Pain is

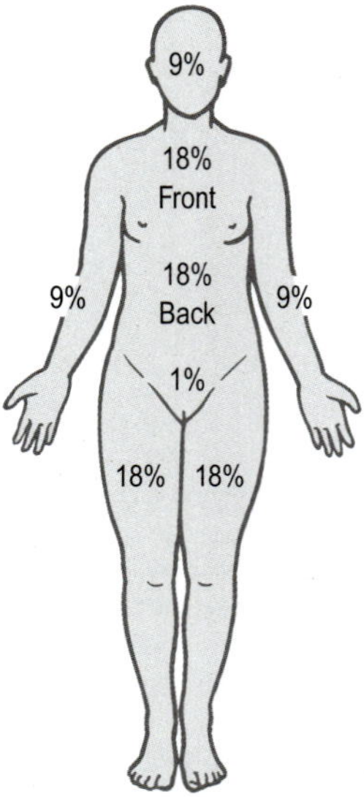

FIGURE 20.6
The 'rule of nines'. A guide to estimating the percentage area of a burn.

characteristic with normal pinprick sensation. Full-thickness burns are charred, or may be white, grey or leathery. They are usually dry. The surface is pain-free, and pinprick sensation is absent.

6. Assess for the presence of circumferential deep dermal and full-thickness burns around the limbs or the chest. Swelling under these burns causes a tourniquet-like effect which threatens ventilation or the vascularity of the limb and indicates urgent escharotomy (incision through eschar) along midaxial lines of the extremities to preserve or re-establish distal blood flow, or across and down the chest to allow expansion (Figure 20.7). Care should be taken to avoid underlying sensitive structures.
7. Keep the patient warm. Loss of skin interferes with thermoregulation, combined with widespread exposure from assessment. Patients rapidly become hypothermic, which can contraindicate urgent surgery due to the risk of bleeding and cardiorespiratory arrest.
8. Pain relief. Frequent small doses of i.v. morphine should be given.
9. Obtain a history as part of a secondary survey: source of burning, e.g. fire or scald; duration of contact, indoors or outdoors; contact with any toxic gases; first aid given.
10. Tetanus cover is mandatory. Prophylactic antibiotics are not usually indicated. Common causes of sepsis are *Staphylococci, Streptococci* and *Pseudomonas*. Antibiotics should be given on the basis of culture and sensitivity.

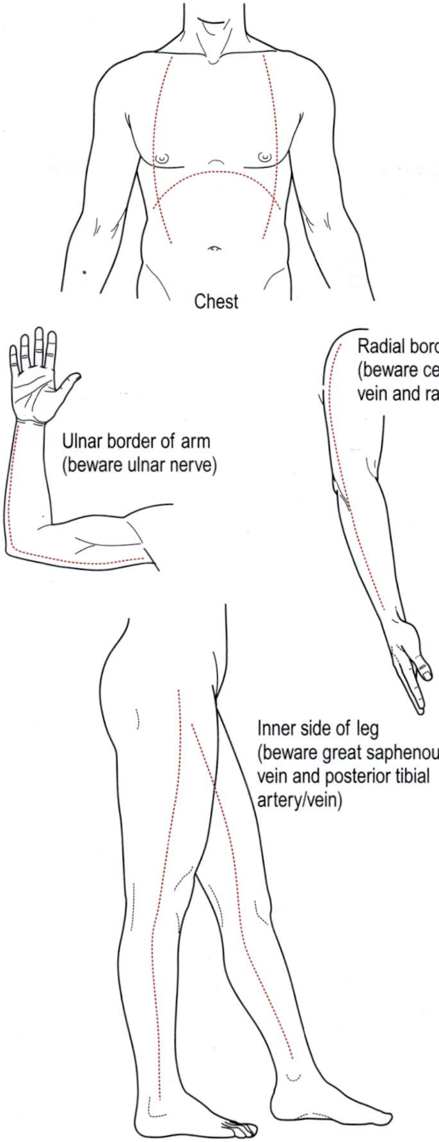

FIGURE 20.7

Lines of escharotomy placement.

HINTS AND TIPS

FLUID RESUSCITATION FOR MAJOR BURNS

Hypovolaemic shock occurs from plasma loss. Intravenous fluids should be given if the burn is >15% TBSA (10% in the child). The rate of fluid replacement may be guided by the Parkland formula:

Weight (kg) × 2–4 mL × TBSA (%) = mL of crystalloid (Ringers Lactate or Hartmann's) over 24 h

where one-half is given over the first 8 h **from the time of the burn** and the second half over the subsequent 16 h.

Children also require maintenance fluids with one-half or one-fifth normal saline. Vital signs and urine output should be monitored hourly to guide adjustments to infusion rate. Increased rates may be required in the presence of inhalation injury or electrical burns.

Aside from resuscitation-level burns, indications for referral to a specialist burns unit include burns involving the face, hands, eyes, genitalia and perineum; electrical or chemical burns; smoke inhalation or inhalation of other toxic fumes; suspicion of nonaccidental injury.

Urine output indicating adequate fluid resuscitation

$$\text{Adult} = 0.5 - 1\,\text{mL}\,\text{kg}^{-1}\text{h}^{-1};\ \text{Child} = 1.0 - 1.5\,\text{mL}\,\text{kg}\,\text{h}^{-1}$$

Curreri formula for daily calorific requirement in burns

$$\text{Adult} = 25\,\text{kcal}\,\text{kg}^{-1} + 40\,\text{kcal per percent burn};\ \text{Child} = 40 - 60\,\text{kcal}\,\text{kg}^{-1}$$

Early Management of Burns

If the patient is otherwise stable, for major burns (>15% TBSA) this is best performed on admission in an operating theatre under general anaesthesia (GA) with a high ambient temperature to prevent heat loss. Excision of deep burns at this stage is important, as it reduces the incidence of later 'burn shock' caused by lipopolysaccharide (LPS) complex that is released from degrading dermis; also operative blood loss is less in the first 24 h post burn because inflammation is less at this stage. Facial burns are scrubbed clean. Burnt hair is shaved to expose burnt scalp. Burns are dressed with liquid paraffin.

The remaining burn is scrubbed clean and involved/surrounding hair is shaved. After skin preparation and draping, the burn is re-assessed for depth. Full-thickness and deep dermal burns appear dry, whereas superficial burns with an intact blood supply exude fluid. Dry areas are marked and infiltrated with subdermal tumescence containing adrenaline to prevent blood loss and bupivacaine for analgesia. The deep burn is excised by tangential shaving with a Watson knife until a healthy bleeding bed is reached.

Once the burn is excised, either the wound can be dressed for split-skin grafting at a later date once the patient is more stable and warmer, or if otherwise stable, available donor sites (commonly the thighs) can be harvested for split-skin grafts that are typically meshed, applied to the burn wound and dressed. If there is lack of availability of donor skin to cover the whole wound, cadaveric allograft skin or synthetic skin substitutes may be used temporarily, to be later covered with skin graft once the donor sites have re-epithelialised.

Superficial partial-thickness (SPT) burns (blistered, pink, blanching, sensate, wet) can be covered with a skin substitute, or dressed with silver sulfadiazine or a variety of other options to allow re-epithelialisation from the skin appendages over the ensuing 3 weeks.

Less extensive burns (<15% TBSA) may be dressed and await assessment for conservative or surgical management at an appropriate time. Skin grafting of deep burns should have been performed by 21 days, after which the scar outcomes are poorer.

The Systemic Effects of Major Burns

Burns over 20% TBSA cause systemic inflammatory response syndrome (SIRS), which can lead to acute respiratory distress syndrome (ARDS) (particularly in the context of inhalation injury), cardiac output suppression, renal impairment, multiorgan failure, immunosuppression, bowel stasis and a catabolic response. Stress gastric ulcers (Curling's ulcers) are relatively rare in major burns since the routine adoption of early enteral feeding via a nasogastric tube. This also maintains nutrition and prevents bacterial translocation and gut stasis. Prophylactic H_2 receptor antagonists can also be given for gastric protection. Major burn patients are therefore initially managed in the context of a critical care unit.

Multidisciplinary Care and Follow-up

Burns are managed in a multidisciplinary setting including specialist nurses, dieticians, anaesthetists, occupational therapists, physiotherapists and clinical psychologists. Continued scar care and physiotherapy are central to successful return to function. The long-term management of patients with burns scarring is complex and involves all these disciplines as the scars mature over 2 years. Secondary revision using a variety of techniques such as skin grafting or local flaps may be necessary.

HAND INJURIES

The hand is a sophisticated tool. It enables us to interact with and manipulate our world. Upper limb specialists manage upper limb reconstruction and/or restoration of function following brachial plexus injuries, congenital anomalies, compression neuropathies, vasculospastic disorders, tumours, trauma and arthropathies in the hand and wrist. Some common elective hand conditions (Dupuytren's disease, trigger finger, carpal tunnel syndrome) are outlined in the Orthopaedic section (Ch. 18). Hand injuries and infections should be referred to a specialist hand surgeon, usually a plastic or orthopaedic surgeon. Expert care is necessary from the outset to preserve or restore function. Here, an approach to traumatic hand injury and infections is covered.

Principles of Management of Hand Trauma

First Aid

- Stop any bleeding by direct pressure. Never apply a tourniquet.
- Apply a clean, dry, nonadherent dressing.
- Do not bandage tightly.
- Save any avulsed or severed digit in a clean container. Place the digit in a separate bag on ice (a bag of frozen peas will suffice). Do not cover in ice, in case the part gets frozen.

AT HOSPITAL

History

- Age, occupation, hobbies, hand dominance, any pre-existing anomaly or injury
- The exact details of the injury – how it occurred, when it occurred, where it occurred
- Tetanus prophylaxis status and allergies
- General medical history.

Examination (Compare With Contralateral Hand)

- Look:
  - Lacerations, skin loss and viability of loose flaps or distal part
  - Gross contamination
  - Swelling, erythema or discharging pus
  - Deformity – fractures, dislocations
- Feel:
  - Tender, warm, cool
  - Presence of pulses
  - Presence of sensation in median, ulnar and radial nerve distributions
- Move:
  - Systematically move all hand and wrist tendons against resistance
  - Note pain elicited by passive and active movements
- Other injuries.

Investigations

- X-ray for presence of fractures or foreign bodies
- Ultrasound scan for radiolucent foreign bodies, equivocal exam of tendon integrity.

Prophylaxis Against Infection. Use tetanus prophylaxis and antibiotics in the presence of open hand wounds or infections.

SURGERY

Approach to the Hand Wound. Under tourniquet control, the wound is sharp debrided to bleeding healthy tissue, irrigated with saline and explored for integrity of structures running through the zone of injury. Damaged structures (bones, nerves, vessels, tendons and ligaments) are repaired. The skin is sutured or the injury covered with a skin graft or flap of soft tissue and the hand splinted and elevated. Physiotherapy regimes depend on the structures injured.

Tendon Injury. These are broadly divided into flexor and extensor tendons. Inability to actively flex a digit or the wrist against resistance following a laceration or sudden hyperextension force suggests division or avulsion to one or more of the flexor tendons and indicates surgical exploration. A similar situation exists for extensor tendons with regard to loss of extension after dorsal laceration or hyperflexion. Pain on active movement may suggest partial division that can later rupture and indicates exploration.

Anatomical Classification by Zones of Extensor Tendon Injury

Zones in the digit: (In the finger even numbers are over bone, odd numbers over a joint).

Zone I: Overlying distal interphalangeal joint (DIPJ)

Zone II: Between proximal interphalangeal joint (PIPJ) and DIPJ

Zone III: Overlying PIPJ
Zone IV: Between metacarpophalangeal joint (MCPJ) and PIPJ
Zone V: Overlying MCPJ
Zone VI: Between extensor retinaculum and MCPJ
Zone VII: Under extensor retinaculum
Zone VIII: Proximal to extensor retinaculum

Zones in the thumb

Zone I: Overlying IPJ
Zone II: Overlying proximal phalanx
Zone III: Overlying MCPJ
Zone IV: Overlying metacarpal
Zone V: Overlying carpus

Flexor Tendon Injury Zones: Verdan Classification

Fingers' zones

1. Distal to flexor digitorum superficialis (FDS) insertion (therefore includes flexor digitorum profundus alone)
2. Proximal A1 pulley to FDS insertion ("No man's land" – Bunnell)
3. Distal margin of carpal tunnel to just proximal to A1 pulley
4. Within the carpal tunnel "Enemy territory"
5. Distal forearm musculotendinous junctions to proximal carpal tunnel

Thumb Zones

1. Distal to IPJ
2. Overlying proximal phalanx, i.e. A1 pulley to IPJ
3. Thenar eminence
4. As above
5. As above

Repair is affected by a variety of grasping or locking suture techniques that are designed with the linear fibre constitution and slow healing nature of tendons in mind. In the case of flexor tendon repair, the hand is protected in a splint for 6 weeks, after which further rehabilitation may continue for a further 6 weeks (totalling 3 months off heavy manual work). Active tendon motion exercises are commenced soon after surgery to encourage strong tendon union and prevent scarring adhesions between the tendon and its surroundings. At 2 weeks post-op, the tendon repair is at its weakest therefore patient compliance is vital to prevent a repair rupturing.

Nerve Injury. Traumatic nerve (sensory digital nerves, mixed nerves e.g. median/ulnar) divisions can be coapted under the operating microscope using fine epineural sutures. Traumatised ends are trimmed to healthy fascicles that are aligned prior to repair. If the nerve is under too much tension, it may require a nerve graft, favourable donor sites including lateral/medial cutaneous nerve of the forearm or sural nerve for larger nerve defects. Nerve regrowth through the distal part is dependent on several factors, including age. The older the patient, the less likely distal nerve function will recover.

Vessel Injury. Divided hand/digital veins and arteries are repaired using microvascular techniques under the operating microscope. Successful restoration of flow is less likely in vessels crushed over a significant area than sharp lacerations. In such cases, excision of the crushed vessel is required and replaced with a vein graft harvested from the volar forearm.

Bone Injury. Fractures are treated according to general orthopaedic principles.

- If the fracture is open, it requires washout and closure.
- Is the fracture reduced? If not, it requires reduction. If it cannot be reduced by closed manipulation, it will need an open reduction.
- If it is reduced, is it stable? If so, it can be protected from displacement in an external splint. If not, it will require fixation.

Fixation in hands is commonly achieved with percutaneous K-wires or with plates and/or screws under intraoperative X-ray guidance.

Paediatric Epiphyseal Fractures: Salter and Harris Classification of Growth Plate Injury

Type I: Shearing of epiphysis from metaphysis
Type II: Epiphysis separated taking a small fragment of metaphysis
Type III: Epiphysis intra-articular fracture. No interference with epiphyseal plate
Type IV: Vertical displaced fracture through epiphysis, growth plate and metaphysis
Type V: Compression fracture. No evident injury of epiphysis or metaphysis

SECONDARY RECONSTRUCTIVE SURGERY. High-energy trauma or debridement of necrotic structures secondary to severe infection or burns may result in extensive soft tissue loss, indicating secondary reconstruction of hand components. Once the wound has been controlled, missing structures are reconstructed using bone, tendon or nerve grafts or transfer of neighbouring tendons. Soft tissue cover may require flap reconstruction.

Reimplantation of Severed Part. Simultaneous two-team approach to perform sharp debridement of devitalised tissue, irrigation with saline and identification of arteries, veins, nerves and tendons in both parts. First stabilisation of bones, then repair of tendons, arteries, veins and nerves to reimplant digits. Never close incision under tension. Skin graft may be necessary. Light dressings and splintage in the position of function. Elevation to prevent oedema. Physiotherapy.

REHABILITATION. This should start as soon as possible. A painful, stiff hand should be avoided. Appropriate early treatment is wasted unless early physiotherapy and occupational therapy are instituted. Career counselling may be appropriate.

HAND INFECTIONS

The incidence and severity of hand infections have decreased in the past two decades owing to earlier presentation and more appropriate treatment with antibiotics. The gross infections of the palmar spaces seen in the preantibiotic era are rare today. However, they should be recognised and treated appropriately to avoid long-term or permanent disability to the hand. Care should be taken with hand infections in patients with already compromising conditions, e.g. steroids, immunosuppressive therapy, diabetes, rheumatoid arthritis and other collagen diseases and patients with poor peripheral circulation, e.g. Raynaud's phenomenon.

Paronychia (Whitlow)

In this condition, pus accumulates between the cuticle (eponychium) and the nail matrix. The pus tracks round the nail margin or under the nail. The causative organism is usually *Staphylococcus aureus*. In chronic cases, *Candida* may be responsible. In the acute case, spontaneous rupture may occur. If it is treated early, antibiotics and rest may suffice. Often surgical drainage is required. Incision is through the nail fold. Removal of the base of the nail may be necessary if pus is trapped beneath it. If fungus is located, long-term oral antifungal agents may be used or the nail may be avulsed followed by application of a topical antifungal agent as the nail regrows.

Pulp Space Infection (Felon)

This is a surgical emergency. The origin of the infection is usually a minor penetrating injury. Pressure builds up in the pulp space with oedema and suppuration, and the terminal branches of the digital vessel may thrombose owing to pressure from the pus. Necrosis and osteomyelitis of the terminal phalanx may result. Treatment is by surgical decompression and drainage via a longitudinal incision over the point of maximum tenderness. Antibiotics should be given.

Suppurative Tenosynovitis

This is a surgical emergency. This is most common in the flexors of the fingers and thumb. Organisms reach the tendon sheath either from a direct puncture wound or by extension from an undrained pulp space infection. An exudate, which becomes purulent, forms in the sheath and, if untreated, may result in tendon adhesions in the sheath that leads to permanent stiffness and discharge and infect the palmar spaces.

Symptoms and Signs. Kanavel's signs consist of a fusiform, swollen digit; tenderness over the entire sheath; digit held in a semiflexed position; pain on passive movement.

Treatment. In early presentations with low suspicion, a trial of i.v. antibiotics, rest and elevation may be commenced; however, there should be a low threshold to proceed to operative exploration if there is no improvement, the history and examination findings are unequivocal or pus is present at presentation. The tendon sheath should be opened proximally and distally, a fine catheter passed down the sheath and irrigation with saline carried out. Rest, elevation and systemic antibiotics should be given. Active exercises should be undertaken as pain subsides.

Deep Palmar Space Infection

This is rare and may arise as a result of penetrating trauma, infection of a callosity, or as a complication of suppurative tenosynovitis. The infection occurs in the space deep to the flexor tendons but superficial to the interossei. The deep palmar space is divided into two by a septum attached to the third metacarpal. The space medial to the septum is the midpalmar space, the space lateral is the thenar space.

Symptoms and Signs. Oedema of the dorsum of the hand. The skin is looser here, and the swelling initially forms on the dorsum of the hand, although the infection is on the palm. Ballooning of the palm or thenar eminence. Acute throbbing pain. Fingers held flexed. Attempts at extension painful. Pain on pressure over affected space. Fever. Malaise.

Treatment. Incision and drainage. The midpalmar space is drained by an incision in the web space between the fourth and fifth or third and fourth metacarpal heads. The thenar space is opened by an incision posteriorly in the web space between the thumb and index finger. Rest. Elevation. i.v. antibiotics.

Bites

Most human 'bites' are the result of teeth and knuckles coming into contact in a fight. They frequently become infected, always with oral commensals, including anaerobic bacteria. Dog bites are common and usually cause more extensive injury than human bites.

Symptoms and Signs. Obvious with dog bites. Check for teeth marks on the hand, particularly the knuckle (metacarpophalangeal joints) area after fights, frequently extensor tendons may have been lacerated, presenting with a lag of the finger, and the tooth may have entered the joint predisposing to septic arthritis. Oedema, cellulitis and frank suppuration may be apparent with delayed presentation.

Treatment. Antibiotic and tetanus prophylaxis. Explore all wounds where the skin is breached for damaged underlying structures such as tendons. Remove foreign bodies or tooth fragments and wash out open joints. Take swabs for bacteriology. With extensive dog bites, excise any ragged areas of skin. Avoid primary closure in infected wounds. Elevate the hand postoperatively. If nerves or tendons are damaged in an already infected wound, delayed repair is more appropriate.

Classification of Congenital Limb Malformation

I. Failure of formation of parts
II. Failure of differentiation of parts
III. Duplication
IV. Overgrowth
V. Undergrowth
VI. Congenital constriction ring syndromes
VII. Generalised skeletal abnormalities

Moreover, there are subclassification of each group, but this is beyond the scope of this book.

COSMETIC (AESTHETIC) SURGERY

When a patient seeks cosmetic surgery, the surgeon must assess the degree of concern that they express regarding the feature in question, and whether or not surgery will be truly beneficial. In many cases, the patient seeks surgery to change their attributed features, the appearance of ageing or the physical symptoms that this process creates. In some cases, a formal psychological assessment may be appropriate prior to surgery particularly if the surgeon detects a disproportionate concern with bodily features. The decision to operate on prominent ears in a child who is the subject of taunts at school can be straightforward, whereas the decision to alter the facial appearance of a young woman simply because she does not like the way she looks is more difficult.

Reconstructive Breast Surgery

Reconstruction Following Mastectomy

This may be carried out at the same time as a mastectomy or several months later. If the skin and soft tissue is adequate, the breast can be primarily reconstructed with a silicone implant. A tissue expander (see above) may be necessary to create a skin envelope under which a prosthesis can be inserted. If there has been extensive surgery or irradiation, reconstruction importing vascularised tissue is required. A pedicled latissimus dorsi musculocutaneous flap is most commonly used to cover an implant, but free and pedicled flaps from the abdomen, based on the rectus abdominis muscle blood supply, or from the buttock or thigh can also be used. Symmetrisation with reduction of the contralateral breast, and reconstruction of the nipple and areola may be carried out at the time of reconstruction or at a later stage.

Augmentation Mammaplasty

INDICATIONS. Small breasts (developmental or involutional after pregnancies); breast asymmetry with hypoplasia of one breast.

Treatment. By insertion of silicone implants. Implants may be placed in the subglandular plane between the breast and the underlying pectoralis major muscle or subpectoral (under pectoralis major) via a submammary, periareolar or axillary approach.

Complications. Infection. Haematoma. Development of a firm capsule around the prosthesis may lead to distortion of the breast and discomfort. Silicone gel may leak out of the implant. There is no evidence that silicone prostheses increase the incidence of carcinoma.

Reduction Mammaplasty

INDICATIONS. Abnormally large breasts may cause backache, neck ache, intertrigo. Interfere with active sports. Taunts and sexual harassment.

Treatment. Several techniques are described. All involve removal of breast tissue and skin with transposition of the ptotic nipple and areola to a higher level. Care must be taken to preserve the blood supply to the nipple. In very large breasts a free nipple graft may be required. The satisfaction rate among patients is high.

Complications. Haematoma, infection, nipple or fat necrosis, asymmetry, dysphasia or paraesthesia, breast-feeding problems.

Gynaecomastia

Treatment is by liposuction and/or excision of breast tissue to restore the normal breast contour, preserving the nipple. A circumareolar incision is used when possible.

Other Types of Surgery

Rhinoplasty

This is correction of congenital or acquired nasal defects. It may be carried out for cosmetic or functional reasons (breathing difficulties). Controlled nasal bone fracture is combined with excision or augmentation of varying amounts of bone and cartilage. The operation can be carried out through intranasal incisions (closed rhinoplasty). Alternatively, a columellar incision can be made extending along the inferior edges of both lower lateral (alar) cartilages, then the skin is raised off the dorsum of the nose to access the bony and cartilaginous framework of the tip and dorsum for augmentation, reduction or realignment procedures (open rhinoplasty).

CLASSIFICATION OF NASAL ANATOMY

1- Upper third: Nasal bones
2- Middle third: Upper lateral cartilages (lie posterior to nasal bones and alar cartilages)
3- Lower third: Lower lateral (alar) cartilages

Important terms in rhinoplasty

Bony vault: Area overlying the nasal bones
Cartilaginous vault: Area overlying the upper lateral cartilages
In fracture: Medial movement of nasal bones to correct an open roof deformity
Infratip lobule: Area from the tip to the start of the columella
Lobule: Area overlying the alar cartilages

Nasal length: Distance between the nasofrontal groove (root of the nose) and nasal tip

Open roof deformity: The flat, wide appearance of the dorsum after removal of a dorsal

Hump without in fractures

Out fracture: A fracture which mobilises nasal bones prior to in fracture

Soft triangle: Nasal rim that doesn't contain cartilage separating the dome from nostrils' border

Supratip: Area just above the domes of the alar cartilages

Tip defining points: Most prominent areas of nasal tip: domes, supratip, columella break point

Tip projection: Distance from the nasal spine to the nasal tip

Ears

A child with prominent ears may be taunted at school. The operation should be carried out at about 7 years, as the ear cartilage has undergone 85% of its growth by this time. This can be done using sutures placed posteriorly to draw the ear back, or moulding the underlying cartilage through anterior scoring to recreate a deficient antihelical fold.

Blepharoplasty

This is used to modify the appearance of the ageing eyelids by excising the excess upper and lower eyelid skin and herniating fat and through upper and/or lower lid skin incisions. Removal of too much skin from the lower eyelid may result in ectropion (out-turned lower eyelid) with a watery eye that is difficult to correct.

Face Lift (Rhytidectomy)

This is used to treat the 'ageing' face and or neck. There are various techniques commonly employed that excise excess skin of the face and neck and excise or tighten the underlying fascial suspension – the superficial musculoaponeurotic system. Excess skin is excised at hair-bearing areas, thus hiding the suture line. The skin of the face and neck are tightened, smoothing out wrinkles and giving a more youthful appearance. Complications include haematoma, skin necrosis, infection and damage to branches of the facial nerve and great auricular nerve.

Classification of Facelift Techniques

1- Skin lifting alone
2- Skin and superficial musculoaponeurotic system (SMAS)/ platysma
3- Deep plane: composite flap of skin and SMAS MACS lift: minimal access cranial suspension surgery
4- Midface suspension
5- Nonendoscopic subperiosteal facelift
6- Endoscopic facelift

Abdominoplasty

This is excision of redundant abdominal skin and fat. It is indicated in patients who have undergone weight loss and in women who have had repeated pregnancies where there are redundant skin folds and a lax anterior abdominal wall. For some minor or moderate degrees of tissue laxity, a limited transverse lower abdominal excision may be sufficient (combined with umbilical transposition). When the operation is carried out after bariatric surgery or after massive weight loss, a 'fleur-de-lys' excision pattern is used leaving an inverted T-shaped scar, or the excision is continued around the back (belt lipectomy).

Huger Classification of Zones of Arterial Supply to the Abdomen

Zone I: Deep superior and inferior epigastric arteries
Zone II: Superficial epigastric, superficial external pudendal, superficial circumflex iliac systems
Zone III: Segmental perforators: intercostals, subcostal, lumbar arteries.

Liposuction

This is carried out for the removal of localised deposits of fat, e.g. hips, thighs, buttocks through small incisions by cannulae of varying diameter attached to a vacuum system. It is not indicated for generalised obesity and is therefore not a weight-reduction procedure. Cannulae are inserted through remote stab incisions and the subcutaneous fat removed through a series of tunnels using suction. Complications are rare, including uneven contouring and infection. Temporary numbness and bruising may occur. Occasionally, when large amounts of fat are removed, significant fluid replacement is required to prevent hypovolaemia.

Classification of Liposuction Technique According to Subcutaneous Infiltration Volumes

1- Dry– No infiltrate
2- Wet– 200–300 cc infiltrate per treated area
3- Superwet– 1 cc infiltrate: 1 cc aspirate
4- Tumescent– 2–3 cc infiltrate: 1 cc aspirate

Filler Injections

These are used for correcting minor irregularities of skin contour, e.g. static wrinkles on the face. A variety of filler materials are available, biological and synthetic, and include autologous fat and dermis, hyaluronic acid, poly-L-lactic acid, and bovine collagen.

CLEFT LIP AND PALATE

Cleft lip occurs in 1:750 live births. Cleft palate occurs in 1:2000 live births. In half the affected children, cleft lip and cleft palate occur together. Cleft lip may be complete or incomplete and it may occur unilaterally (70%) or bilaterally (25%) or, rarely, in the midline. A unilateral cleft lip usually occurs on the left. Clefts of the palate may be unilateral and usually affect the soft palate and posterior third of the hard palate. They may be complete, incomplete or submucous. Bilateral clefts usually affect the soft and hard palate.

Primary palate (cleft lip, prepalatal). – Structures of the primary palate are those anterior to the incisive foramen. They include the lip and alveolus. The nasal tip cartilages and floor of the nose may also be involved.

Secondary palate (cleft palate, palatal). – Structures of the secondary palate are those behind the incisive foramen. They include the hard palate, soft palate, and uvula.

The incisive foramen. – This occurs where the lateral maxillary bones meet the premaxilla in the midline and is just behind the upper front incisors.

Symptoms and Signs. Cleft lip and/or palate may be detected during routine antenatal ultrasound scan; however, cleft lip is obvious at birth. Cleft palate is discovered on routine inspection soon after birth or may be discovered when difficulties occur with feeding. Beware missing a submucous cleft in which the palate initially appears intact. Late presentation may occur with speech and hearing difficulties.

Treatment. The problem and its treatment must be explained to the parents. Cleft care is coordinated via a network of specialist centres, and paediatricians refer to a cleft care nurse who sees the patient and their parents urgently. Isolated cleft lip babies can normally breast- and bottle-feed successfully. In cleft palate, feeding may be a problem. Sucking may be difficult, making breastfeeding and bottle-feeding a problem. Swallowing is normal. Feeds may be delivered to the back of the tongue via a spoon or pipette or using a bottle with a specialised teat. Feeding in the upright position prevents regurgitation.

Classification of Timings of Cleft Lip Repair

- Traditional "10s": 10 lbs, 10 weeks, 10 gdL^{-1} haemoglobin
- Neonatal < 48 h
- Conventional: 3/12-lip and anterior palate, 6/12 remaining hard and soft palate
- Other regimes: Delaire – 6–9/12 – lip and soft palate, 12–18/12 remaining hard palate

The aims of surgery are to achieve an intact lip, alveolus and palate and to permit normal speech and dentition, and to address the associated nasal deformity. The timing of operations on cleft lip and palate remains controversial. Although some surgeons are now carrying out neonatal lip repair, the majority would undertake primary lip repair from 10 weeks. The methods of lip repair are numerous, but the principles involve realignment and repair of the orbicularis oris muscle, supplementing the deficient medial mucosa and philtrum with skin and mucosal tissues from the lateral side. Operation on cleft palate should be undertaken before the child starts to articulate sounds. This is normally around 9–12 months. The aims of treatment of cleft palate are:

- To close the cleft, thus separating nasal and oral cavities
- To ensure adequate length of the soft palate, allowing separation of the nasopharynx and oropharynx on phonation.

Various relaxing or plastic procedures may be necessary to achieve this.

Prognosis. A good cosmetic result is normally achieved in closing cleft lip. With cleft palate 15–20% may require a pharyngoplasty due to velopharyngeal incompetence (abnormal nasal escape during speech, nasal regurgitation of fluids). All children need speech therapy. Occasionally, secondary procedures may be required such as secondary alveolar bone grafting at 9–11 years and corrective rhinoplasty around the age of 16 years.

SKIN AND SOFT TISSUE

The skin is the largest organ of the body. It has many functions including structural support whilst allowing flexibility, sensitivity for interaction with the outside world, thermoregulation, prevention of water loss, cosmesis, vitamin D production, physical defence against environmental trauma/radiation and immune defence against microorganisms. There are many skin disorders which fall under the realm of the

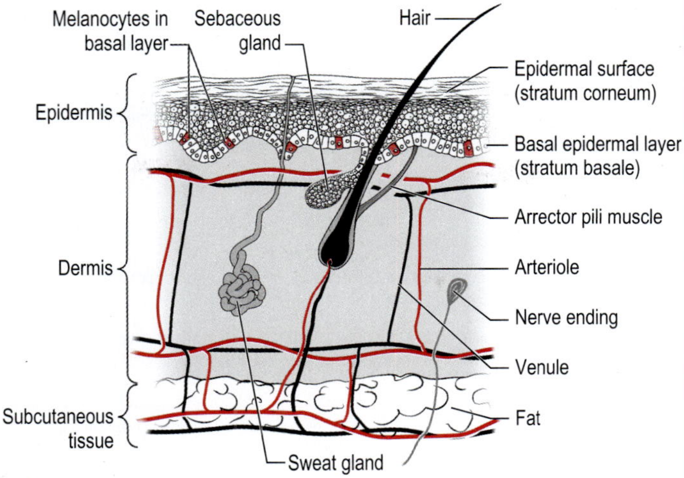

FIGURE 20.8

Cross-section of normal skin.

dermatologist; there are those which are a manifestation of underlying systemic disease. This chapter outlines the skin and subcutaneous lesions relevant to the surgeon in practice. A schematic cross-section of the skin to demonstrate the relationships between the layers is illustrated in Figure 20.8, and a summary of the lesions described can be seen in Table 20.1.

Epidermis – Benign

Skin Tags (Pedunculated Papillomas)

These small polypoid lesions occur in adults, most frequently on the trunk, neck, axilla and groin. They may catch on clothes and bleed, and are often cosmetically unacceptable. They are removed by excision under local anaesthetic.

Warts (Verrucae Vulgaris)

These are caused by papovavirus and usually occur in the second decade of life. They are common on fingers, hands and soles of feet (*verrucae plantaris*). Plantar warts may be very painful. Resolution of warts may occur spontaneously. Treatment may be by curettage, freezing with liquid nitrogen or application of keratolytic agents.

Seborrhoeic Keratoses

These are found in elderly patients and are often multiple, well-demarcated raised 'stuck on' lesions with varying degrees of pigmentation. It may be difficult to differentiate from malignant melanoma if deeply pigmented. Treatment is to leave alone or treat by surgical excision or curettage.

Keratoacanthoma

This is a nodular lesion with a central crater containing a keratin 'plug'. They progress rapidly in 2 weeks to 2 months. Probably of viral aetiology, they often show

TABLE 20.1

'SURGICAL' SKIN LESIONS

Benign	
Epidermis	Pedunculated papilloma, wart, seborrhoeic keratosis, keratoacanthoma
Dermis	Pyogenic granuloma, fibrous histiocytoma, keloid
Appendages	Furuncle, carbuncle, hidradenitis suppurativa, sebaceous cyst, dermoid cyst, pilonidal sinus
Subcutaneous	Lipoma, neurofibroma
Melanotic	Intradermal naevus, blue naevus, compound naevus, Spitz naevus, congenital naevus
Vascular	Campbell de Morgan spots, haemangiomas, capillary/venous/arteriovenous/lymphatic malformations, spider naevi, glomus tumours
Premalignant	
Epidermis	Actinic (solar) keratosis, Bowen's disease, erythroplasia of Queyrat (penis)
Malignant	
Epidermis	Basal cell carcinoma, squamous cell carcinoma
Dermis	Kaposi's sarcoma, secondary deposits
Appendages	Sebaceous carcinoma (rare), sweat gland carcinoma (rare)
Subcutaneous	Liposarcoma, neurofibrosarcoma
Melanotic	Malignant melanoma
Vascular	Angiosarcoma (rare)

spontaneous regression. Occasionally, they are difficult to distinguish from squamous cell carcinomas (SCC). Treatment is by excision biopsy to exclude SCC.

Epidermis – Premalignant

Actinic (Solar) Keratoses

These are rough, scaly epidermal lesions on sites of exposure to the sun; 10–20% undergo malignant change. The diagnosis is confirmed by biopsy and then the lesion is excised. Topical chemotherapy with 5-fluorouracil cream has been used in patients with multiple lesions.

Bowen's Disease

Intraepidermal squamous cell carcinoma (carcinoma *in situ*). A well-defined erythematous plaque with occasional crusting, it occurs in the fourth to sixth decade and may be associated with the presence of internal malignancy. Diagnosis is confirmed by a biopsy. Treatment is by excision, cryotherapy, curettage, topical 5-fluorouracil or photodynamic therapy. Intraepidermal carcinoma may occur on the glans penis and is then called erythroplasia of Queyrat and appears as a reddish-brown velvety plaque.

Leukoplakia

Leukoplakia consists of a thickened white patch on a mucous membrane. It can occur on the vermillion border, oral mucosa and the vulva. It occurs due to chronic irritation.

In the mouth, this is usually due to sunlight but can occur due to dentures. Approximately 20% will show dysplasia and may progress to carcinoma. Erythroplasia is a red patch and always represents in situ carcinoma.

Epidermis – Malignant

Basal Cell Carcinoma (Rodent Ulcer)

Basal cell carcinoma arises from the basal keratinocytes of the epidermis. It is common in the middle-aged and elderly. Slow growing and locally invasive; it very rarely metastasises. Frequently found on skin exposed to sunlight, the commonest area is the face above a line drawn from the angle of the mouth to the lobe of the ear. Other predisposing factors include immunosuppression, radiotherapy, xeroderma pigmentosum and naevus sebaceus.

There are several different types:

- Nodular – most common, starts as a nodule that ulcerates and develops a rolled edge with a pearly appearance and local telangiectasia.
- Superficial – presents as red scaly patches.
- Morphoeic or sclerosing – forms a flat spreading plaque; it has a fibrous stroma and may cause distortion, i.e. around the eyelids.
- Gorlin's syndrome – autosomal dominant condition associated with multiple basal cell carcinomas, dental cysts and a splayed 12th rib; radiotherapy will convert the basal cell carcinoma to a much more aggressive form and is thus contraindicated.

Differential diagnosis includes seborrhoeic keratoses and malignant melanoma. Treatment options include surgical excision (with a 3–5 mm margin) or radiotherapy. Cure rate is high when treated early and adequately. Larger defects may require reconstruction using the principles of the reconstructive ladder.

Squamous Cell Carcinoma

Squamous cell carcinoma arises from keratinocytes in the epidermis. This may grow rapidly. It metastasises via lymphatics and rarely via the bloodstream. Exposure to sunlight may be a causative factor. It can also develop in areas of Bowen's disease and erythroplasia of Queyrat. Other causative factors include chemical burns, chronic ulcers (e.g. Marjolin's ulcer, i.e. malignant change in a chronic venous ulcer), irradiation dermatitis.

It starts as a lump, which ulcerates with bleeding and discharge. The edge of the ulcer is characteristically raised and everted. Local lymph nodes may be involved. Differential diagnosis includes keratoacanthoma, basal cell carcinoma, amelanotic malignant melanoma, pyogenic granuloma, traumatised seborrhoeic wart. Diagnosis is confirmed by biopsy. Treatment is by wide excision (with a 5–10 mm margin) or radiotherapy. Block dissection of regional lymph nodes is required if these are affected. Large defects may require reconstruction with skin grafts, local or free flaps as described above.

Classification of Treatment Options for Non-Melanoma Skin Cancers

1- Surgical excision,
2- Curettage and cautery,
3- Mohs micrographic surgery,
4- Cryotherapy,
5- Radiotherapy

Melanocytic Lesions – Benign and Premalignant

Melanocytes are present within the dermis and epidermis with similar numbers in all races, which differ in melanin production. At birth, most melanocytes are situated in the basal layer of the epidermis. Melanin is transferred in melanosomes to keratinocytes to form a melanin cap over the cell nucleus protecting the contents from the damaging effects of UV irradiation.

Freckle (Ephelis)

Related to sun exposure, they consist of an increase in pigment from melanocytes but no increase in the number of melanocytes.

Solar Lentigo

Occur in areas of sun-damaged skin, especially on the hands and face. They consist of an increase in the number of melanocytes producing normal amounts of pigment. There is no atypia.

Naevi (Figure 20.9)

A naevus is defined as an increased number of melanocytes in an abnormal position producing normal or increased amounts of melanin. Over the next few decades, some will migrate to the dermis. Melanocytes within the dermis have no malignant potential as they have lost their ability to divide.

The position of melanocytes can give rise to a number of pigmented lesions:

- Melanocytes in the basal layer form a simple lentigo or *mole*.
- Melanocytes at the dermoepidermal junction form a *junctional naevus*. These appear as either a macule or papule and are brown, smooth and hairless. They develop at or around puberty and can occur anywhere, including the hands and the soles of the feet. A small percentage may turn malignant but this comprises the vast majority of malignant melanomas.
- Fibroblast migration may draw some melanocytes into the dermis, leaving some at the dermoepidermal junction. This forms a *compound naevus*. It is clinically indistinguishable from an intradermal naevus. It does, however, have malignant potential.
- As a naevus matures in the late 30s, an *intradermal naevus* is formed, all the melanocytes lying in the dermis. Clinically they appear as a well-defined papule. They are brown or flesh-coloured and often hairy. They have no malignant potential.

SPITZ NAEVUS. Benign lesions, usually seen in children and young adults. Clinically they appear as pink, dome-shaped nodules. Histologically, they can be difficult to differentiate from malignant melanomas.

HALO NAEVUS. Benign lesion. Clinically it appears as a lesion surrounded by an area of depigmentation secondary to invasion of lymphocytes. This phenomenon can occur in malignant melanomas and is thus an important differential diagnosis.

BLUE NAEVUS. Consists of melanocytes in the dermis. They form lesions with a slate-blue colour. There are two types:

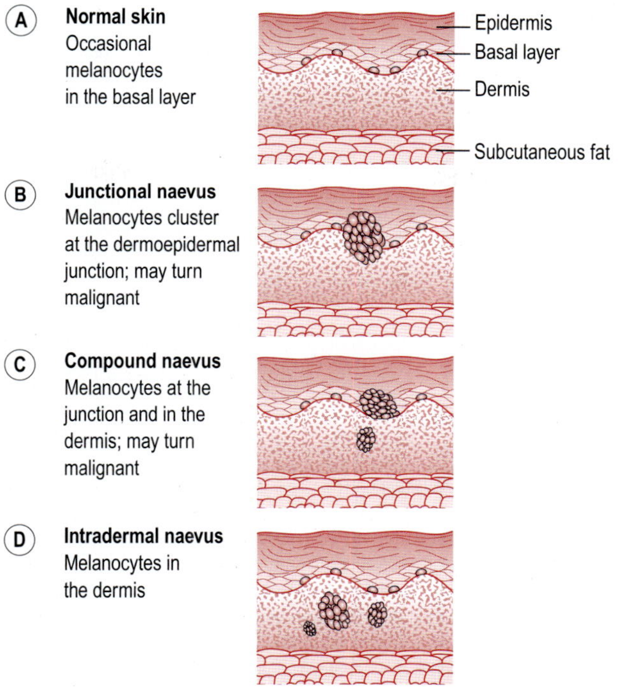

FIGURE 20.9

Pathological varieties of naevus (mole): (**A**) normal skin, (**B**) junctional naevus, (**C**) compound naevus and (**D**) intradermal naevus.

Common. Benign lesion often seen in the head or hands. More common in women and usually seen in women in their 40s.

Cellular. More common in women. More than 50% occur in the sacrococcygeal/ buttock area. They are benign, but malignant transformation may occur.

Congenital Naevi. May be single or multiple. One important variant is the giant pigmented naevus. These lesions are >20cm in diameter and are flat, pale brown and hairless or lumpy, black and hairy in appearance. Malignant melanoma may develop, usually in the teenage years. Management is usually by excision. This may require extensive plastic surgical reconstruction due to tissue loss.

Lentigo Maligna. Also known as Hutchinson's freckle. It occurs on sun-damaged skin in the elderly. It is an irregular flat brown-black lesion. It may increase in size over many years and it consists of an abnormal proliferation of atypical melanocytes in the dermo-epidermal junction. It is essentially malignant melanoma in situ. Development of invasion and therefore malignancy is usually heralded by the development of a pigmented nodule within the lesion. Confirmed by incision biopsy, treatment is by excision.

Malignant Melanoma

More than 13000 cases of malignant melanoma are diagnosed annually in the UK. They may occur anywhere on the skin or on the retina, oesophageal mucosa or anus. Malignant melanomas can arise in pre-existing naevi or *de novo*.

Signs of malignant change in a mole include:

- Change in size, shape or deepening of colour
- Irregular border
- Bleeding or ulceration
- Itching.

Predisposing factors for malignant melanoma include:

- Fair skin
- History of intense sun exposure and sunburn
- Family history
- Multiple naevi
- Dysplastic naevus syndrome.

Classification

Superficial Spreading Melanoma. 60%. This is the commonest type of melanoma. In males it occurs most commonly on the back; in females most commonly the legs. Prognosis tends to be good, as growth is predominantly radial rather than vertical (this correlates to a reduction in the level of invasion).

Nodular Melanoma. 30%. Found on the trunk, they appear as raised nodules, often with ulceration. The growth is almost entirely vertical, thus these tumours have a poor prognosis.

Lentigo Maligna Melanoma. 7%. Arises from lentigo maligna. Occurs in the elderly, i.e. 60–70 years. Tends to have a good prognosis and has low metastatic potential.

Acral Lentiginous Melanoma. 1%. Rare. Occurs on the soles, palms and under nails (subungual).

Amelanotic. 1%

Desmoplastic. 1%. Spread of melanoma occurs by local growth and infiltration. Lymphatic spread occurs early. Bloodstream spread occurs in almost any organ, particularly the liver, brain and lung.

STAGING. A number of different classifications may be used to stage the level of invasion – this links directly with prognosis. Classifications are as follows:

- Breslow thickness – <1mm, 1–2mm, 2–4mm and >4mm
- Clarke's level:
  - I Epidermis
  - II Papillary dermis
  - III Junction of papillary and reticular dermis
  - IV Extends to reticular dermis
  - V Subcutaneous tissue.
- American Joint Committee on Cancer:
  - Tis Melanoma in situ
  - T1 ≤1.0mm
  - T2 1.01–2mm

- T3 2.01–4mm
- T4 >4.0mm
- N1 1 node
- N2 2–3 nodes
- N3 ≥4 nodes
- M1 Metastatic disease.

(These are further subdivided dependent on further prognostic variables).

Treatment

1. Should be managed within a multidisciplinary team (MDT) setting. Confirm the diagnosis and depth of invasion. Occasionally a malignant melanoma is clinically obvious, but lesions may need to be confirmed by excisional or incisional biopsy.
2. The mainstay of treatment is surgical. Initial excision should be performed with an adequate clearance margin. Following removal of the lesion, histology will confirm the diagnosis and allow the measurement of Breslow thickness.
3. After measuring the Breslow thickness, further surgery may be needed. A tumour of <1mm in thickness requires a 1-cm excision margin. Tumours of greater depth may need a wider margin, but margins over 3cm confer no survival benefit.
4. In patients with involved nodes, a regional lymph node dissection should accompany the removal of the lesion. In patients with no clinical involvement, the management is controversial. As many as 20% of T2/T3 patients may have metastases. Accurate staging is assisted by radiolabelled probe/dye-directed sentinel node biopsy.
5. Chemotherapy is of little value in primary disease. Isolated limb perfusion may be used in local recurrence.
6. Radiotherapy and immunotherapy have been used but are strictly palliative.

Prognosis. Favourable factors include early diagnosis, a depth of penetration of <1mm and melanoma in a radial growth phase. Unfavourable factors include lymph node and distant metastases at presentation, increasing depth of penetration, ulceration and presence of vertical growth phase. If the disease is confined to the primary site and has a penetration of <1mm, then a 5-year survival of 90% may be expected. With lymph node metastases this is reduced to 30%, and with distant metastases patients rarely survive for 1 year.

Dermis – Benign

Pyogenic Granuloma

This is a dark red nodule of exuberant granulation tissue and polymorphs. There is rapid initial growth, often at the site of trauma. Occasionally, the surface may ulcerate and then must be distinguished from amelanotic melanoma. Treatment is by excision.

Fibrous Histiocytoma

This is a well-circumscribed deep reddish-brown tumour. On inspection, it may be mistaken for a malignant melanoma. However, palpation reveals a hard consistency due to the dense fibrous stroma. Treatment is by excision.

Keloid

This is an abnormal scar characterised by excessive deposition of collagen beyond the boundaries of the wound itself and is covered by normal epithelium. It must be distinguished from a hypertrophic scar in which the wound becomes broad and raised – the latter usually settles within 6 months. Keloid may increase after 6 months. Black Africans and the young are particularly affected. It may follow burns. Treatment is by intralesional injection of steroid, excision (recurrence is common), pressure garment therapy, applying silicon-impregnated dressings; or for refractive, problematic lesions, radiotherapy after excision is an option.

Classification of Scar Assessment

Vancouver Burn Scar Assessment Scale (Summarised)

	Score
Pigmentation	0–2
Vascularity	0–3
Pliability	0–3
Height	0–3

Global Acne Scarring Classification. Grade 1: Macular

Erythematous, hyper, or hypopigmented flat marks.

Grade 2: Mild

Mild rolling, small soft papular.

Grade 3: Moderate

More significant rolling, shallow boxcar, mild to moderate hypertrophic or papular scars.

Grade 4: Severe

Punched out atrophic (deep boxcar), ice pick, bridges and tunnels, marked atrophy, dystrophic significant hypertrophy, or keloid.

Dermis – Malignant

Kaposi's Sarcoma

These are raised purplish nodules. Initially they are usually single, but gradually multiple nodules occur and may ulcerate. It is the commonest tumour to develop in patients with AIDS; 90% are in male patients. The solitary nodule should be excised. Local radiotherapy or cytotoxic therapy is useful for multiple lesions.

Metastatic Carcinoma

Small, hard, painless skin nodules may occur. Skin secondaries are commonest with cancer of the breast, lung, bowel and melanoma. In most patients, the primary will be obvious or will already have been treated. Ulceration of the secondaries may occur. Biopsy confirms the diagnosis. Treatment is given that is appropriate for metastatic disease for that particular tumour, e.g. tamoxifen in carcinoma of the breast.

Others

Malignant dermal tumours such as dermatofibrosarcoma protuberans (DFSP) are relatively rare and fall outside the scope of this chapter.

Skin Appendages – Benign

Boil (Furuncle)

This is an infection in a hair follicle usually caused by *Staph. aureus*. It can occur in any part of the body but is more common in the head, neck, axilla and groins. Diabetes, immunosuppression and general debility are predisposing conditions. Any patient presenting with boils should have their urine tested for sugar.

Usually, they heal when pus has discharged. Antibiotics should be avoided except in the following situations:

- 'Dangerous' areas of the face, i.e. between the orbit and angle of the mouth where venous drainage is into the cavernous sinus – cavernous sinus thrombosis may occur.
- Multiple boils with surrounding cellulitis in diabetics and immunosuppressed patients where septicaemia is a risk.

Carbuncle

An infection which dissects through the dermis and subcutaneous tissues to form connecting channels, some of which open to the surface. There is considerable induration and pus discharges through the sinuses. The back of the neck is a common site. Treatment is with antistaphylococcal antibiotics, e.g. flucloxacillin, with desloughing and adequate drainage of the abscesses if necessary.

Hidradenitis Suppurativa

A chronic disease of skin and subcutaneous tissue in apocrine gland-bearing areas, e.g. axilla, groin, perineum and perianal areas. The involved area is indurated, fibrotic and inflamed with sinuses draining pus. *Staph. aureus* is the usual organism grown but occasionally coliforms may be cultured. Treatment is initially by antibiotics. Abscesses are incised and drained. Advanced cases may need wide excision with or without skin grafting. Severe perianal disease may require a diverting colostomy prior to skin grafting.

Sebaceous Cysts

These are common on the scalp, face, neck and back and are soft or firm and spherical. They contain cheesy sebaceous material, which may become infected and discharge. They are attached to the skin and a punctum is usually seen at the point of attachment. Treatment is by excision under local anaesthetic.

Dermoid Cysts

These may be congenital or acquired.

Congenital. They are formed in intrauterine life when skin dermatomes fuse and present at birth or a few years after. They are most common in head and neck, e.g. outer end of eyebrow (external angular dermoid). Treatment is by excision. Midline dermoid cysts should be radiologically assessed to exclude intracranial extension.

Acquired. These are implantation dermoids. A piece of skin is forcibly implanted into the dermis as a result of trauma. They are common on fingers. Treatment is by excision.

Pilonidal Sinus

This chronic infection in the sinus is caused by penetration of hairs into skin and subcutaneous tissues. Infection leads to pilonidal abscesses. The sinus leads to a cavity filled with hair and granulation tissue. Common sites include posteriorly in the midline over the sacrococcygeal area and natal cleft (usually hirsute males with sedentary occupations); between the fingers in hairdressers; occasionally umbilicus, axilla and nipple. Differential diagnosis includes perianal fistulae, hidradenitis suppurativa, simple boils. Treatment includes:

- Deroofing the track, removing the hairs and packing; the surrounding skin should be shaved until the sinuses have healed.
- Injection of the sinuses with methylene blue, followed by wide excision of all tracts until no dye is seen and either packing, primary suture or reconstruction of large defects using local flaps can be carried out under GA.
- For pilonidal abscesses, incising, curetting and packing.

Skin Appendages – Malignant

There are malignant tumours that can arise from all of the skin appendages e.g. sebaceous carcinoma, sweat gland carcinoma. On the whole these are rare but aggressive and fall outside the scope of this chapter.

HINTS AND TIPS

WHAT TO DO WITH A SKIN LESION

Small benign-appearing skin lesions, e.g. skin tags, sebaceous cysts that will close directly without distorting features (lip, eyelid, eyebrow, etc.):

- Simple excision with narrow margin

Small lesions of malignant appearance that can be adequately excised with appropriate surgical margins and not distort features or require reconstruction.

- Excision biopsy with appropriate margin

Lesions or ulcers requiring exclusion of malignancy or vasculitis where excision would cause distortion of features, or require reconstruction.

- Incision biopsy or punch biopsy

For confirmed malignant lesions.

- Wide excision of adequate margin and depth ± reconstruction

Radiotherapy for basal cell carcinoma may be an alternative to surgery, especially in sites where skin preservation is important.

Subcutaneous Tissue – Benign

Lipoma

This is a common, benign tumour of fatty tissue. It is soft, lobulated and pseudofluctuant, and the overlying skin appears normal. It is slow growing. Treatment is by excision. Multiple lipomas may occur. These need to be distinguished from neurofibromata by biopsy of at least one lesion. Occasionally, there may be multiple tender lipomas on the trunk (Dercum's disease). Treatment of lipoma is by excision, which is curative. Liposarcomatous change may rarely occur in a benign lipoma.

Neurofibroma

These are benign tumours arising from the connective tissue element of peripheral nerves. They are often multiple and may be asymptomatic, but if closely related to the nerve the patient may get paraesthesia in the distribution of the nerve. Biopsy of one lesion may confirm the diagnosis. If neurofibromata are multiple, congenital and familial, the condition is known as neurofibromatosis. Occasionally, malignant change to neurofibrosarcoma occurs (see below).

Subcutaneous Tissues – Malignant

These fall under the category of soft tissue sarcoma (e.g. liposarcoma), of which there are more than 50 histological subtypes including those of synovium, muscle, nerves, blood vessels, bone and gut. They have a variety of prognoses and management depends on type, stage and grade. They are best managed in an MDT setting of surgeons, oncologists, pathologists, radiologists and allied professionals with a specialist interest.

HINTS AND TIPS

SARCOMAS

The presence of a soft tissue lump should raise suspicion of sarcoma if it:

- Has a diameter >5 cm
- Has a history of rapid growth
- Is fixed to deep tissues
- Is painful or tender.

If these criteria are met, then an urgent referral to a sarcoma MDT would be advised. Initial management, under advice, may involve a magnetic resonance imaging scan and a diagnostic punch or incisional biopsy of the mass through an incision/track that would be excised in any subsequent elective extirpative surgery. Computerised tomography staging to detect possible systemic metastases may also be recommended.

SARCOMA CLASSIFICATION BY TISSUE OF ORIGIN

Skin

- Dermatofibrosarcoma protuberans (DFSP)
- Malignant fibrous histiocytoma (MFH)
- Atypical fibroxanthoma (AFX)

Fat

- Liposarcoma

Fibrous tissue

- Fibrosarcoma

Muscle

- Smooth:– Leiomyosarcoma
- Striated: – Rhabdomyosarcoma

Blood vessel

- Angiosarcoma,
- Kaposi sarcoma

Lymph vessel

- Lymphangiosarcoma

Bone

- Osteosarcoma

Cartilage

- Chrondrosarcoma

DISORDERS OF THE NAILS

Ingrowing Toenail (IGTN)

A common condition, it usually appears on the great toe, particularly the lateral side. Caused by a combination of tight shoes and paring the nail downwards into the nail fold rather than cutting it transversely. The sharp edge of nail then grows into the nail fold producing ulceration, infection and granulation tissue.

Treatment

Noninfected. Give advice on correct cutting of nails, i.e. transversely. Avoid tight, pointed shoes. Tuck a pledget of cotton wool soaked in mild antiseptic under the corner of the nail to lift it out of the soft tissue. Soak feet in warm water regularly.

Infected. With mild infection, it may be possible to adopt the above regimen in addition to the administration of antistaphylococcal antibiotics. If this fails, carry out the following:

- Simple nail avulsion with curettage of infected granulation tissue under local anaesthetic. Antistaphylococcal antibiotics should be administered.
- Wedge excision. Lateral or medial nail and nail bed are removed together with granulation tissue and germinal matrix. Liquefied phenol may be applied to the germinal matrix to ensure complete removal.
- Zadik's procedure. This is reserved for recurrent IGTN. The nail is avulsed and the germinal matrix completely excised after raising a skin flap to expose it. To ensure complete removal of the germinal matrix, liquefied phenol is applied after protecting the skin. The nails should not regrow after this procedure.

Complications. Recurrence may occur. This is common after simple avulsion. Spikes of nail may occasionally regrow after a Zadik's procedure. Infection may occur, and it is appropriate to give a course of antistaphylococcal antibiotics prophylactically. Osteomyelitis and septic arthritis may occur after Zadik's procedure.

Onychogryphosis

This is a 'ram's horn' deformity of the toenail. The nail thickens and curls over the end of the toe as it grows. Common in the elderly, it may follow trauma to the nail in the younger patient. It can be treated by either cutting the nail with bone forceps or grinding the nail down. Avulsion is always followed by recurrence. Zadik's operation is curative.

Nail Bed Lesions

Haematoma. There is a history of trauma, e.g. trapping, or dropping a heavy object on the nail. Very painful. A haematoma is evacuated by piercing the nail with a red-hot paper clip. Small haematomas following trivial injury may closely simulate subungual melanoma. Haematomas grow out with growth of the nail. If there is any doubt, biopsy should be carried out.

Melanoma. Subungual malignant melanoma is not uncommon. The lesion does not grow out with the nail. Biopsy is necessary. If the diagnosis is confirmed, amputation of the digit is indicated.

Subungual Exostosis. This nearly always affects the great toe. It occurs in adolescents and young adults. It lifts the overlying nail and causes deformity. Diagnosis is confirmed by radiograph. Treatment is to remove the nail and excise the underlying bony nodule.

Glomus Tumour. See below.

LESIONS OF VASCULAR ORIGIN

Campbell de Morgan Spots

These are small bright red spots containing capillaries and connective tissue. They are rare before the age of 40 and increase with age. They are of no serious significance. Patients should be reassured and the lesions left alone.

Benign Vascular Tumours

HAEMANGIOMAS (STRAWBERRY NAEVI). These benign vascular tumours commonly grow rapidly in the first few months of life; are red, soft, compressible fleshy lesions that commonly involute; 50% of haemangiomas have resolved by 5 years of age. Haemangiomas that ulcerate and bleed, obscure vision or hearing, or interfere with speech development may require treatment with propranolol, steroids or excision, otherwise they are treated expectantly during involution.

GLOMUS TUMOUR. Glomus bodies occur in the subcutaneous tissues of the limbs – especially the fingers, toes and nail bed. They are small arteriovenous communications associated with muscle and nerve (angioneuromyoma). Clinically, they are small, raised, bluish-red lesions. They are painful and exquisitely tender if pressed. Treatment is by surgical excision.

Malignant Vascular Tumours

These fall under the category of soft tissue sarcoma (e.g. angiosarcoma – see above).

Vascular Malformations

CAPILLARY MALFORMATIONS (PORT-WINE STAINS). These are flush with the skin and occur on the face, lips and buccal mucosa. They can become more thickened during life and are reddish-blue in colour. If the lesion is small, surgical excision may be attempted. Larger lesions are cosmetically distressing. Sclerosing agents and lasers have been used. Advice on the use of cosmetic preparations may be the most appropriate. Lesions in the 5th cranial nerve dermatome (ophthalmic division –VI) may be seen in association with meningeal involvement (Sturge–Weber syndrome), which may cause focal epilepsy. Similar lesions may be seen in Klippel–Trénaunay syndrome.

VENOUS MALFORMATIONS, ARTERIOVENOUS MALFORMATIONS (AVM). Grow in proportion with the child's growth. High-flow lesions (AVM) can present as pulsatile masses with bruits and may progress to high-output cardiac failure – after investigation of extent by angiography, treatment is by a combination of radiologically guided sclerotherapy and excision if symptomatic.

Lymphatic Malformations. Can be macrocystic (cystic hygroma) or microcystic and localised or involve whole limbs, leading to lymphoedema and limb hypertrophy. Associations with AVM (Parkes Weber syndrome) and capillary malformations (Klippel–Trénaunay syndrome) are recognised. Treatment is usually conservative as lesions often recur after excision.

Congenital Haemangiomas. These are classified into:

1- RICH: Rapidly involuting congenital haemangioma
2- NICH: Non-rapidly involuting congenital haemangioma

Some common examples of them include:

Pyogenic granuloma:– A rapidly growing proliferation of vascular tissue

Kasabach–Merritt phenomenon:– An invasive vascular tumour associated with platelet trapping, profound thrombocytopenia giving rise to an increased risk of intracranial, pleural-pulmonic, intraperitoneal and gastrointestinal haemorrhage. It is associated with Kaposiform haemangioendothelioma

Chapter 21

Paediatric Surgery

Richard J. England

CHAPTER OUTLINE

This chapter will cover some of the paediatric surgical emergencies that arise in the newborn, the more common paediatric surgical problems presenting at outpatient departments and common paediatric surgical emergencies.

ALIMENTARY TRACT EMERGENCIES IN THE NEWBORN

Oesophageal Atresia

There are five main types of oesophageal atresia, the commonest (85%) of which is a blind-ended, upper oesophagus associated with a tracheo-oesophageal fistula involving the lower oesophagus (Figure 21.1A). Pure oesophageal atresia (Figure 21.1B) alone (without tracheo-oesophageal fistula) exists in 8% of cases. The other types are extremely rare. In some cases there is only a short gap between the blind-ended upper oesophagus and the distal oesophagus, while in others there is a long gap. The incidence of oesophageal atresia is approximately 1:3000 births. There is a high incidence of associated anomalies described by the acronym VACTERL:

- **V**ertebral anomalies (e.g. hemivertebrae)
- **A**norectal anomalies (e.g. imperforate anus)
- **C**ardiac anomalies
- **T**racheal anomalies (e.g. fistula, tracheomalacia)
- **E**sophageal anomalies
- **R**enal anomalies
- **L**imb anomalies (e.g. radial aplasia).

Symptoms and Signs. Association with maternal polyhydramnios (diagnosis may be suspected antenatally – ultrasound features of polyhydramnios and diminished or absent foetal stomach bubble). Dribbling of saliva, inability to swallow feeds, production of frothy mucus, choking, cyanotic attacks, aspiration pneumonia.

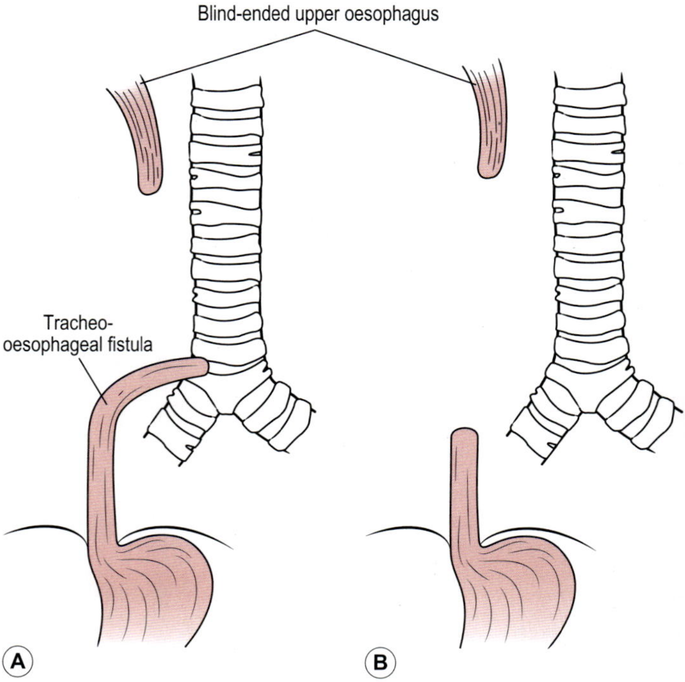

FIGURE 21.1

Types of oesophageal atresia. (**A**) Oesophageal atresia with distal tracheo-oesophageal fistula – the commonest with an incidence of 85%. (**B**) Isolated oesophageal atresia with an incidence of 8% – note the long gap between the proximal and distal oesophagus.

HINTS AND TIPS

Oesophageal atresia (± tracheo-oesophageal fistula) should be considered whenever a baby develops feeding and respiratory difficulties in the first few days of life.

Investigations

- Pass an orogastric tube – it will arrest at the obstruction.
- Chest X-ray (CXR) including neck; to see the position of tube at obstruction: aspiration pneumonia.
- AXR: gas in stomach and intestine will indicate the presence of a tracheo-oesophageal fistula.
- Echocardiogram: to look for cardiac abnormalities and position of aortic arch before repair.

Treatment. Rehydration. Treat any chest infection. Keep upper oesophageal pouch empty by continuous aspiration. Urgent surgical ligation of the tracheo-oesophageal fistula and correction of atresia by primary end-to-end anastomosis of the oesophagus is carried out for the 'short gap' form. If primary repair is not possible, e.g. with the 'long gap' form, a gastrostomy is performed to feed the baby until it has grown sufficiently to perform a delayed primary anastomosis. Sequential lengthening techniques such as the Fokker technique may be tried in some centres, otherwise a cervical oesophagostomy with subsequent oesophageal substitution using either stomach or colon is required.

If the condition is suspected antenatally, the baby should be delivered somewhere with ready access to a paediatric surgical unit.

Prognosis. Survival is over 97%. Neonates with cardiac anomalies or very low birth weights have a higher mortality.

HINTS AND TIPS

If possible, obtain an echo before operating. Cardiac anomalies occur in approximately 20% of cases. If the aortic arch is lying abnormally on the right side, consider performing the thoracotomy on the left side instead. The anatomy will be reversed but the arch will not be obscuring the oesophagus!

Duodenal Atresia

This occurs in 1:6000 births. The common bile duct may open proximal or distal to an atresia. There is an association with Down's syndrome and congenital heart disease.

Symptoms and Signs. Associated with maternal polyhydramnios. Vomiting in first few hours of life usually bile-stained.

Investigations

- Antenatal diagnosis is possible with USS.
- AXR shows 'double bubble' sign, i.e. gas bubble and fluid level on each side of upper abdomen owing to gas in stomach and proximal duodenum (Figure 21.2).

Treatment. Rehydration. Urgent surgery. Duodenoduodenostomy, i.e. a side-to-side or diamond-shaped anastomosis between proximal and distal duodenal segments.

Prognosis. Mortality depends on associated abnormalities and is higher with Down's syndrome and cardiac anomalies. Late complications can occur, and long-term follow-up may be required.

Small Bowel Atresia

The incidence varies worldwide from 1:400 to 1:3000 live births. It may occur at any level and may be multiple. It is now accepted to be linked to a vascular accident during development.

Symptoms and Signs. Bilious vomiting. Abdominal distension. Visible peristalsis.

Investigations. AXR: multiple distended bowel loops depending on level of obstruction.

Treatment. Rehydration. Urgent surgery. Resection of areas of atresia or stenosis with end-to-end anastomosis.

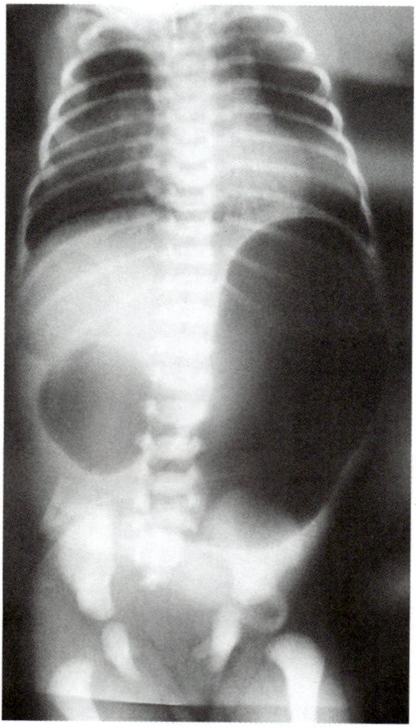

FIGURE 21.2
Duodenal atresia. AXR with 'double bubble' gas sign and no gas pattern beyond the duodenum.

Malrotation and Volvulus

In the first trimester, the midgut herniates outside the abdominal cavity but returns at the end of the third month, rotating as it does so. Several rotational abnormalities may result. Obstruction may consequently be the result of a variety of causes, from peritoneal bands to volvulus of the midgut. The mesentery of the small bowel normally stretches from the duodenojejunal flexure in the left upper quadrant to the caecum in the right iliac fossa. Malrotation can result in the duodenojejunal flexure and caecum not being fixed retroperitoneally, resulting in the attachment of the base of the midgut mesentery being very narrow as it is not secured at either end. As a result of this, the whole of the midgut can twist around its own blood supply with resulting ischaemia. This is a malrotation volvulus which requires emergency laparotomy. Failure of normal rotation invariably occurs in patients with exomphalos and diaphragmatic hernia.

Symptoms and Signs. Bile-stained vomiting. Tenderness and abdominal distension may occur later. The symptoms are similar initially to duodenal atresia. However, volvulus will lead to venous and subsequently arterial obstruction, gut infarction and consequent potential short bowel syndrome.

Investigations

- USS to identify superior mesenteric vein/artery relations – the position of the vein and artery in relation to one another changes with rotation.

- Contrast meal: abnormally placed duodenojejunal junction.
- Contrast enema: may show abnormally placed caecum but the latter may also be normal in position.

Treatment. Time-Critical Transfer to Paediatric Surgery Centre. Emergency laparotomy. Right upper quadrant transverse incision. Untwist the volvulus. Divide Ladd's bands. Tease out mesenteric base to prevent recurrence. Excise any gangrenous bowel and re-anastomose bowel if conditions optimal.

Meconium Ileus

This occurs in 15% of patients with cystic fibrosis. Meconium becomes inspissated in the terminal ileum with soft meconium above associated with distended proximal small bowel.

Symptoms and Signs. Infant born with distended abdomen. Bilious vomiting. Meconium is not passed and the rectum is empty.

Investigations

- AXR: dilated loops of bowel with soap bubble appearance of inspissated meconium. *In utero* perforation will produce flecks of calcification visible on X-ray.
- Gastrografin enema will show an empty colon and may relieve the obstruction by refluxing into the terminal ileum and 'loosening' the meconium.
- Prenatal diagnosis may be made with USS.
- Postnatal confirmation of cystic fibrosis by genetic analysis, sweat test or immunoreactive trypsinogen on Guthrie card newborn screening test.

Treatment. Simple meconium ileus may resolve with enemas alone. Some 50% may have associated atresia, perforation or volvulus and then laparotomy is required. The terminal ileum is opened and the inspissated meconium washed out. A temporary ileostomy may be required.

Complications. Meconium peritonitis. May occur *in utero* or postnatally. The chemical peritonitis resulting is treated by peritoneal lavage and repair of the perforation. The mortality rate is 10%.

Anorectal Abnormalities

These occur with an incidence of 1:5000 births. Management depends on accurate definition of the abnormality.

Symptoms and Signs. Infant fails to pass meconium. Perineal inspection reveals imperforate anus with or without a fistula to anterior structures in male or female. There may be associated genitourinary/cardiac or spinal abnormalities (VACTERL association, p. 521).

Investigations

- USS/Echo: assess for associated malformations.
- Perineal inspection helps to decide management in most cases.
- Prone lateral shoot-through X-ray can occasionally demonstrate rectal gas close to a marked anal dimple.

Treatment. Low perineal fistula or membranes can be treated by a simple anoplasty. More complex anomalies should be managed with a divided sigmoid colostomy. This allows further evaluation prior to a more complicated reconstructive procedure that is also protected by the colostomy.

Necrotising Enterocolitis (NEC)

This is an ischaemic disorder of the intestine of the newborn. The aetiology of the disease is unknown, but bacterial infection, hypoxia and umbilical artery cannulation have been implicated. It is more common in premature infants, and 'epidemics' have occurred on neonatal intensive therapy units, suggesting an infective aetiology. There is some evidence that probiotics and breast milk can help prevent NEC.

Symptoms and Signs. Abdominal distension with tenderness, bilious aspirates, blood, mucus per rectum. Unwell premature baby.

Investigations

- Raised CRP, low platelets
- AXR shows distension of bowel.
- Later, a diagnostic radiological sign is intramural gas indicative of bowel wall necrosis.
- Free gas confirms intestinal perforation. Gas outlining the abdominal structures gives a 'football sign' appearance on X-ray.

Treatment. This is initially nonoperative unless perforation occurs. Resuscitation includes i.v. fluids and NG suction together with i.v. broad-spectrum antibiotics. Feeds are withheld and the baby is given TPN via a peripheral long line. Supportive intensive care may be required.

Laparotomy is required if there is evidence of perforation or failure of patient to improve on medical treatment. Gangrenous bowel is excised with anastomosis or temporary stoma.

Prognosis. The mortality rate is high in severe cases. Stricture may develop in healing bowel and present later.

Diaphragmatic Hernia

This occurs with an incidence of 1:4000 births. A hernia may occur through the foramen of Bochdalek, i.e. a defect in the pleuroperitoneal canal; through the foramen of Morgagni, between the xiphoid and costal margin; through a deficiency in the central tendon; or through a congenitally large oesophageal hiatus. Herniae through the foramen of Bochdalek are most common. Normal development of the ipsilateral lung is impaired and that of the contralateral lung may also be impaired.

Symptoms and Signs. May be diagnosed by prenatal USS. Presents with respiratory distress at birth. Apex beat displaced. Bowel sounds in chest. Scaphoid abdomen if the hernia is large and most of the bowel is in the chest.

Investigations

- CXR/AXR: mediastinal shift, abdominal viscera in thorax; lack of intestinal gas pattern in abdomen (Figure 21.3).

Treatment. If diagnosed antenatally, a few high-risk pregnancies may be considered for foetal surgery. Standard care is to electively intubate at birth. Advanced neonatal ventilation techniques such as 'gentle ventilation', nitric oxide and high-frequency oscillation may be required to combat pulmonary hypertension. Severe cases may be referred for Extra-Corporeal Membrane Oxygenation (ECMO). When ventilation is adequate and the patient is haemodynamically stable, closure of the defect is undertaken. May require prosthetic patch.

Prognosis. Mortality is high, especially with large defects, and is due to consequences of pulmonary hypoplasia. Use of a patch increases risk of recurrence.

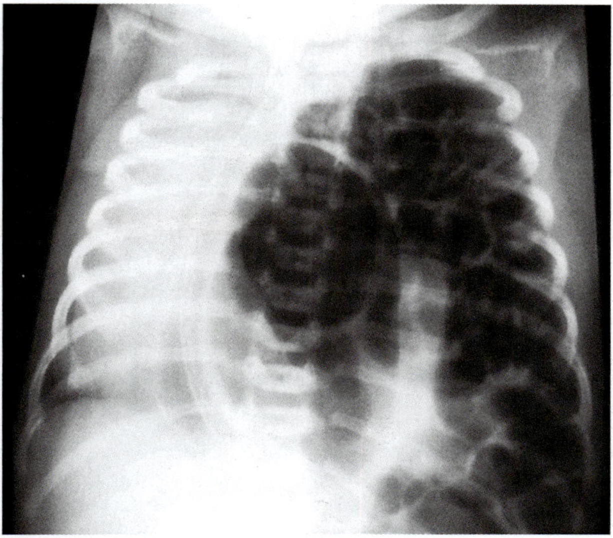

FIGURE 21.3

CXR of a neonate with a left diaphragmatic hernia. Note the hypoplastic lungs, mediastinal shift to the right, and gas in abdominal viscera in the left chest.

Hirschsprung's Disease

This occurs in 1:5000 births. There is a defect in the parasympathetic ganglia in the submucosal and myenteric plexus of the bowel wall. The aganglionic segment is present for a varying distance upwards from the anus and always involves the rectum. Rarely it affects the whole colon. The peristaltic waves stop at the affected segment and the proximal bowel becomes dilated and hypertrophied. The aganglionic segment remains contracted. It is more common in males than females.

Symptoms and Signs. Delayed passage of meconium in the newborn period. However, late presentation can occur, especially with short segment involvement, when it presents in infants and older children with constipation and abdominal distension. Digital rectal examination may demonstrate an empty rectum, which feels 'tight' on the examining finger.

Investigations

- AXR: multiple dilated loops of bowel
- Rectal biopsy shows absence of ganglion cells.
- Contrast enema may demonstrate the transition zone but is unreliable.

Treatment

1. If the baby is healthy, and only rectosigmoid Hirschsprung's is suspected, it may be managed by regular rectal washouts to clear the bowel followed by a pull-though operation, avoiding a colostomy if possible.

2. If the baby is ill or if a longer segment Hirschsprung's is suspected, then management is by initial defunctioning colostomy using frozen section specimens to ensure the stoma is 'ganglionic'. This can be followed several months later by the pull through operation combined with reversal of stoma.

Prognosis. Some infants develop Hirschsprung's enterocolitis which can be life threatening. Long-term outcomes are variable with a high incidence of constipation or faecal incontinence which require bowel management.

ABDOMINAL WALL DEFECTS

These occur with an incidence of 1:4000 births. There are two types, gastroschisis and exomphalos. Aetiology is unknown.

Gastroschisis

In this condition, there is a defect in the abdominal wall immediately adjacent to the umbilicus but the abdominal wall itself is completely formed. Coils of gut have no protective covering and are thick, oedematous and matted together. The diagnosis is obvious at birth.

Treatment. Primary closure of the defect may be possible after decompressing the gut and returning it to the peritoneal cavity. However, it may be necessary to avoid abdominal compartment syndrome, by reducing the bowel gradually using a silo technique before closure. A silo can be a preformed silicone device which has a flexible ring that is inserted beneath the fascial defect. The bowel is suspended within the silo and gradually compressed into the abdomen over a few days. Alternatively, a silo can be constructed from mesh and sewn to the fascia around the exposed viscera. It may be weeks or months before normal gastrointestinal (GI) motility is restored – long-term TPN may be required. Occasionally an intestinal atresia occurs necessitating further surgery.

Exomphalos

In this condition, the opening is at the umbilicus. The umbilical cord coverings continue into a sac, which covers the visceral protrusion. Chromosomal abnormalities, heart defects and also genitourinary malformations frequently occur.

Treatment. This is by either primary closure or staged repair. Larger defects can be managed with a mesh silo or conservatively by allowing the sac to epithelialise using dressings and bandaging.

Rare Abdominal Wall Defects

These include bladder exstrophy, cloacal exstrophy and prune belly syndrome.

Umbilical Hernia

See Chapter 13 p. 230.

ALIMENTARY TRACT PROBLEMS IN OLDER INFANTS AND CHILDREN

Congenital Hypertrophic Pyloric Stenosis

The aetiology of this condition is unknown. Progressive hypertrophy of the circular muscle of the pylorus occurs. The condition affects boys more than girls, being four times more common in boys, and occurs with an incidence of 1:4000 births. The first-born male child is most commonly affected. There is a familial tendency, especially on the maternal side.

Symptoms and Signs. The infant thrives for the first 3–4 weeks of life and then presents with projectile vomiting after feeds. The vomit is nonbilious. The infant is usually hungry and eager for further food after vomiting. Wasting is rare nowadays, but weight loss and dehydration are presenting features.

Diagnosis. This can be clinical by performing a test feed and palpating the thickened pylorus. In many units ultrasound diagnosis has superseded clinical palpation. The thickness of the muscle can be measured and absence of pyloric opening can be visualised.

HINTS AND TIPS

The test feed is a dying art! It is worth practising, as it can save time waiting for an ultrasound. Let the mother hold the baby in her lap and feed the baby. The abdomen is inspected for visible peristalsis passing from left to right across the epigastrium. Palpation is carried out during feeding for the classical 'olive'-shaped lump, which is felt deep to the right rectus muscle in the RUQ. Ensure the tips of your fingers dip under the liver edge. Aspirate the stomach with a nasogastric tube if it is too distended. Never sit facing the infant during this examination. You may experience the full impact of the projectile vomit!

Treatment. Ramstedt's operation (pyloromyotomy). This is an elective operation and should be carried out only after correction of any dehydration and the classical hypochloraemic hypokalaemic metabolic alkalosis. The stomach is emptied via an NG tube. Originally the operation was described using a right transverse abdominal incision. Generally, now it is performed either laparoscopically or via a supraumbilical incision. The serosa of the pylorus is then incised longitudinally along its anterosuperior border. The incision is deepened by splitting the thickened muscle until the mucosa pouts out, relieving the obstruction.

Complications. Postoperative recovery is rapid. There should be no mortality. Morbidity relates to accidental mucosal perforation or incomplete division of the thickened muscle.

Intussusception

This is the invagination of a portion of intestine into its lumen (Figure 21.4). It is commoner in children than adults. The peak incidence is between 6 and 9 months, although it may occur any time between 3 months and 3 years and occasionally in those younger and older than this age range. Most cases are ileocolic, but ileoileal and ileoileocolic may occur. In most cases, the aetiology is presumed to be due to hypertrophied Peyer's patches, but polyps, Meckel's diverticulum or intramural haematomas (Henoch–Schönlein purpura) may be contributory.

Symptoms and Signs. An otherwise healthy child presents with colicky abdominal pain and vomiting. The child often screams, draws up its knees to its chest and goes pale with an attack of colic. In between bouts of pain, the child appears normal. A first stool passed after onset of the pain may be normal, but 30% of subsequent stools contain blood and mucus, the so-called 'redcurrant jelly stool'. Palpation of the

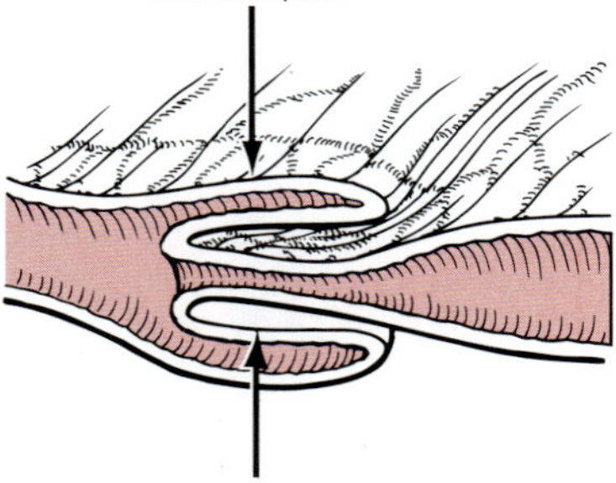

FIGURE 21.4
An intussusception.

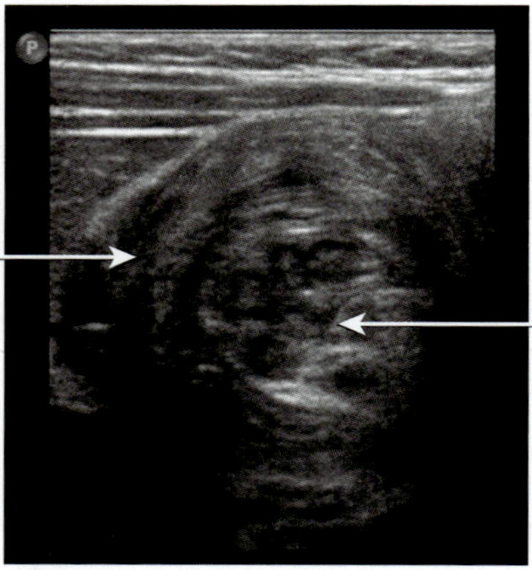

FIGURE 21.5
Ultrasound showing the typical target sign appearance of an ileocolic intussusception.

abdomen reveals a palpable sausage-shaped mass in the line of the colon. An empty RIF may be apparent on palpation as the swelling moves into the upper abdomen with peristalsis. PR examination may reveal blood or mucus. Occasionally, the apex of the intussusception may be palpable per rectum.

Investigations

- AXR may show abnormal gas distribution and signs of small bowel obstruction.
- Ultrasound is diagnostic and shows target sign (Figure 21.5).
- Air enema with X-ray screening.

Treatment. The child should be adequately resuscitated and given analgesia. The intussusception may be reduced by performing a pneumatic or hydrostatic reduction, monitoring the pressure applied and observing the reduction under X-ray screening. Barium should not be used as there is a risk of perforation.

Operation is required in patients with peritonitis, radiological signs of perforation, or failure of pneumatic reduction. Delayed presentation is a relative indication for surgery. At operation, the intussusceptum is reduced by gentle retrograde reduction, squeezing the apex out of its containing bowel. Traction should not be applied to the proximal bowel. If the bowel cannot be reduced or is gangrenous, resection is required.

Prognosis. Recurrence occurs in 1–2% after surgery but there is a 10% risk of recurrence after nonoperative treatment.

Obstructed Inguinal Hernia

This is a common cause of surgical admission in boys under the age of 2 years. It may also occur in girls when bowel or ovary may become irreducible. It is associated with a patent processus vaginalis. There is a higher incidence in premature babies. The condition may be bilateral.

Symptoms and Signs. A parent usually notices a tense lump in the groin of the crying child. Examination reveals an irreducible lump, which may extend into the scrotum.

Treatment. Analgesia may be given and a gentle attempt made to reduce the hernia. If the hernia does not reduce, surgical repair should be undertaken. If infarcted bowel is found, this must be resected. If the hernia does reduce, surgical repair should be delayed for 24–48h to allow oedema to resolve. It is prudent to electively repair inguinal herniae in neonates as soon as possible.

Acute Appendicitis

This is dealt with more fully in Chapter 15. Certain points, however, are relevant to appendicitis in children. The condition is rare under the age of 6 months. The stool is liquid and the appendiceal lumen relatively wide. Therefore, acute obstructive appendicitis is rare. It does, however, occur and may present with diarrhoea and vomiting and consequently be mistaken for gastroenteritis. Careful and repeated examination is therefore essential.

Mesenteric Adenitis

This is enlargement of mesenteric lymph nodes caused by an adenovirus infection. *Yersinia enterocolitica* has also been implicated. It affects young children and adolescents. Usually there is a preceding history of URTI, with sore throat and cervical lymphadenitis. Essentially, mesenteric adenitis is inflammation of Peyer's patches with secondary mesenteric lymphadenitis. The fever is usually higher than that of appendicitis, often 38–39°C. The abdominal pain is more diffuse, and examination reveals shifting tenderness rather than sharply localised tenderness in the RIF. Headache and mild photophobia may occur. These rarely occur in appendicitis. The WCC is usually raised, but there is a relative lymphocytosis rather than neutrophil leukocytosis as seen in acute appendicitis. Ultrasound may show multiple lymph nodes with absence of features suggesting appendicitis. Treatment is symptomatic.

Constipation

This is a common problem in children. The child is usually afebrile and relatively well, despite the abdominal pain which may be relieved by a macrogol laxative disimpaction regimen.

Urinary Tract Infections (UTIs)

There is abdominal pain and high pyrexia associated with dysuria, frequency and cloudy urine. Right pyelonephritis or cystitis may be mistaken for appendicitis. An FBC reveals neutrophil leukocytosis. An MSSU and microscopy reveal cells and organisms. Beware the presence of cells alone. Pelvic appendicitis may irritate the bladder, producing frequency and pyuria, but organisms will be absent on microscopy. Beware the presence of organisms *alone*, as it may be due to contamination from the foreskin or vulva. Treatment of UTI is with appropriate antibiotics. Further investigation is with USS.

Lower Lobar Pneumonia

In this condition, pain may be referred via the thoracic nerves to the lower abdomen. Right lower lobar pneumonia may refer pain to the RIF and be mistaken for acute appendicitis. It is important to observe the breathing pattern and auscultate the chest. Anteroposterior and lateral CXR will confirm diagnosis.

Testicular Torsion (→ Ch. 17)

> **HINTS AND TIPS**
>
> The pain from testicular torsion may radiate to the iliac fossa. The child may be embarrassed to draw attention to scrotal symptoms. Always examine the scrotum in a child with abdominal pain.

Crohn's Disease

Acute regional ileitis may occur in children.

Gynaecological Problems

Remember pregnancy may occur in very young girls. Onset of periods may be associated with acute lower abdominal pain. Ovulation can cause midcycle abdominal pain. Torsion of ovarian cyst or ovarian dermoid may occur (see Ch. 23).

CHRONIC AND RECURRENT ABDOMINAL PAIN

A common problem in children of school age, and many are referred to general surgery clinics. Occasionally the pain has a nonorganic basis. Organic causes include chronic constipation, Crohn's disease, UTIs, hydronephrosis, peptic ulceration. Gallstones are becoming more common in older children but may also be associated with haemolytic anaemia at any age. If the child has had previous abdominal surgery, adhesions should be considered. Chronic and recurrent abdominal pain in children may need to be jointly managed with a paediatrician and a paediatric surgeon.

> **HINTS AND TIPS**
>
> Assessing young children with abdominal pain is not easy. History-taking, and examination especially, requires a gentle approach and patience. Distraction is an important tool, as palpating the abdomen of a crying child is of no use. If this is the case, come back later. Blood tests may worsen this fear and contribute little. Ultrasound examination can be useful, especially in older girls. However, in young children the appendix is often not visible, although signs of significant inflammation or free fluid may be apparent unless it is performed very early in the course of the illness.

INFANTS WITH JAUNDICE

Neonates often develop physiological jaundice starting about 2 days after birth and lasting up to 2 weeks. Persistent jaundice beyond the first 3 weeks of life requires investigation. The two most common surgical causes are biliary atresia and choledochal cysts.

Biliary Atresia

This occurs with an incidence of 1:25,000 live births. The aetiology is unknown. It appears to develop after birth.

Symptoms and Signs. Presents from 2 weeks to 4 months. Usually a healthy child with persistent jaundice. Pale stools. Dark urine. Later hepatosplenomegaly, ascites. Without treatment, death from liver failure occurs within 2 years.

Investigations

- LFTs
- USS: obliterated ducts, shrunken or absent gallbladder
- Liver biopsy: bile duct proliferation with hepatocellular necrosis
- Isotope scan demonstrates absence of bile drainage.
- Diagnostic laparotomy with operative cholangiography – if a normal duct system is demonstrated, hepatitis should be suspected as a diagnosis
- α_1-antitrypsin deficiency and cystic fibrosis must also be excluded.

Treatment. If an extrahepatic duct can be found, a Roux loop of jejunum is anastomosed to it – this is called correctable biliary atresia. Usually extrahepatic ducts cannot be found, and a portoenterostomy (Kasai procedure) is necessary. Patent ducts are exposed in the porta hepatis and a Roux loop anastomosed to it. Intrahepatic biliary atresia (total absence of intrahepatic ducts) requires liver transplantation.

Prognosis. Optimal prognosis is achieved if Kasai is performed by 8 weeks of age. This is dependent on early recognition and transfer to a hepatobiliary centre. Initial clearance of jaundice can be achieved in 50–60% of patients, but only 45% will survive without liver transplantation at 10 years.

Choledochal Cyst

Cystic dilatation of the bile ducts is usually extrahepatic involving the common bile duct. The aetiology is unknown.

Symptoms and Signs. It occurs between 3 months and adult life. More common in females. Pain, jaundice, abdominal mass.

Investigations

- LFTs
- USS
- Magnetic resonance cholangiopancreatography (MRCP)/ endoscopic retrograde cholangiopancreatography (ERCP).

Treatment. Excision of CBD with Roux loop hepaticojejunostomy this may be performed with laparoscopic or robotic assistance. Severe forms with involvement of the intrahepatic ducts require liver transplantation. Residual CBD can develop malignancy.

ABDOMINAL MASSES IN CHILDHOOD

An abdominal mass is an uncommon reason for surgical referral in children. (For causes→Table 21.1.)

Symptoms and Signs. In addition to the mass, failure to thrive, nausea, vomiting, weight loss, abdominal pain, constipation, diarrhoea. Anaemia. Jaundice. Uraemia. UTI symptoms. Spontaneous bruising.

Investigations

- FBC
- ESR
- U&Es
- LFTs
- Urinalysis: 24-h urine (VMA in neuroblastoma)
- α-Fetoprotein (tumour marker for teratoma and hepatoblastoma)
- AXR
- CXR (metastases)
- USS: solid-v-cystic lesions

TABLE 21.1

ABDOMINAL MASSES IN CHILDHOOD

Gastrointestinal System	
	Pylorus (infantile pyloric stenosis) Constipation (faecal masses) Intussusception Crohn's disease
Hepato-Pancreatico-Biliary System	
Liver	Biliary atresia Portal hypertension
	Metastases Hepatitis Hepatoblastoma
Bile duct	Choledochal cyst
Pancreas	Pseudocyst
Genitourinary System	
	Hydronephrosis Nephroblastoma (Wilms') Bladder (urethral valves) Ovarian tumour or cyst
Other	
	Neuroblastoma Lymphoma Splenomegaly Retroperitoneal sarcoma Teratoma Other rare malignancies, e.g. primitive neuroectodermal tumour, rhabdomyosarcoma

- Computerised tomography (CT) scan: solid-v-cystic spread
- Magnetic resonance imaging (MRI): Tissue characterisation, central nervous system (CNS) involvement
- Bone scan, bone marrow aspirate
- Biopsy.

Treatment. This is of the underlying cause.

ABDOMINAL MALIGNANCIES IN CHILDHOOD

The commonest are neuroblastoma and nephroblastoma (Wilms' tumour). Neuroblastoma is the commonest extracerebral malignant solid tumour in children. Wilms' tumour accounts for about 10% of all the childhood tumours.

Abdominal Neuroblastoma

This is a highly malignant tumour arising from the neural crest. The commonest site is the adrenal gland. It occurs in children under the age of 5; 70% occur under 1 year. Metastases occur early.

Symptoms and Signs. Abdominal mass, failure to thrive, fever, anorexia, nausea, vomiting, diarrhoea. Metastases occur to liver, orbit, skull, long bones, spinal canal. Abdominal mass has a hard irregular surface and tendency to cross midline with vascular encasement.

Investigations

- AXR: calcification
- USS: solid lesion
- CT or MRI: size, site and metastases, and demonstrates displaced kidney
- 24-h urine VMA and HVA grossly elevated
- Tumour biopsy and or bone marrow aspirate: histological and cytogenetic tests.

Treatment. Localised tumours are excised. Unresectable primary and metastases require combination chemotherapy. Irradiation may be necessary. In neonates, tumour regression may be permanent. The older the child, the worse the prognosis.

Nephroblastoma (Wilms' Tumour)

This is an embryonic tumour of the kidney. The majority occur in the first 3 years of life. Less than 5% are bilateral. Metastases occur to the liver, lungs and regional nodes.

Signs and Symptoms. Abdominal mass, pain, haematuria, weight loss, fever. May be associated with abnormalities of the GU tract, Beckwith–Wiedemann syndrome and aniridia.

Investigations

- USS: solid tumour, vascular extension into renal vein and IVC
- CT (Figure 21.6) or MRI: size, site, metastases.

Treatment. Surgical resection before or after chemotherapy depending on protocol followed. Additional chemotherapy and radiotherapy depending on the stage; 80–90% chance of cure. If the condition is bilateral, partial nephrectomy may be possible following extended chemotherapy.

RECTAL BLEEDING IN CHILDREN

This is not an uncommon problem. Causes include fissure-in-ano, rectal polyps, rectal prolapse, Meckel's diverticulum, intussusception and blood dyscrasia.

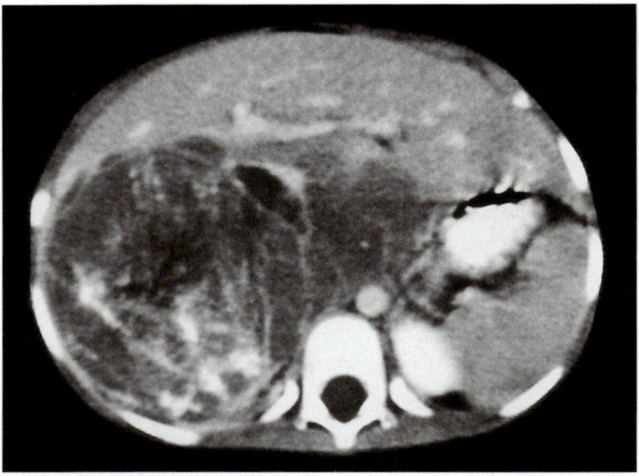

FIGURE 21.6
An abdominal CT scan of a child with an abdominal mass. There is an extensive nephroblastoma (Wilms' tumour) of the right kidney.

Fissure-in-Ano

Constipation causes a split in the mucosa of the anal canal. It is usually painful on defaecation. A vicious circle occurs with worsening constipation owing to fear of defaecation. There is blood on the stool and toilet paper. The fissure is often in the midline, usually posteriorly. Treatment involves explanation of the condition to the parent. Lactulose or a macrogol laxative helps to soften stool, and local anaesthetic is applied before and after defaecation. Most cases settle on this regimen. Persistent bleeding may require diltiazem cream or botulinum toxin injection to the sphincter. An examination under anaesthetic may be required to rule out other causes.

Polyps

In addition to bleeding, polyps may prolapse on their stalk if they are low enough in the rectum. Occasionally they may twist and auto-amputate and are passed PR. Occasionally they may precipitate intussusception. Treatment is by excision. If they are in the rectum, this may be done under GA using a proctoscope, the stalk being cut with diathermy. Higher polyps can be snared at colonoscopy.

Rectal Prolapse

This usually occurs around 2 years. Most cases settle spontaneously. Straining at stool precipitates the condition initially, which may then occur every time the child defaecates. There may be an underlying abnormality, e.g. spina bifida, previous anoplasty for imperforate anus or cystic fibrosis. Prolapse may involve the mucosa only or may involve the full thickness of the rectum.

Symptoms and Signs. Usually prolapse occurs with defaecation and returns spontaneously. The prolapsed mucosa may ulcerate and bleed.

Treatment. May settle spontaneously with toilet training and laxatives to relieve constipation. Persistent mucosal prolapse may be treated by submucosal injection of a sclerosant such as hypertonic saline or phenol. Rarely rectopexy may be required.

Meckel's Diverticulum

This is a remnant of the vitellointestinal duct which was attached to the umbilicus and is found on the antimesenteric border of the terminal ileum about 60 cm from the ileocaecal valve in an adult and proportionately nearer in a child. Rarely, this may bleed if it contains gastric mucosa, which produces acid and ulcerates the adjacent small bowel mucosa. Either bright red or dark red bleeding can occur, depending upon the degree of haemorrhage. Abdominal pain is usually absent. The presence of gastric mucosa in a Meckel's diverticulum may be demonstrated by a technetium scan. Treatment is by excision.

Intussusception

(See p. 529.)

NECK LUMPS IN CHILDREN

The general management of lumps in the neck is dealt with in Chapter 8. However, lumps in the neck are common in children, the most common cause being due to reactive lymphadenitis secondary to tonsillitis. The other causes of lumps in the neck in children are shown in Table 21.2.

Symptoms and Signs. Child may otherwise be well. Malaise. Pyrexia. Lethargy. Weight loss. Bruising. Bleeding. Rash. Cough. Signs of URTI, tonsillitis, inflamed tympanic membrane. Examine head and neck thoroughly for sites of primary lesion (infective or neoplastic). Check for lymphadenopathy elsewhere. Check for hepatosplenomegaly.

TABLE 21.2

LUMPS IN THE NECK IN CHILDHOOD

Anterior triangle	Lymph nodes: • Primary infection, e.g. atypical mycobacterium, TB, toxoplasmosis • Secondary infection, e.g. lymphadenitis • Primary tumours, e.g. Hodgkin's, leukaemia • Secondary tumour – rare Thyroglossal cyst Dermoid cyst Goitre Submandibular gland Branchial arch remnant
Posterior triangle	Lymph nodes Cystic hygroma (lymphangioma) Sternomastoid tumour Parotid swelling

Investigations

- FBC
- ESR
- U&Es
- LFTs
- TFTs (goitre)
- Paul–Bunnell
- Toxoplasmosis screen
- Mantoux
- CXR
- USS of lump
- CT: lump, spread.

Treatment. This is of the underlying disorder.

Chapter 22

Organ and Tissue Transplantation

Badri M. Shrestha • Teresa Diago Uso

CHAPTER OUTLINE

Transplantation has developed from an experimental procedure over 60 years ago to an established therapeutic option for most types of end-stage organ failure. Transplantation improves survival rates, improves the quality of life and is cost effective. The undergraduate is unlikely to need a great knowledge of transplantation but should understand the terms used, how to approach the family regarding organ donation, which organs it is possible to transplant, the types of immunosuppression used and the general complications of immunosuppression. It is particularly important to understand that opportunistic infections can arise in immunosuppressed patients and that advice regarding patient management should always be sought from the transplant unit, particularly for infective episodes.

CLASSIFICATION

This depends on the relationship between donor and recipient.

Autograft. Tissue is transferred from one area of the body to another in the same individual, e.g. skin grafts and kidney for renovascular disease.

Isografts. Tissue is transferred between genetically identical individuals (e.g. monozygotic twins).

Allografts. Tissue is transferred between genetically dissimilar individuals of the same species (e.g. deceased donor renal transplants).

Xenografts. Tissue is transferred between species. The only clinically applicable xenografts at the present time are porcine skin grafts in human burns victims and cardiac valves. Current research projects are trying to expand the use of xenograft, for example an isolated report of heart transplant from porcine donor was recently performed with poor outcomes.

ORGAN AND TISSUE DONORS

Organs and tissues may be obtained from:

- Deceased donors – donation after brain death (DBD; heart beating donors) or donation after circulatory death (DCD; nonheart beating donors)
- Living donors

Exponential increase in the demand for organs resulted in increased gap between organs available and patients waiting for an organ. While in the East world 90% of the transplants are living donors, only around 20% are living donors in the West, where the efforts to increase the donor–recipient gap was placed on split livers, domino and extended criteria including donors after cardiac death.

Deceased Donors

Donation After Brain Death (DBD)

Brainstem Death

A brain death donor is a donor deceased by neurologic criteria, the remaining of the decease organ donors are deceased by circulatory death (donor after circulatory death). Brain death is the complete and irreversible cessation of cerebral and brainstem function. This is covered in detail in Chapter 19.

General Criteria (→ Table 22.1). As the decease organ shortage is becoming more severe, it was realised that ideal requirements for selection of organ donors were not feasible. Selection criteria for solid organ donors have therefore recently been extended. Organs that long ago would not have been considered for transplantation are currently

TABLE 22.1

GENERAL CRITERIA FOR DECEASED DONORS

Brainstem Dead With Intact Circulation
Cause of death: • Cerebral trauma • Cerebral haemorrhage • Hypoxic brain injury • Primary cerebral tumour (histologically proven) • Cardiac arrest with brain death
Absolute Contraindications (NHSBT UK Guidelines 2011)
• Cancer with evidence of spread outside affected organ (including lymph nodes) within 3 years of donation (however localised prostate, thyroid, in situ cervical cancer and nonmelanotic skin cancers are acceptable) • Active melanoma • Choriocarcinoma • Active haematological malignancies (myeloma, lymphoma, leukaemia) • Definite, probable or possible causes of human TSE, including CJD and vCJD, individuals whose blood relatives have had CJD, other neurodegenerative diseases associated with infectious agents • TB: active or within 6 months of start of treatment • Malaria: if not fully treated • Meningoencephalitis for which no infection has been identified • HIV disease (but not HIV infection)

CJD, Creutzfeldt–Jakob disease; TSE, transmissible spongiform encephalopathy.

being used, bringing in a new class of organ donor termed 'ECD' formerly known as 'extended criteria donor'. For example, a kidney ECD is any brain-dead donor aged >60 years or donor aged >50 with two of the following conditions: a history of hypertension; a terminal serum creatinine level >1.5, or death resulting from a cerebrovascular accident. Selection of liver, heart and heart/lung donors depends on size match with the recipient and/or crossmatch, depending on the organ. Although in the past no attempt was made to match other than on blood group compatibility with these organs, nowadays blood type-incompatible transplantation has been successfully attempted.

Obtaining Permission for Deceased Organ Donation. This varies from country to country. Laws allowing consent for organ donation differ from country to country, and, therefore, donation rates also vary widely. However, the basic principles are listed below.

1. A potential donor should be identified by the consultant in charge of the patient.
2. Contact may be made with a transplant team prior to establishment of brainstem death to assess if the donor is suitable for organ donation.
3. The first set of brainstem death criteria is carried out. If they are satisfied, the question of organ donation may be raised with the relatives. Consent should not be obtained until two sets of brainstem death criteria have been obtained.
4. If the relatives wish to know more about what is involved in transplantation, the Transplant Coordinators will speak to them and explain the details.
5. Blood is taken for tissue typing, blood group, HIV and hepatitis B and C screening, CMV and EBV.
6. Confidentiality must always be maintained.
7. Bereavement counselling and follow-up support should be arranged for the family; the Transplant Coordinators can also help with this.

Donation After Circulatory Death (DCD)

This type of organ donation applies to renal, liver, pancreas, lung and heart transplantation; tissues such as heart valves, corneas, bone, can also be removed from this type of donor. The distinction between a DBD and DCD donor lies in the mode of death. DBD donors usually die from an intracranial catastrophe (→Table 22.1), the mode of death being classified as 'brainstem death'. In DCD donors, the patient dies from a circulatory arrest, their death being classified as a 'circulatory death'. A warm ischaemic time of less than 40 min is desirable but depends on the organ. There are five types of DCD donors (Maastricht criteria). They may be classified as *controlled* (cardiac arrest is anticipated and gives time for organisation of necessary resources; category III) or *uncontrolled* (donor dies without warning, thus the ischaemic time is longer as resources are not readily available; categories I, II and IV). The groups of DCD donors are classified as follows:

I. Dead on arrival at hospital
II. Unsuccessful resuscitation
III. Awaiting cardiac arrest
IV. Cardiac arrest in brainstem dead patient
V. Unexpected cardiac arrest in patients in an ITU

HINTS AND TIPS

There is a gross shortage of organ donors around the world. If you think a patient is a suitable donor, speak to your consultant in the first instance. Then discuss the patient's potential for donation with the Specialist Nurse Organ Donation (SNOD) before making any approach to those close to the patient. Be in a position to supply the clinical details to the SNOD. A multidisciplinary team (MDT) will then be responsible for planning the approach and discussing organ donation with those close to the patient. The MDT should include the medical and nursing staff involved in the care of the patient, led throughout the process by an identifiable consultant; the SNOD; and, where relevant, a local faith representative.

Living Donors

This type of organ donation relates mainly to renal and liver transplantation, although it is now possible to transplant segments of pancreas, segments of small bowel and lobes of lung from living donors. For example, at the present time, more than 45% of renal transplants in the UK are carried out from living donors owing to the shortage of deceased donors. Living donation, like deceased donation, is regulated by the Human Tissue Authority (HTA) under the Human Tissue Act 2004 in UK.

Categories of living donation established under the Act are:

1. Directed (i.e. the organ is directed to a known recipient):
   a. Genetically related (formerly living related)
   b. Emotionally related (living unrelated)
   c. Paired
2. Nondirected (i.e. the organ is for a recipient whose identity is unknown as with deceased donation):
   a. Domino
   b. Altruistic

Directed

Genetically and Emotionally Related. This is donation to a known person, i.e. brother to sister, parent to child, husband to wife or between friends. Under the Human Tissue Act, the approval process is the same for directed genetically and directed emotionally related organ donation. Both will be dealt with by a local independent assessor who is trained and accredited by the HTA and who will assess all donor/recipient pairs and, where the requirements have been met, will give approval for the transplant to proceed.

Paired Donation. This relates to circumstances where a close relation, friend or partner is fit and able to donate but kidney transplant may not be possible or be associated with high risk due to blood group incompatibility, positive crossmatch or combination of both. That couple can be matched to another couple in a similar situation so that both individuals in need of a transplant receive a well-matched organ.

Nondirected

Domino. This is when a patient with a metabolic disorder receives a new liver and that liver is transplanted to another recipient. For example, a patient with familial amyloidosis.

ALTRUISTIC. This is when a person offers to donate an organ to anyone who might benefit, i.e. a complete stranger. Before such organ transplants are undertaken, it is essential that all medical, surgical and psychiatric assessments necessary to ensure fitness to donate have been completed. The independent assessor must be satisfied that all procedures have been fully complied with before any application for a nondirected altruistic donation is sent to the HTA panel for approval.

Independent Assessors

Independent assessors are trained persons, i.e. medical consultants or someone of equivalent registered professional status, independent of the transplant team. They are trained to approve all living organ donations, both directed and nondirected. The role of the independent assessor is to act on behalf of the HTA in an altruistic capacity and to satisfy the requirements of the Human Tissue Act.

Work-up for a Living Donor

For a genetically related donor, there are three potential histocompatibility matches:

- 'Perfect match' (2 haplotype match): all antigens match. There is a 25% chance of this occurring.
- 'Half match' (1 haplotype mismatch): half the antigens match. There is a 50% chance of this occurring.
- 'No match': no antigens match. There is a 25% chance of this occurring. In the past it was rare to use such a donor but it is now clear that the results from a 'no-matched' live related donor are almost as good as those from a well-matched deceased donor.

The following sequence is undertaken (and/or additional work-up depending on organ type):

- Identify a potential donor.
- Give full explanation of procedure and risks.
- Medical and surgical history, physical examination, social history
- Take blood for blood group, tissue typing and cross match to identify compatibility.
- Urinalysis: exclude proteinuria, haematuria, infection
- CBC, BMP, ESR, U&Es, creatinine, LFTs, glucose, hypercoagulable work-up
- Infection screen: HAV, HBV, HCV, HIV, CMV, EBV, TB
- Creatinine clearance, glomerular filtration rate (GFR) via ^{51}Cr-ethylenediaminetetraacetic acid (^{51}Cr-EDTA)
- Autoimmune disorders work-up
- Chest X-ray (CXR), computerised tomography (CT) chest/abdomen– magnetic resonance cholangiopancreatography (MRCP; if liver)
- Cardiac testing: EKG/ ECHO
- Cancer screening
- Anaesthesia, bioethics and psychiatry evaluation.

For example, in the case of renal transplant, if all of the above are satisfactory, the patient undergoes a CT angiography and urography to assess the renal vasculature and to check for any abnormality in the excretory system. It is ideal that at least one kidney should have a single renal artery to anastomose to the recipient's internal iliac artery (end-to-end) or to the recipient's external iliac artery (end-to-side). Although kidneys with multiple arteries can be used in deceased donor transplantation as they can be removed with a Carrel patch of aorta, clearly this is not the case with a living donor. However, with living donors it is possible to use kidneys with multiple arteries, e.g. two equal-sized arteries may be anastomosed in a double-barrelled fashion before being anastomosed to the recipient's arteries, or a small polar artery may be anastomosed to the side of the main renal artery.

If angiography and urography are normal, the donor–recipient pair will be referred to the independent assessor who will send a report to the clinician responsible for the donor and a copy to the HTA indicating that the transplant may go ahead.

Living Donor Nephrectomy (LDN)

Laparoscopic or robotic removal of kidney has become a routine where the kidney is removed through a 6–10cm suprapubic incision once the mobilisation and division of the blood vessels and ureter is completed. Open nephrectomy is reserved for cases where previous abdominal surgery has led to adhesions making access to the kidney unsafe. LDN has resulted in less pain, shorter hospitalisation, a reduced duration of convalescence and better cosmesis, compared with the open flank approach. LDN is done through transperitoneal or retroperitoneal approach, which can be either total or hand-assisted.

COMPLICATIONS OF LDN. These include: bleeding; wound infection; chest infection; urinary tract infection, persistent wound pain and incisional hernia; ileus, pneumothorax, DVT; pulmonary embolism and mortality (1:3000–6000). The donor should be warned that if subsequently they develop trauma to, or a tumour in, their one remaining kidney, they may require nephrectomy and dialysis themselves.

Tissue Typing and Crossmatch

ABO COMPATIBILITY. In the past, ABO compatibility has been essential. However, currently, ABO-incompatible transplants are being carried out with good success (see below.)

HISTOCOMPATIBILITY MATCHING HLA are encoded on the short arm of chromosome 6; these code for the antigens involved in transplant rejection. Class I molecules consist of HLA-A, B, and C; class II molecules consist of HLA-DP, DQ and DR. HLA-A, B and DR are generally considered the most important, a perfect match at the DR locus being associated with improved graft survival in deceased donor renal transplants. Each locus is highly variable and thus gives rise to numerous combinations. The HLA matching of patients is expressed as the HLA 'mismatch' – this describes how well-matched the kidney is and the mismatched HLA molecules are relevant to rejection. Despite complete HLA matching, even in twin transplants, rejections do occur due to immune response to non-HLA antigens.

Some examples of HLA matching are given below:

1.	A6, A3	B27, B15	DR3, DR15 Donor
	A2, A3	**B7, B8**	**DR3, DR12 Recipient**
2.	A1, A24	B8, B44	DR4, DR15 Donor
	A1, A3	**B27, B15**	**DR4, DR15 Recipient**

In example (1) the recipient is a 1–2–1 mismatch. In example (2) the recipient is a 1–2–0 mismatch.

Cytotoxic Crossmatch. The recipient's blood is tested for cytotoxic antibodies against antigens on donor T lymphocytes using either complement-dependent lymphocytotoxicity or flow cytometric crossmatch techniques. If such antibodies are present, they would lead to hyperacute antibody-mediated rejection and destroy the transplanted kidney. Therefore, a negative crossmatch is desirable. Pretransplant crossmatch is performed routinely for kidney and pancreas transplants and in selected recipients of heart transplants. Prospective crossmatch is not necessary for liver transplants.

ABO-Incompatible and Positive Crossmatch Living Donor Kidney Transplantation

The presence of anti-A/B blood group antibodies and donor-specific antibodies (DSA) has been considered a contraindication to transplantation for the risk of hyperacute rejection. Currently, kidney transplants between ABO-incompatible donors and recipients and recipients with DSA and positive crossmatch are carried out by removing the antibodies pretransplantation, by either immunoabsorption or plasmapheresis, until a low level of antibody (1:8) is reached. The patient then receives rituximab (anti-CD20 monoclonal antibody against B cells) or intravenous immunoglobulin. Induction with antithymocyte globulin or basiliximab in combination with tacrolimus, mycophenolate mofetil (MMF) and prednisolone followed by maintenance with last three drugs has produced a 1-year graft survival of over 95%. Frequent monitoring of antibody levels, low threshold for biopsy and aggressive treatment for antibody-mediated rejection is needed for good outcome.

ORGAN PRESERVATION

Organs are perfused with a balanced salt solution, e.g. University of Wisconsin or HTK solution at 4°C, and are stored surrounded by the same solution in sterile bags, which in turn are surrounded by crushed ice. Nowadays, most of the organs are also preserved by hypothermic or normothermic perfusion machines. This is ideal for marginal donors and DCD donors.

SITTING OF THE TRANSPLANT

Orthotopic. The organ is situated in the place where the diseased organ had been, e.g. heart and liver transplantation.

Heterotopic. The new organ is placed in a different site from the native organ, e.g. renal transplantation – the kidney is placed in the iliac fossa.

REJECTION

There are four types of rejection.

Hyperacute

This occurs with ABO incompatibility or preformed cytotoxic antibodies. It occurs on the operating table (hours or minutes post organ implantation). It is caused by the presence of pre-existing antibodies in the recipient that recognise antigens in the donor organ. This irreversible damage causes thrombosis and graft necrosis. In the case of the kidney, it is seen to be flaccid, cyanotic and eventually thrombosis. Nephrectomy is required, often at the time of transplantation or within 24h. The incidence of this type of rejection is decrease thanks to pre-transplant screening for antibodies to donor tissues.

Note that due to organs shortage, nowadays ABO-incompatible transplant can be carefully performed.

Accelerated Acute Rejection

Rapid onset within a few days after transplantation. It results from prior sensitisation to HLA antigens.

Acute Rejection

This is the most common form of rejection, and the majority occur within 3 months of transplantation. Two distinct types are seen:

Cell-Mediated. The recipient T lymphocytes are activated in response to the alloantigens and attack the organ causing damage, which is predominantly cell mediated and usually easily reversible by appropriate treatment (see below).

Antibody-Mediated. Antibody-mediated rejection is being increasingly recognised due to routine monitoring of antibodies directed against the mismatched HLA antigens. Complement activation and injury to the vascular endothelium leads to more severe injury to the allograft, which requires more intensive treatment.

Chronic Allograft Injury. Chronic allograft rejection is the commonest cause of late graft loss which results from the interplay of immune and nonimmune factors. It is an insidious form of rejection that leads to graft destruction over the course of months or years. It is related to either vascular damage or parenchymal damage causing fibrosis. For example, in renal transplant clinical manifestations include proteinuria, hypertension and progressive deterioration of renal function. Histology shows interstitial fibrosis, tubular atrophy, glomerulosclerosis and obliterative arteriolopathy. Management includes use of least nephrotoxic immunosuppressive drugs, control of hypertension and proteinuria with ACE inhibitors.

IMMUNOSUPPRESSION

All transplant patients require immunosuppression for life, although clinical studies for transplant tolerance are in progress. Large doses are given in the perioperative period (induction immunosuppression), but these are gradually scaled down to maintenance dose over a few months post-transplant. Polyclonal (ATG) or monoclonal antibodies (basiliximab) are being used routinely as induction agents in combination with other agents such as corticosteroids, antiproliferative drugs, e.g. azathioprine and MMF, CNIs, e.g. ciclosporin and tacrolimus, and mTOR inhibitor, e.g. sirolimus and everolimus. Rejection episodes are treated with pulsed doses of methylprednisolone, polyclonal (ATG) or monoclonal (rituximab) antibodies. The immunosuppressive agents are tailored to the individual recipient based on the degree of HLA-mismatches, sensitisation, graft function and drug tolerance. The most commonly used regimen includes basiliximab, tacrolimus, MMF and prednisolone combination.

Corticosteroids

Prednisolone is usually used in combination with CNI and antiproliferative agents. It has multiple anti-inflammatory effects, as well as immunosuppressive effects, the latter mainly the result in inhibition of cytokine (IL-1 and TNF-α) production and nonspecific effects on cell-mediated and humoral immunity. A high dose of prednisolone is given during transplantation (1000 mg i.v. followed by usually 0.3 mg/kg body weight/day), which is gradually decreased, and stopped depending on the organ. Pulsed doses of methylprednisolone are an effective treatment for acute rejection episodes. The side effects of corticosteroid include cushingoid features, hypertension, peptic ulceration, poor wound healing, acne, easy bruising, osteoporosis, myopathy, cataracts, stunted growth, pancreatitis, avascular necrosis of bone, hyperglycaemia and diabetes.

Antiproliferative Drugs

These include azathioprine, which was the first widely used immunosuppressive drug, and the newer drug, MMF. Azathioprine is metabolised to 6-mercaptopurine by the liver, and this in turn inhibits DNA and RNA synthesis by interfering with purine metabolism. In so doing, it inhibits proliferation of lymphocytes in response to antigenic stimulation and impairs antibody response. Side effects include nausea and vomiting, rashes, agranulocytosis, leukopenia, hepatic dysfunction, malignancy (especially skin malignancies and lymphoid tumours). MMF has a greater effect than azathioprine in preventing rejection, the active compound being mycophenolic acid. It blocks the proliferation of T and B cells by the reversible inhibition of the enzyme inosine monophosphate dehydrogenase (IMPDH). This enzyme is involved in the synthesis of guanosine nucleotides, which are required for DNA and RNA synthesis; lymphocytes are preferentially affected as other cells have salvage pathways. The main side effects of MMF include haematological effects (anaemia and leukopenia) and gastrointestinal (GI) effects, particularly abdominal pain, diarrhoea and, in some cases, GI haemorrhage. The GI side effects are managed by reducing the dosage.

Calcineurin Inhibitors

These include ciclosporin and tacrolimus. Cyclosporin is a fungal metabolite that inhibits the enzyme calcineurin, thereby preventing the dephosphorylation and translocation of the nuclear factor of activated T-cells (NF-AT), which is essential for IL-2 gene transcription within the nucleus. This prevents IL-2 production, which is essential for the proliferation and clonal expansion of cytotoxic T lymphocytes. It has considerably improved the results of organ transplantation since its introduction in 1983. The dose is titrated to trough level in the blood. Side effects include nephrotoxicity, hypertension, hirsutism, tremor, gingival hyperplasia, hepatotoxicity, hyperlipidaemia and gout. Tacrolimus is more potent than cyclosporin and has a similar mechanism of action to cyclosporin. Tacrolimus is proven to be more effective in reducing the incidence of acute rejection and prolonging the graft survival, compared with ciclosporin. This has led to a wider use of tacrolimus in solid organ transplantation. The side effects of tacrolimus are similar to those of ciclosporin except that there is a lower incidence of hirsutism and gingival hyperplasia with tacrolimus, but it is more neurotoxic and diabetogenic compared with ciclosporin. The incidence of BK polyoma virus has increased with the use of tacrolimus.

mTOR Inhibitors

Sirolimus and everolimus are potent immunosuppressive agents that block T-cell proliferation by inhibiting the mTOR, which is essential for activation of S6 kinase and progression of cell cycle from G1 to S phase. Sirolimus, in combination with ciclosporin, has reduced acute rejection rate significantly and has proven useful in the management of CAI. Side effects include thrombocytopenia, hypercholesterolemia and hypertriglyceridemia, mouth ulcers, wound dehiscence and lymphocele.

Polyclonal Antibodies

Polyclonal antibodies are produced by immunising horses or rabbits with human lymphoid tissue/thymocytes. The resulting immune sera are then harvested. Two types are used:

- Antilymphocyte globulin (ALG)
- Antithymocyte globulin (ATG).

They can be used for induction of immunosuppression and the treatment of rejection. Severe depletion of both T and B lymphocytes occurs following their administration through complement mediated and antibody-dependent cellular cytotoxicity. Complications include anaphylaxis and a high incidence of viral infection, particularly CMV.

Monoclonal Antibodies

Monoclonal antibodies in clinical use are:

- Anti-CD3 (cluster of differentiation-3) antibodies – OKT-3
- Anti-IL-2 receptor (IL-2R) antibodies – basiliximab and daclizumab
- Anti-CD20 antibody – rituximab.

OKT-3 is directed against the CD3 antigen of T lymphocytes, binding leading to a reduction in the number of CD3+ T lymphocytes in the circulation. OKT3 was used for induction immunosuppression and in the treatment of steroid-resistant acute rejection, and its use has been discontinued due to severe side effects resulting from the release of cytokine following lympholysis such as fever, hypotension, pulmonary oedema and fatal myocardial depression. Administration of antihistamines, steroid and antipyretic is needed to ameliorate these manifestations. There is a higher incidence of herpes virus reactivation, opportunistic infections (cytomegalovirus and fungi) and Epstein–Barr-associated lymphoproliferative disorders and B cell lymphomas.

Anti-IL-2R antibodies (basiliximab and daclizumab) bind to the IL-2 receptor and thus inhibit IL-2 mediated responses. They are given preoperatively in combination with ciclosporin and prednisolone as a routine and have proven to decrease acute rejection. They are not effective in the treatment of acute rejection. Side effects have not been reported.

Anti-CD20 monoclonal antibody (rituximab) is used in transplants involving ABO incompatibility. It is also used as induction therapy in highly sensitised patients prior to kidney transplantation and as rescue agent to treat antibody-mediated rejection. The symptoms related to cytokine release are minimal.

Currently, proteasome inhibitor (bortezomib), co-stimulation blocker (belatacept), JAK-3 inhibitor (tasocitinib), protein kinase-C inhibitor (sotrastaurin), anti-C5 monoclonal antibody (eculizumab) anti-leucocyte function action inhibitors (natalizumab and efalizumab) and TNF-α inhibitor (infliximab) are also used.

SPECIFIC ORGANS

Kidney Transplant

Recipient. Over 50% of patients with chronic kidney disease are suitable for transplantation. Severe compromise of the cardiovascular system is the main reason for unsuitability for a transplant. Some diseases may recur in the transplant kidney, e.g. mesangiocapillary glomerulonephritis, focal segmental glomerulosclerosis and IgA nephropathy. If malignancy was the cause of renal failure, e.g. bilateral nephrectomy for Wilms' tumour or renal carcinoma, a period of time should be allowed for recurrence to occur. If it does not occur within that time period, then the patient is reassessed for transplantation.

Donor. HLA typing is essential. Ideally, crossmatch should be negative. Kidneys can be safely kept for 36h, and occasionally up to 48h. Recently perfusion machines can extend the perfusion time.

Operation. This is heterotopic, the kidney being placed extraperitoneally in either the RIF or the LIF. The renal vein is anastomosed to the external iliac vein. The renal artery is anastomosed either end-to-end to the internal iliac artery or end-to-side to the external iliac artery. The ureter is anastomosed to the dome of the bladder. Some 80% of kidneys from DBD donors function immediately; 20% show delayed function due to ATN and require dialysis until the kidney begins to function.

Diagnosis of Rejection

- Clinical: general malaise, fever (rare), increased weight, decreased urine output
- Laboratory: increased serum creatinine, decreased creatinine clearance
- Radioisotope scan: MAG3 scan shows reduced perfusion
- Biopsy: core biopsy with a Tru-Cut needle. This is the Gold Standard.

Complications

Early

- Vascular – bleeding, renal artery thrombosis, renal vein thrombosis
- Urological – ureteric leak and ureteric necrosis
- Lymphocele
- Acute rejection – occurs in approximately 20% of patients
- Primary nonfunction (the kidney never functions)
- Delayed graft function.

Late

- Chronic allograft injury
- Vascular – renal artery stenosis
- Urological – ureteric stenosis (obstruction)
- Recurrent disease
- Infections (see below)
- Malignancy (see below).

Results

- 90–95% 1-year graft survival and 70–80% 5-year survival

HINTS AND TIPS

Patients who have had renal transplants frequently appear in undergraduate final OSCE examinations, especially for abdominal examination. It is therefore important to know that kidney transplantation is a heterotopic transplant and is placed in either the right or the left iliac fossa. Therefore, if you locate a smooth, fixed swelling deep in either iliac fossa underlying a surgical incision, either a Gibson's incision or a J-shaped (hockey stick) incision, it is likely to be a transplanted kidney. A further clue to the diagnosis is that the patient may have a pre-existing arteriovenous fistula for dialysis (usually in the upper limb), other abdominal scars suggesting previous continuous ambulatory peritoneal dialysis, or a scar on the neck after parathyroidectomy for secondary or tertiary hyperparathyroidism.

Liver Transplant

RECIPIENT. Indications for liver transplantation include: Fulminant hepatic failure following hepatitis or drug overdose. Extrahepatic biliary atresia or hypoplasia. Inborn errors of metabolism including (alpha-I antitrypsin, Crigler-Najjar disease, glycogen storage disease, Wilson's disease, hemochromatosis, familial amyloidotic polyneuropathy and other). Sclerosing cholangitis. Hepatic vein thrombosis (Budd-Chiari). Cirrhosis including (alcohol, biliary cirrhosis, chronic active hepatitis (A, B, C, non A, non B, auto-immune; congenital biliary cirrhosis, cryptogenic cirrhosis, hemochromatosis, alpha-I antitrypsin deficiency, NASH). Tumour with strict criteria (HCC, cholangiocarcinoma and colorectal metastasis).

DONOR. Blood group match (ABO incompatibility in process). No HLA undertaken in cadaveric donors, and cytotoxic crossmatch taken but used only to assess post-transplant risk of rejection and adjust IS. Size compatibility is important. Cold preservation for up to 15h using HTK or University of Wisconsin solution, and new normothermic perfusion machines are currently in use allowing longer preservation time. Liver reduction or split techniques have been developed based on segmental anatomy of the liver such that parts of adult livers may be used in paediatric and adult patients. Living related liver transplantation may also be undertaken, using right lobe, left lobe or left lateral segment.

Operation. This is an orthotopic operation. The recipient's liver is removed. The donor vena cava is anastomosed to the recipient vena cava above and below the liver (Conventional technique) or a common cuff fashioned between the right, middle and left hepatic veins can be anastomosed to the donor vena cava (Piggyback technique). The portal vein is anastomosed end-to-end. The donor hepatic artery is anastomosed usually to the common hepatic artery of the recipient. End-to-end biliary tract anastomosis is performed.

Diagnosis of Rejection. Elevation of liver enzymes. Biopsy.

Complications

EARLY

- Vascular – bleeding, hepatic artery thrombosis, hepatic artery stenosis and portal vein thrombosis. Outflow.
- Biliary – biliary leaks and strictures
- Acute rejection
- Primary graft nonfunction – rare.

LATE

- Chronic rejection –'vanishing bile duct syndrome'
- Recurrent of primary disease
- Infections (see below)
- Malignancy (see below).

Results

- 1-year graft survival depends upon the underlying liver disease. For chronic liver disease the 1-year graft survival is in excess of 90% but for fulminant hepatic failure is lower.
- 5-year graft survival is around 70%.

Some individuals have lived for more than 25 years after liver transplantation. Late graft loss is less common than for other forms of solid organ transplantation. About 20% of liver transplants at 5 years post-transplant appear to accept their liver grafts with low need for continuing immunosuppression.

Heart and Heart/Lung Transplant

RECIPIENT. End-stage heart disease with survival of 1 year unlikely, e.g. viral myocarditis, cardiomyopathies, severe IHD. Heart and lung transplants are usually carried out for cardiac problems associated with pulmonary vascular hypertension. The four possible lung transplant operations are heart/lung, double lung, sequential single lung or single lung transplantation. The procedure used depends upon the lung condition. The commonest causes for lung transplantation in general are cystic fibrosis, bronchiectasis, primary pulmonary hypertension, emphysema and idiopathic pulmonary fibrosis.

DONOR. Blood group match. HLA or cytotoxic crossmatch not required but ideal when possible. Size compatibility important. A safe time limit for cold ischaemia for the heart used to be 4–6h, again now modified with the new perfusion machines. The lungs are less tolerant of ischaemia than the heart. The lungs are usually ventilated with 80% oxygen and kept semi-inflated if storage.

Operation

Heart. This is an orthotopic operation, the recipient's heart being removed. The recipient pulmonary veins are anastomosed to the left atrium and the recipient right atrium to the donor right atrium. The aorta and pulmonary arteries are anastomosed end-to-end to the corresponding recipient vessels. The operation is carried out on cardiopulmonary bypass.

Lung. The technique depends upon whether it is a double lung transplant, sequential single lung transplant, or single lung transplant. A single lung transplant offers the advantage of maximum use of donor organs and relative technical simplicity. Cardiopulmonary bypass is not required. The main disadvantage of the single lung transplant is that there is only a limited amount of lung tissue and complications may result from the remaining diseased lung. The operation is therefore unsuitable for infective lung conditions such as bronchiectasis or cystic fibrosis.

Diagnosis of Rejection

Heart. Cardiac arrhythmias. Regular endomyocardial biopsies via forceps inserted via the external jugular vein and guided to the endocardium under radiographic control.

Lung. Acute rejection is characterised by fever, lethargy, hypoxia and infiltrates on CXR. The diagnosis is confirmed by biopsy (bronchoscopic and transbronchial).

Complications

Heart. Cardiac arrhythmias and death. Sepsis. Chronic rejection with small vessel disease and recurrent angina.

Lung. Late complications include infection, obliterative bronchiolitis and malignancy.

Results

Heart, Heart/Lung

- 85–90%- 1-year graft survival
- 75% 5-year graft survival.

Lung

- 80% 1-year graft survival
- 50–60% 5-year graft survival.

Pancreatic Transplant

RECIPIENT. These are juvenile-onset diabetics with recurrent hypoglycaemic unawareness, who have concomitant renal failure and require kidney transplantation in addition. The aim is to prevent the development of other microangiopathic complications. The kidney and pancreas from the same donor are usually transplanted simultaneously, one organ into the RIF, the other into the LIF. The use of pancreatic transplantation alone to attempt to prevent the complications of diabetes is increasing.

DONOR. Blood group match. No history of diabetes. No family history of diabetes. Normal blood sugar.

Operation. This is usually a heterotopic transplant; the pancreas being placed in either the right or the left iliac fossa. The majority of pancreatic transplants are whole pancreatic transplants with bladder or enteric exocrine drainage. The pancreas is removed with a duodenal segment, the latter being anastomosed to the bladder or the terminal ileum. The vascular anastomoses are based on the splenic artery, superior mesenteric artery and portal vein. These are anastomosed to the iliac vessels.

Diagnosis of Rejection. Blood labs. Isotope scans. Reduction in urinary amylase where the pancreas is drained into the bladder. Biopsy.

Complications. Bleeding, graft thrombosis, graft pancreatitis, pancreatic fistulae, perigraft collections, fibrosis.

Results. According to the expertise of the centre where the transplant is carried out, there is a 50–80% 1-year graft survival. In centres with considerable experience of pancreatic transplantation, where the pancreas and kidneys are transplanted simultaneously the 1-year graft survival is 80%, with a 5-year graft survival of 75%. Where pancreas transplantation alone is carried out, the 1-year graft survival is only around 50%.

The poor results and complications have encouraged an attempt to transplant isolated islets of Langerhans. These are injected via the portal vein into the liver. Encouraging results are being reported.

Small Bowel Transplant

The main indication is intestinal failure (usually from short bowel syndrome or dysmotility) where complications secondary to TPN have developed, i.e. no vascular access. The surgical technique may be via an isolated intestinal graft (superior mesenteric artery and vein anastomosed to the recipient aorta and IVC, respectively, the intestine being anastomosed to the native bowel and the distal end brought out as a stoma). Alternatively, a liver–intestine graft may be carried out. A few cases of living donation have been reported. The main complications are graft thrombosis, rejection, sepsis and GVH disease. Graft survival is around 65% at 1 year.

GENERAL COMPLICATIONS

These include infection and malignancy.

Infection

Infection post-transplant may be dangerous and life threatening and is related to use of immunosuppression. Infections may be bacterial, viral, fungal or protozoal. These include:

- *Bacterial*, e.g. coliform urinary tract infections, septicaemia, chest infections, e.g. *Staphylococcus aureus*, tuberculosis
- *Viral*, e.g. herpes simplex (cold sores on lips), herpes zoster, CMV; the latter giving rise to pneumonia, encephalitis and deterioration of graft function and BK polyoma virus leading to interstitial nephritis and ureteric strictures
- *Fungal*, e.g. oral, oesophageal and vaginal candidiasis, aspergillosis, *Pneumocystis carinii*
- *Protozoal*, e.g. toxoplasmosis.

Management of Infection. When a transplant patient develops a fever and rejection has been excluded, aggressive investigation should be undertaken to elucidate the cause. Investigations include swabs of wound discharge, urine cultures, sputum cultures, blood cultures, viral studies, CXR, USS, CT scan, bronchoscopy, bronchial washings, lung biopsy. Treatment may have to be started on a 'best guess' basis. Appropriate therapy should be started as soon as laboratory confirmation of the diagnosis has been obtained. In severely ill patients with overwhelming infection, immunosuppressive drugs should be reduced or stopped until the infection is under control. Prophylaxis against CMV with valganciclovir and *Pneumocystis* with co-trimoxazole for high-risk transplant recipients is routine.

HINTS AND TIPS

A temperature in a transplant patient is potentially serious until proved otherwise. What may be a simple infection may become serious because of immunosuppressive therapy. All patients with pyrexia should be referred to the transplant unit for appropriate blood tests, swabs and X-rays before commencing treatment. Early diagnosis and specific therapy of opportunistic infections are the cornerstone of successful management. The general rule is to be aggressive in pursuing a specific microbiological diagnosis in immunocompromised patients. Invasive diagnostic tests may be required. A specific diagnosis avoids the potential toxicity of giving blind broad-spectrum antibiotics, e.g. nephrotoxicity, drug interactions and the potential for *Clostridium difficile* colitis.

Malignancy

The incidence of malignancy is increased in all immunosuppressed transplant patients, and therefore long-term follow-up is mandatory. Primary cancers develop in 5% of all recipients. There is a 100-fold increase compared with age-match controls. Altered immunity with depressed tumour surveillance is an aetiological factor.

Skin cancers are the most common, followed by post-transplant lymphoproliferative disorder (PTLD). In ciclosporin-treated patients, PTLD occurs earlier in the post-transplant patient than with steroid and azathioprine therapy. Other cancers occur more commonly in transplant patients than in the general population.

Malignancy in transplant patients should be treated by standard methods. A decision to withdraw immunosuppression as part of the treatment of cancer is difficult. In general, patients with localised disease should be continued on immunosuppressive therapy, while the development of metastases is an indication for withdrawal of immunosuppression. However, decisions must depend on a careful consideration of the individual case.

LONG-TERM FOLLOW-UP OF TRANSPLANT PATIENTS. Any patient who has had a transplant should be followed up long term by the transplant unit. Patients remain on immunosuppression for life, and long-term complications may develop. Surveillance for development of malignancies is important. Other important factors involve prompt and appropriate treatment of infection; advice on vaccination procedures (live vaccine should never be given to immunosuppressed patients); contact with infectious disease; travel abroad; pregnancy.

Chapter 23

Gynaecology and Obstetrics

Paul Timmons • Alastair McKelvey

CHAPTER OUTLINE

Many causes of both acute and chronic abdominal pain in women are gynaecological in origin though differentiation from gastrointestinal pathology can be challenging. Exclusion of potentially life or organ-threatening diagnoses such as ectopic pregnancy or ovarian torsion is crucial in the acute setting.

ECTOPIC PREGNANCY

Defined as the inappropriate implantation of the fertilised ovum outside of the uterine cavity, ectopic pregnancy affects 1% of all pregnancies and typically (~95%) arises in the fallopian tube; however, it may also occur in the ovary, cervix, abdominal cavity or even the uterine scar from a previous caesarean section. Risk factors include history of previous ectopic pregnancy, pelvic inflammatory disease (PID), smoking, pelvic surgery and assisted-reproductive-techniques such as in vitro fertilisation (IVF); however, most women have no discernible risk factors. Use of intrauterine contraceptive devices (IUCDs) are often quoted as a risk factor though this is somewhat misleading – as effective contraceptives, overall IUCDs prevent unwanted pregnancy, but where a patient has a positive pregnancy test and an IUCD in situ, ectopic pregnancy should be excluded. Pregnancy should be a primary consideration in *all* women of reproductive age presenting with abdominal pain and exclusion of ectopic pregnancy is a priority with a positive pregnancy test – although the majority present insidiously, a ruptured ectopic pregnancy is a life-threatening emergency which requires urgent gynaecological assessment and surgical management.

Symptoms and Signs. Pelvic pain localised to either the right or left iliac fossa in a woman with a positive pregnancy test is the typical presentation. Pain occurs as the developing conceptus outgrows the fallopian tube and gradually worsening pain will precede rupture in most cases. Timing of onset is variable though typically around 6–7 weeks' gestation. Pain may occur in isolation or alongside vaginal bleeding and occasionally, changes in bowel habit.

HINTS AND TIPS

Remember that in the early stages, gestation is calculated from the *first* day of the *last* menstrual period (LMP), even though conception cannot yet have taken place. Ensure this is clarified as patients may offer an estimated gestation based on their own perception of when conception occurred which may differ from the LMP date by up to several weeks.

Rupture of the fallopian tube may be the presenting feature and is characterised by diffuse, peritonitic abdominal pain with haemodynamic compromise and/or hypovolaemic shock. Intra-abdominal haemorrhage may trigger diaphragmatic irritation which causes the classic symptom of referred shoulder-tip pain.

Investigations

Beta-human chorionic gonadotrophin (β-HCG) is first line in all women and any positive result raises the possibility of ectopic pregnancy. Where there is diagnostic uncertainty, repeated levels after 48 hours are useful – in intrauterine pregnancy, β-HCG approximately doubles every 48 hours while in ectopic pregnancy a 'suboptimal' rise (defined as <67% in 48 hours) is suggestive.

USS (transvaginal) looking for an adnexal mass, intraperitoneal free-fluid and the absence of an intra-uterine pregnancy.

FBC may show a fall in haemoglobin (Hb) though similarly may be normal if taken shortly after bleeding begins.

Laparoscopy is the gold standard as it enables simultaneous diagnostic confirmation and treatment.

Treatment

- **Conservative**: a small number of stable patients can be considered for expectant management, as spontaneous abortion may occur in ectopic as in intrauterine pregnancy. Careful case selection and follow-up are essential.
- **Medical**: systemic methotrexate may be suitable for stable patients with a small ectopic mass, no evidence of rupture/leakage, low β-HCG levels and a willingness to engage with longer-term follow-up.
- **Surgical**: laparoscopic salpingectomy (removal of the fallopian tube) is the gold standard, though laparotomy may be required if there is hypovolaemic shock. Salpingostomy (removal of the conceptus with conservation of the tube) may be considered where future fertility is a concern (e.g. if the contralateral tube is missing or damaged). This carries a significant increased risk of recurrent ectopic pregnancy and women should be counselled accordingly.

OVARIAN DISEASE

Ovarian Cysts

'Ovarian cyst' is the common term for a wide range of ovarian pathologies. These includes serous-fluid or blood-filled 'true' cysts, though also solid masses including benign germ-cell tumours (dermoid cysts) as well as malignant lesions. The full classification of ovarian cysts is complex and beyond the scope of this chapter, however there are broadly applicable principles of investigation and management.

Symptoms and Signs. Many ovarian cysts do not cause symptoms and are encountered incidentally during pelvic examination, imaging or intra-operatively. Pain may occur due to pressure effects on the surrounding viscera or from a secondary event such as torsion or cyst rupture, releasing irritant fluid or blood into the peritoneal cavity. Larger cysts may cause symptoms which manifest over a longer, such as menstrual irregularity, dyspareunia or changes in bowel and bladder habit.

Clinical examination may reveal a palpable mass in the lower abdomen. Detection of ascites raises the possibility of a malignant cause.

Investigations

FBC may demonstrate a low Hb in the presence of malignancy or cyst haemorrhage. WCC may be elevated in torsion.

Tumour markers should be measured where appropriate (complex cysts in pre-menopausal women and all cysts in post-menopausal women). An elevated **Ca125** is suggestive of, though not specific for, malignancy. Others including **β-HCG**, alpha-feto protein (**AFP**) and carcinoembryonic antigen (**CEA**) may be of value in the diagnosis of germ-cell tumours.

USS (either abdominal or transvaginal) is the first line imaging investigation in most cases of suspected ovarian pathology.

Magnetic resonance imaging (MRI) may provide additional information on larger or more complex cysts.

Computerised tomography (CT) is used to assess extent of disease (including local and metastatic spread) where malignancy is suspected.

Treatment. Highly dependent on underlying pathology as well as the symptom profile, age of patient, desire for future fertility and suspicion of malignancy. Simple cysts will often resolve spontaneously in time, though larger or complex, solid cysts are more likely to require surgical treatment, generally by way of laparoscopic or open cystectomy. Oophorectomy (removal of the whole ovary) may be required in some cases and patients should be counselled around this in all cases where surgical treatment of a cyst is planned.

Ovarian Cancer

The poor prognosis associated with ovarian cancer is often due to delay in presentation and most diagnoses are made in the advanced stages of the disease.

Symptoms and Signs. In early disease, often nonspecific, if present at all, while advanced disease may be characterised by abdominal pain, bloating, back pain, increased urinary frequency, constipation, abnormal vaginal bleeding and weight loss. Examination may reveal an abdominal mass and/or ascites.

Investigations

Ca125 tumour markers and pelvic ultrasound are first line in suspected cases with CT reserved for staging where these are suggestive.

Tissue diagnosis is usually not made until the time of surgery or from **cytology** on a sample of ascitic fluid where appropriate.

Treatment. Highly variable, depending on stage at presentation. Early disease may be amenable to surgery (oophorectomy) while complex debulking procedures may be necessary in advanced disease.

Chemotherapy is commonly employed both as an adjunct to surgery and in isolation.

Ovarian Torsion

A common cause of acute pelvic pain in women of all ages requiring a high index of suspicion and swift diagnosis as delays can may to loss of the ovary which can have devastating consequences for fertility prospects in younger women.

The ovarian artery (a branch of the abdominal aorta) runs in the infindibulopelvic ligament connecting the ovary to the pelvic side wall – occlusion by torsion leads to infarction and the release of inflammatory mediators.

Signs and Symptoms. Onset of pain is usually acute though may manifest as a worsening of existing chronic pain in those with an existing symptomatic cyst. Severe nausea and vomiting are common. Examination usually reveals a diffusely tender abdomen with a focus of more severe pain over the affected ovary which may be palpable. Guarding and/or rebound tenderness may be present.

Investigations

Diagnosis relies on both clinical assessment and pelvic **USS** appearances of an enlarged or cystic ovary. Normal ovarian appearances are generally exclusionary as torsion of a normal ovary is very rare. Reliable detection of torsion itself on USS requires a high degree of operator experience and should not be depended upon where the history and findings are otherwise suggestive.

Inflammatory markers (**WCC** and **CRP**) may be elevated where there is delay in presentation though are often normal in the acute phase.

Treatment. Laparoscopic detorsion of the ovary is first line management unless there has been significant delay and appearances suggest necrosis or superimposed infection – there is increasing evidence of reperfusion and sustained ovarian function in most cases.

Concurrent cystectomy may be considered, though is often deferred as the ovarian tissue is likely to be more friable.

ENDOMETRIOSIS

Characterised by the presence of endometrial tissue outside the endometrial cavity, the precise aetiology of endometriosis, a common disorder affecting as many as 10% of reproductive-age women, remains uncertain.

Symptoms and Signs. Correlation between disease severity and symptomology is poor, and endometriosis may be an incidental diagnosis at laparoscopy in asymptomatic women. Severe dysmenorrhoea is characteristic, though dyspareunia, dyschezia and subfertility are also common. There may be rectal bleeding or haematuria in disease involving the bowel/bladder respectively.

Examination may be unremarkable, though nodular thickening of the uterosacral ligaments in the posterior fornix may be felt on vaginal examination in women with advanced disease. Uterine mobility may be limited, and a pelvic mass is occasionally felt. Ovarian endometriosis typically manifests as an endometriotic cyst.

Endometriosis outside the pelvis or abdominal cavity is rare, though described, and may cause bizarre symptoms corresponding to location such as haemoptysis and pneumothorax in pulmonary endometriosis.

Investigations. Conventional imaging such as USS or MRI are of limited value in assessment and the diagnosis can only be conclusively made by way of direct visualisation at **laparoscopy**.

Treatment

Pain control with usual **analgesia**. Hormonal therapy including combined oral contraceptives and progesterone IUCD are often used initially, though some require ovarian suppression with GnRH analogues.

Laparoscopic excision or ablation (energy including diathermy and LASER) of focal lesions can offer medium-to-long term relief.

Hysterectomy and/or **oophorectomy** in severe cases once childbearing complete.

UTERINE FIBROIDS (LEIOMYOMA)

Fibroids are benign tumours of uterine smooth muscle (myometrial) origin. Present in up to 40% of women, they are more common in women of Afro-Caribbean ethnicity and those with a family history.

Symptoms and Signs. Often asymptomatic though can cause heavy, painful and/or irregular menses. Abdominal/pelvic discomfort can arise secondary to pressure on surrounding structures (e.g. bladder or rectum) which may also carry associated symptoms such as polyuria or urgency.

Larger fibroids may be palpable on abdominal examination though are seldom painful.

Investigations

- **FBC** to exclude anaemia where menorrhagia is the primary concern
- Pelvic **ultrasound** is first line, though **MRI** can provide useful information in some cases.

Treatment

- Conservative: small, asymptomatic fibroids do not necessarily require treatment
- Medical: GnRH analogues may be used to shrink fibroids prior to surgery
- **Surgery**: options include myomectomy, hysteroscopic resection and uterine-artery-embolisation where uterine preservation is desired. Hysterectomy when family complete.

PELVIC INFLAMMATORY DISEASE (PID)

PID is a generic term for inflammation of the pelvic organs, usually with an infective aetiology. Sexually transmitted infections (STIs) such as *Chlamydia Trachomitis* or *Neisseria Gonorrhoea* are the most common causes though infection secondary to termination of pregnancy, childbirth and use of IUCDs also carry a risk of ascending infection.

Symptoms and Signs. Lower abdominal/pelvic pain usually accompanied by malodourous vaginal discharge and irregular bleeding. There may also be pyrexia and other symptoms of general malaise. Examination usually elicits focal/diffuse abdominal tenderness and there may be a palpable mass. Cervical motion tenderness is usually present.

Investigations. Inflammatory markers are usually elevated (**WCC/CRP**). High vaginal and endocervical **swabs** should be collected for microscopy and culture plus a comprehensive **STI screen**. Pelvic **USS** may be normal or demonstrate a tubo-ovarian abscess.

Treatment. Depends on severity and clinical condition. Systemically well patients may be suitable for outpatient therapy with oral antibiotics (depending on local sensitivities) covering *C. Trachomitis* and *N. Gonorrhoea*. Systemically unwell patients, or where there is evidence of a pelvic abscess, should be admitted for i.v. therapy and consideration of surgical drainage.

ABDOMINAL TRAUMA IN PREGNANCY

Trauma in pregnancy is not uncommon (7% of pregnancies), and pregnant woman are at increased risk of domestic abuse (including violence) and suicide (violent methods more likely in pregnancy). Joint care by Trauma and Obstetric teams (including an obstetric anaesthetist) is important. A systemic approach is key, with prioritisation given to securing the airway, then addressing breathing, before moving to assess circulation. In advanced pregnancy (>20 weeks), displacement of the uterus is necessary to improve venous return to the heart. Cervical immobilisation and spine control may be required if there is a suggestion of high-velocity injury. Assessment of the foetus comes after the primary survey of the mother and is then followed by the secondary maternal survey. Healthy, young pregnant women can lose a large amount of blood before showing overt evidence of haemodynamic collapse. Systolic pressure is generally maintained until 30–40% of circulating volume has been lost, therefore active consideration should be given to restoring normovolaemia (rather than adopting hypotensive resuscitation, which the foetus is unlikely to survive). Resuscitation in cardiac arrest in advanced pregnancy (over 20 weeks amenorrhoea) includes perimortem caesarean delivery, to reduce aortocaval compression by the gravid uterus).

Key Principles

ABC first
Uterine displacement
Cervical/spinal immobilisation as appropriate
Early fluid resuscitation
Maternal 1^0 survey, then Foetal assessment, then 2^0 survey
Joint management with Trauma team, Obstetricians, Anaesthetists and Midwives

Surgical Abdominal Emergencies in Pregnancy

Just as clinicians assessing women of childbearing age with abdominal pain should consider the possibility of pregnancy (including labour), so those assessing pregnant women presenting with abdominal pain, should be open-minded about the possibility of a nonobstetric cause.

Changes in anatomy and physiology can alter the presentation and response to acute abdominal conditions, making it difficult to distinguish between obstetric and surgical causes. The location of pain can be different, due to organ displacement (e.g. appendicitis). Maternal adaptation to blood loss can mask concealed haemorrhage until blood loss is critical (e.g. splenic artery aneurysm). In the UK, approximately three pregnant women die annually from intra-abdominal pathology. Use of a modified early obstetric warning scoring system (MEOWS) is important in identifying the deteriorating pregnant patient. Placental abruption or uterine rupture (in a woman with a scarred uterus) can mimic an acute abdomen.

History can still help differentiate between causes.

Acute pain. *Persistent pain* – Ruptured structure (ectopic, uterus, spleen, aneurysm, gastrointestinal (GI) perforation)

Colicky pain – obstructed structure (intestinal, ureteric, gall stones).

Gradual and increasing pain. Inflammatory causes (appendicitis, fibroid degeneration, pancreatitis, diverticulitis, liver oedema)

A general clinical examination as well as a focused obstetric and foetal assessment by CTG can help differentiate obstetric (rigid/tender uterus, pathological CTG and/or vaginal bleeding) from surgical problems (normal CTG, soft nontender uterus, normal vaginal findings). Bedside ultrasound can detect large volumes of intraperitoneal fluid or blood but is not reliable in excluding placental abruption or uterine rupture.

Investigations

Blood tests

A moderate leucocytosis is normal in pregnancy, as is an elevated Alk Phos and an elevated D Dimer

A WCC over 15 is significant, as is an elevated CRP, raised ALT or raised amylase.

Imaging (remember uterine displacement)

Formal radiology USS is useful in assessing the kidneys but is of weaker diagnostic value in appendicitis and other GI pathologies because of the enlarged uterus, where MRI is superior (provided the patient is stable enough). CT is sensitive and specific but involves a high dose of radiation to the foetus and mother, and a senior discussion should take place before performing CT for this reason.

Treatment. Will depend on cause, but the principle of offering the standard treatment (including surgery), with appropriate modification to consider the pregnancy, is key. When the pregnancy is close to term, consideration of early delivery (e.g. with renal obstruction) can sometimes alleviate pathology.

Index

Page numbers followed by '*f*' indicate figures, '*b*' indicate boxes, and '*t*' indicate tables.

B

D

G

H

I

N

O

P

Q

R

S

T